Plastic and Reconstructive Surgery

Oxford Specialist Handbooks published and forthcoming

General Oxford Specialist Handbooks

A Resuscitation Room Guide
Addiction Medicine, 2e
Day Case Surgery
Perioperative Medicine, 2e
Pharmaceutical Medicine
Postoperative Complications, 2e
Renal Transplantation

Oxford Specialist Handbooks in Anaesthesia

Anaesthesia for Medical and Surgical Emergencies
Cardiac Anaesthesia
Neuroanaethesia
Obstetric Anaesthesia
Ophthalmic Anaesthesia
Paediatric Anaesthesia
Regional Anaesthesia, Stimulation and Ultrasound Techniques
Thoracic Anaesthesia

Oxford Specialist Handbooks in Cardiology

Adult Congenital Heart Disease
Cardiac Catheterization and Coronary Intervention
Cardiac Electrophysiology and Catheter Ablation
Cardiovascular Computed Tomography
Cardiovascular Magnetic Resonance
Echocardiography, 2e
Fetal Cardiology
Heart Failure, 2e
Hypertension
Inherited Cardiac Disease
Nuclear Cardiology
Pacemakers and ICDs
Pulmonary Hypertension
Valvular Heart Disease

Oxford Specialist Handbooks in Critical Care

Advanced Respiratory Critical Care
Cardiothoracic Critical Care

Oxford Specialist Handbooks in End of Life Care

End of Life Care in Cardiology
End of Life Care in Dementia
End of Life Care in Nephrology
End of Life Care in Respiratory Disease
End of Life in the Intensive Care Unit

Oxford Specialist Handbooks in Infectious Disease

Infectious Disease Epidemiology

Oxford Specialist Handbooks in Neurology

Epilepsy
Parkinson's Disease and Other Movement Disorders, 2e
Stroke Medicine

Oxford Specialist Handbooks in Oncology

Practical Management of Complex Cancer Pain

Oxford Specialist Handbooks in Paediatrics

Paediatric Dermatology
Paediatric Endocrinology and Diabetes
Paediatric Gastroenterology, Hepatology, and Nutrition
Paediatric Haematology and Oncology
Paediatric Intensive Care
Paediatric Nephrology, 2e
Paediatric Neurology, 2e
Paediatric Radiology
Paediatric Respiratory Medicine, 2e
Paediatric Rheumatology

Oxford Specialist Handbooks in Pain Medicine

Spinal Interventions in Pain Management

Oxford Specialist Handbooks in Psychiatry

Child and Adolescent Psychiatry
Forensic Psychiatry
Medical Psychotherapy
Old Age Psychiatry

Oxford Specialist Handbooks in Radiology

Interventional Radiology
Musculoskeletal Imaging
Pulmonary Imaging
Thoracic Imaging

Oxford Specialist Handbooks in Surgery

Cardiothoracic Surgery, 2e
Colorectal Surgery
Gastric and Oesophageal Surgery
Hand Surgery
Hepatopancreatobiliary Surgery
Neurosurgery
Operative Surgery, 2e
Oral and Maxillofacial Surgery, 2e
Otolaryngology and Head and Neck Surgery
Paediatric Surgery
Plastic and Reconstructive Surgery
Surgical Oncology
Urological Surgery
Vascular Surgery, 2e

Oxford Specialist Handbooks in Surgery

Plastic and Reconstructive Surgery

Henk Giele
Consultant Plastic, Reconstructive and Hand Surgeon,
Oxford Radcliffe NHS Trust, UK and Nuffield
Orthopaedic Centre NHS Trust, UK and
Honorary Clinical Senior Lecturer,
University of Oxford, UK

and

Oliver Cassell
Consultant Plastic and Reconstructive Surgeon,
Oxford Radcliffe NHS Trust, UK and
Honorary Clinical Senior Lecturer,
University of Oxford, UK

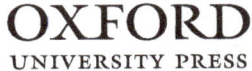

OXFORD
UNIVERSITY PRESS

Great Clarendon Street, Oxford, OX2 6DP,
United Kingdom

Oxford University Press is a department of the University of Oxford.
It furthers the University's objective of excellence in research, scholarship,
and education by publishing worldwide. Oxford is a registered trade mark of
Oxford University Press in the UK and in certain other countries

© Oxford University Press, 2008

The moral rights of the authors have been asserted

First published 2008
First published in paperback 2016

All rights reserved. No part of this publication may be reproduced, stored in
a retrieval system, or transmitted, in any form or by any means, without the
prior permission in writing of Oxford University Press, or as expressly permitted
by law, by licence or under terms agreed with the appropriate reprographics
rights organization. Enquiries concerning reproduction outside the scope of the
above should be sent to the Rights Department, Oxford University Press, at the
address above

You must not circulate this work in any other form
and you must impose this same condition on any acquirer

Published in the United States of America by Oxford University Press
198 Madison Avenue, New York, NY 10016, United States of America

British Library Cataloguing in Publication Data

Data available

Library of Congress Cataloging in Publication Data

Data available

ISBN 978–0–19–263222–7 (flexicover: alk.paper)
ISBN 978–0–19–878478–4 (Pbk.)

Printed in Great Britain by
Ashford Colour Press Ltd, Gosport, Hampshire

Links to third party websites are provided by Oxford in good faith and
for information only. Oxford disclaims any responsibility for the materials
contained in any third party website referenced in this work.

Foreword

The Oxford Handbook series has established itself as a byword of quality in medical education and *Plastic and Reconstructive Surgery* is overdue.

Like the Sunday paper the familiar proven format makes for intuitive, easy reading and rapid homing to subjects of interest. This recipe-style cookbook has a British flavour different from the staple American full plate diet and the menu has been compiled by two renowned local plastic surgical chefs, Henk Giele and Oliver Cassell. They point out that this is a collation of current thoughts gleaned from multiple authors and articles, 'research rather than plagiarism', and in this sense it is not nouvelle cuisine but low fat and rich in vitamins and essential minerals.

Just as the British forefathers of plastic surgery had strong Antipodean connections, so too do these latter day teachers. Giele is Australian and Australian trained, while Cassell is British with fellowship and research training in Australia. I had the privilege of getting to know them personally as both elected to train with me at St Vincent's Hospital and the Bernard O'Brien Institute in Melbourne and to complete post graduate degrees through Melbourne University. I would have boasted that I 'taught them all they know' until I browsed through the manuscript. How embarrassing. This is a veritable encyclopaedia totalling almost 1000 pages designed for the pocket, a book lover's PC. The book will not only serve the needs of medical students, plastic surgical trainees, and trained surgeons but also those of us who still have the humility to realize how little we ever knew.

Both authors are, appropriately, consultant plastic surgeons at the Oxford NHS Trust hospitals and each brings special qualities to the task. Giele the charismatic teacher with a special expertise in hand and musculoskeletal reconstruction and Cassell the equally good communicator with broad interests in plastic surgery including skin cancer, head and neck, and breast microsurgical reconstruction. Both have academic training and interests.

The chapters on plastic surgery science; anatomy; and drugs and tools are exceptional and this core knowledge is rarely presented in such an accessible format in plastic surgery texts and difficult to dissect from journals. The sections that overlap with other disciplines are also novel and timely. Skin pathology and dermatology, head and neck and ENT, and burns surgery are all areas where there has been a creeping concession by some surgical units that these are lost and now 'no go', but the complete plastic surgeon must be able to participate knowledgably in the decision making process of referrals and not be merely a manual labourer contracted to fill holes dug by others. The inclusion of the wrist in hand surgery recognizes that the plastic surgical derived upper limb surgeon must be equal to his orthopaedic counterpart.

Reading the scope of this book confirms the belief that plastic surgery is truly the general surgery of today. By no means trivial pursuit but the platform on which all surgery should be based. My old general surgery chief used to mock that 'the only difference between plastic surgery and general surgery was 10 days', the difference between a good and a bad haircut or more clearly stated the difference between primary and secondary healing. Good design based on an understanding of blood supply coupled with meticulous repair are the cornerstones of primary wound healing. This is the stock and trade of the good plastic surgeon and this book in its very first chapter recites the plastic surgeons' creed—Gillies' golden rules, later expanded by Millard.

At the risk of being accused of plagiarism myself, I quote what I believe was Oscar Wilde's comment, although I cannot find the source, 'I know of many book collectors who only seek out the first edition; I would much rather wait for the second edition to confirm that it is worth reading.' Giele and Cassell's handbook is new off the rank but I am sure it is destined for many editions. This work is too good and too interesting for it not to become one of the Oxford Handbook stable's prized bloodlines.

Wayne Morrison,
Professor of Surgery,
St Vincent's Hospital,
University of Melbourne and Head of Plastic and
Reconstructive Surgery,
Director, Bernard O'Brien Institute of Microsurgery,
Melbourne

Acknowledgements

'Copying one person's work is plagiarism, copying lots of people's is research.'

In producing this book we have 'copied' many people's work. Like much in medicine, little is original, and where we have expressed our experiences and preferences these have arisen from lessons learnt from patients, nurses, therapists, registrars and, of course, from the always constructive criticism of our surgical colleagues. We thank our patients, trainees, surgical trainers and colleagues in Australia, Paris (HG) and the UK who put us on the right path and honed and developed our skills.

Plastic surgeons have the great benefit of working closely with other specialists. In our case we are appreciative of the education and stimulation provided by our colleagues in orthopaedics, infectious diseases, oncology, dermatology, head and neck, general surgery, neurosciences, anaesthetics, radiology, and pathology.

We would like to thank our parents for their encouragement and support of all our endeavours, and also our wives for their love and patience (they knew what they were getting themselves into, as the commencement of this book predated them)!

Thanks to all the contributors who took on a selection of topics when our energy was starting to flag. We apologize for editing the contributions in some cases beyond recognition. We accept full responsibility for the errors within the book and would be grateful if they could be pointed out at errors@what-about.me.uk.

Thanks also to Josephine (Miss Moneypenny), Alison, Jocelyn, Jenry, and Sue for all their secretarial support and organization. Thanks must go to the illustrator Suzy Adams who interpreted sometimes sketchy diagrams into digital clarity. Thanks also to the editorial and production staff at OUP who have exhibited incredible patience. Without them of course the book would not exist.

Thanks most of all to the readers. We hope they find this book as educational to read as we did to write.

Henk Giele
Oliver Cassell

Introduction

Plastic and reconstructive surgery is an exciting surgical speciality. Unlike other areas, plastic surgery is a speciality based mainly on techniques rather then pathologies or anatomical zones. This makes plastic surgery difficult to define and understand. It remains the last true general surgical speciality in treating patients of all ages, in all anatomical areas, with the whole gamut of pathologies from acquired to zoonotic (congenital, degenerative, traumatic, infective, and neoplastic are the main patient providers). This diversity means that plastic surgery interfaces with more medical, surgical, and allied health specialities than any other field. This diversity also occurs at a level in that multiple solutions are possible for every patient's problem, allowing analytical procedure selection, constant improvement, and innovation.

This handbook attempts to give useful information about the disorders and treatments managed by plastic surgeons. The format follows that of the Oxford Handbook Series, with each subject covered in note format. Operative techniques and preferences may differ amongst surgeons, and in many cases there are no right answers; however, the challenge for every surgeon is continually to think critically, use all their perceptive faculties to diagnose each patient, and select each operation based on personal experience and the latest evidence, always trying to do the best for each patient. We hope that this handbook condenses the core information and stimulates readers to delve deeper.

The book is organized to aid learning. Diseases are discussed under the following headings **D**efinition; **I**ncidence; **A**etiology; **G**eneral clinical presentation and classification; **N**atural history; **O**ptions; **S**urgery; **E**ffect of treatment/surgery. You may have noticed that this produces the acronym DIAGNOSE. Surgical techniques are presented by description, indication, principles, technique, complications, and outcome.

Contents

Contributors *xi*
Detailed contents *xiii*
Symbols and abbreviations *xxvii*

1	Plastic surgery science	1
2	Embryology	61
3	Anatomy and clinical assessment	71
4	Drugs and tools	105
5	Congenital	133
6	Skin	233
7	Eyelid	283
8	Nose, ear, face, mouth	305
9	Head and neck	339
10	Chest	363
11	Abdomen and trunk	383
12	Upper limb	389
13	Lower limb	429
14	Vascular	449
15	Infection	465
16	Tumours	479
17	Trauma	505

18	Metabolic, endocrine, degenerative	631
19	Miscellaneous disorders	643
20	Aesthetic	655
21	Reconstruction	727
22	Flaps	735
23	Appendices	907

Index 931

Contributors

Suzy Adams
(illustrations), London

Lucy Cogswell
Specialist Registrar in Plastic Surgery,
Radcliffe Infirmary, Oxford

Dominic Furness
Specialist Registrar in Plastic Surgery,
Radcliffe Infirmary, Oxford

Simon Heppell
Specialist Registrar in Plastic Surgery,
Radcliffe Infirmary, Oxford

Daniel Morritt
Specialist Registrar in Plastic Surgery,
Radcliffe Infirmary, Oxford

Greg O'Toole
Specialist Registrar in Plastic Surgery,
Radcliffe Infirmary, Oxford

Ankur Pandya
Specialist Registrar in Plastic Surgery,
Radcliffe Infirmary, Oxford

Yu Sin Lau
Specialist Registrar in Plastic Surgery,
Radcliffe Infirmary, Oxford

Marc Swan
Specialist Registrar in Plastic Surgery,
Radcliffe Infirmary, Oxford

Steve Wall
Consultant Plastic & Craniofacial Surgeon,
Oxford Craniofacial Unit

Detailed contents

Contributors *xi*
Symbols and abbreviations *xxvii*

1 **Plastic surgery science** 1
Gillies' principles of plastic surgery *2*
Other aphorisms in plastic surgery *3*
Wound healing: general *5*
Wound healing: factors affecting *8*
Skin basics *11*
Skin healing *13*
Skin grafts *15*
Scars: symptomatic, hypertrophic, and keloid *19*
Bone and bone healing *23*
Bone graft *25*
Distraction osteogenesis *27*
Cartilage *31*
Tendon healing *33*
Peripheral nerve healing *35*
Composite grafts *37*
Fat grafts *38*
Fetal wound healing *41*
Tissue expansion *42*
Delay phenomenon *45*
Topical negative pressure *46*
Pathology basics *48*
Principles of radiotherapy *49*
Sun damage *52*

Microbiology *55*
Clostridia *57*

2 Embryology 61

Embryology of the external genitalia *62*
Embryology of the face *63*
Embryology of the nose *65*
Embryology of the lip and palate *66*
Embryology of the ear *67*
Embryology of the hand *68*

3 Anatomy and clinical assessment 71

Skin vascular anatomy *72*
Head and neck anatomy *74*
Nose anatomy *78*
Eyelid anatomy and physiology *82*
External ear anatomy *84*
Facial nerve anatomy *87*
Hand anatomy: basic *90*
Nerve supply to the hand *97*
Wrist anatomy and examination *99*
Penis anatomy *101*
Parasympathetic nervous system *103*

4 Drugs and tools 105

Local anaesthesia *106*
Blood transfusion *108*
Drugs used in inflammatory arthritis *110*
Oncological drugs *111*
Injectables *112*
Antibiotic prophylaxis in plastic surgery *114*
Thromboprophylaxis in plastic surgery *116*

Dressings *118*
Implants *120*
Smoking and plastic surgery *123*
Leech therapy *125*
Microsurgery *127*
Lasers *130*

5 Congenital 133

Hypospadias *134*
Epispadias–exstrophy complex *138*
Craniosynostosis *141*
Non-syndromic craniosynostosis *142*
Syndromic craniosynostosis *144*
Plagiocephaly without synostosis (PWS) *146*
Surgery for craniosynostosis *147*
Hemifacial microsomia *148*
Romberg's disease *149*
Treacher Collins syndrome *150*
Pierre Robin sequence *152*
Microtia *154*
Branchial clefts *155*
Cleft lip and palate: introduction *156*
Cleft lip repair: unilateral *162*
Cleft lip repair: bilateral *166*
Cleft palate repair *168*
Cleft rhinoplasty *175*
Velopharyngeal incompetence *178*
Palatal fistula *182*
Orthodontics *184*
Alveolar bone grafting *187*
Congenital upper limb anomalies *189*
Radial dysplasia *191*

Ulnar dysplasia *195*
Cleft hand *197*
Camptodactyly *200*
Clinodactyly *202*
Clasp thumb *204*
Trigger digit *205*
Syndactyly *206*
Polydactyly *209*
Thumb duplication *210*
Congenital radial head dislocation *211*
Radioulnar synostosis *212*
Thumb hypoplasia *214*
Brachydactyly *216*
Symbrachydactyly *218*
Macrodactyly *220*
Amniotic band syndrome *223*
Arthrogryposis *224*
Madelung's deformity *226*
Poland syndrome *228*
Toe phalanx non-vascularized transfer *230*
Pollicization *231*
Chest wall deformity *232*

6 Skin 233

Epidermolysis bullosa *234*
Albinism *236*
Pigmented melanocytic lesions *238*
Skin tumours: classification *239*
Melanocytic lesions *240*
Epidermal lesions *240*
Dermal lesions *241*

Naevus cell lesions 242
Special naevi 243
Premalignant 245
Melanoma 246
Non-melanoma 250
Malignant 258

Benign skin lesions
Cysts 268
Fibrohistiocytic tumours 270
Epidermal tumours 272
Sweat gland tumours 274
Hair follicle tumours 276
Vascular tumours 277
Mast cell tumours 278
Port wine stain 279
Pyoderma gangrenosum 281

7 Eyelid 283
Ectropion 284
Entropion 288
Blepharophimosis, ptosis, and epicanthus inversus syndrome (BPES) 290
Anophthalmos and microphthalmia 291
Hypertelorism, epicanthus, telecanthus, and hypotelorism 293
Ptosis 295
Eyelid reconstruction 297
Eyelid reconstruction in facial nerve palsy 302

8 Nose, ear, face, mouth 305
Nasal reconstruction 306
Rhinophyma 314

Ear reconstruction *315*
Facial nerve palsy *318*
Cheek reconstruction *323*
Drooling *327*
Lip reconstruction *329*
Swallowing *336*

9 Head and neck

Tumours of the nasal cavity, sinuses, and nasopharynx *340*
Tumours of the oral cavity, oropharynx, and hypopharynx *344*
Head and neck cancer reconstruction *351*
Salivary gland tumours *354*
Superficial parotidectomy *357*
Neck dissection *359*

10 Chest

Breast cancer *364*
Breast reconstruction *367*
Nipple–areolar complex reconstruction *373*
Chest wall reconstruction *375*
Sternum reconstruction *378*

11 Abdomen and trunk

Abdominal wall reconstruction *384*
Spinal closure *387*

12 Upper limb

Anatomy of extensor mechanism of the fingers *390*
Digital extensor mechanism defects and assessment *392*
Hand infections *394*

Dystonia *400*
Hand tumours *401*
Soft tissue tumours *405*
Vascular tumours *409*
Bone tumours *412*
Metastatic tumours *417*
Upper limb amputations *418*
Ray amputation *420*
Upper limb proximal amputations *421*
Prostheses *422*
Arthrodesis: digital *423*
Examination of the wrist *425*

13 Lower limb

Lower limb trauma *430*
Lower limb ulceration *433*
Pretibial laceration *435*
Diabetic feet *437*
Lower limb reconstruction *442*
Below-knee amputation *445*
Above-knee amputation *448*

14 Vascular

Raynaud's phenomenon *450*
Lymphoedema *453*
Vascular anomalies *457*
Haemangiomas *459*
Vascular malformations *461*

15 Infection

Microbiology *466*
Clostridia *468*

Osteomyelitis *471*
Prosthesis exposure or infection *475*
Necrotizing soft tissue infection *476*

16 Tumours   479

Fibromatoses *480*
Soft tissue sarcoma *481*
Neurilemoma (benign schwannoma) *488*
Neurofibroma *490*
Neurofibromatosis *492*
Lipoma *495*
Axillary dissection *497*
Groin dissection *500*
Sentinel lymph node biopsy *503*

17 Trauma   505

Extravasation *506*
Frostbite *508*
Traumatic tattooing *510*
Degloving injuries *511*
Crush injuries *513*
Compartment syndrome *515*
Fasciotomy *518*
Gunshot and blast injuries *522*

Facial trauma
Facial lacerations *524*
Middle-third facial injuries *527*

Hand trauma
Hand assessment in trauma *533*
Nailbed and perionychial injuries *537*
Flexor tendon injuries *540*

Flexor tendon repair *542*

Flexor tendon avulsion *544*

Flexor tendon rehabilitation *546*

Ring avulsion injury *548*

Boutonnière deformity *549*

Swan-neck deformity *551*

Ulnar collateral ligament injury of the thumb MCPJ *553*

Hand fractures *555*

Complications in metacarpal and phalangeal fractures *570*

Scaphoid fracture *573*

Carpal instability *576*

Distal radius fractures *579*

DRUJ disorders *582*

DRUJ instability *583*

Ulnar head procedures *584*

Triangular fibro-cartilaginous complex (TFCC) disorders *585*

Ulnocarpal abutment syndrome *587*

Brachial plexus injuries *589*

Obstetrical brachial plexus palsy *593*

Sequelae of obstetrical brachial palsy *595*

Volkmann's ischaemic contracture *596*

Peripheral nerve

Peripheral nerve injury *598*

Tendon transfers *600*

Burns

Burns emergency care *602*

Burns fluid resuscitation *604*

Assessment of burns *606*

Escharotomy 610
Pathophysiology of the burn wound 613
Burn infection 616
Burn treatment 618
Burn reconstruction 620
Burns to trunk, genitalia, and head and neck 621
Hand burns 623
Foot burns 625
Chemical burns 626
Electrical burns 628
Non-accidental injury in burns 630

18 Metabolic, endocrine, degenerative 631
Rheumatoid arthritis 632
Scleroderma, CREST syndrome, systemic sclerosis 636
Osteoarthritis 638
Gout 640

19 Miscellaneous disorders 643
Pressure sores 644
Complex regional pain syndrome 647
Hidradenitis 649
Hyperhidrosis 651
Gender reassignment 653

20 Aesthetic 655
Aesthetic surgery 656
Assessment of a patient for aesthetic surgery 657
Facial ageing 660

Breast

Bra and breast sizing 661
Aesthetic breast surgery assessment 662
Breast reduction surgery 664
Breast augmentation 670
Breast ptosis 674
Inverted nipples 677
Tuberous breast 678
Gynaecomastia 679

Skin

Non-surgical aesthetic techniques 682
Skin-lightening methods 685

Facial

Blepharoplasty 686
Brow lift 692
Rhinoplasty 694
Submucous resection 698
Facelift 700
Augmentation of the facial skeleton 704
Genioplasty 706

Body contouring

Body contouring 709
Arm reduction 711
Abdominoplasty 713
Thigh and buttock contouring 717
Medial thigh lift 719
Calf augmentation 720
Liposuction 722

21 Reconstruction — 727

The reconstructive ladder 728
Direct closure (primary intention) 729
Secondary intention 734

22 Flaps — 735

Flaps 736
Flap terminology 739
Classification of flaps 741
Free tissue transfer 743
Lessons in free flap transfers 746
Flap monitoring and care 748
Advancement flaps 750
Pivot flaps 756
Rotation flaps 758
Distant flaps 760
Fascio-cutaneous flaps 762
Muscle flaps 764
Vascularized bone 'graft' 766
Venous drainage in reverse flow flaps 769
Venous flaps 771
Z-plasty 773
W-plasty 776
Rhomboid flap 778
Dufourmental flap 780
Bi-lobed flap 781
Horn flap 783
Banner flap 785
Dorsal nasal flap 787
Nasalis flap 789
Nasolabial flap 791

Cervico-facial flap *793*

Jejunal flap *795*

Omental flap *797*

Lateral arm flap *799*

Medial arm flap *801*

Radial forearm flap *803*

Ulnar forearm flap *806*

Dorsal ulnar flap *808*

Posterior interosseous artery flap *810*

Fingertip flaps *813*

Kite flap *816*

Flag flap *819*

Brunelli dorsal ulnar thumb flap *821*

Neurovascular island flap *823*

Cross-finger flap *826*

Moberg flap *828*

Thenar flap *830*

Dorsal finger flaps *832*

Forehead flaps *835*

Temporalis flap *839*

Temporo-parietal flap *841*

Auriculo-temporal flap *843*

Delto-pectoral flap *845*

Pectoralis major flap *847*

Scapular flap *850*

Parascapular flap *853*

Trapezius flap *855*

Gluteus maximus flap *858*

Rectus abdominis flap *861*

VRAM (vertical rectus abdominis myocutaneous) flap *863*

TRAM (transverse rectus abdominis myocutaneous) flap *865*

DIEP (deep inferior epigastric perforator) flap *868*

Latissimus dorsi flap (and TAP flap) *870*

Serratus anterior flap *873*

Gracilis *876*

Groin flap *878*

DCIA (deep circumflex iliac artery) flap *880*

TFL (tensor fascia lata) flap *882*

Anterolateral thigh flap *884*

Biceps femoris flap *886*

Soleus *888*

Medial and lateral gastrocnemius flaps *890*

Medial plantar flap *892*

Toe transfer *894*

Great toe wrap around flap *896*

Fibula flap *898*

Sural flap *901*

Leg fascio-cutaneous flaps *903*

23 Appendices

Classifications *908*

Staging and survival of common cancers *914*

Eponymous syndromes *915*

Eponymous procedures *923*

Flap bibliography *924*

Bibliography *925*

Major plastic set *927*

Index 931

Symbols and abbreviations

📖	cross reference
>	greater than
≥	greater than or equal to
<	less than
≤	less than or equal to
=	equal to
#	fracture
~	approximately
5-FU	fluorouracil
5-HT	serotonin
ABCD	airways, breathing, circulation, and disability
ABG	arterial blood gas
ABG	alveolar bone grafting
ABPI	ankle brachial pressure index
ACE	angiotensin-converting enzyme
ACh	acetyl choline
AD	autosomal dominant
ADH	antidiuretic hormone
ADM	abductor digiti minimi
AER	apical ectodermal ridge
AH	abductor hallucis
AIA	anterior interosseous artery
AJCC	American Joint Committee on Cancer
AKA	above-knee amputation
AMC	arthrogryposis multiplex congenita
AP	anteroposterior
APB	abductor pollicis brevis
APL	abductor pollicis longus
APS	annals of plastic surgery
APTT	activated partial thromboplastin time
APUD	amine precursor uptake and decarboxylase
AR	autosomal recessive
ARDS	adult respiratory distress syndrome
ASA	American Society of Anesthesiologists
ASAP	as soon as possible
ASD	atrial septal defect

ASIS	anterior superior iliac spine
ATA	anterior tibial artery
ATLS	acute trauma life support
ATN	acute tubular necrosis
ATP	adenosine triphosphate
AV	arteriovenous
AVN	avascular necrosis (bone)
BAPN	beta-aminopropionitrile
BAPS	British Association of Plastic Surgeons (now BAPRAS)
BAPRAS	British Association of Plastic, Reconstructive and Aesthetic Surgeons
BCC	basal cell cancer
BKA	below-knee amputation
BMI	body mass index
BMP	bone morphogenic protein
BOA	British Orthopaedic Association
BP	blood pressure
BPB	brachial plexus block
BPI	brachial plexus injury
BR	brachioradialis
BSA	body surface area
CABG	coronary artery bypass grafts
cAMP	cyclic adenosine-3',5'-monophosphate
CEA	cultured epidermal autograft
CIA	carpal instability adaptive
CIC	carpal instability combined
CID	carpal instability dissociative (proximal row)
CIND	carpal instability non-disssociative
CL	cleft lip
CLP	cleft lip and palate
CMCJ	carpometacarpal joint
CMV	cytomegalo virus
CN	cranial nerve
CNS	central nervous system
COC	combined oral contraceptive
COPD	chronic obstructive pulmonary disease
CP	cleft palate
CP	compartment pressure
CPP	capillary perfusion pressure
CPR	cardiopulmonary resuscitation
CRP	c-reactive protein
CRPS	complex regional pain syndrome
CT	computed tomography

CVA	cerebral vascular accident
CVP	central venous pressure
CXR	chest X-ray
DCIA	deep circumflex iliac artery
DCIS	ductal carcinoma *in situ*
DDH	developmental dysplasia of the hip
DEB	dystrophic epidermolysis bullosa
DFSP	dermatomafibrosarcoma protruberans
DIA	dorsal interosseous artery
DIC	disseminated intravascular coagulation
DIEP	deep inferior epigastric perforator
DIPJ	distal interphalangeal joint
DISI	dorsal inter calated scaphoid instability
DMSA	$^{99m}Tc(V)$-dimercaptosuccinic acid
DMSO	dimethylsulphoxide
DRUJ	distal radioulnar joint
DVT	deep vein thrombosis
EAM	external auditory meatus
EBS	epidermolysis bullosa simplex
EBV	Epstein–Barr virus
ECG	electrocardiogram
ECRB	extensor carpi radialis brevis
ECRL	extensor carpi radialis longus
ECU	extensor carpi ulnaris
EDC	extensor digiti communis
EDM	extensor digiti minimi
EDQ	extensor digiti quinti
EGF	epidermal growth factor
EI	external intercostal
EIP	extensor indicis propius
EJV	external jugular vein
ENT	ear, nose, and throat
EPB	extensor pollicis brevis
EPL	extensor pollicis longus
ESR	erythrocyte sedimentation rate
FBC	full blood count
FCR	flexor carpi radialis
FCU	flexor carpi ulnaris
FDB	flexor digitorum brevis
FDG-PET	[^{18}F]fluorodeoxyglucose positron emission tomography
FDI	first dorsal interosseous
FDM	flexor digiti minimi

FDMA	first dorsal metatarsal artery
FDP	flexor digitorum profundus
FDS	flexor digitorum superficialis
FGF	fibroblast growth factor
FLPD	flashlamp pulsed dye (laser)
FNA	fine-needle aspiration
FNAC	fine-needle aspiration cytology
FPB	flexor pollicis brevis
FPL	flexor pollicis longus
FTSG	full-thickness skin graft
GA	general anaesthetic
GIST	gastrointestinal stromal tumour
GIT	gastrointestinal tract
GKI	glucose, potassium, and insulin infusion
GTN	glyceryl trinitrate
Hb	haemaglobin
HBV	hepatitis B virus
HIV	human immunodeficiency virus
HLA	human leucocyte antigen
HP	hard palate
HPV	human papilloma virus
HRT	hormone replacement therapy
ICU	intensive care unit
IEA	inferior epigastric artery
IFSSH	International Federation of Societies for Surgery of the Hand
IHD	ischaemic heart disease
IJV	internal jugular vein
IL	interleukin
ILVEN	inflammatory linear verrucous epidermal naevus
IMA	internal mammary artery
INF	interferon
INR	international normalized ratio
IPJ	interphalangeal joint
IPPV	intermittent positive pressure ventilation
ITU	intensive therapy unit
IUCA	inferior ulna collateral artery
IV	intravenous
IVF	*in vitro* fertilization
JEB	junctional epidermolysis bullosa
JXG	juvenile xanthogranuloma
K	potassium
KGF	keratinocyte growth factor

LA	local anaesthetic
LCIS	lobular carcinoma *in situ*
LEN	linear epidermal naevus
LFT	liver function tests
LMWH	low molecular weight heparin
LN	lymph node
LNC	linear naevus comedonicus
LSN	linear sebaceous naevus
MABP	mean arterial blood pressure
MACS	minimal access cranial suspension lift
MAGPI	meatal advancement and glanuloplasty incorporated
MCPJ	metacarpophalangeal joint
MDT	multidisciplinary team
MED	minimal erythema dose
MFD	mandibular facial dysostosis
MM	malignant melanoma
MPNST	malignant peripheral nerve sheath tumour
MPS	mucopolysaccharides
MRI	magnetic resonance imaging
MS	multiple sclerosis
MTPJ	meta-tarsal phalangeal joint
MVA	motor vehicle accident
Na	sodium
NAC	nipple–areola complex
NAI	non accidental injury
ND	neck dissection
NF1 (2)	neurofibromatosis type 1 (2)
NG	nasogastric
NGF	nerve growth factor
NICH	non-involuting congenital haemangioma
NSAID	non-steroidal anti-inflammatory drug
NTOM	nerve territory oriented macrodactyly
NVB	neurovascular bundle
OA	osteoarthritis
OBPP	obstetrical brachial plexus palsy
OCP	oral contraceptive pill
OPG	oral pantomogram
ORIF	open reduction–internal fixation
ORL	oblique retinacular ligament
PD	Parkinson's disease
PDGF	platelet derived growth factor
PE	pulmonary embolus

PEG	percutaneous endoscopic gastrostomy
PIA	posterior interosseous artery
PIPJ	proximal interphalangeal joint
PL	palmaris longus
PMN	polymorphonuclear leucocytes
POP	plaster of Paris
PQ	pronator quadratus
PTA	posterior tibial artery
PTT	prothrombin time
PUCA	posterior ulna collateral artery
PVD	peripheral vascular disease
PWS	plagiocephaly without synostosis
PWS	port wine stain
qds	four times daily
RCL	radial collateral ligament
RICH	rapidly involuting congenital haemangioma
ROM	range of motion
RP	Raynaud's phenomenon
RSTL	relaxed skin tension lines
RTA	road traffic accident
SBE	sub-acute bacterial endocarditis
SCC	squamous cell cancer
SCIA	superficial circumflex iliac artery
SCIV	superficial circumflex iliac vein
SCM	sternocleidomastoid
SFS	superficial fascia system
SGAP	superior gluteal artery perforator flap
SLE	systemic lupus erythematosus
SLNB	sentinel lymph node biopsy
SMAP	superficial musculo-aponeurotic plane
SMAS	superficial musculo-aponeurotic system
SMCP	submucous cleft palate
SMR	submucous resection
SP	soft palate
SSD	silver sulfadiazine
SSG	split skin graft
SUCA	superior ulna collateral artery
SVC	superior vena cava
TAP	thoracodorsal artery perforator
TAR	thrombocytopenia absent radius syndrome
TATA	total anterior teno-arthrolysis
TB	tuberculosis

TBSA	total body surface area
TCL	transverse carpal ligament
tds	three times daily
TES	transthoracic endoscopic sympathectomy
TFCC	triangular fibrocartilage complex
TFL	tensor fascia lata
TGF	transforming growth factor
THR	total hip replacement
TKR	total knee replacement
TMJ	temperomandibular joint
TNF	tumour necrosis factor
TNM	tumour, nodes, metastases
TPFF	temporo-parietal fascia flap
TRAM	transverse rectus abdominus myocutaneous
TS	thymidylate synthase
TVP	thrombo-venous prophylaxis
U&E	electrolytes–12 channel
UCL	ulnar collateral ligament
UCL	unilateral cleft lip
US	ultrasound
UTI	urinary tract infection
VACTERL	vertebral, anal atresia, cardiac, tracheo-esophageal fistula, renal and limb anomalies
VATER	vertebral, anal atresia, tracheo-esophageal fistula, & renal anomalies
VBG	vascularized bone graft
VCs	venae comitantes
VEGF	vascular endothelial growth factor
VFTF	venous flow-through flap
VISI	volar inter calated scaphoid instability
VPC	velopharyngeal closure
VPI	velopharyngeal incompetence
VRAM	vertical rectus abdominus myocutaneous
VSD	ventricular septal defect
VTE	venous thrombolic event
WCC	white cell count
WHO	World Health Organization
XM	cross match (blood)
XR	X-ray/radiograph
ZPA	zone of polarizing activity

Laplace's law: $P = T/R$ (pressure = tension in wall/radius), so as the radius increases less pressure is required to overcome tension. Relevance in sudden increase in size of ganglia, aneurysms.

Chapter 1

Plastic surgery science

Gillies' principles of plastic surgery *2*
Other aphorisms in plastic surgery *3*
Wound healing: general *5*
Wound healing: factors affecting *8*
Skin basics *11*
Skin healing *13*
Skin grafts *15*
Scars: symptomatic, hypertrophic, and keloid *19*
Bone and bone healing *23*
Bone graft *25*
Distraction osteogenesis *27*
Cartilage *31*
Tendon healing *33*
Peripheral nerve healing *35*
Composite grafts *37*
Fat grafts *38*
Fetal wound healing *41*
Tissue expansion *42*
Delay phenomenon *45*
Topical negative pressure *46*
Pathology basics *48*
Principles of radiotherapy *49*
Sun damage *52*
Microbiology *55*
Clostridia *57*

Gillies' principles of plastic surgery

'A list of common sense rules setting forth a philosophical guide to Plastic Surgery' (D.R. Millard, *Principilization of Plastic Surgery*)
- Thou shalt make a plan (but keep flexibilities to the plan).
- Thou shalt have a style.
- Honour that which is normal and return it to normal position.
- Thou shalt not throw away a living thing.
- Thou shalt not bear false witness against thy defect.
- Thou shalt treat thy primary defect before worrying about the secondary one.
- Thou shalt provide thyself with a lifeboat.
- Thou shalt not do today what thou canst put off until tomorrow (procrastination principle).
- Thou shalt not have a routine.
- Thou shalt not covet thy neighbour's plastic unit, handmaidens, forehead flaps, Thiersch grafts, cartilage, or anything else that is thy neighbour's.

These principles are to a large extent valid today except for the procrastination principle, which has largely been supplanted by the 'do it all at once' principle—particularly for trauma and to a lesser extent even for cancer reconstruction.

Other aphorisms in plastic surgery

- Life is short, and Art long; the crisis fleeting; experience perilous, and decision difficult. The physician must not only be prepared to do what is right himself, but also to make the patient, the attendants, and externals cooperate.
- It is the most vital part of the flap that undergoes complete necrosis.
- Visibility of the scar is not determined by the length but by the site of the incision.
- A surgical short cut often ends up taking longer.
- A graft has no blood supply but must attain one; a flap has supply but must keep it.
- The surgeon who removes a breast with a malignant tumour should be the mortal enemy of the surgeon who is closing the wound (Halstead).
- Treat the patient not the X-ray.
- We diagnose only things we think about, we think about things we know, we only know things we've studied.
- You can always cut out more, never less.
- An operation is an assault on a person, legalized but still an assault (Walt).
- Even in plastic surgery, where meticulous artistry might be thought to be the first consideration, the best results are obtained by those who think, plan, and prepare, rather than those who perform with the self-conscious skill of the trapeze artist (Ogilvie).
- Worry about the blood loss you hear.
- There is no condition that cannot be made worse by surgery.
- What drugs do not cure, iron may cure.
- It's better to see the outside of an artery before you see the inside.
- Never promise a patient anything that is not in your power to provide.
- A patient is not always right but is never wrong (perhaps uninformed, uneducated or ignorant, but not wrong).
- Watch carefully what you do. Function before beauty (or style).
- The lesser the indication, the greater the complication.
- The patient is the most important person in the operating room.
- Treat every patient as you would like to be treated.
- Faster surgery does not represent better surgery.
- There are three kinds of surgeons: good fast surgeons, bad fast surgeons, and bad slow surgeons.
- The plural of anecdote is not data!
- The likelihood of infection has been determined before the last stitch has been inserted.
- Appose it, don't necrose it.
- A routine/protocol is only a substitute for thought.
- Attention to trifles leads to perfection, and perfection is no trifle.
- Good judgement comes from experience. Experience comes from bad judgement.
- Experience is that which allows you to recognize the mistake the second time around.
- Bleeding always stops.
- Skin is the best dressing (Lister).
- Soap and water and commonsense are the best disinfectants (Osler).

CHAPTER 1 Plastic surgery science

- When talent fails, triumph with effort.
- Better to be lucky than good.
- The harder I work, the luckier I get.
- The better you are, the luckier you get.
- Luck is when opportunity meets preparedness.
- Plan for the worst, deal with the best.
- Aptitude should determine specialization.
- Acknowledge your limitations so as to do no harm and extend your abilities to do the most good.
- Go for broke (always go for the very best, no matter what!).
- No guts no glory.
- Fortune favours the brave.
- Beware that when you have a hammer every thing looks like a nail.
- Do not fit a procedure to a patient just to increase your statistical figures.
- Pink as stink (the preferred colour of flaps in our unit).
- When tissues must be cut, the knife is best (Ogilvie).
- Slice, don't scratch, poke or push.
- Surgeons are judged by 3 As: ability, availability, and affability (Reznikof)
- The most skilful operators are not necessarily the best surgeons, but the best surgeons are rarely average technicians.
- Clinical ego is the patient's enemy… know when to back off and when to call for help.
- Just when you think you have it mastered, it'll turn round and bite you.
- Real surgeons do what's necessary, only the indecisive or inept or egotistical fortify themselves with more delay, investigations or dressings.

'Principles must be questioned, scrutinised, tested and modified. A principle should not be accepted based upon who said it or how it sounds. It is imperative for a competent surgeon to understand the difference between good, sound principles and principles that sound good!' (Chase.)

Wound healing: general

Definition
Wound healing involves three overlapping phases of inflammation, cell proliferation, and remodelling. This produces a scar resulting in a healed wound.

Phases of wound healing
- Inflammatory.
- Proliferative (fibroplasia).
- Remodelling (maturation).

Types of wound healing
- Primary: this occurs in a directly closed wound.
- Secondary: this wound is left open and allowed to heal by contraction and epithelialization.
- Tertiary (or delayed primary healing/closure): a wound which has been left open for several days is then closed primarily. The delay permits swelling or bleeding to diminish.

Systems involved in wound healing
- Vascular changes.
- Coagulation.
- Inflammation.
- Growth factors.
- Collagen synthesis and remodelling.
- Contraction.

Mechanism of wound healing

Vascular changes
The wound causes haemorrhage, initial vasoconstriction, and later vasodilatation with release of inflammatory mediators (histamine, bradykinin, prostaglandins, leukotrienes) and erythrocytes, leucocytes, and platelets. Neovascularization commences, producing granulation tissue

Coagulation (Fig. 1.1)
Haematoma and fibrin bind the wound, stabilizing the wound, adhering platelets, and supporting fibroblast migration. The coagulation and complement cascades are important conductors of inflammation and wound healing. Fibronectin is a glycoprotein found in association with fibrin in the first 24–48 hr of wound healing which helps leucocyte processes and forms the substrate for collagen deposition and organization.

Inflammation
Polymorphonuclear leucocytes (PMNs) and monocytes migrate to the wound within hours, and macrophages after 24–36 hr. The PMNs phagocytose debris and bacteria. The macrophages trigger and modulate fibroblast production of collagen via a wide variety of factors which may act with a dose-dependent relationship. Lymphocytes may inhibit or stimulate collagen synthesis or degradation.

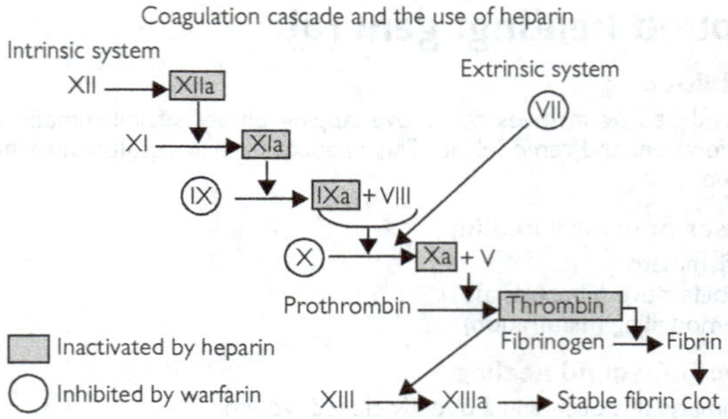

Fig. 1.1 Clotting and fibrinolysis cascades.

Growth factors

Chemotactic factors such as PDGF released on degranulation of the platelets attract fibroblasts, and other cells release PDGF-like substances to prolong the effect. Fibroblast growth factors (FGFs), transforming growth factor beta (TGFβ), and epidermal growth factor (EGF), amongst others, attract and stimulate mitosis in keratinocytes, fibroblasts, and other inflammatory cells. Interleukins (ILs) and tumour necrosis factors (TNFs) activate other cells to synthesize growth factors. Vascular endothelial growth factor (VEGF) does just that, stimulating angiogenesis.

Collagen synthesis, deposition, cross-linking, and remodelling

Under the influence of all of the above, the surrounding fibroblasts (usually from the endothelium of small vessels) proliferate and produce collagen which replaces the haematoma and fibrin. Collagen comprises three coiled polypeptide chains in complicated arrangements. Collagen is manufactured by fibroblasts as a repeating chain of the tripeptide of glycine–proline–hydroxyproline (or hydroxylysine) which is secreted as procollagen and then arranged in the triple helix of tropocollagen. After the amino and carboxy ends are cleaved off, these collagen molecules cross-link into fibrils and fibres with a quarter-length overlay. The type of weave determines the type of collagen. There are at least 10 types, of which types 1 and 3 figure importantly in healing. Type 1 comprises 80% of collagen in skin and tendon. Type 3, which is more elastic, comprises most of the remaining 20% of collagen in skin, mainly found in the papillary dermis and vessels.

The hydroxylation of proline is disturbed in hypoxia and vitamin C and iron deficiency. The hydroxylation of lysine is disturbed in one form of Ehlers–Danlos syndrome. Other forms relate to other aspects of collagen synthesis. Colchicine inhibits the cleavage of the ends of tropocollagen. BAPN and D-penicillamine (lathyrogens) prevent the cross-linking of the collagen bundles.

Collagen is initially disordered, offers little in the way of strength, and is cross-linked and remodelled in response to wound stresses. The remodelling is responsible for the restoration of tensile strength. Strength increases in weeks 3–8 but never reaches normal (only 80% normal). Even at the completion of wound healing continual turnover of collagen occurs with an equilibrium between deposition and removal, as in normal skin. Collagen removal is influenced by collagenases, peptidases, and proteinases. These may be increased by corticosteroids, parathyroid hormone, and colchicines, and inhibited by progesterone.

In addition to collagen, the fibroblasts produce ground substances like the glycosaminoglycans. Hyaluronic acid, chondroitin sulphate, and dermatin sulphate are produced in order and play a role with fibronectin in the organization of collagen fibres.

The type of collagen and ground substance changes as the healing process matures. The numbers of PMNs, macrophages, and fibroblasts diminish. Initially collagen type 3 predominates, but later type 1 becomes predominant. Ground substance initially rich in mucopolysaccharides and glycosaminoglycans returns to normal. Wound healing is complete.

Wound healing: factors affecting

Poor regulation of wound repair leads to 'over-healing' and excessive scar formation (see hypertrophic and keloid scar). However, there are also many factors which may impair wound healing, causing delay in repair or weakening of the eventual scar.

Local factors

Surgical wound handling: Tight closure, rough handling of the tissues, and excessive cauterization are detrimental.

Denervation: These areas are more prone to ulceration; the rate of collagenase activity is also increased.

Infection: Local infection prolongs the inflammatory phase and delays healing. It prevents epithelialization, promotes collagenolytic activity, and leads to haemorrhagic granulation tissue.

Radiation: Causes endarteritis obliterans in the local blood vessels, damages the lymphatics leading to local oedema, and causes permanent fibroblast damage.

Wound oxygenation. Transient low oxygen tension stimulates the healing mechanisms, especially angiogenesis. However, prolonged hypoxia is detrimental. Hyper-oxygenation may stimulate epidermal mitogenesis.

Local tissue ischaemia. Caused by radiation, peripheral vascular disease, diabetes, smoking (local vasoconstriction), and local oedema or haematoma. The resulting hypoxia prevents collagen synthesis.

Wound covering. Healing is improved in a warm and moist environment.

General factors

Drugs. Antimitotic chemotherapeutic agents. Steroids inhibit macrophages and hence fibrogenesis, angiogenesis, and wound contraction. NSAIDs reduce collagen synthesis

Age. Generally slower healing and weaker wounds in the elderly.

Smoking. Reduces arterial oxygen levels because of the high levels of CO.

Vitamin deficiency. Vitamin A promotes epithelialization and wound strength. Vitamin C deficiency leads to immature fibroblasts and defective capillaries in granulation tissue which cause local haemorrhages.

Zinc. This is a component of most enzymes; zinc deficiency retards healing.

Nutritional status. Low albumin levels (<30) are detrimental. Wound healing burns calories. Collagen synthesis needs vitamin A, C, D, zinc.

Temperature. Warmer environmental temperatures result in faster healing and stronger wounds.

Inherited disorders. Pseudoxanthoma elasticum, Ehlers–Danlos syndrome, cutis laxa, progeria, Werner's syndrome, and epidermolysis bullosa, amongst others, impair wound healing.

Acquired disorders. Diabetes (reduces local blood supply and innervation but also affects white cell activity), autoimmune inflammatory disorders.

Growth factors and wound healing

Definition: Growth factors are polypeptides which act on individual cells to promote cell growth, cell proliferation, and cell migration.

Classification and nomenclature: This can be confusing. Growth factors are named after their cell of origin (e.g. platelet-derived growth factor (PDGF)), the cell on which they act (e.g. fibroblast growth factor (FGF)), or their biological function (e.g. keratinocyte growth factors (KGFs)).

Mechanism of action
- Endocrine: produced by a cell in one part of the body and transported in the circulation to a distant cell where it produces its effect.
- Paracrine: acts on an adjacent cell.
- Autocrine: released from and acts on the same cell.
- Intracrine: not released but acts within the same cell.

Function
General Growth factors can produce a significant effect on wound healing even in minute amounts. They act as chemoattractants for macrophages, neutrophils, fibroblasts, and endothelial cells. They promote cell growth and mitosis even of quiescent cells. They have a role in differentiation of stem cells, such as fibroblasts from endothelial stem cells.

Future Trials have been conducted which add growth factors to a wound. Both PDGF and EGF reduce the healing time when added to an optimally treated wound. This suggests that growth factors are an intrinsic but not independent component of wound healing. A general caveat to the use of growth factors is that they work together to exert a combined effect on a wound. It may be that the use of individual growth factors produces inadequate or deficient wound healing rather than the physiological effect of their combined action. Increasing the rate of one aspect of wound healing may have no effect or a detrimental effect on other aspects, such as strength and maturation.

Growth factors in wound healing

PDGF: Potent chemoattractant; mitogen for fibroblasts, smooth muscle cells, and inflammatory cells. Produced by platelets, macrophages, vascular endothelial cells, and fibroblasts, and stimulates the production of fibronectin, hyaluronic acid, and collagenase. Extensively studied in decubitus and diabetic ulcers; accelerates the normal sequences of wound healing. Recombinant PDGF is approved for clinical use in the USA.

TGF-β: Potent chemoattractant produced by platelets, macrophages, fibroblasts, keratinocytes, and lymphocytes with a wide range of actions. Stimulates the growth of fibroblasts. It improves healing of diabetic ulcers.

VEGF: Potent mitogen for endothelial cells. Its role in wound healing may lie in its angiogenic properties.

EGF: Mitogen for fibroblasts produced in large quantities in early phase of wound healing by the platelets. Stimulates production of fibronectin. Early studies on chronic wounds are encouraging but more data are required for confirmation.

FGF: Heparin-bound growth factors produced by fibroblasts, endothelial cells, smooth muscle cells, and chondrocytes, which are mitogens for endothelial cells and function as angiogenic factors. There are no clinical trials to date with FGF.

Platelet releasates: Growth factors that are normally produced and released by platelets in the acute phase (e.g. PDGF, TGF-β, FGF, EGF, platelet factor 4, platelet-derived angiogenesis factor, and β-thromboglobulin) can be purified from peripheral blood and stored. Drawbacks include transmission of infection (unless harvested from patient), and presence of inhibitory factors in releasates. Results from clinical studies have been inconsistent.

Rate of wound healing
Improves if there is a smaller gap between wound edges, no dead space, no haematoma (less wound), no oedema (less distance to travel), good blood and oxygen supply, a well-nourished patient, no infection, no necrotic material to be removed by body (no prolongation of inflammatory phase).

Scar minimization
- Scar is remodelled collagen produced by the healing process.
- The amount of scar generated directly corresponds to the degree and duration of the inflammatory and proliferative phases.
- Minimal inflammation and proliferation results in little scar. Hence atraumatic handling of tissues and closure of all dead spaces, with good approximation of surfaces to be healed, minimizes the extent and duration of the inflammatory response, thus minimizing collagen production and fibroblast proliferation, resulting in better scars.

Skin basics

Skin is the impermeable barrier keeping water in and toxins out; it regulates body temperature, and maintains an awareness of its environment through a system of sensory receptors. It contains glands which secrete pheromones to attract or repel the opposite sex (sweat), tears to moisten the eyes, and fluid to nourish offspring (milk). What is more, it has an enhanced well-developed self-repair mechanism.

Layers of the skin
- Epidermis:
  - Stratum corneum (keratin containing dead cells, cemented).
  - Stratum granulosum (basophilic granules of keratohyalin).
  - Stratum lucidum (glabrous skin).
  - Stratum spinosum (cells with filaments/dendrites/desmosomes).
  - Stratum basale (also known as stratum germinatum) (basal layer).
- Dermis:
  - Reticular dermis.
  - Papillary dermis.

Epidermis
Stratified squamous epithelium mainly comprising keratinocytes with a few other cells. Keratinocytes produce keratin. The epidermis has layers: the basale and spinosum are the Malpighian layer. Melanin is found here.

Keratin
- Covalent cross-linked cystine-linked proteins which are hydrophilic. They are insoluble in water, acids, alkalis, and solvents, and are resistant to trypsin and pepsin.
- Keratin disorders are associated with rapid transit of epithelial cells through the epidermis or an abnormally short basal cell cycle. Keratin disorders include parakeratosis (cornified cells retain their nuclei), dyskeratosis (individual cells are prematurely keratinized), and hyperkeratosis (there is an increase in thickness of the stratum corneum with a thicker layer of keratin-containing cells and acanthosis (pseudo-glandular appearance to the epidermis).

Skin cells
- Include epidermal cells (keratinocytes), melanocytes, Langerhans cells, Merkel cells, and adnexal cells. Langerhans cells and mobile dendritic cells are important in immune function; presenting antigens to T-lymphocytes. Their numbers are reduced in sun exposed areas, and in patients on steroids and cytotoxics.
- Melanocytes are in the basal layer of the epidermis. They have long dendrites that extend to the surrounding keratinocytes. Melanocytes produce melanin and transfer it to the keratinocytes. The number of melanocytes is the same in all races, but melanin production and transfer differ.
- Langerhans cells also have dendrites. Merkel cells are involved in sensation.

Dermis
- Dermis consists of collagen, elastin fibres and ground substance, and has a rich blood supply. Dermis has layers: the subepidermal papillary layer containing tactile corpuscles of Meissner, and under this the reticular dermis containing the hair follicles, adnexal glands, Pacinian corpuscles, and erector pili smooth muscle.
- The Grenz layer is a usually superficial layer of collagen originating from hyperplastic fibroblasts just deep to the basement membrane, which attempts to repair the ravages of ultra violet light. It is this region that is responsible for the regenerative changes seen in dermabrasion or a chemical peel.

Solar damaged skin
Ultraviolet radiation:
- UVC   100–280 nm, blocked by ozone.
- UVB   280–320 nm, blocked by epidermis.
- UVA   320–400 nm, blocked by dermis and subcutaneous tissue.

Visible light has wavelengths >400 nm. The changes caused by solar damage parallel those seen in ageing skin but are accelerated and more severe; they consist of degenerative changes in the epidermis and dermis.

Dermis changes
- Elastosis whereby dermal collagen is replaced by a thickened tangled mass of altered elastic fibres, so that the content of elastic fibres is greater than the normal 5%. This leads to increased stretching of the skin.
- Increased ground substance, especially acid mucopolysaccharides.
- Decreased vascularity replaced by dilated vessels; evidenced by telangectasia.
- Chronic inflammation with patchy perivascular lymphocytes, histiocytes, and mast cells.

Epidermis changes
These are disorderly, giving variably thickened epidermis and thickened, ragged, and blurry basement membrane. Melanocytes may show increased number of cells (hyperplasia) in an uneven distribution giving blotchy skin.

Glands
- *Sweat glands* Can be eccrine or apocrine; eccrine occur on the body and discharge watery inorganic salts, apocrine tend to be in the axilla and groin and discharge organic cellular matter. Compare this with merocrine secretion and holocrine secretion of sebaceous glands. Sweat glands have myoepithelial cells which contract to discharge the sweat under neurological control.
- *Sebaceous glands* Produce sebum, an oily discharge of lipid and degenerate cells.

Hair follicles
Consist of a hair shaft arising from a root, surrounded by an epithelial follicle, associated with a sebaceous gland and an erector pili muscle.

Skin healing

Definition
Skin wound healing involves epithelialization, wound contraction, and extracellular matrix regeneration in three overlapping phases of inflammation, cell proliferation, and remodelling. This produces wound repair resulting in the formation of a scar.

Phases of wound healing
- Inflammatory.
- Proliferative (fibroplasia).
- Remodelling.

Types of cutaneous wound healing
Primary: This occurs in a directly closed wound.
Secondary: This wound is left open and allowed to heal by contraction and epithelialization.
Tertiary (also known as delayed primary healing/closure). A wound that had been left open is closed primarily after several days delay, usually once swelling or bleeding has diminished.

Physiology of cutaneous healing
Epithelialization
The first stage is *mobilization* when cells at the wound edge enlarge, flatten, and lose their attachment to adjoining cells and the basement membrane. This loss of contact inhibition allows the cells at the wound edge to *migrate* across the wound. The cells behind them also undergo this change and flow across the wound. Migration is halted when they meet the cells from the opposite side and contact inhibition is re-established. Cells are replaced by *mitosis* of fixed basal cells away from the wound edge. When the wound is bridged *cellular differentiation* occurs and the normal layers of the epidermis return. Epithelialization starts approx. 12 hr after suturing in a directly closed wound and continues for 7 days.

Dermal repair
Occurs by collagenization as described in general wound healing.

Contraction
This is a function of myofibroblasts. These are more prominent in granulating wounds. The extent of wound contraction is dependent on the number of myofibroblasts present. The contraction of the wound is maintained by collagen deposition and cross-linking.

Wound strength
This reaches approx. 50% at 6 weeks, eventually attaining 70–80% of pre-injury levels 8 weeks after injury. Full strength may take 12 weeks.

Scar minimization

Scar is remodelled collagen produced by the healing process.
- The amount of scar generated is inversely related to the degree and duration of the inflammatory and proliferative phases.
- Minimal inflammation and proliferation results in little scar. Hence atraumatic handling of tissues and closure of all dead spaces with good approximation of surfaces to be healed minimizes the extent and duration of the inflammatory response, thus minimizing collagen production and fibroblast proliferation resulting in better scars.

Skin grafts

Definition
A skin graft is a shave of epidermis including a variable thickness of dermis. This graft can be transferred to a distant site (bed) where, once applied, it establishes a blood supply. A split skin graft (SSG) must leave some remaining dermis at the donor site. The epidermal elements in the remaining dermis multiply and re-epithelialize the donor site. A full-thickness skin graft (FTSG) comprises the whole dermis and hence the donor site must be closed directly or itself skin grafted to heal.

Classification
- Autograft: graft removed from and returned to another site on the same individual.
- Isograft: graft taken from a genetically identical donor.
- Allograft: graft from an individual of the same species.
- Xenograft: graft taken from another species.

Uses
Skin cover, biological dressing.

Indications
A skin defect with a well-vascularized bed.

Donor site
Common donor areas
- SSG:
  - Thigh.
  - Medial upper arm.
  - Buttock (especially children).
  - Amputated skin or part (trauma case).
  - Hypothenar emminence or instep (glabrous skin).
- FTSG:
  - Groin.
  - Medial upper arm.
  - Cubital crease.
  - Distal wrist crease.
  - Pre- or post-auricular.
  - Supra-clavicular.

Anaesthesia
GA, LA (small), regional, local anaesthetic creams.

SSG
Methods of graft harvest
- Dermatome.
- Graft knife, e.g. Humby (roller), Watson.
- Scalpel.

Technique
Ensure adequate and even tension on surrounding skin. Lubricate skin (liquid paraffin, Cetavlon, water). Check thickness setting on knife or dermatome. Use a slicing back and forth movement if using a knife to take the graft. The powered dermatome does the to and fro movement automatically, so you only have to advance the dermatome evenly over the skin with constant pressure maintaining skin tension with your hand in front of the advancing machine. Place the graft, skin surface down (shiny side up), onto tulle gras or board. Ensure spread to full extent. The depth of graft depends on the knife setting, degree of pressure exerted when taking the graft, and the tension and thickness of skin.

Types of graft
Sheet (no perforations), perforated (multiple scalpel perforations), or meshed.

Mesh graft: Meshing is controlled placement of holes to allow the skin to spread over a greater surface area. The range is from 1:1.5 to 1:6. Advantages: allows free drainage of blood and exudate, covers a greater surface area, smaller relative donor site, increased edges for re-epithelialization, more comfortable over difficult recipient area. Disadvantages: greater area heals by secondary intention, less aesthetic appearance, harder to apply to wound. Can mesh the skin but leave unexpanded, thus reaping some benefits without the problems.

SSG application
The SSG is applied to the wound which should be as dry (haemostatically) as possible. It is applied shiny side down (epithelial side up). It should be trimmed to fit with minimal overhang. Overhanging SSG overlies water-resistant epithelium and it fails to revascularize and becomes moist and necrotic—a perfect environment for bacterial proliferation! The SSG edges, once trimmed to fit, are secured to the wound edges using sutures, staples, or cyanoacrylate glue welds. The latter is a personal favourite. The SSG should be dressed with paraffin gauze (tulle gras) and the defect packed carefully with moist well wrung out gauze to help compress the SSG to the contours of the bed until the defect is slightly overfilled. This is then covered by gauze and where possible bandaged to help compress the dressing to the bed and reduce shear. In areas which cannot be bandaged, such as the scalp and face, the SSG can be sutured and the dressing sutured to the wound edges with a tie-over 'pressure' dressing of gauze or foam. This secures the dressing but does not produce pressure!

Dressing for the SSG donor site
This should be absorbent, occlusive, able to remain intact for 1–2 weeks, and able to reduce dessication and mechanical trauma. Many different types of dressing have been used. Alginate dressings covered with absorbent gauze and left intact for approx. 10 days are the most popular. Marcaine can be sprinkled onto the alginate for post-operative analgesia. A personal favourite is perforated adhesive tape (Mefix, Hypafix, Fixomull) directly applied and left to drop off.

Healing at the SSG donor site

The area epitheliazes from the margins and from dermal remnants, particularly the hair follicles, sebaceous glands, and sweat glands. These dermal structures are derived from the epidermal cells which invade the dermis in the third month of fetal life. Healing commences under a clot of fibrin and blood within the first 24 hours. Thin SSG donor areas will heal in 7 days. The rate of healing is directly proportional to the thickness of the SSG harvested.

Donor site complications

Pain, delayed healing, infection, hypertrophic scarring, colour mismatch.

Recipient site complications

- Failure to 'take': this is caused by poor bed vascularity, or anything preventing revascularization, such as infection, shear or movement, and the accumulation of blood or fluid between the graft and bed.
- Graft pigmentation.
- Hypertrophic scarring.

Tips

- Overgrafting of the donor with meshed skin, particularly in the elderly, reduces many of the complications.
- When taking a very thin graft, mark the skin surface as it is often difficult to tell the two surfaces apart.
- Graft fixation to the recipient site is most efficiently achieved by drops of cyanoacrylate glue applied to the edges of the SSG as welds.

FTSG

Definition

This is a skin graft that comprises epidermis and all of the dermis.

Classification

As for SSG.

Uses

Classically for defects on the face, scalp, and hand. Also in hypospadias and hand surgery (Dupuytren's contracture, syndactyly, trauma). Defects are smaller and **should have a well-vascularized bed**.

Donor sites

- Post-auricular, pre-auricular, and supraclavicular.
- Any scar.
- Groin, lateral to the femoral artery for non-hair-bearing skin.
- Upper arm, cubital fossa, wrist crease, or medial forearm.

Harvesting

A template of the recipient defect is taken. The shape is transferred to the donor site and is completed to form an ellipse. The shape of the defect is scored into the epidermis only, and the whole ellipse is then excised and the donor site directly closed. The graft may then be defatted further with sharp scissors. Tensioning the graft over the surgeon's finger aids this process.

Graft care
The graft is inset with the dermis side down and trimmed to fit. The FTSG is secured by sutures. Some surgeons reduce graft shear and haematoma by quilting the graft to the bed. Others prefer to secure the dressing over the FTSG using a tie-over dressing. This involves suturing the FTSG to the wound edges with independent sutures which are left long. Once the wound and FTSG are encircled by these long sutures, a dressing of gauze, foam, or, traditionally, acriflavine wool is applied and the suture ends tied to secure the dressing. Many believe that these tie-over dressings exert pressure on the FTSG, thus helping to avoid fluid accumulating under the FTSG and improving graft take. However, these dressing do not exert pressure on the FTSG–wound interface; they merely fix the dressing, reducing shear.

Advantages
Better contour and texture, less pigmentation, potential for growth as the patient grows, less contraction, can transfer dermal structure e.g. hair follicles. More robust.

Disadvantages
Requires better vascularized bed, may have unwanted hair growth, limited supply.

Scars: symptomatic, hypertrophic, and keloid

Definition
Skin scars are the sequelae of the wound healing process following a breach in the epidermis and dermis. The optimal scar is a thin flat pale line in a relaxed skin tension line which does not traverse or contract anatomical boundaries or structures.

Pathophysiology
Scarring is a normal essential reparative response. It becomes pathological if the scar becomes symptomatic in either objective or subjective ways.

The clinical course of a normal scar is that 1–2 weeks following injury the wound appears nicely healed as a thin line. The continuing deposition of collagen often causes the scar to thicken for up to 4–6 weeks after injury. The scar may be red, inflamed, and feel tight and itchy. At the end of the proliferative phase of wound healing, the collagen deposition and resorption is at equilibrium and the wound strength is approximately 50% of normal. From this point on as the scar remodels it should gradually soften, becoming pale and asymptomatic and leaving a fine scar at 12–18 months after injury. Wound strength approaches normal at this stage.

Massage with a simple cream once the wound is fully healed helps to soften and desensitize the scar. Reassurance and information with regard to the natural history of scar will help the patient

Symptomatic scars

Classification of scars is descriptive
Scars may be flat, thin, wide/stretched, depressed, trap-door, contracted, hyper- or hypopigmented, raised, hypertrophic, or keloid.

Causes of symptomatic scars depend on
- Wound features: site, size, shape, complexity (e.g. shelving laceration, stellate laceration, multi-planar laceration), and the degree of injury.
- Scar position: crosses relaxed skin tension lines (RSTLs) or anatomical boundaries, flexural creases, close to deformable structures especially apertures.
- Wound management: was it closed directly, grafted, left to heal by secondary intention, closed under tension, closed by deformation?
- Abnormalities of wound healing particularly causing delayed wound healing: wound infection, dehiscence, tension, wound overlap, foreign body including necrotic material, healing disorders including malnutrition.

Scars may be symptomatic by
- Clinical complaints such as erythema, discoloration, pruritis, tenderness, pain, recurrent breakdown, cyst formation, contracture, loss of movement, deformation, widening or closure of apertures.
- Psychological complaints of ugliness, prominence, disturbance of aesthetic boundaries, drawing attention to injury or anatomical areas, and consequent embarrassment or anxiety.

Prevention of symptomatic and hypertrophic scars
When creating a scar ensure placement of the incision along relaxed skin tension lines and tension-free edge-to-edge closure with no dead space and the least possible foreign body introduction. The objectives are to reduce the risk factors for poor wound healing and hence the duration of the inflammatory phase.

In situations where wounds are already created ensure excisional debridement to remove foreign material, with early closure of wounds using flaps and grafts where necessary. Replacement of like with like, and restoration of structures and tissue to their rightful place will also prevent symptomatic scars.

Hypertrophic scars
Definition
Scars that are thickened and raised above the skin surface but remain within their original borders.

Pathophysiology
In essence these wounds heal with an over-proliferative response, producing excessive cells and extracellular matrix components including collagen and ground substance. The collagen is predominantly immature type III and disorganized with a nodular structure. Collagenase production is also increased indicating a generalized increase in wound activity. The epidermal layer is thickened and there is increased vascularity.

Natural history
These scars usually become obvious 1–2 weeks after epithelial closure and usually regress spontaneously (eventually). They are more responsive to treatment than keloid scars.

Epidemiology
They can occur at any age but mainly <20 years, and there is a familial inheritance. Males and females have an equal incidence

Aetiology
Idiopathic or any interference with normal wound healing such as infection, dehiscence, or tension. Chronic wounds or those with an increased inflammatory reaction, wounds not in RSTLs, wounds in areas of high tension such as the anterior chest, shoulders, and anterior neck, and wounds that heal by secondary intention. Those that take longer than 2–3 weeks to heal are more likely to be hypertrophic.

Keloid scars
Definition
These scars are thickened and elevated, and extend or invade beyond the boundaries of the original wound.

Pathophysiology
There is a build-up of collagen due to either excessive production or a relative reduction in degradation. The collagen is composed of larger fibrils laid down in an irregular pattern with less evidence of cross-linking than in normal scars. There are higher levels of soluble collagen and collagenase, indicating greater wound turnover. These wounds are relatively

hypocellular, and the fibroblasts present are phenotypically distinct from those in a normal scar. There is an increase in vascularity.

Natural history
These scars may occur up to a year after trauma or with no defined injury, as well as the usual presentation in the first few months following injury. They reach a specific size and remain at that size for many years without regression.

Epidemiology
These are most common at age <30 years. There is a significant familial incidence and they are 5–15 times more common in blacks and twice as common in Chinese and Japanese than in whites.

Aetiology
Genetic relationship, but actual cause unknown, hormonal (exhibit rapid growth during pregnancy and puberty and resolve after the menopause) and poor wound healing due to infection, dehiscence, tension, and trauma.

Location
Keloids most commonly occur on the face, earlobes and anterior chest.

Management of symptomatic, hypertrophic and keloid scars

Assessment
Take a history of the wound and the patient to assess the cause of the wound and patient predisposition to poor scars, including family history. Particularly identify any scar features which contributed to it becoming symptomatic that are potentially reversible.

Examination
Decide whether the scar is keloid, hypertrophic, or just symptomatic. Assess for signs of activity (inflammation, redness) or pigmentation. Check the site, orientation, and consequence of the scar. Examine any other scars to assess predilection of patient to scar poorly.

Investigations
Pretreatment photographs.

Conservative management
Allow the scar to settle for a year or until pale. Symptoms may be controlled by:
- Pressure: applications include elasticated pressure garments for trunk and limbs, facemasks, and clip earrings for ear lobes. Ideally, the pressure should exceed normal capillary pressure (24 mmHg). Pressure applications are applied when the wound is fully healed and need to be worn for 18–24 hr/day for 4–6 months to show their effect. The mode of action may be due to the pressure or increase in heat under the garments, or a combination of the two. Collagenase activity is increased and wound metabolism is decreased, leading to an early maturation of the scar.
- Silicone gel: this needs to be applied after full healing for 12–24 hr/day for 2–3 months before any benefits are seen. Some patients react to the gel with inflammation, rashes, and skin breakdown. The mode of

action is unknown, but factors such as pressure, wound hypoxia, increased skin temperature, hydration, or a direct chemical effect of silicone have been suggested. Success rates of over 80% for hypertrophic scars and 35% for keloid scars have been reported. Other occlusive materials such as hydrogels have been trialled with similar success rates to silicone.
- Tape: tape placed longitudinally along the wound post closure for 2 months has prevented hypertrophic scarring. The mode of action is thought to be due to the reduction in tension across the scar, and possibly the effect of occlusion.
- Corticosteroids: intralesional triamcinalone. In adults 20 mg/cm scar to a maximum of 120 mg. In children up to the age of 5 years maximum dose of 40 mg and from ages 5–10 maximum dose is 80 mg. A course of four injections is given every 4–6 weeks and the response is monitored. Intraoperative injection followed by a course if used in conjunction with surgery. Side effects are pain on injection, hypopigmentation, crystalline deposits, telangiectasia, and atrophy. Mode of action is to reduce collagen levels either by increased activity of collagenase due to a reduction in wound α_2-macroglobulin content or reduced collagen deposition due to a reduction in fibroblast activity. Steroids also reduce inflammation, resolving the pruritis and tenderness.
- Medication: topical vitamin A (retinoic acid) inhibits fibroblast production and vitamin E reduces fibroblast number. 5-Fluorouracil inhibits cell division, penicillamine prevents collagen cross-linking, and colchicine increases collagenase activity. Interferon and cyclosporin A have also been used.
- Laser: can reduce pigmentation and inflammation.

Surgical management
- Surgery should be reserved until the scar has matured unless it is causing a contracture. Revision surgery should consider the causes of the abnormal scar and prevent their recurrence. Options include scar excision and better surgical closure, serial excision (staged excision of the scar allowing adjacent skin relaxation between stages; used if the scar is too wide for single-stage complete excision and direct tension-free closure), break-up of the line of the scar or realignment along RSTL or anatomical boundaries. The latter two options may require Z-plasty, W-plasty, other flaps, or grafts.
- The patient should be warned that surgery may result in a worse scar.
- In symptomatic or hypertrophic scars arising from a wound complication or crossing RSTLs, excision and reorientation can result in a good scar. Excision of a keloid scar or a scar arising from an uncomplicated wound without adjunctive therapy gives recurrence rates of up to 80%. However, recurrence rates and outcomes can be improved by surgery and adjunctive treatments such as:
  - Radiation: five or six doses of 15–20 Gy external beam radiation or by local application (brachytherapy).
  - Steroids: success rates of approx. 75% have been quoted for surgery and steroid therapy. This may be further enhanced with added pressure or silicone.

Bone and bone healing

Types of bone
- Endochondral: in the axial skeleton and the limbs.
- Intramembranous: in the facial skeleton, cranial vault, and clavicle.

Bone zones
- Articular.
- Subchondral.
- Metaphyseal.
- Diaphyseal.

Composition
Bone has an outer dense cortex and an inner spongy cancellous component. The cortex is covered in periosteum on its outer surface and endosteum on its inner surface. The main cells are osteoclasts which resorb bone, osteoblasts which produce the unmineralized bone matrix (osteoid), and osteocytes which are osteoblasts surrounded by mineralized (mature) matrix. The matrix is organic, consisting of connective tissue components similar to skin, and inorganic, comprising calcium salts, the most significant of which is hydroxyapatite. The cortex is made up of osteocytes surrounded by their mineralized matrix. The cancellous component consists of trabeculae which are similar in structure to cortical bone and form the framework surrounding the marrow-filled spaces.

Blood supply
The external blood supply comes via the nutrient vessel direct from the adjacent artery or via the periosteum. The cortex is penetrated by Volkmann's canals which contain vessels that anastomose with those of the Haversian canals. Individual osteocytes are supplied by canaliculi from the Haversian vessels. A longitudinal blood supply comes via the bone marrow, which is also a supply of osteoprogenitor cells for wound healing.

Physiology
Bone changes constantly during skeletal growth (modelling). Bone continues to turn over in adult life (remodelling) where a balance between osteoclast resorption and osteoblast production is achieved (coupling).

Bone healing
Bone healing follows the same general wound healing processes of inflammation, proliferation, and repair, followed by remodelling. The first two phases take 6–8 weeks and remodelling takes months to years.

Like cutaneous wounds, bone can be described as having primary and secondary healing. Most bone heals by secondary healing.

Primary bone healing (also known as osteonal healing as occurs from osteocytes directly)
This occurs when the fracture is rigidly fixed and the bone ends are very close together and do not move. Osteoblasts from the bone ends produce matrix and the fracture heals with minimal inflammatory reaction

and callus. This process may take longer than secondary healing and is essentially similar to the remodelling of bone that occurs in adult life.

Secondary bone healing
Can be intramembranous (subperiosteal) or endochondral (external callus). Both contribute bone to the fracture site. The more movement at the site, the more endochondral bone is formed. It is very easy to be confused by terminology.
- **Intramembranous** bone formation (so called as it resembles how bone is formed in the skull, *not* because it only forms bone in these areas) occurs when committed osteoprogenitor cells from periosteum, muscle, and marrow form osteoblasts. These produce osteoid and progress on to mature bone.
- **Endochondral** bone formation (so called as it resembles bone formation at the epiphyseal growth plate) occurs by:
  - Induction and inflammation. Clot fills the fracture site and the usual inflammatory reaction is elicited. Osteoclasts derived from the marrow and circulating monocytes commence to remove the dead bone. Uncommitted mesenchymal cells differentiate into osteoblasts and chondroblasts following stimulation by factors such as hypoxia, electronegativity, inflammatory mediators, and growth factors (e.g. BMP). By the fourth day the clot is replaced with granulation tissue as vascularization occurs.
  - Soft callus. As the osteoclasts continue to consume the dead bone, chondroblasts lay down a colloid matrix (chondroid). The chondroid starts to calcify.
  - Hard callus (7–14 days). The osteoclasts commence to break down the calcified chondroid and osteoblasts lay down osteoid to replace it. This calcifies to form the hard callus which becomes disorganized woven bone.
  - Remodelling. The woven bone is remodelled into lamellar bone and a medullary canal is established. Wolff's law of remodelling in response to stress, possibly due to electromagnetic forces, holds.

The whole process is under mediation by local factors such as proteoglycans, BMP, osteocalcin and systemic factors such as calcitonin and parathyroid hormone.

Generally bone is formed by the intramembranous method on the periphery of the fracture and by the endochondral formation in the centre of the fracture.

Bone healing is stopped by reducing blood supply (by cooking with the drill/saw, stripping periosteum, and traumatizing surrounding soft tissue), instability, or by introducing infection.

Bone graft

Bone graft is the process of transferring bone from one site to another to augment healing or replace loss of bone substance. As in all grafts, the bone graft has to be vascularized by its bed. A bone flap bearing its own blood supply will heal in the same way as a fracture. By comparison, a bone graft incorporates in a similar sequence to that of fracture healing but three additional events occur.

- **Osteo-induction** is the ability of the autograft to stimulate osteoblast differentiation from progenitor cells at the recipient site. Osteo-inducing factors emitted from the graft include BMP.
- **Osteoconduction** is the influence that the autograft exerts on cells already committed to osteogenesis, thus promoting the process of creeping substitution.
- **Creeping substitution** is the process by which vascular tissue invades the graft and osteoblasts lay down the new bone.

Classification

Autologous bone graft, or allograft: autologous bone graft, has the optimal osteoconductive, osteo-inductive, and osteogenic properties and is biocompatible. However, it is limited in quantity.

Types of bone graft

Cortical bone grafts Osteoclasts remove the necrotic Haversian systems, thus increasing the porosity of the graft. Vascularization is slow, starting at the end of the first week and taking up to 8 weeks. At approx. 12 weeks osteoblasts lay down new bone, entrapping any remaining foci of necrotic cortex, thus leaving a mixture of new and old bone. The grafted area remains weaker than normal for 1–2 years.

Cancellous bone grafts In contrast, these start with osteoblast laying down new bone and complete osteoclastic absorption of foci of necrotic graft. Revascularization is generally completed by 2 weeks and the area goes on to complete repair of normal strength.

Cortico-cancellous bone grafts have the benefits of cancellous grafts with the structural support and integrity of cortical grafts.

Membranous bone grafts are more resistant to absorption and revascularize faster than endochondral bone.

Vascularized bone flap in which the ends heal like a fracture site. It should be used to cover gaps greater than 6 cm in patients where growth of the area is important, in a compromised poorly vascularized bed, and where rapid healing or instant relative strength is required. This may be a free tissue transfer or transferred on a defined pedicle. It may comprise bone only (e.g. fibula, iliac crest) or bone and surrounding muscle or skin (e.g. radial forearm skin and radius).

Factors influencing bone graft survival
Recipient site Ideally in a non-irradiated non-scarred tissue bed with a good blood supply.
Graft orientation With the periosteum towards the soft tissue and the cancellous component in contact with host bone.
Periosteum This influences revascularization and enhances new bone formation.
Fixation Rigid fixation allows vessel in-growth. The graft survives longer with greater weight and volume.
Mechanical forces: Force transmission or graft loading enhances bone formation and minimizes resorption.
Inlay versus onlay Inlay bone graft usually is more rigidly fixed and loaded compared than onlay.
Surgical: Air exposure, saline, and some antibiotics reduce the cellular viability of the graft. Therefore wrap the graft in a blood-soaked swab. Avoid dead space around the graft and keep each fragment less than 5 mm^2.

Bone substitutes
Compare these with autologous bone graft. Consider the substitutes properties under the categories:
- Genic: has capacity to form bone itself.
- Inductive: stimulates new bone but can not produce by itself.
- Conductive: passive scaffold.
- Biocompatibility

Osteogenic materials
Composite material. Hydroyapatite loaded with bone marrow stromal fibroblasts that will differentiate.

Osteoinductive materials
Demineralized bone matrix contains BMPs which stimulate cells to become osteoblasts. BMPs are a subset of the transforming growth factor-β super-family which includes TGF-β.

Osteoconductive materials
Most bone substitutes are scaffolds which do not produce bone or stimulate its production from surrounding tissue. However, they are replaced by creeping substitution.

Distraction osteogenesis

Distraction osteogensesis is the formation of new bone after creation of an osteotomy by controlled gradual distraction of the fracture ends. Initially described by Alessandro Codivilla (1904) but developed by Gavril Ilizarov (1954).

General principles

External fixation of the bone to be distracted. A fracture is created by osteotomy, which is distracted as it heals by using the fixator. As the fracture gap is distracted, bone healing is stimulated. The new bone formation is intra-membranous with no cartilaginous intermediate.

Distraction osteogenesis techniques

- Distraction lengthening.
- Acute lengthening + interpositional bone graft.
- Bone transport (to close a non-union create a distant osteotomy and transport the segment of bone to close and heal the non-union site creating bone at the new osteotomy site).

Bone generation

The principle is that slow controlled seperation of healing bone ends results in a 'tension stress effect' leading to increased cell activity, increased vascularity, and increased collagen type 1 production. Within a week a fibrous bridge of dense longitudinally aligned collagen fibres is formed. In the subsequent week bone spicules form at the edges of the osteotomy, extending into the fibrous interzone. This is called the primary mineralization front. This progressively extends to close the gap, with remodelling and maturation of the bone it leaves behind as it progresses. This bone eventually becomes lamellar.

A longitudinal section through a osteogenic site will show the following zones:

- Bone with osteotomy site then maturing bone zone.
- Bone remodelling zone.
- New bone formation zone.
- Fibrous inter-zone.
- New bone formation zone.
- Bone remodelling zone.
- Bone with osteotomy site then maturing bone zone.

Process steps of distraction osteogenesis

- Operation to apply fixator and create osteotomy.
- Latency period.
- Distraction.
- Consolidation.
- Removal of fixator.
- Optional steps: bone graft interposition.

Operative technique

- External fixator/distractor device placed first.
- Longitudinal periosteum split.

- Osteotomy (preferably corticotomy only preserving endosteal blood supply) by low-energy method.
- Check distraction possible; then close gap to <1 mm.
- Close periosteum.
- Wound closure.

Latency period
- Wait 7 days; then commence distraction.

Distraction period
- Regular frequent distraction 0.25 mm four times a day.
- Pin site care.
- Weekly X-ray.
- Use affected part to maintain function.
- Physiotherapy to maintain joint and tendon mobility.

Consolidation period
Period between the end of distraction to the removal of the fixator. Remove the fixator when:
- There is neocortex on three of four sides on AP and lateral X-ray.
- When the period exceeds twice the duration of distraction.

Remove fixator
- May not need anaesthetic.
- After removal of devices, X-ray 6/52, 3/12, 6/12, 9/12, and 12/12.
- Can also assess regenerate by ultrasound.

Factors affecting new bone formation
- Patient variables:
  - Age (children twice as fast as adults).
  - Bone.
  - Blood supply.
  - Health.
- Fixation stability:
  - ↑ bone if ↑ stability.
  - Ring better then uniplanar fixator.
  - Longitudinal wire better then none.
- Type of osteotomy:
  - Corticotomy to preserve periosteum and endosteal supply.
  - Subperiosteal corticotomy better than dividing periosteum.
  - 'Low-energy' division techniques; use osteotomes rather than saw.
  - Uni/bi/trifocal osteotomies—the less the more bone formation.
- Site of osteotomy:
  - Metaphyseal better than diaphyseal.
- Latency period:
  - Optimal period is 5–7 days.
  - Avoid acute inflammatory phase.
  - Shorter delay in children, longer in the aged.
  - Not too long (>14 days) or will not be able to distract (premature consolidation).
  - Avoid an immediate distraction gap as healing may fail to initiate.

- Rate and frequency (rhythm) of distraction:
  - 1 mm/day is best.
  - ↑ frequency of distraction better (60 > 4 > 1 per day).
  - Regular rhythm better than random.
  - ↓ In older.
  - Reduce rate in hand.
  - ↓ Rate as gap length increases or as new bone formation width narrows, especially in narrow bones.
  - 1 mm/day in very frequent regular increments is also better for soft tissues and angiogenesis.

Indications

Bone loss or deficit particularly if small and covered with a good well-vascularized soft tissue envelope. Bone sufficiently long to insert fixator. Bone well vascularized.

- Craniofacial:
  - Mandibular hypoplasia.
  - Distraction of midface, orbits.
- Hand and upper limb:
  - Digital hypoplasia.
  - Thumb reconstruction.
  - Bone loss or hypoplasia in forearm.
- Lower limb:
  - Bone loss in trauma or tumour.

Contraindications

- Non-compliant patient/family.
- Unstable home environment.
- Unstable skin and soft tissue.
- Infection.
- Small bone fragments.
- Age <6–12 years.

Advantages

- Avoids morbidity of bone graft.
- Distracts the soft tissues as well so no soft tissue envelope limitation.

Disadvantages

- At least two operative procedures., one to create the 'fracture' and apply the distracting fixator and another to remove the fixator. In practice there may be other procedures to adjust the fixator, re-fracture the bone, apply bone graft, and treat complications.
- Lengthy process.
- Soft tissue distraction causes scar and other complications.

Complications

- Early:
  - Pin injury to soft tissues.
  - Pin site infection.
  - Pin loosening.
  - Device failure.

- Late:
  - Bone pin site infection.
  - Distraction neuropathy.
  - Ischaemia.
  - Contractures from distraction or lack of movement.
  - Scars.
  - Fibrosis of soft tissues.
  - Pain.
  - Premature fusion of osteotomy.
  - Non-union.
  - Malunion.
  - Fracture of new bone.

Bone graft may be needed if the regenerate is poor or if the goal is rapid soft tissue and bone distraction with interposition bone graft rather then osteogenesis.

Distraction lengthening in the hand

In 1970 Matev used distraction osteogenesis for thumb metacarpal lengthening for thumb amputation reconstruction (in teenagers). The lengths achievable by this technique are:
- Metacarpal   34 mm
- Proximal phalanx   17 mm
- Middle phalanx   23 mm

Soft tissue distraction has been used to correct radial dysplasia and syndactyly to facilitate surgery.

Distraction osteogenesis in craniofacial surgery

Continues to evolve but is now commonplace for correction of mandibular deformity. Seems to have fewer complications than in the limbs, presumably because of the better blood supply. Now being applied to move orbits, midface, hard palates, and zygomas.

Advances
Automated distractors which continually distract, giving embryonic type growth with little fibrosis, faster bone growth, and better soft tissues.

Debates
Role of tobacco and NSAIDs in inhibiting bone formation.

Cartilage

Composition
Cartilage cells (chondrocytes) secrete a matrix of chondromucoprotein, elastin, and collagen which surrounds them and has a significant water content. The exact content of the matrix depends on the type of cartilage. The cartilage is covered by a vascular layer of perichondrium.

Growth
This occurs by mitosis of younger chondrocytes and differentiation of perichondrial cells into chondrocytes. Cartilage stops growing in adults and becomes harder, eventually calcifying.

Types
- Hyaline covers articular surfaces of bones and forms the costal, alar, and airway cartilages.
- Elastic cartilage is more flexible and makes up the external ear.
- Fibrocartilage provides strong support in the intervertebral discs and where tendons insert into bone.

Nutrition
There is no intra cartilagenous blood supply. Nutrients and oxygen diffuse through the matrix.

Healing
In children cartilage has the ability to regenerate from chondrocytes and perichondrium. This is much reduced in the adult, although still occurs from the perichondrium and the defects tend to fill with fibrous tissue.

Cartilage grafts
Classification Autograft, allograft, xenograft.

Immunogenicity Cartilage is weakly immunogenic because of the barrier to chondrocytes created by the weakly antigenic matrix. Most cartilage grafting is autograft, as allograft and xenograft have a generally poorer outcome probably because of rejection.

Uses Nasal, auricular, craniofacial, and joint reconstruction; nipple fabrication.

Donor site Concha (good for nasal tip and ala; also used for joint resurfacing); nasal septum (best for nose reconstruction); costal cartilage (good for nasal dorsal defects needing structural support). (See Fig. 1.2.)

Recipient site The cartilage undergoes no change; hence elastic cartilage remains elastic etc. It is nourished by diffusion.

Technical features Cartilage may be carved or moulded by scoring (Gibson effect). (See Fig. 1.3.) Its survival is enhanced if transferred with perichondrium.

Other autografts Perichondrial graft has been shown to regenerate cartilage. Tissue cultured cells within an injectable matrix are being investigated.

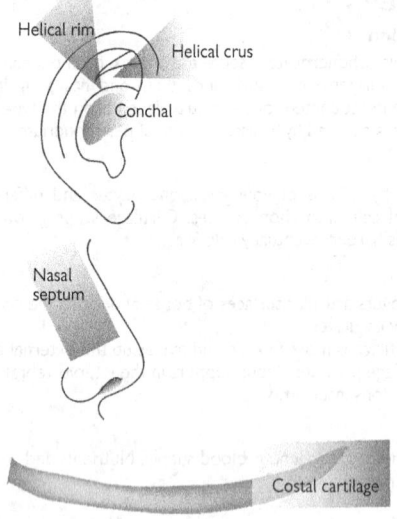

Fig. 1.2 Sources of cartilage grafts.

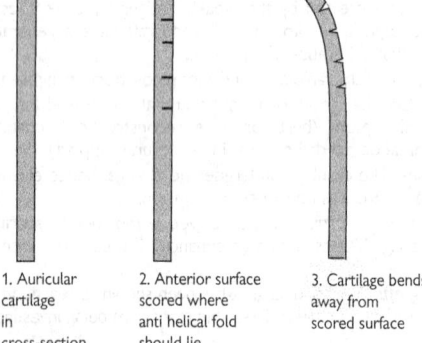

1. Auricular cartilage in cross-section
2. Anterior surface scored where anti helical fold should lie
3. Cartilage bends away from scored surface

Fig. 1.3 Gibson effect.

Tendon healing

Introduction
A tendon is composed of collagen and connects muscle to bone or other structure. It may be surrounded by paratenon or sheath, and on the palm and fingers is enclosed by bursae.

Blood supply
- Mesotenon on the dorsal surface supplies in the forearm and palm. These condense into vinculae that enter the deep side of the flexor tendons proximal to the interphalangeal joints.
- Longitudinal internal supply between the tendon fascicles.

Nutrition
- Perfusion via the vascular supply.
- Diffusion via synovial fluid which bathes the tendons.

Healing
See Wound healing.

Inflammation (0–6 days)
Blood clot, fibrinous material, and inflammatory cells are deposited between the tendon ends. Epitenon cells from the tendon surface migrate and differentiate into fibroblasts. Fibroblasts and inflammatory cells also migrate from peritendinous structures, creating adhesions.

Proliferation (6–28 days)
Collagen produced by fibroblasts (peak level at 2 weeks). Tendon revascularizes.

Remodelling (28 days–4 months)
Peritendinous adhesions break down. Collagen fibres orientate longitudinally. Gradual gain in strength to normal at 9 months.

Debate: intrinsic versus extrinsic healing
Controversy over whether collagen production comes from tenocytes, found in endotenon or paratenon in or on the tendon (intrinsic), or from fibroblasts originating from the surrounding tissue (extrinsic). Originally it was believed that tendons relied on fibroblast proliferation from the peritendinous structures, meaning that tendons had to heal by forming fibrous bridges to the surroundings. These were called adhesions as they prevented free movement. Lundborg showed that tendons could heal without extrinsic adhesions even when suspended in synovial fluid. The relative importance of both elements is debated, but current techniques of post-operative management rely heavily on intrinsic healing with early tendon movement to reduce adhesion formation, with the goal of improving the long-term functional result. This dependence on intrinsic healing has led to debate regarding the importance of tendon sheath repair to retain nourishing synovial fluid around the repair site and limit adhesions.

Factors affecting healing
See Wound healing factors. Controlled stress and mobilization of the tendons. Palmar suture placement is recommended to minimize the impact of grasping sutures on the blood supply, which is mainly dorsal.

Relevance
As inflammatory changes occur, softening and loss of tendon structural integrity mean that the strength of the repair diminishes. This is at its lowest at 14–21 days as inflammation peaks and before considerable fibroplasia has occurred. During this period care needs to be taken not to overstress the repair. Stress is an important component of later therapy to encourage collagen deposition and alignment to strengthen the tendon.

Peripheral nerve healing

Anatomy

The nerve is comprised of multiple neurons. Each neuron has a cell body and an axon. The axon consists of a single nerve fibre containing many neurofibrils. Each axon is ensheathed by a Schwann cell, a neuroectodermally derived cell which produces the phospholipid myelin coating to the axon.

Peripheral nerves have three distinctive supportive connective tissue sheaths. The endoneurium, which is composed mainly of fibroblasts collagen and ground substance, surrounds each nerve fibre. The perineurium surrounds the fascicles, whilst the nerve itself is covered by the perineurium.

The vascular supply may be intrinsic or extrinsic. The extrinsic supply comes from segmental arteries, including muscular perforators and periosteal vessels, via a mesoneurium and ramifies on the epineurium. Branches from the epineurium connect with the intrinsic supply, which exists in all layers of the nerve.

Nerve healing

This is characterized by initial degeneration followed by regeneration.

Degeneration

This continues for up to 14 days post injury. Distal (Wallerian) degeneration is from the site of injury to the termination of the nerve and commences initially with axoplasmic condensation (0–2 days). The myelin disintegrates, and this and the axon are cleared by pluripotential Schwann cells (3–14 days). Towards the end of this phase the perineurium starts to break down. Proximal degeneration is to the last preserved internode. The end organ starts to degenerate once neuronal stimulation ceases.

Wound site

This initially fills with blood clot, followed by Schwann cell proliferation filling the defect and fibroblasts from the connective tissue layers laying down collagen.

Regeneration

This commences after a variable latent period (approx. 24 hr). The neuron undergoes central chromatolysis and tubulin (nerve protein) production increases, with an associated decrease in the concentration of nerve transmitter substances. Proximally the cut end bulges and forms a growth cone. Branches sprout from the cone and enter the Schwann cell scar. The successful branches find an endoneurial tube and continue down the nerve.

Distally, Schwann cells pack remaining endoneurial sheath. They accept advancing buds and remyelinate the advancing axons. Collagen is being laid down external to the basement lamina, thus progressively narrowing the internal diameter of the nerve fibre.

Regeneration is promoted by neurotrophic factors, such as nerve growth factor and laminin, and neurotropic changes in the external environment of the nerve which guide nerve growth.

Speed of healing

All figures vary. Usually, after a latent period of 24–48 hr, the nerve grows through the scar at 0.25 mm/day. Once in the distal endoneurial tube, growth rate is approx. 1 mm/day. An advancing Tinel's sign should be elicited at 6 weeks–3 months at the latest. Muscle can be innervated up to 3 years post injury but the result at approx. 18 months is usually final.

Factors affecting nerve healing

Patient Age <6 years, 2PD <6 mm; age 6–20 years, 2PD = age; age >30 years, 2PD >30 mm if median or ulnar is divided. Cooperative patient has better results.
Injury Mechanism of injury. Best to worst: sharp laceration–crush–stretch–blast.
Level of injury Proximal worse than distal.
Degree of injury See nerve repair. Complete division with gap formation has the worst prognosis.
Bed Ischaemic area around the repair is no good.

Management

Timing Earlier the better.
Surgical technique Gentle handling. No gap and no tension with the minimum number of sutures. Epineural repair recommended.

Post-operative care

Relieve discomfort, protect muscle from deforming forces, mobilize joints, and protect non-sensate skin (Sunderland). During recovery splinting and sensory re-education are useful.

Composite grafts

Definition
Two or more tissue components

Classification
By tissue grafted.

Indications
- Alar rim using skin and cartilage from the helix.
- Nipple using contralateral nipple.
- Eyelid using full-thickness eyelid–tarsal grafts or nasal mucosa and septum.
- Dermal fat for contour defects

Graft take
There is minimal plasmatic imbibition. Blood flow is established on the third or fourth post-operative day.

Classically go through colour changes: white, (grey-)blue, then pink over a 7–10 day period as the graft is initially ischaemic, then receives some blood but is blue because of poor flow and cyanosis, and becomes pink as circulation develops.

Technical factors
- Maximum diameter is 1–1.5 cm from nearest well-vascularized edge.
- Some surgeons pre-excise the wound bed and leave for 10 days prior to grafting.
- Cooling of the graft (5–10°C), when initially inset may improve take.

Fat grafts

Fat has been used as graft since the late 1800s.

Fat graft healing theories
- Host replacement theory:
  - Fat in cells taken up by histiocytes which replace fat cells.
- Cell survival theory:
  - Fat cells survive if revascularized.
  - Histiocytes remove dead cells and fat.
  - Means large volumes resorb more, as slower and poorer revascularization.

Fat graft healing
- Inflammation (first 3 days).
- Revascularization (4–7 days) with increased inflammatory cells and foreign body giant cells seen.
- Fat degeneration, depending on revascularization (2–3 months).
- Fat stabilization (after 1 year). Fat that survives this long persists.

Autogenous fat graft

Definition
- Fat.

Indications
- Contour defects—small.
- Depressed scars.
- Gliding cover for nerves or tendons.
- Space filler
  - To fill frontal sinus when obliterated.
  - To prevent bone healing as in epiphysiolysis/ correction synostosis.

Donor sites
- Abdomen wall.
- Adjacent to incision/operating site.
- Any scar.
- Groin.
- Lateral gluteal area.
- Gluteal fold.

Technical factors
- Overcorrect the defect by 20–30% to counter reabsorption.
- Fix the graft securely.
- Better to use multiple small grafts then one big one.

Advantages
- Autograft.

Disadvantages
- Resorption.
- Fat necrosis leading to discharge.

Free dermal fat grafts

Definition
- Dermis, denuded of epidermal covering, and its underlying fat.

Indications
- Contour defects.
- Depressed scars.
- Gliding cover for nerves or tendons.
- Space filler:
  - To fill frontal sinus when obliterated.
  - To prevent bone healing as in epiphysiolysis/correction synostosis.

Donor sites
- Any scar.
- Groin.
- Lateral gluteal area.
- Gluteal fold.

Technical factors
- Overcorrect the defect by 20–30% to counter reabsorption.
- Fix the graft securely.
- Some debate on whether it is best inset with dermis up or down.
- Careful haemostasis.

Advantages
- Autograft.

Disadvantages
- Resorption.
- Cyst formation.
- Fat necrosis leading to discharge.

Fat flaps

Definition
- Fat but vascularized by axial vessel.
- Dermal fat, fat, or omentum.
- Pedicled or free.

Indications
- Contour defects—large.
- Depressed scars.
- Gliding cover for nerves or tendons.
- Prevent healing of transverse carpal ligament.

Donor sites
- Free (groin, gluteal area, omentum).
- Pedicled (hypothenar fat pad flap).

Technical factors
- No resorption as well vascularized.
- Fixation can be difficult in areas subject to gravity, especially if fat alone transferred.

Advantages
- Autograft.

Disadvantages
- Size changes with weight gain or loss.

Fat injection

Definition
- Fat initially harvested as part of liposuction procedure has been used to treat contour depressions since 1983.
- Coleman technique involves concentration of fat cells by centrifugation and use by injecting tiny globular amounts in different areas and in different planes.

Indications
- Contour defects:
- Usually small facial defects.
- Depressed scars.
- Penile augmentation.
- Vocal cord augmentation.
- Sphincteric incontinence augmentation.

Donor sites
- Any fatty area.

Technical factors
- Harvested by syringe suction using 10 mL syringe and gentle suction.
- Syringe then centrifuged 3000 rpm for 2 min.
- Concentrated fat cells collected and injected gently using 18 gauge needle.
- Must over-correct.

Advantages
- Autograft.

Disadvantages
- Resorption.

Complications
- Uncommon except for resorption.
- Arterial occlusion at site of injection leading to blindness, stroke, skin necrosis (reportedly can occur after as little as 0.5 mL injected on nasal bridge!).
- Fat emboli and stroke.

Fetal wound healing

Introduction
Scarless healing in the human fetus was first noted in the late 1970s. Further study has shown fetal wounds to heal by a process of regeneration rather than repair. There are many controversies and much ongoing research in this area

Intrinsic factors
Inflammatory phase
The fetal wound contains very few inflammatory cells and this phase is absent in the fetus.

Proliferative phase
This is controlled by the fibroblast and the epidermis. This is characterized by hyaluronic acid deposition and the laying down of organized type 3 collagen, which persists in the wound. Myofibroblasts exist in the wound but contraction is absent.

Remodelling
As the fetal wound repairs by regeneration, a remodelling phase is not seen.

Growth factors
Controversies exist, but TGF-β and β-FGF appear to be absent in fetal wounds.

Oxygenation
The fetus is relatively hypoxic compared with the postnatal human.

Extrinsic factors
Environment
The fetus is bathed in amniotic fluid, which is rich in growth factors, hyaluronic acid, and fibronectin. It provides a warm sterile environment for wound healing and inhibits fibroblast contraction. However, studies of fetal wound healing without amniotic fluid show the same scarless result.

Timescale
Fetal wounds heal rapidly, usually within 5–7 days. This is thought to be due to the faster deposition of fibronectin and the amount of hyaluronic acid in the wound.

Trimester
All third trimester wounds heal with a scar. Earlier gestation healing depends on the wound size. Wounds less than 9 mm in diameter heal scarlessly in the first trimester, as do smaller wounds in the second trimester. Larger wounds heal with a scar regardless of gestational age.

Tissue variation
Bone, skin, and palatal mucoperiosteum appear to heal scarlessly in the fetus. Tendon and nerve heal with a scar.

Tissue expansion

Definition
Tissue expansion is the increase in surface area of tissue brought about by mechanical means. The term is frequently used to describe a specific plastic surgical technique involving placing an expander under the tissue to be expanded and then gradually expanding the expander.

Tissues expanded
Skin, fascia, muscle and experimentally nerve.

Physiology
The skin expands by a process of creep and stress relaxation. Creep is the time-dependent plastic deformation of any material or tissue in response to constant stress. Stress relaxation occurs when the force required to stretch the skin to a given length gradually decreases over time. The extra skin in tissue expansion comes from creep and stress relaxation but also recruitment from surrounding skin, new growth, and compression/thinning of the skin. The epidermis thickens because of cellular hyperplasia and has an increased rate of mitosis. The dermis thins and there is fragmentaion of elastic fibres. Fat loss occurs and is permanent. Muscle may have some temporary decrease in bulk but there is no loss of function. With the exception of fat, the parameters return to normal after expander removal.

A capsule with four zones forms around the expander: inner zone of macrophages; central zone of fibroblasts and myofibroblasts orientated parallel to the implant surface; transitional zone containing collagen; outer zone of vessels and collagen. The vascularity of expanded skin is better than normal and shows a similar picture to flap delay.

Uses
- Expand local tissue adjacent to a defect or lesion.
- Expand tissue adjacent to a flap or full-thickness skin graft donor site and hence permit closure.
- Expansion of the flap itself.

Indications
Expansion works best when there is a firm bony base below the expander. Hence it is best suited to breast reconstruction, scalp defects, and baldness, and less so to limb, neck, and abdomen.

Technique
Planning
Site selection for best tissue match: solid base to expand against, preferably with a suprafascial plane, and with good quality skin and soft tissue. Avoid if compromised by previous scars, trauma, infection, poor vascularity, or risk of recurrence of malignancy. Plan eventual flap and incisions before expander placement. Choose appropriate shape expander with a base size at least twice the size of the defect (2.5 better). Measure the circumference of the part of the body using reliable landmarks. Measure the size of the defect. Planned expansion will be the addition of the two

measurements to create a new circumference. The defect may increase in size with expansion so this measurement will need adjustment. For confidence over-expand requirements by 15%. Estimate expander size required using formula. However, expanders can be safely inflated to multiples of their stated volume.

Equipment

Expanders are silicon 'bags' connected to an injection port by tubing. The bags may be textured or smooth, have a firm or pliable base, be any shape or size, or be custom made. The port is small and non-expansile with a firm base. It is placed subcutaneously at a distance from the expander, in an accessible but inconspicuous spot. Uncommonly ports may be within the expander or placed externally. Saline is injected into the port and fills the expander.

Incision

- A distant radially placed incision, so that expansion forces act longitudinally rather than across the incision scar.
- Through an incision that will be incorporated in the definitive reconstruction.
- A W or V incision within the lesion, with the point(s) of the V (W) aiming away from the expander site.

Procedure

Wide blunt dissection ensuring that the expander is well away from the suture line. Initial dissection should create a tunnel which then opens into the expander placement space. This will reduce tension at the incision site. The expander can then be rolled into a cigar shape and inserted through the tunnel to unfold in the expander space. Intra-dermal sutures are used to support the incision.

Inflation: at time of placement to reduce dead space, ensure correct orientation of the expander and commence expansion. Include 1–2 mL of methylene blue to colour the fluid within the expander as this will increase confidence of correct placement of the injection needle (by checking for blue coloured drawback after needle insertion) on future expansion. Remove some of the initial expansion fluid to reduce tension. Check capillary return of the overlying skin. Beware tight dressings and bandages compromising skin circulation.

At 1–2 weeks post-operatively check incision healing, expander tension, and vascularity, and commence inflation if appropriate. Inflate with Normal saline using 23 gauge needles to minimize port leakage. Inflate until the patient complains of discomfort or capillary refill diminishes over the expander; then remove a few millilitres. Repeat weekly until the desired size. Ideally, smaller inflations every 3 days are better but are less practical. EMLA cream over injection ports reduces discomfort. Rapid expansion can be achieved with a constant infusion pump. Expansion may take 4 weeks to 4 months.

Removal and flap: incorporating incision in flap design and including expander capsule in the flap. Diathermy can be used against the expander without perforating it. The surrounding fibrous capsule can cause contour deformities, especially at the edges, and can be excised or left to resolve.

Risks and complications
- Infection and extrusion are the most common. If these occur early the procedure should be abandoned. Later cases can be treated with antibiotics and dressings and expansion may continue.
- Haematoma, seroma, implant rupture, rotation or loss of port, necrosis of overlying skin, pain, neurapraxia, erosion of bone, muscle, and fat.
- Widening of scars.
- Failure to expand.

Advantages
- Local skin with good colour, texture, and hair match.
- Sensate.
- Absence of donor.
- Simple and reliable.

Disadvantages
- See complications.
- Inconvenience to patient.
- Unsightly as expands.
- Pain of injection.
- Failure to achieve sufficient tissue.

Tips
Check that the expander inflates satisfactorily prior to placement in the patient.

Delay phenomenon

The delay phenomenon is seen in flap delay. Flap delay is a term used to indicate that the flap is developed and transferred in more than one stage to ensure its vascular safety by division of part of the vascular supply or drainage of the flap 1–3 weeks prior to definitive raising of the flap. The delay phenomenon is the increase in flap size or length that can be successfully raised following a delay procedure.

Most blood flow (97%) is for thermoregulation, not nutrition (3%). Normal skin blood flow is 15 mL/min/100 cm^3 tissue. With vessel dilation, flow increases to 90 mL/min/100 cm^3. Skin only needs 1–2 mL/min/100 cm^3 to survive. The limits of a vascular territory are defined as that area of skin that can survive if raised on that vessel alone. The flow at the limits of the territory is less than 1–2 mL/min/100 cm^3. If the flow can be increased, the territory increases. Flow can be increased by increasing flow in existing vessels by increasing perfusion pressure or vasodilation, by capturing new vessel territories by the opening of 'choke vessels', or by neovascularization. However, delay operates by more complex mechanisms than purely by increasing flow, size, and number of supplying blood vessels. Delay also conditions the tissue to survive on less nutrient flow.

Delay is created mechanically by dissection which reduces blood flow in the dissected plane, creating relative ischaemia and therefore hyperaemia. This encourages blood flow along the longitudinal or undissected plane.

Mechanism of delay

- Vascular reorganization by:
  - Mechanical disruption of transverse vessels.
  - Longitudinal orientation of vessels.
  - Opening of choke vessels.
  - Angiogenesis mediated partly by chemoattractants and partly by change in tension.
- Vasodilation secondary to:
  - Inflammatory mediators.
  - Sympathectomy.
- Reactive hyperaemia secondary to relative ischaemia and oxygen free radicals, anaerobic metabolites, and acidosis.
- Acclimitization to hypoxia.

Tissue expansion utilizes the delay phenomenon as the pocket formation can reorganize the vessels and the mechanical forces and relative ischaemia from expansion increases the vascularity of the expanded flap.

Topical negative pressure

Definition
The use of vacuum-assisted drainage to remove fluid from a wound surface, using a foam interface to distribute the negative pressure evenly across the wound.

Principles
- Applying subatmospheric pressure to an open wound increases blood flow to the wound bed and increases the rate of granulation tissue formation.
- This effect is maximal with intermittent negative pressure of 125 mmHg.
- Removing fluid from the wound surface may reduce oedema, and removes bacteria and inflammatory mediators.
- The wound margins are gently drawn together, aiding the wound contraction process.

Indications
- Acute or chronic wounds including burns, traumatic and surgical wounds, and pressure sores.
- Contraindicated in wounds containing malignancy, infection, untreated osteomyelitis, and non-enteric fistulae, and over eschar.
- Should not be applied directly to blood vessels or organs.
- Has been used as an SSG dressing for difficult wounds to assist SSG take.

Method
The following describes use of the VAC™ system, which delivers a controlled negative pressure which can be set to be intermittent or continuous.
- The wound is cleaned and necrotic tissue debrided; this may need to be done in theatre with a general anaesthetic.
- For open body cavities, organs should be covered with autologous tissue or a suitable synthetic alternative.
- A piece of sponge is cut to fit the wound approximately (or multiple pieces are laid in the wound).
- The sponge is placed within the wound and a drainage tube placed over it. If the tube has circumferential holes, another piece of sponge should be put over the top of the tube.
- The whole is covered with an adhesive transparent waterproof dressing which overlaps the surrounding skin, and a seal created with the skin and the drainage tube.
- Alternatively, the transparent dressing is placed directly on the sponge; a hole is cut in it; and a suction tube with a flat adhesive end (TRAC™ pad) is stuck over the hole.
- The suction tubing is attached to a further length of tubing with a cannister at one end.
- The cannister slots into the VAC™ unit.
- The VAC™ unit is set to provide the desired negative pressure.

- The foam should collapse within the wound; leaks can be patched with more of the transparent dressing.
- Hydrocolloid dressings such as Duoderm can be used on the surrounding skin to protect it from the foam or to help the transparent dressing to seal.
- Application of a sticky fluid such as friar's balsam to the surrounding skin helps the transparent dressing to adhere.

Post-dressing care
- The transparent dressing allows observation of the wound margins for signs of infection.
- KCI advises changing the dressing every 48 hr, or more often in infected wounds.
- The draining fluid is rich in proteins. If drainage is copious, check albumin and give nutritional supplements as indicated.

Complications
- Fluid shifts.
- Failure to create a seal.
- Failure to progress to definitive surgery.

Pathology basics

- *Hyperplasia* is organized controlled increase in the number of cells.
- *Dysplasia* is a disorganized uncontrolled increase in the number of cells with loss of uniformity and loss of architectural organization, i.e. pleomorphic hyperchromatic nuclei, increased mitoses at abnormal levels.
- *Anaplasia* is dedifferentiation of structure and function of cells with marked pleomorphism, very large nuclei, and marked increase in numbers of mitoses.
- *Hamartoma* is localized overgrowth of mature cells with abnormal organization.

Principles of radiotherapy

Definition
Radiotherapy is the therapeutic use of ionizing radiation for the treatment of malignant disorders.

Physics
- External beam radiotherapy.
- Linear accelerator in which electrons are accelerated by microwaves and then hit tungsten, producing high energy X-rays. These deposit maximum dose a few centimetres below the skin.
- Ionizing beams can also be produced with neutrons or protons.
- High-energy X-rays and other rays are biologically indistinguishable.
- Electron beam therapy has limited penetration.

Basis of radiation therapy
- Radiation consists of packets of energy (photons) which interact with molecules to cause ionization, releasing electrons. The injury can be:
  - Direct injury.
  - Indirect injury which occurs when the released electrons produce secondary damage by production of oxygen free radicals. Indirect injury is oxygen dependent.
- The radiation effect is mainly through DNA damage.
- Non-repairable DNA leads to chromosomal changes.
- Cells can function but the damage prevents mitosis.
- Rapidly dividing cells with high turnover are most affected, which exploits the difference between tumour and normal cells.

Cell susceptibility
This depends on:
- Intrinsic cell radiosensitivity.
- Oxygen tension (the higher the better).
- Position of cell in mitotic cycle.
- Radiation dose:
  - The unit of absorbed dose of radiation is the Gray (Gy).
  - 1 Gy = 1 J kg.
  - 1 Gy = 100 rad.

Tolerance
Tolerance of normal tissue limits radiation dose (e.g. lungs, 20 Gy; single lobe, 60 Gy).

Fractionation
The practice of dividing the total dose and administering it over a number of weeks, usually six. Benefits are:
- Allows recovery of tissue such as CNS and lungs
- Rapidly proliferating tissues repopulate such as skin and GIT.
- Hypoxic areas become better oxygenated.
- Successive doses eliminate equal fractions of tumour cells.

Planning
Plan to provide the maximum dose to the smallest volume which will encompass the tumour—target volume. The target volume consists of:
- Macroscopic tumour volume.
- Biological margin 5–10 mm.
- Technical margin.

Plans need to consider:
- Localizing the tumour (by preoperative images, post-operative scarred area).
- Radiotherapy delivery (single field, opposing fields, or complex multifields; weighting of beams; wedge-shaped filters).
- Patient immobilization to maximize consistency (laser to monitor patient alignment, plastic shell to hold patient's position reproducibly).
- Homogenous distribution to target volume, avoiding non-target healthy tissues.
- Tissue tolerance vs. predicted tumour cure dose:
  - Children.
  - Elderly.
  - Previous surgery.
  - Vascular disease.

Role of radiotherapy
- Primary treatment:
  - Bladder, laryngeal cancers.
  - Radiosensitive tumours.
  - Inoperable tumours.
  - High morbidity and mortality from surgery.
  - Unfit for surgery.
- Adjuvant:
  - Tumour spill.
  - Lymph node metatastasis.
  - Locoregional control.
- Palliation:
  - Bone metastasis.
  - Spinal cord compression.
  - Brain metastasis.
  - SVC obstruction.
- Systemic (isotope or external beam):
  - <4 Gy.
  - 8–10 Gy + bone marrow transplant.
  - Leukaemias.

Complications
Cellular damage to normal tissues:
- Determined by cell turnover time (14 days skin, 5 days GIT).
- Severity and recovery depends on stem cell damage.
- Recovery often complete.

Radiation effects

Acute
- Occur during therapy or within 2–3 weeks.
- Loss of taste, xerostomia, loss of apetite, weight loss.
- Upper GIT oesophagitis.
- Lower GIT vomiting, diarrhoea, ulceration, and bleeding.
- Cranial irradiation somnolence.
- Gonadal damage oligospermia or sterility depending on dose.
- Depletion of parenchymal or connective tissue (thyroid gland is depleted of follicular cells, kidney is depleted of renal tubular cells).
- Skin erythema, tanning, desquamation (dry or moist).

Chronic
- Occur any time after therapy.
- Caused by microvascular changes or stem cell depletion.
- Vascular damage by damage to endothelium and connective tissue.
- Poor wound healing.
- Tissue atrophy.
- Loss of hair, sweat and sebaceous gland function.
- Telangectasia.
- Ulceration.
- Fibrosis.
- Strictures.
- Lymphoedema.
- Osteoradionecrosis.
- Neuropathy: myelitis, plexitis, neuritis.
- Cardiac damage leading to myocardial infarction after internal mammary radiation.
- Secondary malignancy:
  - Acute leukaemias (3–10 years after irradiation for Hodgkin's disease).
  - Risk solid tumours (10% after 20 years).
  - Risks worse if radiotherapy and chemotherapy, especially cyclophosphamide and vincristine.

The future

Accelerated radiotherapy
- Multiple daily fractions; less recovery time for tumour cell proliferation and normal cells.
- Reduced treatment time.

Hyperfractionation
- Smaller daily doses over conventional treatment time.
- Reduces late tissue damage.
- Similar tumour response.
- Theoretically allows dose escalation.

CHART (continuous hyperfractionated accelerated radiotherapy)
- Neutrons and heavy ion therapy.
- Produced by cyclotrons.
- Damage to DNA is by a non-oxygen-dependent mechanism, which means that hypoxic areas are equally susceptible.

Sun damage

Radiation
Radiation from the sun is electromagnetic. Electromagnetic radiation is the general name for different types of energy, including visible light, ultraviolet, infrared, X-rays, gamma rays, and radio and microwaves.

Only a small proportion of the total solar radiation reaches the Earth's surface. Most is blocked by dust, moisture, and the ozone layer. The solar spectrum at sea level is 290–3000 nm. The longer wavelengths are visible light and infrared. It is the shorter-wavelength UV light which causes trouble.

UVA: 320–400 nm
This is partly responsible for chronic photo-damage. The longer wavelength penetrates deeper into the dermis and has influence at the cellular level. UVA stimulates melanogenesis without appreciable thickening of the stratum corneum.

UVB: 290–320 nm
This is the erythematogenic band. 295 nm is most potent. Stimulates melanin production and epidermal thickening. It is photo-carcinogenic.

UVC: 200–290 nm
This is the germicidal band. It is blocked by the ozone layer. It is potently photo-carcinogenic. It also arises from artificial sources including arc welding and germicidal lamps in the laboratory.

Radiation effects
The effects depend on the intensity, duration, and frequency of the radiation, coupled with the sensitivity of the recipient. Sun exposure has, in general, three main acute effects: erythema, photosensitivity, and immunological alterations.

Erythema
Erythema is the most clinically apparent component of the sunburn reaction, which also includes damage to basement membrane and DNA, transient disturbances in DNA, RNA, and protein synthesis, and elaboration of many cytokines and inflammatory mediators.

The minimal erythema dose (MED) is the minimal amount of energy needed to produce a uniform clearly demarcated erythema response, usually at 24 hr. The erythema action spectrum (or relative effectiveness of different wavelengths) is proposed to be a good approximation of the action spectra for most other photobiological events in human skin, including tanning, carcinogenesis and photo-ageing.

4 MED produces a painful sunburn and 8 MED a blister reaction.

Photo-sensitivity
Photo-sensitivity is a generalized term applied to an abnormal skin reaction of the human skin to sun exposure, mostly due to sensitization by toxic compounds or drugs.

Immunology alteration

Immunology alteration by UV radiation is well documented locally and systemically in mice. In humans, acute exposure alters the balance of T cells and depresses natural killer cell activity against melanoma target cells. In chronic exposure epidermal Langerhans cells decrease by 20%–50%.

Photocarcinogenesis

- The relationship between UV radiation exposure and the development of SCC is very high, based on many epidemiological studies. UV radiation in laboratory animals has definitely shown the carcinogenic effect of UVR. Those patients who have had PUVA treatment (UVA plus psoralens) for psoriasis have up to a 12-fold increased chance of developing skin cancer. Sufferers of xeroderma pigmentosa (lack of capacity for nuclear DNA repair after UV radiation damage) develop large numbers of skin cancers.
- BCCs have a less clear association with UV exposure.
- Melanomas arise in less sun-exposed areas in almost half of cases, suggesting immunosupression or even release of melanocyte-stimulating factors to act on melanocytes in covered areas.

UV radiation is a complete carcinogen, in that it is a initiator and promoter. The molecular basis of photo-carcinogenesis is unknown.

Photo-ageing

This refers to changes in the skin resulting from repeated sun exposure, rather than to the passage of time alone. It is also known as premature ageing or dermatocheliosis.

The clinical signs of photo-ageing are coarseness, wrinkling, mottled pigmentation, laxity, telangiectasia, purpura, atrophy, and fibrotic depigmented areas (pseudo-scars). Later, there are pre-malignant and then malignant changes on the habitually exposed areas. Other conditions include dryness, seborrhoeic keratoses, acne rosacea, senile comedones, superficial varicose veins, pterygia, arcus senilis, etc.

Cigarette smoking (>10/day for >10 years) promotes photo-ageing, best seen on the lips.

Histology of ageing

Light microscopy shows changes. Solar elastosis affects the dermis, where abnormal dermal connective tissue is synthesized with the staining qualities of elastic tissue under light microscopy (basophilic). There is loss of the fibrillar structure of collagen (disorganized or 'chopped spaghetti appearance'). There are occasional macrophages. The epidermis is thin with loss of granular cell layers. The stratum corneum is usually unchanged. Grading of photo-ageing depends on the severity of the changes.

Factors affecting the severity of photodamage

- Skin type: Fitzgerald's classification.
- Pigmentation:
  - There is a genetically determined tanning reaction. This is acute and delayed. The acute reaction occurs in dark-skinned persons, arises 6 hr after burn, and rapidly fades. Benefit unclear. Due to photo-oxidation of melanin.

- The delayed reaction is due to stimulation of melanogensis and is apparent after 72 hr. In black skin there is much more melanin and more epidermal granular cell layers.
- Acclimatization: epidermal thickening and increased pigmentation occurs after sun exposure but the benefit is unclear.
- Geographical factors:
  - There are geographical and seasonal variations in UV radiation. Sand, snow, and concrete reflect up to 85% of UV radiation. UV radiation penetrates water. You burn faster in summer, at noon, closer to the equator, at a higher altitude (intensity at 5000 feet is 20% greater than at sea level). Also increased by high humidity, high wind, and warmer temperature.
- Sun protection:
  - Shade–thin cloud decreases by 30%.
  - Beach umbrella–decreases by only 50% because of reflected light.
  - UV-rated clothing–wet T-shirt allows 20% UV penetration.
  - Sunscreens are topical preparations that decrease the deleterious effects of UV radiation by absorption, reflection, or scattering. Need broad spectrum (UVA/UVB).

Sun protection factor (SPF)

The ratio of the amount of UVB energy required to produce a minimal erythema reaction through a sunscreen product film to the amount of energy required to produce the same erythema without any sunscreen application (Schulz). SPF 15 is a 92% UV filter. In mice sunscreens produce dramatic reductions in photo-ageing effects such as dermal damage and photo-carcinogenesis. Estimated that regular SPF 15 usage in the first 18 years of life will decrease the chance of non-melanoma skin cancer by 80%.

Sunscreens

Physical
These work by totally blocking the sun by scatter and reflection. Insoluble pigments dispersed in sun screen film; they interfere with perspiration and may be cosmetically unacceptable.

Chemical
Oil/water-soluble chemicals which are completely dissolved in the film on the skin. They act by absorbing radiant energy before it reaches the epidermis and re-emitting it at a lower energy level.

Tanning accelerators and salons
No evidence that a protective tan is any better than that acquired by sun baking. No evidence that UVA psoralens can induce tanning without photo-ageing and the carcinogenesis risk is at least the same as sun baking.

Microbiology

Leprosy

Organism
Mycobacterium leprae (Hansen's bacillus–Norwegian, 1873).

Pathology
M.leprae is infectious, particularly in children; adults have poor infection transmission. *M.leprae* has a predilection for neural tissue, particularly the peripheral nervous system. The bacilli enter via the endoneural blood vessels and attach to cells. The subsequent histological changes in the nerves depend on the immune status.

Classification
- Tuberculoid leprosy occurs in those with good immunity. Phagocytes become epithelioid cells leading to nerve destruction and intra-neural granulomas.
- Lepromatous leprosy occurs in those with poor immunity. The phagocytes do not destroy the bacilli but carry them away, giving widely disseminated lesions but not as much nerve damage (onion skin perineurium).
- Border-line leprosy causes epithelioid cell granulomas in a more diffuse pattern than tuberculoid leprosy.
- Indeterminate leprosy.

Diagnosis
Clinical evidence of nerve or dermal involvement (plaques).

Investigation
Microscopy for acid-fast bacilli (Ziehl–Neelsen stain), lepromin.

Treatment
- ?Isolate patient.
- Medical treatment—dapsone/rifampicin.
- Surgical management of paralysed muscles and complications arising from paralysed muscles and anaesthetic skin.

Pasteurella multocida
Small genus in the group *Bacillus*; common in cat and dog bites

Treatment
Debridement, penicillin.

Pseudomonas aeruginosa (pyocyanea)

Organism
Gram-negative anaerobic bacteria producing two pigments: a greenish yellow fluorescein and blue-green pyocyanin. *P.aeruginosa* likes moist conditions. Other *Pseudomonas* species include *Pseudomonas pseudomallei*, which gives melioidosis, and *Pseudomonas putrefaciens*, which infects ulcers and gives off the hydrogen sulphide smell.

Pathology
Causes the blue-green pigmentation of bandages, dressings, and wounds. Infects necrotic ulcers and eschars; likes wounds with reduced vascularity. Occasionally prevents skin graft take.

Treatment
Topical application of acetic acid or Milton's solution was popular. This has been replaced by the use of silver sulphadiazine (SSD).

Staphylococcus spp

Organism
Staphylococcus spp, Gram-positive bacteria.

Pathology
Pathological conditions caused by *Staphylococcus aureus* include impetigo (superficial skin), furunculosis (acute necrotizing infection of hair follicle), caruncles (many communicating furuncles), folliculitis (infection of the hair follicle ostium), and scalded skin syndrome. It is the most common organism causing wound infections and bone and joint infection.

Classification
- Coagulase negative: usually *Staphylococcus epidermidis*.
- Coagulase positive: most common *Staphylococcus aureus*.

Treatment
- *Medical*: flucloxacillin, first- and second-generation cephalosporins; IV vancomycin or teicoplanin may be needed for resistant strains.
- *Surgical*: do not forget that debridement of necrotic tissue or drainage of abcesses must be performed.

Streptococcus spp

Organism
Streptococcus spp: Gram-positive coccus.

Pathology
Responsible for many skin infections and can be blamed for failure of skin graft take! Two classifications:
- α-haemolytic, i.e. *Strep.viridens*—partial green haemolysis;
  β-haemolytic, i.e. *Strep.pyogenes*—complete haemolysis;
  γ-haemolytic i.e. *Strep.faecalis* (group D)—no haemolysis.
- A separate classification goes from group A to group O, where group A = *Strep.pyogenes*, group D = *Strep.faecalis*.

Clinical conditions secondary to *Streptococcus* include skin infections such as erysipelas (superficial skin), cellulitis (subcutaneous), impetigo, injury to skin vessels secondary to circulating erythrotoxin (scarlet fever), and allergic hypersensitivity to *Streptococcus* antigens producing vasculitis and conditions such as erythema nodosum. Other conditions include SBE and glomerulonephritis. Streptococcus is implicated as one of the organisms involved in necrotizing fascitis.

Treatment
- *Medical*: penicillin.
- *Surgical*: debridement of necrotic tissue is essential for control.

Clostridia

Family of Gram-positive bacilli which cause numerous common infective diseases.

Clostridium welchii (perfringens)

- Cellulitis: serious septic process of subcutaneous tissue characterized by:
    - Crepitant cellulitis which spreads rapidly along fascial planes.
    - Pain.
    - Grey-reddish-brown discharge.
    - Results in thrombosis.
    - Skin necrosis and fat necrosis.
- Myositis or gas gangrene: similar to cellulitis but more severe:
    - Spreading gangrene and profound toxaemia.
    - Gas + crepitus in muscles.
    - Soft swollen dark red muscle.
    - Foul-smelling brown watery exudates with bubbles of gas.
    - Illness and prostration out of proportion to fever.

Peptostreptococcus, bacteroides, and coliforms may also produce gas gangrene.

Management

- Resuscitation.
- IV penicillin.
- Surgical debridement.
- ± Fasciotomies ± amputation.
- ± Hyperbaric oxygen therapy.

Clostridium tetani

Anaerobic Gram-positive rod; spore bearing. Causes tetanus, produced by powerful exotoxin. Fatal in 40–60%. Incubation 4–21 days.

Tetanus-prone wounds are those that have devitalized tissue with the reduced oxygen environment necessary for the organism. These are usually complex or crush deep wounds with contamination and denervation.

- Prodrome:
    - Restless.
    - Headache.
    - Jaw stiffness.
    - Intermittent tetanic contractions in region of wound within 24 hr.
- Tetanus:
    - Tonic spasm of skeletal muscles.
    - Trismus, risus sardonicus = classical facial distortion.
    - Episthotonos and rigidity; tonic contraction may result from even very minor stimuli.
    - Respiratory arrest may occur during convulsions.
    - Painful contractions associated with tachycardia.
    - Increased salivation and sweating.

Management
- Prevention:
  - ADT ± tetanus immunoglobulin.
- Surgical and medical:
  - Surgical debridement of wound, source of infection.
  - Local + IV tetanus antitoxin if established.
  - IV ABs.
  - Reduce external stimuli (quiet dark room, no visitors).
  - Control seizures with benzodiazepines.
  - ICU—circulatory and respiratory support.
  - Usually die from aspiration, pneumonia, and respiratory arrest.

Tetanus prophylaxis
- Check patient's current immunization record. If he/she has been immunized and had entire immunization course then no further tetanus prophylaxis required. There used to be a 10 year recommendation, in that if no booster had been received in the last 10 years then administer tetanus prophylaxis. However, this has been extended beyond 10 years to indefinitely. In a very tetanus prone wound or if in doubt give prophylaxis.
- Prophylaxis includes surgical debridement of the wound to remove dead and dying (anerobic) tissue!
- Tetanus toxoid in the form ADT or tetanus toxoid adsorbed is always given if immunization status unknown or incomplete course.
- Additionally consider tetanus immunoglobulin in the non-immunized patient in a tetanus prone wound.
- Contraindication is previous hypersensitivity to tetanus toxoid. Consider immunoglobulin (passive immunization).

Clostridium botulinum
- Botulism: acute poisoning from ingestion of toxin produced by C.botulinum.
- Characterized by progressive descending muscle paralysis.
- Block neuromuscular transmission in cholinergic fibres either by release of ACh or binding ACh at its site of release in the presynaptic clefts.
- (Home canned foods)
- Several strains A–G
- Symptoms:
  - Ocular: diplopia, blurry vision photophobia.
  - Bulbar: dysphonia, dysarthria, dysphagia.
  - Muscular extremities: symmetric salivation.

Investigation
- Inject stool or serum in mice—see if they die.

Management
- Symptomatic.
- Antitoxin.

Clostridium difficile
Produces a toxin destructive to intestinal mucosa, leading to pseudomembranous colitis.

Clostridial species
- *C.welchii*
- *C.tetani*
- *C.botulinum*
- *C.difficile*
- *C.bifermentans*
- *C.histolyticum*
- *C.fallax*
- *C.septicum*
- *C.sordelli*
- *C.novyi*

Chapter 2

Embryology

Embryology of the external genitalia 62
Embryology of the face 63
Embryology of the nose 65
Embryology of the lip and palate 66
Embryology of the ear 67
Embryology of the hand 68

Embryology of the external genitalia

The embryological hindgut and allantois (a diverticulum form the yolk sac) meet in the shared cloaca at the caudal end of the embryo. The cloacal membrane closes the distal end of this cavity.

In the third week, mesenchymal cells migrate around the cloacal membrane to form a cloacal fold on either side of the membrane, and a genital tubercle anterior to it. The cloacal membrane migrates caudally.

In the sixth week, a urorectal septum grows from the dorsum of the allantois towards the cloacal membrane, dividing it into the urogenital membrane anteriorly (sealing the urogenital sinus) and the anal membrane posteriorly. The urogenital sinus will subsequently form the bladder and urethra, and part of the anterior vaginal wall. The cloacal folds divide into urogenital folds anteriorly and anal folds posteriorly. The urogenital folds are destined to become the labia minora of the female, or the midline scrotal raphe of the male. Genital or labioscrotal swellings develop lateral to the urogenital folds, and will become the rest of the scrotum or labia majora. The urogenital membrane breaks down in the sixth week, allowing communication between the endoderm of the urogenital sinus, and the ectoderm of the urogenital folds.

Sexual differentiation of the external genitalia to the male phenotype occurs regardless of sex under the influence of testosterone, converted to the more potent dihydrotestosterone by 5-alpha-reductase. In the eleventh week, the genital tubercle elongates to form the phallus. The urogenital folds enlarge around the endoderm of the most ventral part which initially forms a urethral plate and then sinks into the phallus to become the urethral groove. The urogenital swellings unite the ventral part to the anus, to form the scrotum, and fuse along the length of the phallus to the glans to create the penile urethra. The distal glandular part of the urethra is formed later in the thirteenth week by inward migration of ectodermal cells.

Also in the thirteenth week, the labioscrotal swellings migrate around the ventral aspect of the penis. The testes do not descend into the scrotum until about the seventh month.

Embryology of the face

Development of the face begins towards the end of the third week of gestation. At this stage the neural folds have fused to form a neural tube and this tube has folded on itself to create a primitive head. The caudal part of the neural tube is separated from the cardiac prominence by a primitive mouth, the stomodeum. Differential growth of the most cranial neural tube forms a central fronto-nasal prominence, which grows down from its caudal end, and six paired branchial arches, which grow medially. The first branchial arch develops two swellings: the maxillary and mandibular prominences. By the fourth week, the stomodeum is surrounded by, from above down, the central fronto-nasal prominence; paired maxillary prominences; and paired mandibular prominences.

The fronto-nasal prominence is destined to form the forehead, nose, and the central upper lip. The maxillary prominences will form the cheeks, maxillae, and lateral upper lips. The mandibular prominences become the lower lip, chin, and mandible. The remaining branchial arches (2–6) form the lateral and anterior walls of the primitive oropharynx.

The branchial arches decrease in size from above down, and the sixth is not actually visible externally. Each arch contains a cartilage precursor, an artery, a nerve, and muscle and gives rise to specific structures in the head and neck (See Table 2.1). Between the arches are branchial grooves, where the branchial ectoderm and pharyngeal endoderm are separated by only a thin layer of mesoderm. Again, these give rise to specific structures. The first pouch forms the ear canal and middle ear cavity. The second becomes the palatine tonsillar fossa. The third and fourth form parathyroid and thymus tissue; the third forms the inferior parathyroid, which therefore migrates inferiorly past the fourth pouch derivative. The fourth pouch also forms the thyroid gland. The fifth pouch forms the ultimobranchial body and the calcitonin-producing C cells of the thyroid gland.

By the eighth week, the face has acquired a more human appearance, with the pharyngeal pouches obliterated. The maxillary and mandibular processes have fused and the lips and jaws are well defined. The fronto-nasal process lengthens vertically, and the eyes migrate medially. This 5 week period is crucial for facial embryogenesis, and errors in this period may lead to significant deformity. Failure of obliteration of a branchial groove gives rise to a branchial fistula, sinus, or cyst, the most common being a remnant of the second groove.

CHAPTER 2 Embryology

Table 2.1 The contents of each arch and the structures derived

Arch	Artery	Nerve	Muscle	Cartilage precursor	Skeletal structures
First (mandibular)	Maxillary	Trigeminal	Muscles of mastication	Quadrate, Meckel's	Greater wing of sphenoid, incus, malleus, maxilla, zygoma, squamous temporal bone, mandible
Second (hyoid)	Stapedial in embryo cortico-tympanic in adult	Facial	Muscles of facial expression, posterior belly digastric, stylohyoid, stapedius	Reichert's	Stapes, styloid process, hyoid (lesser cornu, upper body)
Third	Part of internal and common carotid	Glosso-pharyngeal	Stylo pharyngeus	Third arch	Hyoid (greater cornu, lower body)
Fourth	Aortic arch, innominate and right subclavian, distal part of pulmonary	Superior laryngeal branch of vagus	Pharyngeal constrictors	Fourth arch	Laryngeal cartilages
Fifth and sixth	Proximal part of pulmonary; ductus arteriosus	Recurrent laryngeal branch of vagus	Intrinsic of larynx	Sixth arch	Laryngeal cartilages

Adapted from *Grabb & Smith's Plastic Surgery*, Lippincott–Raven, Philadelphia, PA, 1997.

Embryology of the nose

At the end of the fourth week, bilateral olfactory (nasal) placodes appear at the inferolateral corners of the fronto-nasal process. Medial and lateral nasal prominences develop adjacent to each olfactory placode. These thicken and the olfactory placodes deepen into olfactory pits and enlarge to form the nasal sinuses. Initially, an oronasal membrane separates the nasal and oral cavities, but when this breaks down they become one. The stomodeum, the primitive oral cavity, is now continuous with the cavity. The bilateral maxillary processes grow medially towards the lateral nasal prominences.

During the sixth week, the medial nasal prominences fuse into a single globular process that will eventually become the nasal tip, columella, prolabium, frenulum, and primary palate. As this occurs, the nasal septum grows down from the medial nasal processes and fronto-nasal prominence. The lateral nasal prominences will become the alae of the nose.

As the paired maxillary prominences grow towards the lateral nasal processes, they are initially separated by a naso-optic furrow. During fusion of these prominences, a cord of epithelium, the nasolacrimal ridge, sinks into the mesenchyme. After birth, it will canalize to form the nasolacrimal duct, connecting the conjunctival lacrimal sac with the lateral nasal wall.

At the end of the sixth week, the maxillary processes fuse with the medial nasal prominences to encircle the nostrils. The floor of each nasal cavity still connects with the stomodeum, and awaits development of the palate to separate mouth from nose.

The conchae develop from swellings in the lateral walls of the nasal cavities. Diverticulae from the nasal cavities expand into the sphenoid, ethmoid, frontal, and maxillary bones to form the paranasal sinuses. However, this occurs much later in development: the maxillary sinuses develop in the third month and the ethmoid develops in the fifth month. The sphenoid and frontal sinuses do not appear until after birth; at 5 months and 5–6 years, respectively. All the sinuses continue to enlarge into adolescence, and are responsible for much of the difference in shape between the child and adult face.

Failure of fusion of maxillary and lateral nasal prominences gives rise to a Tessier 3 facial cleft which runs along the course of the nasolacrimal duct.

Embryology of the lip and palate

The primitive mouth or stomodeum appears in the third week of embryological development. It is surrounded by five primordia (swellings of neural crest derivation): the central fronto-nasal prominence superiorly, and paired maxillary and mandibular prominences laterally.

Over the next four weeks, medial and lateral nasal prominences develop in the fronto-nasal prominence (see nose embryology), move towards the midline, and fuse. The medial nasal prominences form the tuberculum of the upper lip and the primary palate or premaxilla, in which the upper four incisor teeth will develop. The remainder of the upper lip is formed by fusion of the maxillary prominences with the medial nasal prominences. The surfaces of the medial nasal and maxillary prominences are covered with epithelium which forms a transient nasal fin as they fuse. The nasal fin breaks down by apoptosis, and failure of this process can result in a cleft lip. Fusion of the upper-lip elements is not complete until the seventh week. The philtral ridges, normally prominent in neonates, are formed from thickened dermis and dermal appendages. In the fetal alcohol syndrome, the upper lip is flattened.

The lower lip is formed earlier, in the sixth week, by fusion of the bilateral mandibular prominences. Clefts of the lower lip are rare, which may be because it fuses earlier in development.

The secondary palate (so called because it develops after the primary palate) consists of the hard palate, posterior to the incisive foramen, and the soft palate. In the seventh week, lateral palatal processes project from each maxillary prominence into the oral cavity. At this stage, the primitive mouth is almost filled by the developing tongue. Therefore the palatal processes point downwards and lie on either side of the tongue. During the eighth week, over a period of only a few hours, the palatal shelves elevate into a horizontal position. The lateral palatal shelves fuse with one another and with the nasal septum from anterior to posterior. Therefore the mildest form of cleft palate is a bifid uvula.

The exact mechanism by which the palatal shelves elevate is not known. One theory involves the hydration of glycosaminoglycans. It appears that depression of the tongue is an important part of the process. In the eighth week, the embryo's head lifts up, allowing the jaw to open; deficient amniotic fluid may impede jaw movements. Fetal swallowing may be important. Retrognathia due to delayed mandibular development, as seen in the Pierre–Robin sequence, forces the tongue to sit high in the mouth, delaying palate elevation.

Embryology of the ear

Internal ear

In the fourth week of embryological development two otic placodes appear as thickening lateral to the hindbrain. Each placode invaginates to form an otic pit, the mouth of which closes, resulting in an otocyst. Diverticulae grow from the cyst to form the utricle, saccule, semicircular canals, and cochlea. The mesenchyme surrounding the inner ear forms a cartilaginous otic capsule, which later ossifies and becomes the bony labyrinth.

The auditory tube and tympanic cavity develop from an invagination of the first branchial groove, the tubo-tympanic recess. The dorsal end of the first arch cartilage (Meckel's cartilage) ossifies to form the malleus and incus of the middle ear. The dorsal end of the second arch cartilage (Reichert's cartilage) ossifies to form the stapes of the middle ear and the styloid process of the temporal bone.

External ear

During the sixth week, six mesenchymal swellings (hillocks) surround the first branchial cleft. The first three hillocks arise from the first branchial arch, and the second three arise from the second arch. Over the next 2 weeks these hillocks grow and merge to form the auricle. The hillocks of the first arch become the tragus, helix, and the cymba concha; those of the second arch become the antitragus, antihelix, and concha cavum. The ear is initially located inferior to its normal position and lies in a horizontal plane. As the face develops, it gradually moves to a more cephalic position and rotates clockwise.

Patients with microtia or other developmental anomalies of the external ear may have a caudally placed ear. As the external and internal ear structures develop relatively independently of one another, deformities of the external ear are not necessarily associated with inner ear anomalies and hearing may be possible.

Embryology of the hand

Morphogenesis

Hand and upper limb morphogenesis occurs in the fourth to sixth weeks of gestation, initiated by fibroblast growth factors. The limb bud develops along three axes on the trunk:
- Proximal-distal.
- Anterior-posterior.
- Dorsal-ventral.

Limb specification occurs in seven cell divisions, corresponding to the eight segments of the limb. The humerus is the first, the radius and ulna are the second, the proximal carpal row is the third, etc.

Proximal-distal axis

This is controlled by the mesenchymal connective tissue, which lays out the proximal-distal sequence of muscle, vessels, and nerves. Experiments in grafting limb buds to different areas of the body result in limb development based on the tissues normally found at the recipient site.

The *apical ectodermal ridge (AER)* interacts with the underlying mesenchyme to produce the proximal-distal pattern. The AER is an anterior-posterior linear thickening of ectoderm at the leading edge of the limb bud. Destruction of the AER prevents further limb development, resulting in a transverse reduction defect whose level depends on the time of destruction.

The AER influences the mesenchymal cells immediately beneath by secretion of an anti-differentiation factor (fibroblast growth factor 4, FGF-4). These undifferentiated cells are in the *progress zone*. Cells outside the reach of the secreted anti-differentiation factor automatically differentiate. The increased length of time that cells remain in the progress zone and the number of cell divisions determines their development into more distal structures. Delay in cells leaving the progress zone explains the pattern of phocomelia with a hand sitting on a humerus.

HOX-d genes are involved in proximal-distal patterning, perhaps by confirming the differentiation of the cells.

Anterior-posterior axis

In the posterior part of the limb bud an area of mesenchyme called the zone of polarizing activity produces a factor which codes for posterior structures. The gradient of the diffusible factor is responsible for differentiation into anterior and posterior structures. The factor (possibly a bone morphogenic protein) is unknown, but is probably under the influence of sonic hedgehog protein produced by the sonic hedgehog gene.

Dorsal-ventral axis

A similar diffusible protein probably explains the differentiation into dorsal and ventral structures. The protein originates from the dorsal ectoderm and is associated with the wnt 7a (wingless) gene.

Development

The formation of bone, cartilage, and neurovascular and other structures occurs in weeks 7–12. Mesenchyme differentiates into a cartilage anlage, which is invaded by blood vessels and forms primary ossification centres.

In the long bones secondary ossification centres develop in the epiphysis on the other side of the growth plate. The growth plate has layers of cells:
- Reserve layer.
- Dividing layer.
- Maturation layer.
- Calcification and hypertrophy layer.

Joints develop as interzones between adjacent cartilage anlage which on movement differentiates into a synovial joint.

The hand forms as a mitten and, under the influence of hormones, apoptosis occurs (week 6–8) between the rays, progressing from distal to proximal and from pre-axial to post-axial. The most common ray involved in syndactyly is the second post-axial ray, indicating this is the last to undergo separation.

Growth

After the preceding stages, structures increase in dimensions in a controlled fashion with modelling and remodelling.

Chapter 3

Anatomy and clinical assessment

Skin vascular anatomy 72
Head and neck anatomy 74
Nose anatomy 78
Eyelid anatomy and physiology 82
External ear anatomy 84
Facial nerve anatomy 87
Hand anatomy: basic 90
Nerve supply to the hand 97
Wrist anatomy and examination 99
Penis anatomy 101
Parasympathetic nervous system 103

Skin vascular anatomy

Vascularity

Cutaneous vascular plexi:
- Epidermal.
- Dermal.
- Subdermal.
- Subcutaneous.
- Prefascial.
- Subfascial.

The most important is the subdermal plexus, which is the basis for the random pattern flaps, and the prefascial plexus which must be retained in the fasciocutaneous flap. These six plexi have multiple anastomoses.

The arterial supply to the plexi comes from a source artery via muscle (musculocutaneous perforators), a defined septum (septocutaneous perforators), or directly (axial and/or perforator). It is worth noting that there are a multitude of classifications and explanations for skin blood supply, with a ready intermix of nomenclature. The simplest of these was put forward by Spalteholtz in 1893 and confimed by the studies of Taylor and Palmer (1987).

- Direct cutaneous arteries: this is the primary supply to the skin. The main role of these arteries is to supply the skin regardless of their route of getting there.
- Indirect cutaneous arteries: the primary role of these vessels is to supply muscles and deep tissues. They are virtually spent by the time they reach the skin and are meant to provide a back-up or secondary supply.

Angiosomes

- Vessels follow the connective tissue framework of the body. Deeply this is bone and more superficially muscle and fascia.
- Vessels radiate from fixed to mobile areas.
- Vessels 'hitch-hike' with nerves.
- A source artery supplies a three-dimensional composite block of muscle, nerve, bone, and its overlying skin. This block is termed an angiosome.
- At the periphery of each angiosome are choke arteries and arterioles which link with adjacent angiosomes. When raising a flap the immediately adjacent angiosome can safely be taken with that flap, but any more distant angiosome may become necrotic.

Vascular physiology

The microcirculation to the skin is controlled at a systemic and local level.
- Systemic:
  - *Neural regulation.* This is mediated via the sympathetic nervous system, with sympathetic adrenergic discharge causing vasoconstriction and withdrawal combined with cholinergic fibres releasing bradykinin causing vasodilation.

- *Humoral regulation*. Circulating hormones can act directly on receptors in the vessel walls and at the arteriovenous anastomoses. Vasoconstrictors are adrenaline, noradrenaline, serotonin, thromboxane A2 and prostaglandin F_2 alpha. Vasodilators include histamine, bradykinin, and prostaglandin E_1.
- Local:
  - *Metabolic factors*. Hypercapnoea, acidosis, hypoxia, and interstitial potassium cause vasodilation and increased blood flow in an attempt to clear them from the local area.
  - *Physical factors*. The myogenic reflex maintains constant skin blood supply in the face of pressure fluctuations. The vascular smooth muscle responds to stretch by active contraction and to release of stretch by contraction. Local hypothermia and raised blood viscosity cause vasoconstriction.

Reference

Taylor GI, Palmer JH (1987). *Br J Plastic Surg* **40**, 113–41.

Head and neck anatomy

Scalp
Layers of the SCALP:
- Skin.
- Connective tissue: contains fat, arteries, veins, and nerves.
- Aponeurosis galea: membranous tendon of occipitalis and frontalis.
- Loose connective tissue: dangerous zone for spread of infections.
- Pericranium (outer cranial periosteum).

The first three layers are connected intimately and move as a single unit.

Arterial supply
Anterior scalp Supratrochlear, supraorbital branches of internal carotid.
Lateral and posterior scalp Superficial temporal, posterior auricular, and occipital branches of external carotid.
The area below the nuchal line is supplied by the perforators from the trapezius and splenius so a skin flap in this area should not be brought below the nuchal ridge.

Venous drainage
Anterior scalp Supraorbital and supratrochlear veins unite to form the facial vein, which unites with the retromandibular vein (anterior branch) to drain into the internal jugular vein. The facial vein communicates with the cavernous sinus via the ophthalmic veins and pterygoid plexus, and so facial infections can cause meningitis or intra-cranial abscess.
Lateral scalp Posterior auricular and retromandibular veins (posterior branch) unite to drain into the external jugular vein. The superficial temporal vein drains into the retromandibular vein.
Posterior scalp Occipital vein drains into the internal jugular vein.

Lymph drainage
Preauricular, mastoid, and occipital, draining into deep cervical nodes.

Nerve supply
Sensory Cervical plexus (C2/3) supplies lesser occipital, greater auricular nerves; trigeminal (C5) supplies auriculotemporal, supraorbital and supratrochlear nerves.
Motor- Facial nerve supplies frontalis and occipitalis.

Clinical relevance
Scalp wounds bleed copiously as they are held open by the dense subcutaneous tissue. Infections in the scalp usually localize in the subcutaneous layer where the numerous fibrous septa prevent the spread of infection. The scalp should be closed in two layers: absorbable sutures to the galea and non-absorbable continuous sutures to the skin to control bleeding. Release incisions on the galea may help close moderate-sized defects. Larger defects may require rotational flaps, which need to overcome the convexity of the cranium as they advance.

Neck

Fascial planes of the neck

Superficial cervical fascia: Thin layer of subcutaneous connective tissue lying between the dermis and deep cervical fascia, containing the platysma, cutaneous nerves, blood vessels, and lymphatics.

Deep cervical fascia: Consists of three layers: investing, pretracheal, and prevertebral fascia. These layers form planes through which tissues can be dissected during surgery. The investing layer helps prevent the spread of abscesses.

Superficial muscles

- *Platysma* Enveloped by the superficial and deep layers of the superficial fascia. It originates from the fascia of the pectoralis major and deltoid to insert in three main areas: anterior fibres to tip of chin (fibres decussate above the hyoid, which forms a muscular sling under the chin, giving it definition); central fibres to mandible; lateral fibres blend with fibres of the risorius and depressor anguli oris.
    - Innervation: facial nerve (cervical branch).
    - Actions: depresses mandible, draws corners of mouth down.
- *Sternocleidomastoid (SCM)* Broad strap-like muscle originating from manubrium (sternal head) and medial third of clavicle (clavicular head) to insert into mastoid process and superior nuchal line. Key landmark dividing the neck into two triangles.
    - Innervation: accessory nerve (spinal root) and C2/3.
    - Actions: flexion and rotation of head towards opposite side (unilateral), neck flexion (bilateral).
- *Trapezius* Flat triangular-shaped muscle originating from the superior nuchal line; external occipital protruberance; spinous processes of C7–T12 to insert into clavicle (lateral third), acromium, and spine of scapula.
    - Innervation: accessory nerve (spinal root) and C3/4.
    - Actions: elevation (superior fibres), retraction (middle fibres), and depression (inferior fibres) of scapula, and consequently rotation of scapula.

Triangles of the neck (Table 3.1)

- *Anterior triangle* Borders: mandible, midline, SCM. It is further subdivided by the digastric and omohyoid muscles into the submental, submandibular, carotid, and muscular triangles.
- *Posterior triangle* Borders: anterior border of the trapezius, clavicle, and posterior border of SCM.

Table 3.1 Triangles of the neck

Triangle	Boundaries	Main contents
Anterior	SCM, mandible, midline	
Digastric/submandibular	Mandible, anterior and posterior bellies of digastric	Submandibular gland and lymph nodes Facial, submental and mylohyoid vessels Hypoglossal and mylohyoid nerves
Submental	Anterior belly of digastric, body of hyoid bone, midline	Submental lymph nodes Anterior jugular vein
Carotid	SCM, posterior belly of digastric, superior belly of omohyoid	Bifurcation of common carotid artery Vagus, hypoglossal, internal and external laryngeal nerves Lymph nodes
Muscular	SCM, superior belly of omohyoid, midline (hyoid bone to jugular notch)	Part of larynx, thyroid and parathyroid Lymph nodes
Posterior	SCM, trapezius, clavicle	Accessory nerve Brachial plexus (supraclavicular part) Occipital, transverse cervical, suprascapular and subclavian arteries Transverse cervical, suprascapular and external jugular veins Cervical plexus and brachial plexus trunks Lymph nodes

Nerves

Cervical plexus
C1–4, lies deep to SCM, emerging from middle of its posterior border to supply skin of the posterior triangle of neck and scalp. Gives off branches:
- C1: no cutaneous supply.
- C2: lesser occipital nerve, cutaneous supply to neck and scalp posterior to ear, superior part of ear, and cheek overlying the parotid gland.
- C3: supplies the cylindrical part of the neck.
- C4: supplies the anterior shoulder down to the sternal angle, top of shoulders, and upper back down to the scapular spine.

Accessory nerve (XI)
Motor nerve to the SCM and trapezius. It is vulnerable in operations within the posterior triangle superficial to the deep fascia, where injury will affect only the trapezius. Surface marking of its course is a line drawn from the upper-third–middle-third junction of the SCM to the middle-third–lower-third junction of the trapezius, about 5 cm above the clavicle.

Phrenic nerve
C3–5, sole motor nerve to diaphragm. Descends in the posterior triangle deep to the deep fascia, obliquely crossing the anterior surface of scalenus anterior from lateral to medial.

Lymphatic drainage of the head and neck

The lymphatic drainage of the head and neck are arranged into superficial and deep chains. They are also grouped into 6 levels often used to describe zones of lymph node clearance in neck dissection.

The superficial nodes are the facial, submental, superficial cervical, post-auricular, occipital, spinal accessory and anterior scalene.

The deep jugular chain extends from the base of the skull to the clavicle and is formed into superior, middle and inferior groups of lymph nodes.

Table 3.2 Lymph node levels and the areas they drain

Levels	Nodes	Drainage
I	Sub-mental and sub-mandibular	Chin, lip, tongue tip, anterior mouth, nose and cheek
II	Upper jugulodigastric	As above, plus face, parotid, ear, tonsils, palate, posterior tongue and pharynx
III	Middle jugular	Naso- and oropharynx, oral cavity, hypopharynx, larynx
IV	Inferior jugular	Hypopharynx, subglottic larynx, thyroid, oesophagus
V	Posterior triangular	Parietal and occipital scalp, nasopharynx, breast, thorax and abdomen
VI	Anterior compartment	Pharynx, trachea, thyroid

Nose anatomy

The nose is a pyramid, with a bony base (frontal maxilla and nasal bones), a firm cartilaginous middle (upper lateral cartilages and septum), and a soft cartilaginous tip (alar).

Primary components or layers of the nose

- Skin coverage:
  - Upper two-thirds (dorsum and sides): thin skin, mobile.
  - Lower third (tip and alar): thicker, firmly adherent to lower lateral cartilages, with many sebaceous glands.
  - The soft triangle is the portion of the alar rim where the columella (medial crus) turns laterally to form the alar (lateral crus); it has no cartilageneous support but is formed by two layers of skin.
- Skeletal support:
  - Upper third (bony): paired nasal bones, frontal processes of maxilla.
  - Middle third: upper lateral cartilages.
  - Lower third: lower lateral (alar) cartilages.

The nasal bones overlap the upper lateral cartilages at the 'keystone' area. The upper lateral cartilages overlap the lower lateral cartilages at the 'scroll' area.

- Lining:
  - Vestibule: keratinized epithelium.
  - Elsewhere: thin mucosal layer.

Nasal musculature

All are supplied by the facial nerve and permit facial expressions by changing the shape of the nose. They include the procerus, depressor septi, levator labii superioris alaeque nasi, dilator nares, compressor narium, and nasalis.

Nasal vasculature

Arterial supply

- External nasal branch of the ophthalmic artery: upper part of nose.
- Dorsal nasal branch of the ophthalmic artery: dorsum and sides of the nose.
- Angular branch of the facial artery: lateral sides of the nose.
- Superior labial artery: alae and columella.
- Infraorbital branch of the internal maxillary artery: dorsum and sides of the nose.

Venous supply

The venous supply parallels the arterial supply. The facial vein makes important connections with the cavernous sinus through the superior ophthalmic vein.

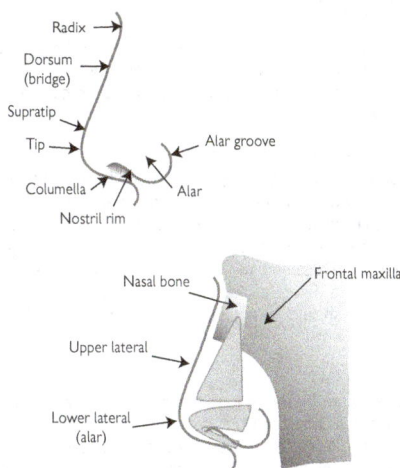

Fig. 3.1 Lateral view of nose and nasal nomenclature; lateral view of nasal skeleton.

Nasal innervation

External nose
- Upper: infratrochlear nerve (ophthalmic branch, CN V).
- Tip: nasociliary nerve or external nasal nerve (maxillary branch, CN V).
- Lateral aspect: Infraorbital nerve nasal branches (maxillary branch, CN V).

Internal nose

The ophthalmic division of the trigeminal supplies the superior half of the septum and the superior anterior quadrant of the lateral nasal wall, and the maxillary division supplies the posterior nose via the palatine nerves and the anterior inferior wall by the infraorbital nerve.

Innervation of the septum is split in two. The superficial half is supplied by the anterior ethmoidal nerve branch of the nasociliary from the ophthalmic division of the trigeminal. This continues to become the external nasal nerve notching the nasal bones. The deep septum is supplied by the nasopalatine nerve, a branch of the sphenopalatine, from the maxillary division of trigeminal.

Innervation of the internal lateral nasal wall is divided into four quadrants. The posterior inferior is supplied by the greater palatine from maxillary division of trigeminal. The posterior superior is supplied by the posterior superior lateral nerve (or short sphenopalatine), a branch of the posterior palatine from the maxillary division of the trigeminal. The anterior inferior is supplied by the anterior superior alveolar nerve, a branch of the infraorbital nerve from the maxillary division of the trigeminal. The anterior superior quadrant is supplied by the anterior ethmoidal nerve from the ophthalmic division of the trigeminal.

Internal nasal valve

The internal nasal valve is formed by the junction of the epithelialized and mucosal vestibule. It governs air entry by dilating or constricting under the influence of the external nasal musculature. It can be disrupted in trauma or surgery.

Nasal subunits/aesthetic units

The nose is divided into nine topographic subunits comprising the dorsum, tip, columella, paired sidewalls, alae, and soft triangles. Each subunit has a characteristic skin quality, unit outline, and three-dimensional contour which must be restored for a nose to look normal following reconstruction. Suture lines are ideally made to correspond with these boundaries to camouflage scars. If a defect encompasses >50% of the subunit, the skin of the entire subunit should be replaced, not just the missing skin of the defect.

Nasal valves

There are external and internal nasal valves. Internal valves are the caudal edge of the upper lateral cartilages as they protrude into the nasal vestibule. These diverge from the septum by approximately 10°–15°. On deep inspiration these valves try to collapse, diminishing the angle and occluding air flow. They are maintained open by the external nasal muscles that attach to the upper lateral cartilages, such as the nasalis. Athletes have taken to wearing an external nasal splint that assists in keeping the nasal valves open to increase air flow and reduce resistance. Collapsed nasal valves can occur with denervation of the muscles (facial palsy) or loss of upper lateral support. Cottle's test is collapse/narrowing of the lower lateral cartilages producing narrowing of the mid-nose on forced inspiration, which can be exaggerated by occluding the nostril. If inspiration is made easier by stretching the cheek laterally, this is a positive test. This can be reconstructed with spreader grafts (Sheen).

Clinical relevance of nasal anatomy

- In nasal reconstruction, tissue loss from each of the three layers of the nose must be identified and replaced with similar material.
- Full-thickness skin graft blends well in the dorsum and sidewalls, whereas a local or regional flap is a better choice for resurfacing the tip or alar.
- Nasal local anaesthetic block requires block of infraorbital nerve, infratrochlear nerve and the dorsal nasal nerves.
- Ensure incisions are along aesthetic unit borders.
- Excisions should be in aesthetic units for optimal aesthetic reconstruction.
- Nasal reconstruction without internal nasal lining undergoes significantly more scar contracture.

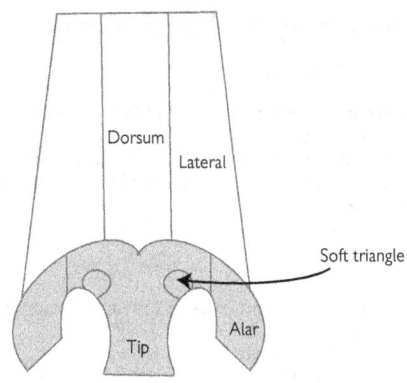

Fig. 3.2 Nasal aesthetic subunits.

Eyelid anatomy and physiology

Eyelid support is provided by:
- Levator.
- inferior suspensory ligament of Lockwood (between inferior oblique/inferior rectus).
- Whitnall's ligament (the thickening of fascia around levator superiorly runs from lacrimal gland capsule to trochlea of superior oblique muscle).
- Lateral canthal tendon.
- Medial canthal tendon.
- Tarsal plates.

Tarsal plates
Thin elongated plates of connective tissue 25 mm long and 1 mm thick:
- Superior is 8–10 mm in height.
- Inferior is 3.8–4.5 mm in height.
- The meibomian glands lie within the substance of the tarsal plate.

Orbicularis oculi
Extends over the orbital margin; overlies the septum orbitale and the tarsus.
- *Orbital portion* originates from the superomedial orbital margin, maxillary process frontal bone, and medial canthal tendon, and inserts medial canthal tendon, frontal process of maxilla, and inferomedial orbital margin.
- *Preseptal portion* has superficial fibres from the orbital margin below the medial canthal tendon and deep fibres from the post-lacrimal crest; together these are responsible for the lacrimal pump mechanism.
- *Pretarsal orbicularis oculi* has a superficial head, which helps form the medial canthal tendon and inserts superio anterior to the anterior lacrimal crest, and a deep head (also known as Horner's muscle) which goes posterior to the lacrimal sac to the posterior lacrimal crest.

Supplied by the facial nerve; vertically running fibres so that vertical incision does not denervate.

Lacrimal pump mechanism
- Closure of the eyelids produces movement of eyelids medially emptying the ampullae and shortening the canaliculi, forcing fluid into the lacrimal sac. In addition, the preseptal muscles produce negative pressure within the lacrimal sac, further drawing fluid into the sac.
- Eyelid opening with relaxation of preseptal muscles allows the elasticity of the lacrimal diaphragm to return the sac to its position of rest, producing positive pressure and thus forcing tears into the nasolacrimal duct.

Orbital septum
- Fascial membrane that separates eyelids from deeper structures.
- Attaches to periosteum at orbital margin (arcus marginalis).
- *Pre-aponeurotic fat* lies below the septum and aponeurosis/lid retractors, so traction or excision of fat here can cause bleeding that extends behind the orbit, causing blindness.
  - Upper lid = medial and central (lacrimal gland lateral).
  - Lower lid = medial central and lateral fat pads.

EYELID ANATOMY AND PHYSIOLOGY

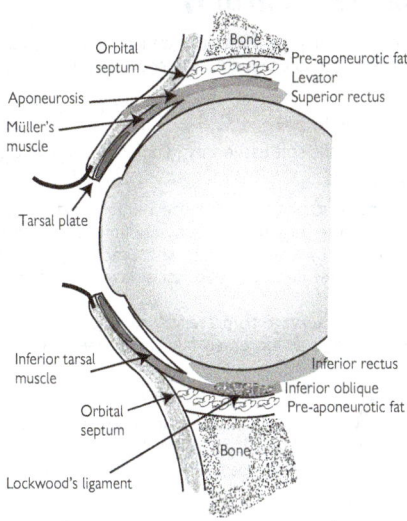

Fig. 3.3 Eyelid anatomy.

Levator palpebrae superioris and Müller's muscle

- Levator palpebrae superiorus (striated muscle) arises from the lesser wing of the sphenoid (above and anterior to optic foramen). It has a triangular shape, with the base inferiorly, which inserts as a broad aponeurosis onto the anterior lower third of the superior tarsus and skin of the upper eyelid (producing the upper eyelid crease). It also has lateral and medial extensions called horns. Note: The aponeurosis blends with the septum for a distance of 3–5 mm above the tarsus.
- Levator is supplied by superior division oculomotor.
- Müller's muscle arises from the deep aspect of the levator muscle and aponeurosis and inserts on the superior border of tarsus. It is supplied by sympathetic nerve fibres and when denervated leads to ptosis of the upper lid in Horner's syndrome.
- The upper eyelid is lifted by the levator and adjusted by Müller's muscle.

Lower lid

- The lower lid moves down 2 mm with extreme downward gaze, partly by the action of a sympathetic innervated muscle similar to Müller's muscle.
- The lower lid has a fascial extension of inferior rectus called the capsulo palpebral fascia which attaches to the orbital septum inferiorly and to the tarsus superiorly with some fibres passing to the fornix.

External ear anatomy

The auricle consists of a single elastic cartilage that is covered on both surfaces with skin and soft tissue. It is anchored in place by muscles and ligaments.

Skin and soft tissue coverage

The components of the soft tissue vary in different areas of the auricle.

Anterolateral ear

Includes the concha, scapha, and their convolutions, extending posteriorly to the helical rim, anteriorly to the tragus, and inferiorly to the antitragus. Formed superficially by very fine skin with practically no subcutaneous fat. Vessels and nerves lie in the thin fascial layer between the skin and perichondrium.

The best plane of cleavage to preserve the vascular layer is under the perichondrium, which is an extremely fine white sheet covering the yellow cartilage.

Posteromedial ear

Thin looser skin, with two layers of subcutaneous fat, between which lies the neurovascular fascia. Deep layer of fat glides easily over the cartilage. Second and equally important vascular layer is the subdermal network.

Lobular

Consists of skin enclosing fat. The skin is vascularized by the subdermal network, and the fat by vessels within the lobe. The fat is so well-vascularized that flaps of lobule fat can be long and narrow

Cartilage

Auricular cartilage is unique elastic cartilage and has no exact equivalent elsewhere in the body. It lies over the bony canal like a funnel and is held in place by tensor muscles and ligaments.

The cartilage is thin and of uniform thickness, covered on both sides by perichondrium. The perichondrium is more adherent to the cartilage along the antihelical curve than in other areas such as the scapha and conchal floor. The cartilage is more dense and fibrous directly under the perichondrium on both sides; this layer is often scratched or abraded to make the cartilage more flexible for reshaping.

Muscles and ligaments

Extrinsic muscles consist of anterior, superior, and posterior auricularis, which extend from the cartilage to the zygomatic arch, epicranial aponeurosis, and mastoid periosteum, respectively. These muscles are innervated by the facial nerve, but in most people can only contract involuntarily. Intrinsic muscles consist of tiny muscles within the pinna itself, which form and maintain the shape of the ear.

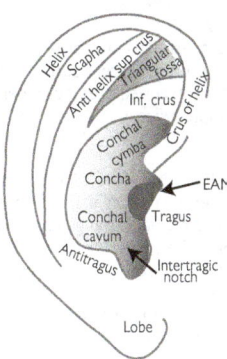

Fig. 3.4 Nomenclature of the external ear.

Arterial supply

This comes from two main branches of the external carotid artery: the superficial temporal artery (anterior) and the posterior auricular artery (posteriorly), which branch extensively in the ear and vary in calibre.

- The superficial temporal artery emerges from the parotid capsule and courses in a plane below the anterior auricular muscle. When it reaches about 1 cm in front of the ear, it gives off three main branches posteriorly:
  - Superior auricular artery—anterior helix.
  - Medial auricular artery—tragus.
  - Inferior auricular artery—lobule.
- The posterior auricular artery supplies the bulk of the blood volume to the ear. It crosses below the great auricular nerve, passing beneath the posterior auricular muscle to give off three main branches in the ear—superior, medial, and inferior. All supply the cranial aspect of the ear, and run in the subcutaneous vascular fascia between the two fat layers.

Venous supply

The veins of the ear follow the arteries. The number of veins per artery varies; frequently there are two or even three. The nerves run superficial to the veins and the arteries deep to them.

Lymphatics

- Concha and tragus: pre-auricular node in front of tragus.
- Scapha and postero-superior helix: mastoid nodes.
- Lobule: parotid nodes.
- Meatus: juxtajugular node anterior to the sternomastoid muscle.

Sensory nerve supply
- Lower half, anterolateral aspect: anterior branch, great auricular nerve.
- Cranial aspect: posterior branch, great auricular nerve.
- Upper anterolateral aspect: auriculotemporal nerve.
- Meatus: vagus ± glossopharyngeal.

Clinical relevance
For local anaesthesia, block the great auricular nerve by subcutaneous injection horizontally inferior to the earlobe in the neck. Then inject anterior to the ear in the auricular facial groove, proceeding over the top of the ear and then down the posterior auricular cephalic groove. Block the vagus by injecting from posteriorly trans-conchal cartilage into the external auditory meatus.

A rich blood supply with great anastomoses between regions means that the ear can survive on even the smallest of pedicles. FTSG will take well on the perichondrium.

The elastic properties of the cartilage and its perichondrium allow shaping by lightly scoring one surface of the cartilage. This breaks the surface tension, allowing the cartilage to bend away from the scored surface in response to the surface tension of the other side. The depth and spacing of the scores modifies the degree and acuteness of curvature. This is called the Gibson effect. It is commonly used to create an antihelical fold when absent in prominent ear correction. Youthful cartilage bends better than older cartilage.

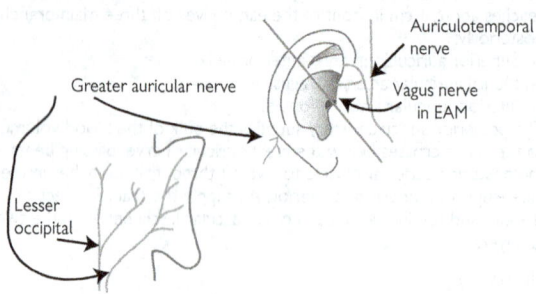

Fig. 3.5 Sensory nerve supply of the ear.

Facial nerve anatomy

The facial nerve is associated with the second branchial arch and its structures.

The nucleus has two parts: an upper branch from crossed and uncrossed fibres supplying the upper face and forehead, and a lower branch from mainly crossed fibres supplying the lower face.

Secreto-motor nerve has a high nerve to muscle ratio (1:8 to 1:50):
- Motor supplies facial muscles.
- Parasympathetics supply:
  - Lacrimal gland (greater superficial petrosal nerve via lacrimal nerve V1).
  - Soft palate taste and nasal glands (greater superficial petrosal nerve via pterygopalatine nerve V2).
  - Taste buds and submandibular and sublingual glands (via chorda tympani and lingual nerve V3).
- Sensory fibres supply:
  - Deep pressure/pain face (greater superficial petrosal nerve).
  - External auditory meatus (via fibres travelling with vagus CN X).

Facial nerve (CN VII) travels with nervus intermedius accompanied by the acoustic nerve (CN VIII) through the facial canal in the temporal bone, and leaves the cranial fossa via the internal auditory meatus. Within the canal it gives off three branches: the greater superficial petrosal nerve (at the level of the geniculate ganglion), the nerve to the stapedius, and the chorda tympani. The nerve occupies 25% of the canal diameter.

It exits the skull at the stylomastoid foramen. Deep to the sternomastoid, the nerve goes anterior to the posterior belly of the digastric, lateral to the styloid process, stylohyoid, external carotid, and external jugular vein, but posterior to the facial vein. It then enters the parotid, splitting it into deep and superficial lobes.

Pre-parotid branches—auricular branch muscular ramii to supply:
- Occipital.
- Auricular.
- Post-digastric.
- Stylohyoid.

Within the parotid gland divides into two main branches and then five terminal branches:
- Temporofacial:
  - Temporal.
  - Zygomatic (largest branch).
- Cervicofacial:
  - Buccal.
  - Mandibular.
  - Cervical (smallest).

There are many and varied interneural connections between these branches especially the zygomatic and buccal.

CHAPTER 3 Anatomy and clinical assessment

The nerve usually lies deep to platysma and enters muscles of facial expression on deep surface (except mentalis, buccinator, and levator anguli superiorus where it enters on their superficial surface; note these are deep muscles and hence dissection in a plane superficial to the facial muscles should be a safe plane).

- Seventeen paired muscles:
    1. frontalis ⎱ elevators of brow
    2. Procerus ⎰
    3. Corrugator supercili
    4. Orbicularis oculi
    5. Dilator nares
    6. Nasalis
    7. Levator labii superioris
    8. Levator labii superioris alaeque nasi
    9. Levator anguli oris
    10. Zygomaticus major ⎱ modiolus
    11. Zygomaticus minor ⎰
    12. Risorius
    13. Depressor labii inferioris
    14. Depressor anguli oris
    15. Mentalis
    16. Orbicularis oris
    17. Buccinator
- One unpaired muscle: platysma.

Danger zones

- Course of temporal branch (line from 1 cm below inter-tragal notch to 1 cm above lateral eyebrow), especially where the nerve changes planes from deep to deep temporal fascia to lie superficial to the deep temporal fascia, but still deep to SMAS/temperoparietal fascia.
- Course of marginal mandibular branch (curved line from 1 cm below inter-tragal notch to commissure extending below midpoint of mandible by 1 cm), especially where the nerve re-ascends to cross the mandiblular border and lies superficial.
- Space between the two lines above anterior to parotid but posterior to line from lateral palpebral angle to commissure where the zygomatic and buccal branches are vulnerable.
- Below ear in posterior mastoid fossa, posterior to the parotid where the main facial nerve is vulnerable.

How to find the facial nerve

Multiple techniques

- Find distal branches and trace posteriorly.
- Find and retract sternomastoid posteriorly; find posterior belly of digastric and follow cranially to mastoid; retract parotid from anterior surface external auditory canal exposing the tragal pointer. The facial nerve lies 1 cm deep and 1 cm anterior inferior to the pointer.

Note that in children the facial nerve lies closer to the surface as the mastoid is not yet developed.

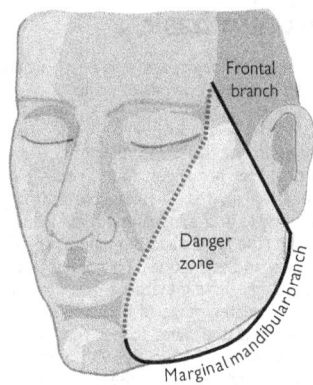

Fig. 3.6 Facial nerve danger zones.

Hand anatomy: basic

Hand anatomy is essential knowledge. It is best to denote the structures by name rather than number to avoid confusion.

Skeleton

There are 27 bones in the hand including the eight carpal bones. five metacarpals, five proximal phalanges, four middle phalanges (not in the thumb), and five distal phalanges. The carpometacarpal joints (CMCJs) are stable and quite immobile in the index and middle fingers, but increasingly mobile in the ring and little fingers and the thumb. The CMCJs allow flexion, with limited abduction and adduction This combination allows circumduction but no rotation. The first metacarpal has a saddle-shaped proximal end, allowing a much greater range of movement. The fifth CMCJ is also relatively mobile, allowing the palm to be 'cupped'. The metacarpophalangeal joints (MCPJs) are hinged joints with a cam effect, i.e. they are loose in extension but tighten up in flexion. The interphalangeal joints (IPJs) are also hinged joints with a slight but opposite cam, being tight in extension but loose in flexion. Note that the MCPs and IPJs are skeletally unstable joints, relying on the joint capsules, ligaments, and tendons for stability.

- The normal range of motion of the MCPJs is 10°–45° of hyperextension increasing from thumb/index to little, with 80°–100° of flexion increasing from thumb to little.
- The normal range of motion of the PIPJs is 0°–15° of hyperextension increasing from little to index, with 90°–110° of flexion increasing from little to index.
- The normal range of motion of the DIPJs is 0°–15° of hyperextension with no real difference between fingers, with 60°–90° of flexion with no real difference between fingers.
- The interphalangeal joint of the thumb moves from 30°–40° of hyperextension to 80° of flexion.

Joint range is measured and recorded in degrees. Functional range is measured by the distance of the pulp from the palm in the fingers, and by the extent to which the thumb can reach across the palm and fingers (Kapandji 0–9).

Fasciae

The flexor retinaculum or transverse carpal ligament is a postage-stamp-sized rectangle of dense fascia which covers the palmar surface of the carpal bones, creating the roof of the carpal tunnel It is attached radially to the scaphoid tubercle and the trapezium ridge, and ulnarly to the pisiform and the hook of the hamate. Nine tendons and the median nerve with their synovial lining pass through the carpal tunnel.

The palmar aponeurosis (fascia) fixes the skin firmly to allow the hand to grip. It is continuous with the flexor retinaculum and palmaris longus proximally; distally it inserts into the flexor tendon sheaths. The palmar

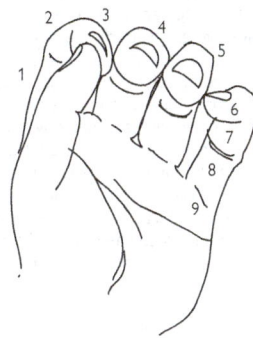

Fig. 3.7 Kapandji assessment of opposition.

fascia has vertical, transverse and longitudinal fibres. The vertical fibres fix the skin, and extend between the metacarpals as the bands of Legue and Juvara at the metacarpal necks. The longitudinal fibres concentrate in the pre-tendinous areas along the lines of tension in each digital ray. The transverse fibres of Skoog lie deep to the longitudinal but superficial to the neurovascular bundles, providing a useful safe dissection plane.

Nerves (Fig. 3.8 and Table 3.3)

The **ulnar nerve** supplies the sensation to the little finger and the ulnar half of the ring finger, and the motor supply to all the intrinsic muscles of the hand except the abductor pollicis brevis and opponens and the radial two lumbricals. It enters the hand under cover on the radial aspect of flexor carpi ulnaris, having given off dorsal and palmar superficial cutaneous branches (these supply the ulnar dorsum of the hand and the hypothenar eminence respectively). It passes superficial to the flexor retinaculum within a loose sleeve of fascia (Guyon's canal). Within Guyon's canal it divides into a superficial sensory branch and a deep motor branch to the hypothenar muscles (abductor digiti minimi, flexor digiti minimi, opponens digiti minimi), all the palmar and dorsal interossei, the ulnar two lumbricals, and the thumb adductor. Although the motor branch frequently leaves the nerve on the nerve's ulnar aspect, it then passes deep to the nerve and curls around the hook of the hamate and into the palm. It is accompanied by the continuation of the ulnar artery as the deep palmar arch.

The **median nerve** passes within the carpal tunnel, entering between the palmaris longus and flexor carpi radialis, superficial to the digital flexor tendons. It supplies sensation to the thumb, index and middle fingers, and the radial half of the ring finger, and a muscular branch to the muscles of the radial thenar eminence. In the distal forearm the median nerve gives a sensory branch (palmar cutaneous branch of the median nerve) which usually passes superficial to the flexor retinaculum to the skin over the thenar eminence and the radial two-thirds of the palm up to the axial line of the ring finger ray. The motor branch usually leaves the median nerve within the carpal tunnel on the nerve's radial superficial aspect. It then emerges on the radial distal end of the transverse carpal ligament and hooks back, heading superficially and radially into the thenar muscles between flexor and abductor pollicis brevis. However, it may exit through the flexor retinaculum, or lie superficial to it, becoming vulnerable to injury in carpal tunnel decompression.

The superficial **radial nerve** passes under cover of the brachioradialis (BR) in the forearm, merging on its dorsal aspect at the junction of the middle third and distal third of the forearm. It then hooks over the aponeurotic border of the brachioradialis (where it may be compressed or irritated, causing Wartenberg's syndrome), dividing into several branches which supply sensation to the skin of the radial dorsum of the hand and digits to the level of the proximal phalanx.

Arteries

The **ulnar artery** runs on the radial aspect of the ulnar nerve, gives off a deep branch, and curves around the palm just deep to the palmar aponeurosis to form the superficial palmar arch. This arch supplies common digital arteries to each web space which divide distally to give proper digital arteries. These lie mid-lateral in the digits, anterior to the nerves.

The **radial artery** gives off the superficial palmar branch 2–3 cm proximal to the wrist. The superficial palmar branch emerges between flexor carpi radialis (FCR) and BR, and crosses very superficially onto the thenar eminence just radial to the scaphoid tubercle. A pulse can be seen or felt here in some individuals. It supplies the thenar muscle and continues on to form the superficial palmar arch with the ulnar artery. The main radial artery, also between FCR and BR, passes deep to abductor pollicis longus (APL) and extensor pollicis brevis (EPB) tendons into the anatomical **snuffbox** (bordered by APL/EPB radially and EPL ulnarly, proximally by the radial styloid, and with the scaphoid on the floor) where it lies with the cephalic vein and superficial radial nerve branches. It leaves between the two heads of the first dorsal interosseous muscle at the base of the first web space and re-enters the palm between the first and second metacarpal bones. It sends digital branches to the thumb and radial side of the index finger (princeps pollicis and indicis), and then curves deep to the flexor tendons to join the ulnar artery to form the deep palmar arch.

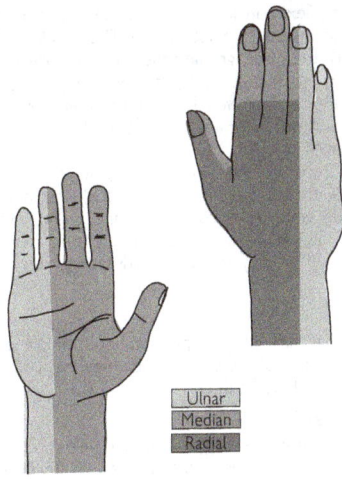

Fig. 3.8 Nerve supply to the hand.

Extrinsic muscles

Flexor tendons
Each finger has a deep flexor tendon (flexor digitorum profundus), inserting onto the palmar base of the distal phalanx. There is also a superficial tendon (flexor digitorum superficialis) which splits, wraps around the flexor digitorum profundus tendon (Camper's chiasma), rejoins, and inserts onto the middle phalanx. The profundus tendon passes from deep to volar through this split and glides smoothly through it. The split serves as a mobile pulley to help restrain the profundus tendon from bowstringing. The thumb has only one flexor (flexor pollicis longus), as it has only two phalanges.

Synovial sheath
All these long flexors are invested in a common synovial sheath between the distal forearm and the palm. In the thumb and little finger the synovial sheath extends all the way to the tendon insertions. This communication between the two digits explains the passage of infection from little finger to thumb or vice versa to form a horse-shoe abscess. The synovial sheaths of the other digits terminate in mid-palm.

Pulleys (Fig. 3.9)
The flexor tendons run in a fibrous tendon sheath which runs from the level of the distal palmar crease to the tendon insertions to bind the tendons down to the bones of the fingers and stop bowstringing. This tendon sheath is cleverly constructed from segments of solid tunnel (annular pulleys) with interlinking collapsible (cruciate pulley) areas which

allow the finger to flex, bringing all the solid segments together to form a continous solid strong pulley in full flexion. The annular pulleys are found over the shafts of the phalanges and the cruciate pulleys over the joints. Destruction of these pulleys reduces flexor tendon glide and allows bowstringing of the tendons, which diminishes their power and excursion (so the fingers will not fully flex). The critical pulleys are the annular pulleys, especially A2 and A4.

In the thumb there are only two annular pulleys (A1 over the base of the proximal phalanx and the A2 over the neck), and in between there is one oblique pulley which runs from the ulnar proximal in the radial distal direction (hence always do an A1 trigger thumb pulley release on the radial side of the A1 pulley to avoid inadvertently dividing the oblique pulley as well).

Vinculae

At the level of the neck of each proximal and middle phalanx vinculae run from the bone side of the tendon sheath to the flexor tendons like a mesentery bringing a blood supply.

Flexor tendon zones (Fig. 3.10)

The pulleys and transverse carpal ligament help divide the hand into zones which are used to describe the levels of flexor tendon injuries. Zone 2 injuries were said to be 'no-man's land' as flexor tendon repairs done in this area had bad results and primary repair was not performed.
- Zone 1: distal to insertion of flexor digitorum superficialis (FDS).
- Zone 2: FDS insertion to proximal end of A1 pulley.
- Zone 3: mid-palm.
- Zone 4: under transverse carpal ligament (TCL).
- Zone 5: forearm.

The thumb does not have zone 3, and zone 1 is distal to the thumb A1 pulley.

Extensors

On the dorsum of the wrist the nine extensor tendons pass through six tunnels/compartments to enter the hand. These contain (from radial to ulnar) two, two, one, two, one , and one tendons:
- First extensor compartment—EPB and APL.
- Second compartment—ECRL and ECRB.
- Third compartment—EPL.
- Fourth compartment—EDC and EIP.
- Fifth compartment—EDM.
- Sixth compartment—ECU.

The dorsum of each digit is wrapped in a wide extensor hood. These receive fibres from the common extensor muscles (extensor digitorum communis) to the fingers, and an additional independent muscle each in the case of the index (extensor indicis proprius) and little fingers (extensor digiti minimi/quinti). These tendons mainly insert into the dorsal base of the distal and middle phalanges and extend the digits. The lateral bands are created by the interossei and the lumbricals (on the radial aspect only) and create flexion at the MCPJ and extension of the IPJs.

HAND ANATOMY: BASIC

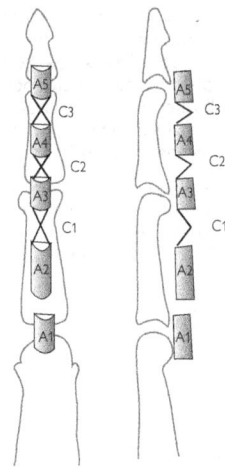

Fig. 3.9 Flexor tendon pulley system.

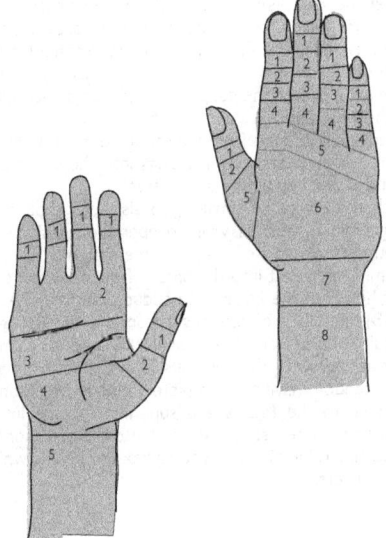

Fig. 3.10 Flexor and extensor tendon zones.

The thumb has three extensor/abductor tendons inserting into the base of each phalanx and the metacarpal. The extensor pollicis longus inserts on the base of the distal phalanx, the extensor pollicis brevis to the base of the proximal phalanx, the abductor pollicis longus to the base of the thumb metacarpal. Abductor pollicis brevis, and adductor pollicis brevis form the lateral bands of the extensor hood of the thumb and in addition to abduction/adduction create extension at the IPJ.

Extensor tendon zones (Fig. 3.10)
Similar to the flexor tendon zones the dorsum of the hand and forearm are divided into zones to aid description of extensor tendon injuries. There are eight zones. The odd numbers lie over joints and the even numbers over bone:
- Zone 1—over DIPJ.
- Zone 2—over middle phalanx.
- Zone 3—over PIPJ.
- Zone 4—over proximal phalanx.
- Zone 5—over MCPJ.
- Zone 6—over metacarpals.
- Zone 7—over wrist joint.
- Zone 8—over forearm.

There are no zones 3 and 4 in the thumb.

Intrinsic muscles

The thenar eminence refers to the bulk of muscles which move the thumb: abductor pollicis brevis, flexor pollicis brevis, and opponens pollicis. They arise from the flexor retinaculum, scaphoid, and trapezium, and insert into the proximal phalanx. All are usually supplied by the median nerve (T1), except the deep head of flexor pollicis brevis which is supplied by the ulnar nerve.

The adductor pollicis arises from the carpal bones and third metacarpal, lying deep to the flexor tendons. It inserts into the proximal phalanx of the thumb, and is supplied by the ulnar nerve.

The hypothenar eminence similarly consists of flexor, abductor, and opponens digiti minimi muscles, which deepen the cup shape of the palm.

Interosseous muscles arise from the metacarpals, filling the spaces between them. They insert into the bases of the proximal phalanges and the extensor hoods of the fingers and adduct (palmar—PAD) or abduct (dorsal—DAB) the MCPJs of each finger from the middle finger.

On the radial side of each flexor profunda tendon, a small lumbrical muscle arises in the palm (the only muscle that arises from a tendon and inserts into a tendon, having a completely mobile origin and insertion). They pass radial to the MCPJs and superficial to the intermetacarpal ligaments (unlike the interossei) and insert into the extensor hood.

The interossei and lumbricals together flex the MCPJs while extending the IPJs of the fingers.

Nerve supply to the hand

Table 3.3 Nerve supply to the hand

Parent nerve	Branch	Sensory	Motor
Median	Anterior interosseous	Wrist and carpal joints	FPL, two radial FDP, PQ
	Palmar cutaneous	Radial palm	Nil
	Muscular recurrent	Nil	APB, FPB, Opponens pollicis
	Palmar digital	Flexor skin, distal dorsal skin, and nail beds of radial 3½ digits	Two radial lumbricals
Radial	–	Nil in hand	ECRL, brachioradialis, brachialis
	Posterior interosseous	Wrist and carpal joints	ECRB, supinator, EDC, EI, EDM, ECU, APL, EPB, EPL
	Superficial	Radial half of dorsum of hand, and dorsum of radial 3½ fingers	Nil
Ulnar	–	Nil in hand	Two ulnar FDP, FCU
	Palmar cutaneous	Hypothenar eminence	Nil
	Dorsal cutaneous	Ulnar skin over dorsum of hand, and dorsal surface of ulnar 1½ digits	Nil
	Superficial branch	Flexor skin, distal dorsal skin and nail beds of ulnar 1½ digits	Nil
	Deep branch	Nil	ADM, FDM, ODM, Two ulnar lumbricals, all interossei, adductor pollicis

Anatomical variants

Martin–Gruber
In 10–20% of people, the median nerve or its anterior interosseous branch may send fibres which connect with the ulnar nerve in the forearm. In 60% of cases, median fibres pass to the ulnar nerve and innervate 'median' muscles; in 35% of cases, median fibres pass to the ulnar nerve and innervate 'ulnar' muscles; in 5% of cases ulnar fibres pass to the median nerve. They are more common on the right.

Riche–Cannieu
Frequent motor crossover between the median and ulnar nerves in the palm, originally described within the substance of FPB. These occur in up to 70% of individuals.

Froment–Robert
Connections between the radial and ulnar nerve have also been reported.

Wrist anatomy and examination

Skeleton

- The wrist joint comprises eight carpal bones, articulating with the radius and ulna proximally and five metacarpals distally, combining in a total of 19 joints.
- The eight carpal bones are arranged either in two rows (proximal and distal) or three columns (radial, central, ulnar).
- The proximal carpal row contains (from radial to ulnar) the scaphoid, lunate, triquetrum, and pisiform. The distal row contains the trapezium, trapezoid, capitate, and hamate.
- The central stable column comprises the capitate and lunate, taking 75% of the forces through the wrist and governing flexion and extension. The radial column contains the scaphoid (interlinking between the proximal and distal rows) and the trapezium and trapezoid, with the others making up the ulnar rotatory column with the triquetrum providing rotation.

Ligaments

Apart from the pisiform, which is considered a sesamoid bone in the course of the flexor carpi ulnaris, there are no muscular or tendinous attachments to the bones of the proximal row. The proximal row moves in response to the compressive and tensional forces in accordance with the shape of the articular surfaces and the ligamentous restraints. These ligaments can be classified into capsular or intra-osseous ligaments. The capsular ligaments are dorsal or palmar. The dorsal ligaments are arranged in a sideways V with the apex ulnar. The palmar ligaments are arranged in a double V with the apex distal, as in the Citroen car logo.

The dorsal ligaments lie within the capsule and comprise the dorsal radio-carpal running from the radius across (with some attachment to) the lunate to the triquetrum and hamate. The distal limb of the V diverges from here, heading radially to the trapezoid and trapezium.

The palmar ligaments are deep to the capsule (intra-capsular) comprising double inverted Vs, with the proximal radial limb formed by the radio-triquetral and the radio-scaphoid-lunate, and completed on the ulnar return limb by the ulno-lunate. The distal V is formed by the radio-capitate on one limb and the capito-tiquetral and the ulno-triquetral on the ulnar limb.

The space of Poirier is the space between the divergent radial limbs of the radio-capitate and the radio-triquetral ligaments, exposing the capito-lunate joint.

Inter-osseous intercarpal ligaments unite the proximal row of carpal bones. These are generally stronger on the dorsum. They are C-shaped on cross-section and open distally. The central portion is the weakest. There are inter-osseous ligaments between each of the distal carpal bones and also in the metacarpal bases.

Surface anatomy

The carpal bones articulate with the radius and the fibrocartilagenous disc (TFCC) covering the distal ulna, at the level of the proximal wrist crease.

The distal wrist crease is at the level of the mid-carpal joint between the scaphoid, lunate, triquetrum, and pisiform proximally and the trapezium, trapezois, capitate, and hamate distally.

The scaphoid and trapezium are palpable in the anatomical snuffbox, running distal from the radial styloid; the pisiform and hook of hamate are palpable in palm distal to the ulna.

The radial styloid, Lister's tubercle, distal dorsal border of the radius, distal radioulnar joint, ulnar head, ulnar styloid, pisiform, and hook of the hamate are all easily felt. The individual carpal bones can also be palpated with manipulation and appropriate positioning of the wrist.

Biomechanics

On wrist flexion, movement mainly occurs at the radio-carpal and mid-carpal joints. The carpal bones, especially the proximal row, are flexed, and on wrist extension the carpus is extended. The proximal row moves passively under the influence of the forces, the shape of the bones, and the configuration of the articular surfaces. Each is intricately linked to the other, such that the disturbance of one link changes the posture and pattern of movement of the carpus. These patterns are reproducible and reflect the forces and resting posture of the carpal bones when not tied by ligamentous attachments. The links are particularly strong with adjacent bones in the rows, and the scaphoid and triquetrum are seen as the link bones completing the 'carpal ring' at the radial and ulnar aspects, and have strong attachments not only with the adjacent bone in the proximal row but also with the distal row.

On wrist radial or ulnar deviation, movement occurs at the radio-ulno-carpal and mid-carpal joints. When the wrist lies in ulnar deviation the proximal row is extended. As the wrist moves into radial deviation the proximal row flexes. By virtue of its shape and articular configuration, the scaphoid flexes most, allowing the distal carpal row to approximate the radius. The distal carpal row and the carpo-metacarpal joints are relatively stable and immobile compared with the proximal joints.

Pronation and supination are chiefly a result of rotation of the radius around the ulna at the distal radioulnar joint (DRUJ). Some limited rotation can occur through the radio-ulno-carpal and inter-carpal joints.

Penis anatomy

The penis has a root, attached to the perineal membrane, and a body. In the root is a central bulb, forming the base of the corpus spongiosum; and two crura which each continue into the corpora cavernosa. The body is formed at the subpubic angle from the paired corpora cavernosa with the penile urethra running through the centre of the corpus spongiosum on the ventral surface. The glans penis is the expanded end of the corpus spongiosum. The normal urethral meatus is slit shaped and emerges at the terminus of the glans.

The corpora cavernosa and spongiosum are surrounded by a tough fibrous sheath termed the tunica albuginea. Trabeculae pass into the corpora cavernosa to divide it into multiple endothelial-lined cavernous spaces, which become engorged with blood upon erection, which interweave with the tunica albuginea. The tunica albuginea separately surrounds each of the corpora, including the glans, but is adherent to its adjacent tunica, forming a fibrous septum between the two corpora cavernosa.

The tunica is surrounded by the deep fascia of the penis (Buck's fascia), a continuation of the deep perineal (Colles') fascia, which attaches to the symphysis pubis by the suspensory ligament of the penis. A central deep dorsal vein, two dorsal arteries, and paired dorsal nerves lie deep to it. Superficial to this are the superficial dorsal veins, and then the Dartos fascia. The skin of the penis is folded back on itself at the neck of the glans to form the prepuce.

Skin and fascial layers

- Skin.
- Dartos.
- Superficial veins, lymphatics, and anterior urethra.
- Buck's fascia—a cylindrical prolongation of Colles' fascia also called the penile fascia.
- Deep artery, veins, and nerves.
- Tunica albuginea of each corpora.

Arterial supply

Arterial supply is via three paired branches of the internal pudendal arteries:

- The artery to the bulb supplies the corpus spongiosum including the glans.
- The deep artery supplies the corpus cavernosum.
- The dorsal artery supplies the skin, fascia, and glans.

The artery of the bulb and the dorsal artery anastomose via the glans.

Venous drainage

Venous drainage is via:

- Venae comitantes, to the internal pudendal veins.
- The deep dorsal vein to the vesico-prostatic venous plexus.
- The superficial dorsal vein drains the dorsal skin into the great saphenous veins.

Lymphatics
- Skin passes to superficial inguinal nodes.
- Glans and corpora lymph drainage goes to deep inguinal nodes. Some glans drainage goes straight to Cloquet's node.

Nerve supply
- Skin: posterior scrotal and dorsal nerve of penis, derived from the pudendal nerves (S2).
- Glans: dorsal nerve of penis.
- Erection: pelvic splanchnic nerves (S2,3) provide parasympathetic supply to enable erection.
- Ejaculation: sympathetic nerves from the superior and inferior hypogastric plexuses (L1).

Parasympathetic nervous system

Introduction
The autonomic nervous system is composed of the sympathetic nervous system and the parasympathetic nervous system. In contrast with the sympathetic nervous system, targets of the parasympathetic nervous system are entirely visceral; there is no supply to the trunk and limbs.

Anatomy
General pattern
In the head and neck, pre-ganglionic fibres arise from a central nucleus and synapse with a post-ganglionic cell body in a peripheral ganglion. From here, post-ganglionic fibres travel to the target organ. Other parasympathetics arise from a central nucleus, but synapse with the post-ganglionic cell in the wall of the viscera supplied. All parasympathetic nerves also carry afferent fibres, mostly relaying pain sensation from the target organ.

Cranio-sacral outflow
- Head and neck parasympathetics supplied by CNs III, VII, IX.
- Heart, lungs, foregut and midgut derivatives supplied by the vagus (CN X).
- Hindgut derivatives and pelvic organs supplied by the pelvic splanchnic nerves.

Head and neck parasympathetics

Table 3.4 Head and neck parasympathetics

Nucleus	Cranial nerve	Ganglion	Target organ
Edinger—Westphal	Occulomotor (3)	Ciliary	Sphincter pupillae, ciliary muscle
Superior salivary	Nervus intermedius (7)	Pterygo-palatine	Lacrimal, nasal, and palatal glands
Superior salivary	Nervus intermedius (7)	Submandibular	Submandibular and sublingual glands
Inferior salivary	Glossopharyngeal (9)	Otic	Parotid gland

Vagal parasympathetics
The vagus (CN X) arises from the brainstem between the olive and the inferior cerebellar peduncle. It exits the skull via the jugular foramen and descends through the neck within the carotid sheath. Cervical cardiac branches here contribute to the cardiac plexi. Both left and right vagi pass posterior to the lung root, and give off branches to the pulmonary plexi. They then break up into several branches to form the anterior and posterior oesophageal plexi, from which the anterior and posterior vagal trunks

emerge to pass through the oesophageal opening in the diaphragm. The anterior vagus gives off a hepatic branch and the posterior vagus a coeliac branch, and the parasympathetic supply to the foregut, midgut, and their derivatives is achieved through these branches.

Pelvic parasympathetics

Several rootlets arise from the anterior surface of the S2, S3, and S4 nerve roots. They pass into the inferior hypogastric plexus, and are distributed to the hindgut derivatives and pelvic viscera along with sympathetic neurons.

Physiology

Table 3.5 Physiology

Target organ	Action
Eye	Constricts pupil, accommodation
Salivary, lacrimal, nasal, and palatal glands	Increases secretion
Heart	Reduces heart rate and contractility of atria
Lungs	Bronchoconstriction, increases secretion
GI tract	Increases smooth muscle contraction, dilates sphincters, increases glandular secretion (e.g. gastric acid)
Bladder	Detrusor contraction
Penis	Erection
Uterus	Variable effects
Sweat glands, arterioles, veins, liver, kidneys, adrenals	No effect

Neurotransmitters

Acetylcholine (ACh) is the neurotransmitter used at both the synapse between pre- and post-ganglionic fibres, and the synapse between post-ganglionic fibres and the target organ. Nicotinic receptors are utilized at the former synapse, and muscarinic receptors at the latter. Co-transmission using a variety of other neurotransmitters (e.g. ATP, 5-HT, nitric oxide) is a general phenomenon.

Clinical relevance

Defects in the head and neck parasympathetics are the most relevant to plastic surgeons. These include gustatory sweating, Horner's syndrome, and drooling.

Chapter 4

Drugs and tools

Local anaesthesia *106*
Blood transfusion *108*
Drugs used in inflammatory arthritis *110*
Oncological drugs *111*
Injectables *112*
Antibiotic prophylaxis in plastic surgery *114*
Thromboprophylaxis in plastic surgery *116*
Dressings *118*
Implants *120*
Smoking and plastic surgery *123*
Leech therapy *125*
Microsurgery *127*
Lasers *130*

Local anaesthesia

Definition
A local anaesthetic (LA) reversibly blocks nerve conduction beyond the point of application, when applied locally in the appropriate concentration.

Pharmacology
Local anaesthetics are classified into amides (lidocaine, prilocaine, bupivicaine) or esters (cocaine, procaine). The mechanism of action is by blocking the Na channel that is responsible for rapid ionic flow allowing propagation of the nerve action potentials. However, the LA can only block the Na channel from within the cell; hence the injected LA has to be a water-soluble injection which becomes lipid soluble, to cross the cell membrane, and then re-ionizes to become soluble in the intra-cellular fluid to be able to block the Na channel from within. Local anaesthetics are free bases when non-ionized and hence become lipid soluble. However, in acid solutions LAs become ionized and water soluble (salts). Hence, LAs are injected in acid water-soluble solutions, which once in the extra-cellular fluid become diluted and less acidic, thus allowing the LA to become non-ionized and lipid soluble and able to cross the lipid cell membrane. Once in the cell, a portion becomes water soluble and able to block the channel. All LAs are vasodilators. Infected inflamed tissue is acidic, which explains why LAs may be less effective or slower acting.

- Pain on administration of LA is due to:
  - Needle pain.
  - Acidity.
  - Cold temperature.
  - Stretch.
  - Anxiety.
- Methods of reducing pain are:
  - Use topical anaesthetics (EMLAs).
  - Smaller gauge needle.
  - Warm the solution.
  - Add bicarbonate to raise the low pH of the LA.
  - Distract the patient (gate control theory).
  - Use sedation.

Dosage
The maximum safe dose of LA depends on the rate, route, and site of injection more than on the mass of drug. However, in a slow injection in the soft tissue, the maximum safe dose of lidocaine is approximately 3 mg/kg plain and 7 mg/kg when mixed with adrenaline. There is 50 mg of lidocaine in 5 mL of 1% solution, which means that, when using a 1% solution 0.3 mL/kg can be administered to the equivalent of 15 mL in a 45 kg patient. When adrenaline is used, this rises to 0.7 mL/kg or 35 mL in a 50 kg patient.

Bupivicaine has a much lower maximum safe dose of 1.8 mg/kg which translates into just under 1 mL/kg of 0.25% solution and just under 0.5 mL per kg of 0.5% solution.

If a mixture of LAs is used there is a possible protective effect but it is probably safer to halve the relative doses.

Toxic effects

- Hypersensitivity: rare to amide LAs but more common with ester LAs; cross-sensitivity with p-amino benzoic acid (sunscreen) and parabens (preservatives).
- Systemic absorption - presents as perioral tingling, paraesthesia and evidence of sympathetic blockade.

Cardiac effects

Cardiac effects are due to the membrane-stabilizing effect and therefore may suppress cardiac dysrhythmias, but lead to a prolongation of action potential duration, increase the refractory period, and slow cardiac conduction seen as QRS changes, brachycardia, hypotension leading to desynchronized ventricular contraction, reduced myocardial contractility and, eventually, VF/asystole. Bupivicaine is more cardiac toxic than levobupivacaine > ropivicaine > procaine > lidocaine.

Neurological effects

LAs are cerebral depressants, but excitation may occur before the generalized depressant effect due to depressing inhibitors, and this may lead to seizures prior to generalized depressant effects resulting in coma and loss of consciousness. Lidocaine neurological toxicity produces peri-oral tingling/numbness, light-headedness, visual or auditory disturbance, muscular twitching, loss of consciousness, seizures, coma, respiratory arrest.

Lidocaine produces neurological symptoms before cardiovascular depression, whereas bupivicaine produces cardiac effects before neurological symptoms. Bupivicaine toxicity may manifest as VF arrest.

Treatment of neurological toxicity consists of anticonvulsants, benzodiazapenes, and ventilatory support as required.

Cardiovascular toxicity is treated by CPR and IPPV, DC shock, adrenaline, and prolonged resuscitation until the LA disassociates (this may take 20–30 min with bupivicaine).

Blood transfusion

Blood transfusion is commonly used in plastic surgery and the proper indication, consent, administration, and recognition and treatment of complications should be known.

Indication
- Symptomatic loss of blood, or occasionally to maintain optimal perfusion of extremities and flaps.
- One unit of blood raises the Hb by approximately 1 g/dl. One unit of packed cells equals 350 mL fluid.
- Use cross-matched blood except in emergencies when O neg blood can be used.
- Consider autologous blood collected preoperatively or intra-operative cell salvage to reduce demand on blood banks and the risk of complications.

Consent
Patients must consent to receive blood products. Consent should include the indications for transfusion, options, side effects, and consequences of refusal.

Administration
Rate of administration depends on the indication. Resuscitation rate is rapid, perhaps under pressure, whereas slow administration is preferred for the management of chronic anaemia. Consider the need for diuretics to avoid fluid overload.

Side effects of transfusion
- Circulatory overload which can occur from the volume of blood transfused.
- The blood itself can cause transmission of infectious diseases (HIV, EBV, CMV, HBV, and bacterial rarely), coagulopathy (including DIC, micro aggregates leading to ARDS), sepsis, and transfusion reactions including allergy, anaphylaxis, non-haemolytic pyrexia, haemolysis (acute or delayed).
- Immune reactions causing allo-immunization or graft versus host disease.
- Metabolic side effects include iron overload (haemosiderosis), hypothermia, citrate toxicity leading to hypocalcaemia, acidosis, and alterations in potassium balance.

Transfusion reactions present with headache, shock, chills, fever, shortness of breath, chest or back pain, haematuria, raised bilirubin, or death.

Treatment

Treatment is to cease transfusion, send the bag and tubing for analysis, and resuscitate, especially volume. Consider diuretics in overload, oxygen, check coagulation status and electrolytes. Treat coagulation and other alterations as required. In anaphylaxis use adrenaline and hydrocortisone.

Other blood products

- Platelets.
- Fresh frozen plasma (FFP).
- Cryoprecipitate.

These do not need to be cross-matched.

Drugs used in inflammatory arthritis

Infliximab (Remicade)
Chimeric IgG1k monoclonal antibody that neutralizes cytokine TNF-alpha and inhibits its binding to TNF-alpha receptor. Reduces infiltration of inflammatory cells and TNF-alpha production in inflamed areas.

TNF-alpha modulates cellular immune responses. Anti-TNF therapies (e.g. infliximab) may adversely affect normal immune responses and allow development of super-infections (more cases of lymphoma were observed in TNF-alpha blockers compared with control groups); may increase risk of reactivation of tuberculosis in patients with particular granulomatous infections; has been associated with lupus erythematosus.

Immunoglobulins, intravenous (Sandoglobulin, Gammagard, Gamimune)
Neutralize circulating myelin antibodies through anti-idiotypic antibodies; downregulate pro-inflammatory cytokines, including INF-gamma; blocks Fc receptors on macrophages; suppresses inducer T and B cells and augments suppressor T cells; blocks complement cascade; and promotes remyelination. May increase CSF IgG (10%).

Cyclophosphamide (Cytoxan)
Alkylating agent that depresses B-cell and T-cell function. Chemically related to nitrogen mustards. As an alkylating agent, the mechanism of action of the active metabolites may involve cross-linking of DNA, which may interfere with growth of normal and neoplastic cells.

Azathioprine (Imuran)
Another drug that may be effective as a steroid-sparing agent. Antagonizes purine metabolism and inhibits synthesis of DNA, RNA, and proteins. May decrease proliferation of immune cells, which results in lower autoimmune activity.

Prednisone
May decrease inflammation by reversing increased capillary permeability and suppressing PMN activity.

Methotrexate (Folex, Rheumatrex)
Antimetabolite that inhibits DNA synthesis and cell reproduction in malignant cells. May suppress immune system.

Oncological drugs

Interferon
- *Definition*: interferon injected systemically or intra-lesionally.
- *Classification*: subdivided into interferon alpha, beta, or gamma.
- *Mechanism of action*: interferons react with cell membrane receptors by entering into the nucleus and depressing cellular genes to produce effector proteins. Their mechanism of action is essentially unknown.
- *Uses*:
  - Approved for the treatment of BCC and metastatic melanoma.
  - BCC management (Greenway): alpha 2b interferon is injected into the lesion at a dose of 1.5 million units three times a week for 3 weeks. This leads to an 80% cure rate. It is only recommended in BCCs smaller than 1 cm.
  - Melanoma treatment with interferon may prolong survival by a few months in those with metastatic disease.
- Side effects: influenza-like symptoms, itch, pain, and leucopenia. Thus interferon is not recommended for the elderly, those with heart, lung, or kidney disease, patients with transplants, or patients who are pregnant.

5-Fluorouracil (Efudix)
- *Definition*: 5-FU is a cytoxic topically applied for 3–4 weeks over pre-malignant skin conditions.
- *Mechanism of action*: fluorinated pyrimidine antimetabolite that inhibits thymidylate synthase (TS) and also interferes with RNA synthesis and function. Has some effect on DNA.
- *Uses*: approved for treatment of BCC and metastatic melanoma.
- *Side effects*: erythema, skin loss, scaliness, blistering, hypo- or hyper-pigmentation.

Imiquimod
- *Definition*: imidazoquinolone; usually 5% cream (Aldara) applied topically.
- *Mechanism of action*: binds to cell surface receptors on macrophages and inflammatory and immune cells and stimulates production of interferon alpha, TNF, and IL-2 (stimulates clonal expansion of T-helper cells and B-lymphocytes which are important for humoral antibody-mediated cell lysis immunity). Produces a T-cell-mediated immune response and pro-inflammatory cytokines.
- *Uses*: treatment of viral infections, non-melanoma skin cancers, lentigo maligna, and keloid scars.
- *Side effects* Hypo -or hyper-pigmentation.

Reference
Greenway HT, *West J Med* 1994 **160**(4): 363.

Injectables

Collagen

A suspension of sterilized fibrillar bovine dermal collagen which is incorporated into tissue but not encapsulated. The collagen telopeptide ends are removed as they are the antigenic immunogenic site of graft species inter-covariability.
- Zyderm 1 is a mix of 95% type 1 and 5% type 2 collagen with saline and lidocaine which contains 35 mg/mL collagen. It is used for fine lines.
- Zyderm 2 contains 65 mg/mL and is used for deeper lines.
- Zyplast is collagen treated with glutaraldehyde making it more stable, with better survival. It is used in thicker deeper dermis.

Injectable collagen is not incorporated but acts as an implant. It only lasts 6–24 months. It shrinks by 30–40% by volume. It may provoke an allergic or immune response of delayed-type hypersensitivity.

Uses

Intradermal or subdermal injection to fill cutaneous defects, lines, and wrinkles.

Complications

- Include a loss of benefit, allergic response (3%), or delayed hypersensitivity.
- Pre-operatively discuss pre-testing, complications, duration of effect, and need for multiple treatments.
- Contraindicated in autoimmune disease., indurated scars, viral pock marks, positive skin test.
- Skin testing is done by injecting 0.1 mL Zyderm 1 intradermally and examining the site at 3 days and 4 weeks. The test is positive if red and swollen. Hypersensitivity is most frequent with the first injection.

Technique

- Zyderm is injected in the superficial dermis in horizontal layers.
- Zyplast is injected into the deep dermis at 45°.
- Use a multiple injection technique with a 30 gauge needle in close spaced intervals. Aim to overcorrect the defect 1.5–2 times with Zyderm but be careful in thin-skinned areas. Do not over-correct with Zyplast.
- Reinject within 6–24 months.
- Zyderm is replaced by host collagen but the collagen is not cross-linked.

Botulinum toxin

Blocks peripheral ACh transmission at the neuromuscular junction by a pre-synaptic action at a site proximal to the release of ACh. Action involves an initial binding step to the pre-synaptic nerve membrane, followed by internalization of the toxin and disruption of the calcium-mediated release of ACh, thus decreasing the end-plate electrical potential causing paralysis. Recovery occurs gradually as new nerve terminals sprout and contact the post-synaptic motor end-plate. This takes 6–8 weeks.

The toxin is produced by *Clostridium botulinum*. Clinically, the disease is called botulism when the toxin is ingested in sufficient quantities to cause respiratory paralysis and death.

Uses

- *Aesthetic*: to reduce wrinkles and frown lines, most commonly around the orbit and glabella.
- *Functional*:
  - **Spasticity**: to reduce muscle contraction and spasticity to allow the affected muscle to be passively stretched without inducing counter-contraction. Such stretch to the muscle fibres and contractile units does have a long-term effect. Used for cerebral palsy, spasmodic torticollis, blepharospasm, and other involuntary muscle contractures such as those that may occur following re-innervation.
  - **Hyperhidrosis**: has been used to reduce sweating in axillae and hands.

Dosage and administration

Varies according to brand and strength (see manufacturer's instructions).

For cerebral palsy use a nerve stimulator to identify the required muscle unit and then inject small volumes. May need to be repeated. Therapy and stretching are an essential component of the treatment.

For blepharospasm, small volumes need to be injected into the junction of the preseptal and the orbital parts of both the upper and lower orbicularis oculi muscles. Glabella muscles are treated similarly. Note that for injections into the upper eyelid the needle needs to be directed away from the eye so as to avoid the levator muscle.

The effect takes 2–5 days to start and then takes 2 weeks to maximum effect. Injections may need to be repeated every 2–3 months.

Risks

- Local weakness in unintended muscles (effect depends on site injected, e.g. at the eye can give ptosis, blurred vision, diplopia, keratitis, dry eye, ophthalmoplegia).
- Pain.
- Bruising.

Antibiotic prophylaxis in plastic surgery

Prevention of endocarditis
- For patients with heart valve lesions, septal defects, patent ductus, or history of endocarditis.
- 'Dermatological' surgery alone does not require antibiotic prophylaxis.

Risk factors for surgical site infection
- Use of implants.
- Long duration of surgery.
- Significant comorbidity (ASA grade >2).
- Immunocompromised patients.
- Poor vascularity (PVD, radiotherapy, diabetes, crush injury).

Operations are classified according to bacterial contamination and likelihood of post-operative infection (Table 4.1).

The SIGN guidelines suggest that antibiotic prophylaxis should be used in:
- Clean-contaminated head and neck surgery.
- Breast surgery.
- Insertion of prosthetic devices.
- Craniotomy.
- Lower limb amputations.

Patients undergoing contaminated or dirty operations should receive appropriate antibiotics as treatment. Excision of an ulcerated skin lesion can be considered 'dirty' under this classification:
- Consider antibiotics for surgery to groin and axilla.
- Animal bite injuries should receive antibiotic treatment.
- Antibiotics are usually given for the duration of catheter insertion in hypospadias repair.
- Patients having leeches applied need prophylaxis against *Aeromonas hydrophilia* for the duration of treatment.
- The choice of antibiotic should be made locally, taking into account local bacterial sensitivities.

A dose should be given prior to surgery or on induction of anaesthesia. Depending on the half-life of the antibiotic used, repeat doses may be needed for prolonged surgery. Antibiotics are not usually continued for post-operative prophylaxis against surgical infection. However, ongoing antibiotics can be used to treat continued infection.

Table 4.1 Classification of operations

Class	Definition
Clean	Operations in which no inflammation is encountered and the respiratory, alimentary, or genitourinary tracts are not entered; there is no break in aseptic operating theatre technique
Clean-contaminated	Operations in which the respiratory, alimentary, or genitourinary tracts are entered but without significant spillage
Contaminated	Operations where acute inflammation (without pus) is encountered, or where there is visible contamination of the wound; examples include gross spillage from a hollow viscus during the operation or compound/open injuries operated on within 4 hr
Dirty	Operations in the presence of pus, where there is a previously perforated hollow viscus, or compound/open injuries more than 4 hr old

Thromboprophylaxis in plastic surgery

Deep vein thrombosis (DVT) presents in approximately 1/1000 people per year. The risk in patients admitted to hospital for major trauma or major surgery is increased 10-fold. All patients undergoing surgery of duration >30 min should be individually assessed for risk of venous thrombolic events (VTEs) and be treated accordingly. In general, mechanical devices and subcutaneous low-dose heparin are combined, omitting heparin on the morning of surgery if a regional block is to be used.

Risk factors for VTEs
- Age >40.
- Obesity.
- Varicose veins.
- Previous venous thromboembolism.
- Thrombophilias or other thrombotic states.
- Hormone therapy (contraceptive, HRT, tamoxifen).
- General anaesthesia (vs regional).

Methods
General
- Early mobilization and leg exercises.
- Adequate hydration.

Mechanical
- Graduated elastic compression stockings.
- Intermittent pneumatic compression devices.

Medical
- Aspirin 150 mg/day started preoperatively and continued for 35 days.
- Subcutaneous low-dose heparin, unfractionated (5000 IU, every 8–12 hr) or low molecular weight heparin (LMWH).
- In order to detect heparin-associated thrombocytopenia, a baseline platelet count should be obtained and platelet count monitored in all patients receiving heparins for 5 days or more.
- Warfarin is a suitable alternative antithrombotic to heparin following heparin-associated thrombocytopenia, once the platelet count has recovered to >100 × 10^9/L.
- Patients on long term oral anticoagulation may continue their medication to achieve an INR of 2.0–2.5, or change to heparin with mechanical prophylaxis.
- Intravenous dextran 40 or 70 is a possible alternative prophylaxis for VTE in high-risk patients undergoing major surgery.

Spinal/epidural block
Advice to avoid vertebral canal haematoma.
- Aspirin: proceed normally.
- UFH: proceed normally but exercise caution, or administer 4–6 hr before block, or delay first dose until after block performed or until after surgery.

- LMWH: administer 10–12 hr before block.
- Warfarin: if INR <1.5 proceed normally; if INR >1.5 delay surgery or consider alternative anaesthetic.

Contraceptive pill, HRT
- Discuss the balance of risks and benefits with the patient when considering stopping these hormones prior to elective surgery.
- Arrange adequate alternative contraception if COC is to be discontinued.
- Consider specific antithrombotic prophylaxis according to overall risk factors.
- Give VTE prophylaxis routinely in emergency surgery.

Dressings

Principles

For a chronic wound to heal, it must pass through the following stages:
- Debridement.
- Vascularization and granulation.
- Epithelialization.

The ideal dressing should have the following properties:
- Mechanical protection for the wound.
- Protect the wound from pathogens.
- Provide a moist environment for the wound.
- Allow gas and fluid exchange.
- Non-adherent.
- Non-toxic and non-allergenic.
- Pain free.
- Allow movement.
- Absorb exudate and avoid maceration.
- Control wound odour.
- Sterile.
- Easy to use—simple infrequent changes, cheap, and in a suitable shape or size.

Table 4.2 Types of dressing

	Biological	Synthetic
Temporary	Allograft, xenograft	'Classical' dressings, antimicrobials
Permanent	SSG, FTSG, cultured epidermal autograft (CEA)	Skin substitutes

Table 4.3 Classical dressings

Dry	Moisture-retaining
Gauze	Pastes, creams, ointments
Bandages	Non-permeable or semipermeable membranes
Meshes, membranes	Alginates
Foams	Hydrocolloids
Adhesives	Hydrogels
	Combination dressings

Table 4.4 Indications for dressings

Wound type	Role of dressing
Dry, black, necrotic	Moisture retention or rehydration
Yellow, sloughy	Moisture retention if dry Fluid absorption if moist ± Odour absorption ± Antimicrobial activity
Clean, exuding, granulating	Fluid absorption ± Odour absorption ± Antimicrobial activity
Dry, low exudates, epithelializing	Moisture retention Low adherence

Implants

Materials
- Bone graft:
  - Autologous.
  - Allograft.
- Cartilage:
  - Autologous.
- Collagen:
  - Autologous.
  - Allograft.
- Alloplast:
  - Metals.
  - Polymers.
  - Ceramics.
  - Monomers.

Autogenous tissue
- Advantages:
  - Vascularized.
  - Biocompatible.
- Disadvantages:
  - Resorption.
  - Donor site.
  - Requires shaping/contouring.
  - Limited tissue.

Alloplastic material
- Alloplast can be soft or hard:
  - Metals (stainless steel, vitallium (cobalt–chromium), titanium).
  - Polymers (silastic, polyethylene).
  - Ceramics.
  - Monomers (methylmethacrylate).
  - Textiles (type of polymer) (proplast, dimethylpolysiloxane (DMPS)).
- Advantages:
  - No donor site morbidity.
  - Limitless source.
  - No operative time to harvest.
  - Biocompatibility.
  - Not physically modified.
  - Inert.
  - Sterilizable/manufacturable.
  - Does not incite inflammatory reaction.
  - Resists mechanical strain.
  - Non-carcinogenic—human carcinogenicity has never been demonstrated from current alloplastic material.

- Disadvantages and contraindications:
  - Defect/area adjacent to or involves bacterially contaminated area (mouth, nose).
  - History of infection.
  - Overlying soft tissue deficiency.
  - Poor vascularity.

Metals (e.g. stainless steel, vitallium (cobalt–chromium), titanium

- Biocompatibility.
- Ion release, electrical current creation.
- Particulate residue.
- Resist corrosion.

Polymers

- More biocompatible (cf. metals).
- Degradation via hydrolysis; therefore hydrophobic polymers will last longer.
- Textiles include Teflon—polymerization of tetrafluorocarbon gas into sheets used for orbital floor reconstruction.
- Polyethylene (Marlex) or polyamide mesh (Supramid).
- Proplast—Teflon fluorocarbon polymer (polytetrafluorethylene carbon; sometimes with white aluminium oxide fibre used as a coating for skeletal implants). Proplast allows in-growth of tissue and is sculpturable, and firm but flexible.
- Porous polyethylene (Plastipore).
- Silicone rubber (Silastic).
- Plastics can be injectible, solid prefabricated, carved, or moulded.

Ceramics (e.g. hydroxy-apatite, tricalcium phosphate)

- Not osteogenic but provide a physical matrix to guide bone regeneration, i.e. osteoconductive.
- Hydroxy-apatite is biocompatible; no cellular response.
- Bone regeneration within the matrix + biodegradation; begins when bone regenerated.
- Rigid fixation.

Monomers (e.g. methylmethacrylate)

- Mix powder into a paste, and contour to defect whilst paste cures; may need securing with wires or sutures.
- Must cool the mould with water while it is setting because the reaction is exothermic (125°C).
- Used for cranioplasty.
- Beware: it shrinks as it sets!

Table 4.5 Complications of implants

Complication	Prevention
Infection	Prophylactic antibiotics, sterile technique
Haematoma	Haemostasis/adrenaline-soaked sponge/compressive tape
Asymmetry and malposition	Care in creating site, size, and shape of pocket
Over-correction	Allow time for oedema resolution and material or base absorption
Extrusion	Ensure good soft tissue cover, layered closure, good pocket, correct size
Nerve injury	Careful dissection with good knowledge of relevant anatomy
Bone absorption	Uncommon, but can occur if the implant is under tension such as over the lower point of mandible; usually self limiting
Under-correction	Careful assessment and procedure

Smoking and plastic surgery

'Giving up smoking is the easiest thing in the world. I know because I've done it thousands of times.' Mark Twain.

- **Background** Smoking is the single greatest avoidable cause of death and disability in the Western world: 50% of smokers will die prematurely because of their habit, losing on average 8 years of life.
- **Incidence** There are 13 million smokers in the UK; although the incidence of smoking has declined in UK adults, it is currently static at ~28%.
- **Quantification** The accepted standard is 'smoking pack years' where one pack-year is equivalent to smoking the equivalent of one pack of cigarettes per day per year (i.e. 40 pack-years could be one pack per day for 40 years, or two packs a day for 20 years).
- **Risks** There is dose–response relationship between heavy smoking, duration of smoking, and early age of uptake of smoking and the risk of developing subsequent smoking-related pathology, which is primarily of a respiratory and cardiovascular nature.
- **Benefits** Smoking may be protective against developing ulcerative colitis. It is also associated with a decreased incidence of Parkinson's disease.

Why quit?

Cessation of smoking has substantial immediate and long-term health benefits for all smokers regardless of age. Those quitting below the age of 35 will have a similar life expectancy to non-smokers. The life expectancy for former smokers exceeds that of continuing smokers. Two-thirds of smokers wish to quit, and about a third try each year, of whom only 2% succeed. Quitting with support doubles the likelihood of success. Quitting gradually is equally effective as quitting abruptly ('cold turkey'). Nicotine replacement therapy (e.g. chewing gum or patches) delivers nicotine far less effectively than a cigarette, thus often failing to satiate the habitual smoker. Nonetheless it almost halves the recidivism rate at 6–12 months (Silagy et al. 1998).

Relevance of smoking to plastic surgery

- **Birth defects** There is a significant dose-related response between maternal smoking whilst pregnant and increased risk of giving birth to a child with a congenital digital anomaly (Man and Chang 2006) or cleft lip and palate (Chung et al. 2000).
- **Delayed wound healing** and other complications:
  - Breast reconstruction with tissue expanders (Becker-type) is associated with an increased wound complication rate in smokers (Camilleri et al. 1996).
  - Smoking is an independent risk factor for the development of post-operative haematoma following face-lift surgery (Grover et al. 2001).
  - In the context of elective abdominoplasty, smoking was associated with an increased risk of wound complications (Manassa et al. 2003).
  - Bilateral breast reduction was also associated with an increased risk of wound complications in smokers (Chan et al. 2006). Interestingly, when questioned post-operatively, 75% of smokers admitted falsely denying smoking in the 4 weeks prior to surgery.
  - Post-mastectomy breast reconstruction.

- **Carcinogenic effects** (e.g. head and neck cancer).
- **Free tissue transfer**:
  - Sarin et al. (1974) demonstrated a marked reduction in human digital artery blood flow following the inhalation of a single cigarette. Patients may be polycythaemic. Peripheral vascular disease and quality of the donor and recipient vessels. Similar results were seen in the thumb (van Adrichem et al. 1992).
  - Chang et al. (2000) examined complication rates in patients undergoing free TRAM flap breast reconstruction. Smokers had twice the incidence of mastectomy flap necrosis than non-smokers, with the risk being greatest in those undergoing immediate reconstruction. Smokers also had more than twice the risk of donor-site complications (e.g. abdominal flap necrosis and hernia) than former smokers or non-smokers. The highest-risk smokers were those with a history of ≥10 pack-years. Interestingly there was no significant increase in the rates of vessel thrombosis, flap loss, or fat necrosis in smokers compared with non-smokers. The authors concluded that smoking more than 10 pack-years is a relative contraindication for free TRAM flap breast reconstruction, and complications could be significantly reduced by quitting smoking at least 4 weeks before surgery.
- **Medical comorbidities** (e.g. COPD) in patients undergoing general anaesthesia.
- **Burns** Smoking in bed is a significant risk factor for house fires.

Pathophysiology

Tobacco smoke contains over 4000 chemicals which put both the smoker and the passive inhaler at risk. Carbon monoxide results in carboxyhaemoglobin formation (5–15% in a smoker versus <2.5% in a non-smoker) which reduces the oxygen-carrying capacity of blood and thus causes local tissue hypoxia. Nicotine causes both physical and psychological addiction, and is as addictive as hard drugs such as heroin. Cigarette smoke significantly increases platelet activation caused by exposure to shear stress, even under normal flow conditions, although nicotine protects against platelet activation (Rubenstein et al. 2004). However, there is no proven adverse effect on the microvascular anastomosis; it has been suggested that the denervated tissue paddle has effectively undergone a surgical sympathectomy which may offer protection from the smoking-induced rise in catecholamine levels.

References

Camilleri IG, Malata CM, Stavrianos S, Mclean NR (1996). Br J Plast Surg 49, 346–51.
Chan LK, Withey S, Butler PE (2006). Ann Plast Surg 56, 111–15.
Chang DW, Reece GP, Wang B, et al. (2000). Plast Reconstr Surg 105, 2374–80.
Chung KC, Kowalski CP, Kim HM, Buchman SR (2000). Plast Reconstr Surg 105, 1448–52.
Grover R, Jones BM, Waterhouse N (2001). Br J Plast Surg 54, 481–6.
Man LX, Chang B (2006). Plast Reconstr Surg 118, 301–8.
Manassa EH, Hertl CH, Olbrich RR (2003). Plast Reconstr Surg 111, 2082–7.
Rubenstein D, Jesty J, Bluestein D (2004). Circulation 109, 78–83.
Sarin CL, Austin JC, Nickel WO (1974). JAMA 229, 1327–8.
Silagy C, Mant D, Fowler G, Lancaster T (1998). Nicotine therapy for smoking cessation. Cochrane Library 1998, Issue 2.
van Adrichem LN, Hovius SE, van Strik R, van der Meulen JC (1992). Br J Plast Surg 45, 9–11.

Leech therapy

Definition
The European medicinal leech (*Hirudo medicinalis*) is an invertebrate annelid. Other species include the Asian medicinal leech (*Hirudo manillensis*) and the Amazon leech (*Hirudo ghilianii*).

History
The first recorded use is by the ancient Egyptians in c. 1500 BCE.

Physiology
Leech saliva contains, amongst other compounds:
- Hirudin, an anticoagulant.
- Hyaluronidase, which facilitates anticoagulant penetration.
- Histamine to maintain vasodilatation.

Indications
The prime indication for leeching is to improve drainage from venously congested tissues (mainly flaps), i.e. those that are dusky blue with a brisk capillary refill and a rapid dark bleed on pinprick. Such congestion may result from the draining vein being too small, thrombosed, or not present, such as when a venous anastomosis was not technically possible.
Typical clinical examples include:
- Distal digital replants where an artery is reconstructed but the vein is not.
- Free flaps where both artery and vein are reconstructed but the venous outflow is inadequate (e.g. a reverse flow flap such as the posterior interosseous flap).
- When arterial inflow exceeds venous outflow (e.g. free auricular flap).
- Venous flaps where venous congestion is the mechanism of nutrition of the flap.

As leeching is used for venous (as opposed to arterial) insufficiency, a typical course of treatment may last for up to 3–5 days, until new vein formation occurs at the margins of the flap. Several leeches may need to be used simultaneously and/or sequentially until the condition of the flap improves.

Contraindications
Their use is contraindicated in cases of arterial insufficiency. They will usually either fail to attach or drop off soon after application. Because of the risk of leech migration, they must be used with care in proximity to body orifices, particularly intra-orally. Close observation during treatment is advised.

Leech care
In the UK leeches are supplied by Biopharm Ltd, Swansea. They are delivered suspended in Hirudo Gel™. Leeches can survive for prolonged periods stored in a refrigerator at 5–25°C. They must be kept away from direct sunlight. Aeration is not necessary. Beware of overcrowding (maximum of 20 leeches per 500 mL container). Leech storage medium consists of water and Hirudosalt™ They must not be stored in distilled water as they depend on the presence of exogenous ions.

Method of use
Gloves are worn and leeches are carefully handled with non-toothed forceps. Alternatively, a section of a Yankauer suction tube can be used as

a bespoke 'leech applicator' (MacQuillan et al. 2002). The skin is prared by shaving excessively hirsute areas and carefully removing any residual alcohol, petroleum jelly, or Betadine by cleaning the treatment area with soap and water. The skin is warmed and pricked with a hypodermic needle at its bluest portion to emit a drop of blood. A gauze swab with a central aperture may be placed over the area of interest—the gauze minimizes the risk of leech migration during the leeching process. Alternatively, with larger sites, a disposable cup with the base removed will act as a 'holding pen' thus preventing an adventurous leech from roaming where it may not be welcome.

The head of the leech is introduced to the blood and it normally attaches (painlessly) and starts to feed immediately. A disinterested leech may be encouraged to attach by the application of a drop of sugar solution to the wound. Once attached, the leech will suck, swell to five to six times its size, and detach from the skin once sated (after approximately 30–60 min). The used leech is normally disposed of by killing it in absolute alcohol and disposing of it in a sharps bin. They should not be flushed down the sluice or lavatory.

After cutaneous contact, leeches leave a characteristic temporary 'Mercedes-type' or inverted Y mark approximately 2–3 mm in diameter. Each of the three jaws accommodates approximately 100 teeth. Since the bite is partial thickness, it does not result in permanent scarring.

Errant leeches should never be forcibly removed. The application of table salt will precipitate a rapid detachment. Traditional bushcraft teaching suggests that a cigarette lighter or match is equally effective, but these are frowned upon in hospitals especially in the presence of oxygen.

Historically, leeches were often reused: by immersing them in sterile hypertonic saline solution, whereupon they regurgitate the imbibed blood, thus enabling them to feed again. Obviously this practice is actively discouraged because of the potential for the transmission of blood-borne viruses.

The anticoagulant effects persist after the leech has detached, and bleeding may occur for some hours (average 10 hr). Thus all patients, particularly young children, must have their haemoglobin levels carefully monitored (i.e. daily FBC) when undergoing prolonged leech therapy. The fluid balance status of the patient must also be closely observed. Excessive bleeding can be remedied by elevation, direct pressure, or local topical thrombin application if necessary. Each leech will imbibe up to 5 mL of blood at a single sucking, and up to 150 mL of blood may be lost in the subsequent ooze.

Prophylactic antibiotics

Aeromonas hydrophila (or *Pseudomonas hirudinis*) exists in an obligate symbiotic relationship within the gastrointestinal tract of the leech. Thus antibiotics should be used in all cases because of the risk of infection with *Aeromonas* species. The rate of infection, resulting in abscess formation and cellulitis, is approximately 2%. In view of beta-lactam resistance, recommended antibiotics include amoxicillin with clavulanic acid or ciprofloxacin. Treatment is continued until wound closure is achieved.

Reference

McQuillan AH, Jones ME, Gault D (2002). *Br J Plast Surg* 55, 540–1.

Microsurgery

Definition
Microsurgery means operating using a microscope with micro-instruments. With the advance of loupe magnification this is now not strictly applied, but microsurgery with magnification should be used for vessels 3 mm or less in diameter. The range of vessels that can be microsurgically anastomosed ranges from 0.3 to 3 mm or more.

Uses
Common technique:
- Vascular: arterial or venous anastomosis or incorporation of a vein graft.
- Lymphatic: lymphatic or lymphatico-venous anastomosis.
- Infertility: reversal of vasectomy and fallopian tube surgery.
- Neural: nerve repair or grafting.

The most common use is for microvascular surgery in replantation, revascularization, and free tissue transfer.

Microvascular anatomy
A vessel has three layers: the intima, the media, and the adventitia. The intima is comprised mainly of the endothelium, the vascular epithelial layer that lines the vessel. The media is composed of connective tissue and muscle, and the adventitia is the surrounding connective tissue layer. The collagen in the media and adventitia, when exposed, causes the greatest platelet aggregation.

Microvascular physiology
Blood flow through a vessel is determined by two factors, the pressure difference across the length of the vessel and the resistance to flow:

$$\text{flow} = \text{pressure difference}/\text{resistance}.$$

Blood flow is essentially laminar with faster flow in the centre and slower flow at the periphery. Any disruption to this produces turbulence, which increases resistance and reduces flow. Causes of turbulence are:
- Obstruction.
- Vessel angulation.
- Branching.
- Vessel redundancy.
- Vessel wall irregularity.

Other factors that increase resistance are increased blood viscosity and reduced vessel diameter.

Control of blood flow under normal physiological conditions is managed by alterations in cardiac stroke volume, heart rate, and peripheral resistance. Control of peripheral resistance may be systemic or local.

Vessel wall healing
Following anastomosis, platelets cover any endothelial breach and a pseudo-intima forms over the first 5 days. Provided that there is no extensive media exposure, the platelets do not progress to fibrin deposition and thrombus but disappear over the first 24–72 hr. By 1–2 weeks a new endothelium has formed. The elastic and muscular layers do not return to their pre-injury state but heal with the deposition of a collagen scar.

Instruments
- **Microscope** Familiarize yourself with the hospital microscope, the focus and zoom adjustment, and your interpupillary distance.
- **Instruments** Jeweller's forceps (5 and 2), vessel dilators, needle holders, scissors, irrigation cannulae or 24 gauge intravenous cannula, microvascular clamps(double and single), and background material.
- **Instrument holding** Classic pencil holding grip with the ulnar border of the hand resting comfortably on the table or a surface built up with sterile drapes.

Technique
Vessel preparation
- Choose recipient vessels with good palpable flow in the region of the defect, which are accessible and preferably dispensible.
- Dissect sufficiently both distally and proximally to prevent acute angles, and for access to apply clamps.
- For end-to-end anastomosis, trim vessels with scissors. If they are cut with some traction towards the terminal end this action will auto-trim the adventitia.
- Remove the arterial clamp and check arterial inflow is adequate. It should spurt at least 30 cm!
- Re-apply the clamps.
- Dilate gently if neccessary and irrigate vessel ends with heparinized saline or Hartmann's solution.
- Trim back adventitia for 1 mm to prevent any adventitial flaps. Check for intimal flaps.
- Make sure vessels are not twisted, kinked, too tight, or too loose.
- For end-to-side anastomoses, trim the flap vessel to reach the side of the recipient vessel. Make an arteriotomy in the side wall of the vessel either by a longitudinal incision or by excising a hole using an arteriotomy forceps and beaver blade.

Anastomotic technique
- Non-absorbable nylon sutures, ranging from 8/0 to 10/0, are the most common. The sutures may be interrupted, continuous, or use the sleeve technique. Sutures are placed through the full thickness of the vessel wall and tied with the knot external.
- Alternative techniques are absorbable sutures, ring clips, glue, laser, and staples.
- Classically, end-to-side anastomoses have one suture placed at either end (heel and toe, at 6 and 12 o'clock) with completion of the back wall followed by the front wall using interrupted sutures.
- End-to-end anastomoses are completed by three popular methods:
  - The triangulation method of Carrel with three key suture placed an equal distance apart followed by suture placement to fill the gaps.
  - Two key sutures (at 6 and 12 o'clock), completing the back wall, and then turning the double clamp to permit front wall suture.
  - A single suture placed in the centre of the back wall. Anastomosis continues around from that always placing the most difficult suture next.

These and other techniques depend on surgical preference and the challenge of the associated anatomy. The deeper or most distant vessel is anastomosed first.

For vessel size discrepancy:
- Cheat in the discrepancy as you suture around the vessel.
- Spatulate the smaller vessel.
- Entubulate or sleeve the smaller vessel.

Good technique
- Gentle handling of the tissues.
- No tension.
- Clean passage of the needle.
- Even bites in depth and spacing.
- Minimal luminal contact.
- Prevention of dessication.

End-to-side anastomosis is indicated in situations where there is considerable size discrepancy or where only one artery is available which is also required for distal tissue viability. The patency rates are similar to those of end-to-end anastomosis. An interposition vein graft may be needed to increase vessel length.

Post-anastomosis
- The clamps are removed in the following sequence:
  - Distal venous.
  - Proximal venous.
  - Distal arterial.
  - Proximal arterial.
- Following clamp removal further sutures may be required if there is an obvious point of leakage.
- Look for a pink flap with capillary bleeding, a full vein, and a pulsatile artery.
- A patency test may be done to confirm flow, preferably downstream from the venous anastomosis as this interferes least with the flap and vessels.
- Check that vessels are not kinked and will not be kinked or compressed by the closure.
- A non-suction drain or suction drain sutured away from the anastomosis prevents haematoma formation around the pedicle.
- Ensure a non-constrictive dressing with an observation window.

Lasers

Laser stands for Light Amplification by the Stimulated Emission of Radiation.

Properties

Laser beams have three main properties:
- **Coherence** Ordinary light is incoherent and consists of light waves radiating in all directions and out of phase with each other. Laser light, on the other hand, has wave patterns that are in phase in time and space with each other.
- **Collimation** A collimated beam is parallel and does not diverge. This has two important impacts on the use of lasers in medicine. There is a minimal loss of power along the beam, and the beam can be focused to intensify its effect or to send it through a slender fibre.
- This allows the vast majority of the generated energy to be collected and intensified into tiny spots for surgical applications.
- **Monochromaticity** This property implies that the light is all of the same wavelength (colour). This application is important in photodynamic therapy where the choice of colour is critical in the process of selective photothermolysis.

Laser machine

A laser machine consists of three important components:
- A collimator which ensures that the light generated is in phase.
- A lasing medium which can be a solid (crystals such as ruby; Nd:YAG (neodymium doped with yttrium aluminium garnet), a gas (CO_2, argon), or a liquid (various dyes used in a tuneable dye laser).
- A delivery system which may be in the form of a fibre-optic or optical lens system.

Lasers are currently named based on the lasing medium used, e.g. CO_2 laser, tuneable dye laser.

Energy concepts

There are some energy concepts which are important in understanding lasers.
- **Power** is a measure of the rate of energy delivered in joules/second (J/sec) and is expressed in watts (W).
- **Power density (irradiance)** is the amount of power that can be focused into a spot and is expressed in watts per square centimetre (W/cm^2).
- **Fluence** combines the concept of power density (spot brightness) with total delivered energy (dosage in joules), and is expressed in joules per square centimetre (J/cm^2).

Mechanism of action

The effects of surgical lasers in the form of vaporization, cutting, and coagulation are based on the effects of heat.

The effects of lasers have been given a broader understanding based on the principle of selective photothermolysis. Selective photothermolysis uses selective absorption of light pulses by pigmented targets such as blood vessels, pigmented cells, and tattoo ink particles to achieve selective thermally mediated injury. Short pulses are used to deposit energy in the targets before they cool off, thus achieving extreme localized heating and tissue destruction.

Table 4.6 Effects of surgical lasers

Temperature (°C)	Visual change	Biological change
36–60	None, warming	Welding
60–65	Blanching	Coagulation
65–90	White/grey	Protein denaturation
90–100	Puckering	Drying
100	Smoke plume	Vaporization, carbonization

Chapter 5

Congenital

Hypospadias *134*
Epispadias–exstrophy complex *138*
Craniosynostosis *141*
Non-syndromic craniosynostosis *142*
Syndromic craniosynostosis *144*
Plagiocephaly without synostosis (PWS) *146*
Surgery for craniosynostosis *147*
Hemifacial microsomia *148*
Romberg's disease *149*
Treacher Collins syndrome *150*
Pierre Robin sequence *152*
Microtia *154*
Branchial clefts *155*
Cleft lip and palate: introduction *156*
Cleft lip repair: unilateral *162*
Cleft lip repair: bilateral *166*
Cleft palate repair *168*
Cleft rhinoplasty *175*
Velopharyngeal incompetence *178*
Palatal fistula *182*
Orthodontics *184*
Alveolar bone grafting *187*
Congenital upper limb anomalies *189*
Radial dysplasia *191*
Ulnar dysplasia *195*
Cleft hand *197*
Camptodactyly *200*
Clinodactyly *202*
Clasp thumb *204*
Trigger digit *205*
Syndactyly *206*
Polydactyly *209*
Thumb duplication *210*
Congenital radial head dislocation *211*
Radioulnar synostosis *212*
Thumb hypoplasia *214*
Brachydactyly *216*
Symbrachydactyly *218*
Macrodactyly *220*
Amniotic band syndrome *223*
Arthrogryposis *224*
Madelung's deformity *226*
Poland syndrome *228*
Toe phalanx non-vascularized transfer *230*
Pollicization *231*
Chest wall deformity *232*

Hypospadias

Definition
Congenital anomaly in which the urethral meatus is abnormally proximal and ventral, on the penis, scrotum, or perineum.

Incidence
One in 100–300 live births; incidence rising in some countries.

Aetiology
Hormonal
Abnormalities in 5-alpha reductase have been found in 10% of patients; androgen receptors have also been found to be abnormal. It is five times more common in boys born from *in vitro* fertilization; this may relate to maternal progesterone treatment during IVF as progesterone competitively inhibits 5-alpha reductase.

Genetic
Monozygotic twin siblings have eight times the risk of hypospadias as singletons. This may be due to competition for human chorionic gonadotrophin *in utero*. Of affected boys, 8% have affected fathers and 14% have affected brothers. If two family members are affected, the risk for a subsequent boy is 22%.

Environmental
Oestrogens have been implicated in animal models, and may be responsible for the increasing incidence.

Classification
According to site of meatus:
- Anterior: glanular or subcoronal, 50% of cases.
- Middle: distal shaft, midshaft or proximal shaft, 20% of cases.
- Posterior: penoscrotal, scrotal or perineal, 30% of cases.

Pathogenesis
Failure of complete fusion of urethral folds which may be due to reduced testosterone stimulation.

Clinical features
- Ventral meatal dystopia: subcoronal position most common.
- Para-urethral sinuses may be present on the glans or shaft.
- Hooded prepuce (98%); however, this is not always the case, and hypospadias may only be found at circumcision.
- Chordee in 15% of anterior but over 50% of posterior cases. Caused by differential growth of the normal corpora cavernosa and abnormal ventral structures; or rarely to fibrous remnants of the undifferentiated corpus spongiosum and fascial layers of the penis which insert into the glans.
- The glans may be flattened, with a groove representing the urethral plate.
- The scrotum may be bifid in very posterior hypospadias.

Nine per cent of cases have associated inguinal hernias and 9% have undescended testis. This increases to 20% and 30%, respectively, for posterior hypospadias. Hypospadias with undescended testis may indicate an intersex state. Urethral valves may be present. Anomalies of the upper urinary tract are rare, unless there are other congenital anomalies. Mild vesicoureteric reflux is not uncommon, but is not treated unless symptomatic (recurrent UTIs).

Untreated, the patient may be unable micturate standing. Chordee may impair sexual function, and if severe, make erections painful. Abnormal cosmesis may also cause psychosexual problems.

Management: medical
Testosterone creams or injections and human chorionic gonadotrophin injections have been used to increase penile size prior to surgery.

Management: surgical
Aims to
- Allow the patient to micturate standing with a normal stream.
- Normal sexual function.
- Natural appearance.

This requires correction of chordee, creation of a neo-urethra; and recreation of a slit-like meatus at the tip of the glans.

One-stage procedures
There are three broad categories.

Urethral advancement
The abnormal urethra is advanced towards its normal position. MAGPI (meatal advancement and glanuloplasty incorporated) is used for a mobile distal meatus; bulbo-urethral dissection may advance the urethra up to 5 cm.

Onlay techniques
A neo-urethra is created using the remaining urethral plate as the ventral wall with a patch of vascularized tissue from elsewhere on the penis as the ventral wall. Mathieu (1932) used ventral penile shaft skin; Elder *et al.* (1987) described a pedicled prepucial island flap.

Inlay techniques
A similar vascularized flap of tissue or a full-thickness skin graft is tubed and inset to form a neo-urethra. Mustardé (1965) used a similar flap to Mathieu; Duckett (1980) used islanded inner prepucial skin; and Harris (1984) used inner prepucial skin for the neo-urethra and outer prepucial skin for the ventral skin cover.

Two stage repair
The repair (Bracka 1995), modified from Cloutier repair, can be performed before 18 months of age, but surgery is best avoided between 18 months and 3 years as the child may be uncooperative. Bracka suggests performing the first stage at 3 years, and the second stage 6 months later.

Stage 1
- GA plus penile or caudal block.
- Erection test: soft latex catheter tourniquet around base of penis; normal saline infiltrated into one corpus cavernosum.
- Surgery performed under tourniquet.
- Inner prepucial full-thickness skin graft harvested.
- Meatotomy performed if necessary.
- Glans split from level of dystopic meatus to dorsal margin of new meatus; corpora cavernosa dissected to level of dystopic meatus.
- Fibres causing chordee divided.
- FTSG inset with tie-over dressing retained for 5 days.
- Catheter for 2 days under antibiotic cover.

Stage 2
- Tourniquet passed.
- U-shaped strip of skin 1.5 cm wide incised to form neo-urethra and tubed around catheter.
- Proximally based flap of prepucial subcutaneous tissue used to waterproof repairs proximal to glans (if there is not sufficient tissue, glans skin can be twisted to offset suture lines).
- Glans repaired.
- Skin of shaft closed and foreskin reconstructed or circumcised.
- Catheter for 5–6 days with antibiotic cover.

Complications

Early
- Haematoma.
- Infection.
- Erections: treated with cyproterone acetate.

Late
- Fistula.
- Meatal stenosis: causes spraying of urine. Treated by meatal revision surgery.
- Urethral stricture: may respond to dilatation.
- Urethral diverticulum: caused by distal outflow obstruction or lack of support to neo-urethra.
- Recurrent chordee.
- Hair in the urethra: hair-bearing skin should not be used to create the neo-urethra as it predisposes to infection. Hair should be ablated, or the skin excised and replaced.
- *Balanitis xerotica obliterans* (BXO) is lichen sclerosis of the male genitalia, of unknown aetiology. It presents as ulceration, progressing to phimosis and meatal stenosis. It is pre-malignant for SCC. It is treated by excision of affected skin, but always recurs if genital skin is used for the reconstruction. Post-auricular skin shows some recurrence; buccal mucosa is the most resistant graft for patients with BXO.

Contentious issues

Over 250 techniques have been described for the repair of hypospadias. These can be broadly classified into one- and two-stage repairs. Proponents of one-stage repair advocate a single-stage operation, which is performed before the child is old enough to remember it. The revision rate is around 10%. The benefit of the two-stage repair is a more versatile procedure, with more reliable results and a more natural-looking meatus. The two-stage repair is technically easier and, because it is so versatile, means the surgeon can master a single technique, rather than needing to learn many one-stage repairs. The long-term outcome of hypospadias repair in terms of psychosexual adjustment is reported to depend more on appearance than on number of operations.

The age at which to operate is also debated, although the period between 18 months and 3 years, when a child is likely to be uncooperative is avoided. Some patient groups advise no surgery until the patient is old enough to request it.

References

Bracka A (1995). *Br J Plast Surg* **48**, 345–52.
Duckett JW (1980). *Urol Clin North Am* **7**, 423–30.
Elder JS, Duckett JW, Snyder HM (1987). *J Urol* **138**, 376–9.
Harris DL (1984). *Br J Plast Surg* **37**, 108–16.
Mathieu P (1932). *J Chir* **39**, 481–6.
Mustardé JC (1965). *Br J Plast Surg* **18**, 413–22.

Epispadias–exstrophy complex

Definition
A spectrum of congenital anomaly thought to arise from the same embryological defect. May include:
- Abnormal position of the urethral meatus on the dorsum of the penis or a bifid clitoris (epispadias).
- Failure of fusion of the anterior abdominal wall and externalization of bladder (bladder exstrophy).
- Externalization of the lower urinary tract and the gastrointestinal tract (cloacal exstrophy).

Incidence
- Bladder exstrophy 3.3/100 000 (male:female 2:1).
- Male epispadias 1/100 000; female epispadias 1/500 000.
- Cloacal exstrophy 1/200 000–400 000.

Aetiology
No risk factors are known, but offspring of patients with exstrophy are 500 times more likely to have this anomaly than the general population (1/70). There is no concordance between dizygotic twins or female monozygotic twins, but 100% concordance between male monozygotic twins.

Classification (by severity)
- Epispadias.
- Bladder exstrophy.
- Cloacal exstrophy.

Pathogenesis
Thought to be due to failure of mesenchymal infiltration into anterior abdominal wall during first trimester. Therefore adjacent cloacal membrane is unstable and ruptures too early, and mesenchyme of genital tubercle and anterior parts of cloacal ridges fails to fuse. If the cloacal membrane ruptures before the urorectal septum is fully formed, the gastrointestinal tract will be involved.

Clinical features
Depend on severity.

Male epispadias
The urethral meatus opens on the dorsum of the penis between the proximal glans and the penoscrotal angle. The penis is short and broad and curves upwards (dorsal chordee). The glans is flattened. The dorsal foreskin is absent. Boys are usually continent with distal epispadias.

Female epispadias
The clitoris is bifid and the labia diverge anteriorly. The dorsal urethra may be open up to the bladder neck. Girls usually have stress incontinence, regardless of the level of the urethral meatus. The vaginal introitus may be narrow. In both sexes, the pubic symphysis may be widened with divergent recti.

Bladder exstrophy
The bladder lies open on the abdomen. Patients usually have vesico-ureteric reflux due to abnormal insertion of the ureters into the bladder. The umbilicus is set low, and the anus anterior. The recti diverge to be inserted onto separated pubic bones. Inguinal hernias are common. In boys, the penis is short and broad and the urethra open dorsally. In girls, the vagina is anteriorly placed.

Cloacal exstrophy
The bladder, vagina, and penis usually lie in two halves. The caecum is open. There is usually an associated omphalocoele. Associated limb or vertebral anomalies are common. Upper urinary tract anomalies are present in a third of patients.

Presentation
May be diagnosed prenatally on ultrasound, but if not is usually apparent at birth. In females, epispadias may only present as urinary incontinence in childhood, and symphysial diastasis as waddling gait.

Management: surgical
Aims:
- Close bladder and abdominal wall.
- Protect renal function.
- Correct incontinence.
- Preserve sexual function.
- Acceptable cosmesis.

Surgical options
- Epispadias may be treated as hypospadias, but on the dorsal surface, or the penis may be dissected into its components and the neo-urethra replaced on the ventral aspect.
- Urinary diversion for bladder exstrophy: used when the bladder plate is too small for direct closure.
- Staged functional closure for bladder exstrophy: the bladder and abdominal wall are closed within 72 hr of birth. If delayed, pelvic osteotomies are used to allow closure. Epispadias is repaired at 12–18 months. This increases bladder resistance, improving capacity. The bladder neck is reconstructed at 4 years and vesico-ureteric reflux is corrected.
- Complete primary repair: the bladder, urethra, and external genitalia are all reconstructed at birth.
- In cloacal exstrophy, the gastrointestinal anomaly is treated as a priority, and vertebral anomalies are treated if required. Pelvic osteotomies are usually needed.

Complications
- Failure of closure or bladder prolapse.
- Loss of renal function: caused by high bladder pressure and vesicoureteric reflux.
- Poor bladder emptying and recurrent infections.
- Malignancy, especially in late-treated bladder exstrophy.
- Reduced fertility in males because of retrograde ejaculation through incompetent bladder neck.

Contentious issues
Whether to reconstruct the urethra primarily in the neonatal period or as a delayed procedure. The former aims to improve long-term bladder function by increasing outlet resistance and therefore encourage bladder growth. It may avoid later procedures to augment the bladder, and later bladder neck reconstruction for continence is less often necessary.

Craniosynostosis

Definition
Craniosynostosis is defined as the premature fusion of one or more of the calvarial sutures occurring *in utero* or shortly after birth.

Incidence
The average incidence for all forms of craniosynostosis is 1 in 2500 live births.

Classification
Craniosynostosis can be classed as either syndromic (where there is a known underlying genetic aetiological cause) or as non-syndromic or isolated synostosis.

Aetiology
- Syndromic synostosis (also known as the craniofacial dysostosis syndromes) has been shown to originate from genetic mutations in the fibroblast growth factor receptor systems or in related systems such as those controlled by the *TWIST* gene.
- Certain forms of syndromic synostosis are not genetically determined, but arise from exposure to teratogens such as sodium valproate.
- Non-syndromic or isolated synostosis is thought to arise as a result of application of mechanical pressure to the involved sutures at a critical point in development.

Pathogenesis
Under normal circumstances the calvarium grows at right angles to every active normal suture. Thus, when a suture fuses prematurely, there is a failure of growth at right angles to the involved suture. In addition, there is a relative compensatory overgrowth at adjacent uninvolved sutures. This combination of growth failure and compensatory excess leads to the classical cranial shapes, which allow predication of the involved sutures.

The following sections give a breakdown of the non-syndromic synostoses as well as the more frequently occurring syndromic conditions.

Non-syndromic craniosynostosis

Sagittal synostosis
This is premature fusion of the mid-line sagittal suture, running anterior-posterior, over the vertex of the skull. Sagittal synostosis is the most commonly occurring synostosis with an incidence of 1 in 5000 live births, and it usually makes up about 50% of a busy practice. The male-to-female ratio is 4:1. The descriptive term used to describe the head shape is scaphocephaly, which literally translates as boat-shaped skull (dolicocephaly is another term that may be used).

As a result of failure of transverse growth the skull is narrow from side to side. Compensatory overgrowth gives the characteristic bossing of the forehead with an occipital bullet. Radiology shows the typical skull shape as well as the absence of the mid-line sagittal suture.

Metopic synostosis
This is premature fusion of the mid-line metopic suture between the two halves of the forehead. This occurs in approximately 1 in 25 000 live births. The male-to-female ratio is 3:1. Constitutes about 10% of an active practice.

Metopic suture synostosis is usually non-syndromic and thought to be a result of mechanical pressure on the developing suture. However, it also occurs in a number of other non-genetic syndromes such as valproate syndrome in epileptic mothers.

Failure of growth at the involved sutures results in a triangular-shaped forehead with inadequate development of the brow. The eyes are relatively close together or hypoteloric. The overall skull takes up a triangular shape with broadening at the back. The descriptive term is trigonocephaly, which literally translates as triangle-shaped skull.

Radiological features usually rely on secondary diagnostic signs, such as the upward elongation and medial rotation of the orbits as well as the relative hypotelorism.

Unicoronal synostosis
This is fusion of one of the two coronal sutures running transversally on the anterior skull. It occurs in approximately 1 in 17 000 live births and constitutes approximately 15% of an average practice. The male-to-female ratio is 1:1.5.

Failure of growth at the involved side causes elevation and posterior rotation of the brow, giving the appearance of an enlarged eye on the affected side. The distance between the eye and the ear on the affected side is shorter than on the unaffected side. Compensatory bossing of the opposite forehead occurs. Likewise, overgrowth of the cheek area inferior to the involved suture causes a distortion of the face, with the nose and the chin rotating away from the involved side. The combination of a flattened brow with prominent cheek when viewed from above is referred to as the 'facial cross'. The resultant craniofacial shape is referred to as plagiocephaly, which literally translates as oblique skull.

Radiological findings on a plain radiograph include absence or sclerosis of the involved suture as well as the pathognomonic upward rotation of the lesser wing of the sphenoid, which on the AP view gives upward and outward peaking of the orbital contour referred to as the harlequin eye sign.

Bicoronal synostosis

This is the premature fusion of both coronal sutures, which occurs either in an isolated state or as part of one of the main syndromes. It occurs in approximately 1 in 150 000 live births and constitutes approximately 5% of a busy practice. The male-to-female ratio is 1:1.5.

Failure of growth at both coronal sutures results in a head shortened in the AP dimension, known as brachycephaly or short skull, as well as a tendency to become vertically high (this is then referred to as turricephaly or tower skull).

Radiological features include absence or sclerosis of the sutures as well as bilateral harlequin eye signs.

Unilambdoid synostosis

This is the rarest of the isolated synostosis conditions. It consists of a premature fusion of one of the lambdoid sutures in the posterior skull. It occurs in approximately 1 in 250 000 live births and constitutes approximately 1% of a busy practice.

Failure of growth at the involved suture and compensatory overgrowth at uninvolved sutures gives a typical posterior skull distortion, in many respects similar to the changes occurring in unicoronal synostosis at the front of the skull. There is distinct flattening over the area of the non-functional suture. The ear on the involved side is slightly retro-displaced compared with the opposite uninvolved side. There is a significant degree of mastoid overgrowth in compensation, giving a bulge behind the involved ear. Compensatory overgrowth at the opposite lambdoid and the sagittal sutures results in a temporo-parietal bossing on the opposite side. The overall result, when viewed from behind, is a windswept skull away from the side of the involved suture.

Syndromic craniosynostosis

(including craniofacial dysostosis syndromes)

All these syndromes generally present with at least one, but usually more, sutures involved. The greater the number of sutures involved the higher the risk of acute raised intracranial pressure. These syndromes, which have typically been known by eponymous names, rely on their associated features (frequently in the limbs) as part of their diagnostic criteria. This was important prior to the discovery of known genetic mutations, which are now used to define the syndromes.

Apert's syndrome

This occurs in approximately 1 in 70 000 live births. It arises as a mutation in *FGFR2* on chromosome 10 at one of two sites: Ser252Trp or Pro253Arg.

The craniofacial features include multiple suture synostoses, usually including the coronal sutures, and later the lambdoid sutures. There is typically an initially enlarged anterior fontanelle. The mid-face and orbits are small, giving relative protrusion of the eyes (exorbitism). The nose tends to be beaky. Patients with *S252W* mutations tend to have cleft palates.

Pathognomonic features of this condition are complex acrosyndactyly of the hands. Associated features include hyperhidrosis and various upper limb anomalies such as elbow fusions.

Crouzon's syndrome

This also occurs in about 1 in 70 000 live births. There are a number of genetic mutations in the *FGFR2* system (however, the *A391E* mutation in *FGFR3* causes Crouzon's syndrome with acanthosis nigricans).

Craniofacial features include bicoronal synostosis with significant turricephaly; variable exorbitism occurs as well as variable mid-facial retrusion. Severe mid-facial retrusion can cause obstructive sleep apnoea (as also occurs in Apert's and Pfeiffer's syndromes). The major diagnostic marker of Crouzon's syndrome, other than the genetic mutation, is normal hands.

Pfeiffer's syndrome

This occurs in 1 in 120 000 live births and is also caused by diverse mutations of *FGFR2* on chromosome 10.

Pfeiffer's syndrome tends to have the worst pan-synostotic features with major calvarial distortion, raised intracranial pressure, and major exorbitism (the severe end of the scale is often referred to as Kleeblattschadel or clover-leaf skull). Pfeiffer's syndrome patients frequently have major exorbitism and significant obstructive airway problems. The diagnostic features are large thumbs and big toes.

Muenke's syndrome

A more recently discovered entity is the *P250R FGFR3* mutation on chromosome 4. This occurs in approximately 1 in 30 000 live births. If looked for, it can be found in approximately 30% of what were previously thought to be non-syndromic unicoronal or bicoronal synostoses.

An interesting factor in this condition is that it does not have any pathognomonic facial or limb appearances. The only feature that is recognized as more frequently occurring is infra-temporal bulging. This is also very variable.

Cranial front-nasal dysplasia

This occurs in 1 in 120 000 live births. It arises as a result of a mutation in the *EFNB1* gene system on the X chromosome. Interestingly, although it is X-linked, virtually all the patients described to date have been female.

The condition consists of coronal synostosis, which can be very asymmetric. The eyes are very widely spaced (hyperterlorism) and the nose tends to be short. The palate is high and arched with a constricted alveolar arch. Other diagnostic features include wiry curly hair and a tendency to longitudinal cracking of the nails. The clavicles and shoulder girdle, as well as the breasts, tend to be slightly hypoplastic.

Saethre–Chotzen syndrome

This arises from either a mutation or a deletion of the *TWIST1* gene on chromosome 7. It occurs in 1 in 80 000 live births. The synostotic element can be variable. Most frequently this is bicoronal, but occasionally it can be single-suture unicoronal synostosis.

Other features include a low hairline, eyelid ptosis, slightly small ears with a transverses crus across the concha, and variable soft tissue syndactyly (usually mild) of the fingers.

Other syndromes

There are many rare syndromic associations with synostosis that are outside the remit of this book.

Plagiocephaly without synostosis (PWS)

(deformational/postural/positional plagiocephaly)
External forces applied to the infantile skull either intrauterine or postpartum can cause a mechanical distortion of the skull without any synostosis. This is a well-recognized entity that occurs in both the anterior skull, where it must be differentiated from unicoronal synostosis, and the posterior skull, where it needs to be differentiated from the rare unilambdoid synostosis. In general, most cases have a degree of both anterior and posterior distortion at the same time.

By far the most common attributed aetiological factor (particularly in posterior plagiocephaly) is the practice since 1992 of having children sleep supine (the 'back to sleep' campaign) which has been shown to significantly decrease the incidence of sudden infant death syndrome.

The deformation present in plagiocephaly without synostosis tends to be a relatively symmetrical skewness resulting in a parallelogram-shaped skull when viewed from above. The anterior flattening is on the opposite side of the skull to the posterior flattening. The brow on the anterior flat side is pushed downwards, giving the appearance of a slightly small eye inferiorly displaced (as apposed to the enlarged and upward displaced brow in unicoronal synostosis). The ear positions are reciprocally displaced. The eye-to-ear distances on the two sides remain the same. In the posterior skull there is flattening in the occipital area, but no compensatory bulging of the mastoid, and no compensatory overgrowth of the opposite temporo-parietal area. Some cases present with marked central flattening over the lambda.

Natural history

PWS appears to have a specific natural history. A degree of flattening may be present at birth, but it is frequently only noted at about the age of 6–8 weeks at the first check-up. Careful positioning, as well as the concept of 'tummy time' (where children are deliberately placed on their stomachs whilst awake), may prevent deterioration, but it is not infrequent for progressive flattening to occur over a period of 3–4 months until the child is capable of sitting unsupported and therefore spending less time with pressure on the back of the head. Progressive rounding out then occurs which, in the experience of the four major craniofacial units in the UK, achieves a level of social acceptability without the need for any intervention. (this implies that, whilst perfect symmetry may not be achieved, the residual flattening is not of a degree to be noticeable or to cause comment/teasing under normal circumstances).

Helmet therapy has become very topical recently in the UK. This consists of a customized helmet worn for 23 hr a day. It needs regular monitoring and potential adjusting. The only available trials published in the literature indicate that rounding out does occur. There are no controlled randomized trials comparing non-treatment with treatment, and currently there is no evidence in the literature to prove that helmet therapy achieves any long term results superior to non-intervention.

Surgery for craniosynostosis

In general, surgery is directed at the cranium, primarily with a planned programme of addressing the lower orbits and the mid-face at a slightly later stage. (However, there has been a swing back towards combined cranial and midface procedures in combination with distraction.)

Indications

- To treat established raised intracranial pressure.
- To prevent the development of raised intracranial pressure.
- To protect the eyes.
- To protect the airway.
- To treat any established deformity.
- To prevent further deformity occurring.

Timing of surgery and surgical options

Emergency surgery in the form of a calvarial release or the insertion of a shunt for hydrocephalus may be required for acute raised intracranial pressure. A tracheostomy may be required for airway protection, and either a tarsorrhaphy or urgent orbital surgery may be required for eye protection.

In the absence of indications for emergency surgery, calvarial surgery is performed at about the age of 1 year in most units, although there has been a swing to early monobloc or a related split-level fronto-facial advancement in syndromic children before the age of 1 year.

In syndromic children who have a significant progression of turricephaly, the option of an early posterior release exists. This is felt to decrease the anterior driving forces and make fronto-orbital advancement remodelling easier to perform at a later date. Fronto-orbital advancement and remodelling is usually performed at the age of 1 year in cases of metopic synostosis and unilateral and bicoronal synostosis.

Sagittal synostosis is treated by modification of strip craniectomy with lateral barrel staving, usually in the first 6 months of life. Children who present later or who have a marked early deformity can be treated with a total or subtotal calvarial remodelling procedure (there are a variety of designs for this).

Mid-facial hypoplasia, obstructive sleep apnoea, and exorbitism are addressed by mid-facial surgery. Traditionally this has been performed via the Le Fort III technique with the insertion of a bone graft. More recently (last 8–10 years), mid-facial distraction techniques have allowed larger advancements and are relatively more stable at an earlier age. Distraction osteogenesis has also reduced the infection rate associated with monobloc or modified monobloc techniques, and therefore there has been a swing back to earlier monobloc or affiliated techniques.

When the children are approaching completion of their growth, facial re-contouring procedures at an appropriate level (bimaxillary surgery, Le Fort I and III, and facial bipartition type procedures) are offered to try and improve the aesthetic appearance of the face. Onlay techniques with either autogenous tissue, or alloplastic material (particularly around the hypoplastic malar areas and the forehead) are also offered.

Hemifacial microsomia

(craniofacial microsomia, first and second branchial arch syndrome)

Introduction
A congenital underdevelopment of the structures of the middle and lower face similar to Romberg's disease, but mainly skeletal, not progressive, and a different age group. 'Unilateral craniofacial microsomia' designates the unilateral form of the disease and 'bilateral craniofacial microsomia' describes the bilateral form.

Genetics
The genetic component is ill defined and, with a few exceptions, there is no proven genetic link. There is a type of craniofacial microsomia known as Goldenhar syndrome in which a strong autosomal dominant (AD) transmission has been identified.

Aetiopathogenesis
Various theories have been proposed for the causation of hemifacial microsomia.
- Mesodermal deficiency theory (Veau).
- Stapedial artery deficiency theory: this artery provides a temporary vascular supply for the precursors of the first and second branchial arches. A vascular deficiency caused by abnormalities in the development of this artery during fetal life may contribute to impaired development of the first and second branchial arches.
- Haematoma theory (Poswillo): the induction of haematoma formation in embryonic life by the administration of triazene and thalidomide correlated with the size of the defect. This tied in with the development of this anomaly in the offspring of patients who had been administered thalidomide during their pregnancy.

Incidence
- Varies from 1/4000 to 1/5500.
- Male to female ratio 2:1.
- Laterality of involvement: although the cases of unilateral craniofacial microsomia far outnumber the bilateral cases, close examination even in unilateral involved patients reveals mild but definite involvement of the 'normal/unaffected' side.

Pathology
Hemifacial microsomia is characterized by variation in the degree and extent of involvement. Three main anatomical components are involved in this syndrome: the ears, the mandible, and the maxilla. The problem also extends to the soft tissues and the adjacent bony components of the skull base. The predominant deformities are those of the jaws and the ear.

Jaws
The predominant deformity is that of ipsilateral mandibular hypoplasia. The ramus may be either short or a small remnant, giving the appearance of being almost absent. The chin is deviated to the involved side. There may

be compensatory changes on the uninvolved soft tissues and the skeleton of the opposite 'uninvolved' side. There is an occlusal cant towards the involved side. Pruzansky has graded the degree of mandibular deformity:
1 Minimal hypoplasia.
2 Varying degrees of hypoplasia of the entire system; body and ramus may be small; condyles may be flattened; the glenoid fossa may be shallow or deficient; the condyle may just hinge on a flattened infratemporal surface.
3 The ramus may either be absent or thinned to a thin lamina of bone.

Facial asymmetry becomes more obvious during the years of growth and the mandible tends to deviate laterally and upwards towards the more affected side. Other components of the skeletal system may be involved in the form of hypoplasia of the mastoid process, a smaller and shortened styloid process, underdevelopment of the zygoma, and possibility of microphthalmos. Vertebral (hemivertebrae/fused vertebrae/spina bifida/scoliosis) or rib abnormalities are common.

Ear Hypoplasia or micotia is common, as are ear tags.

Soft tissues Lateral facial cleft or unilateral macrostomia, facial hypoplasia.

Muscles of mastication These are absent or hypoplastic.

Nerves The facial nerve may be absent or weak and other cranial nerves may be affected.

Management
- Pre-surgical orthodontics.
- Mandibular surgery to correct length, mobility and occlusal cant by osteotomy, graft or distraction.
- Soft tissue correction by closure of macrostomia and soft tissue augmentation.
- Ear reconstruction.

Romberg's disease

(progressive hemifacial atrophy)

Incidence
- <20 years,
- Male-to-female ratio 1.5:1.
- 95% unilateral.

Aetiology
- Subcutaneous atrophy then bone/cartilage loss.
- ? due to vasomotor trophoneuritis.
- Sympathetic disturbance either ablation or stimulation.
- The disease 'burns out' after 2–10 years.

Management
- Delay until disease is burnt out.
- Skeletal reconstruction by onlay bone grafts or implants.
- Soft tissue reconstruction by grafts or flaps.

Treacher Collins syndrome

This is a congenital condition presenting at birth as bilateral mandibulo-facial dysostosis (MFD) producing a 'fish-like' facial appearance, described by Berry in 1889, Treacher Collins in 1900, and Franceschetti and Klein in 1949. The condition also fits the Tessier craniofacial cleft classification as bilateral 6,7, and 8 clefts.

Incidence
One in 25 000–50 000.

Genetics
AD: varied penetrance; male and female equal incidence. Treacher Collins gene: 5q31.3–q33.3 (Jabs 1991). More common with increased paternal age.

Aetiology and embryology
The cause is unknown but the main theories are:
- Neural crest cell injury or defect given that neural crest ectoderm forms craniofacial soft tissue, cartilage, bone, and teeth. MFD has been shown in animal studies resulting from vitamin A neural crest injury.
- Failure of differentiation of branchial arch mesoderm interferes with facial bone development.
- Stapedial artery hypoplasia causes facial ischaemia.
- Defective facial bone ossification.

Clinical presentation
- Bilateral condition affecting first and second branchial arch structures. The extent of the deformity is present at birth and remains fairly stable during growth.
- Zygoma and mandible hypoplastic, with class 2 malocclusion.
- Sideburns displaced anteriorly.
- Eyes: anti-mongoloid slant, coloboma of lower lids, medially absent eyelashes.
- Downward beaking of the nose.
- Macrostomia.
- Ears: variable deformities, commonly microtia but may be complete agenesis.
- Associated features: mental retardation 5%; deafness (>90% have at least moderate hearing loss); vertebral anomalies; cleft palate/velopalatine insufficiency; clubfoot; frontalis agenesis; choanal atresia very rarely.
- Hypoplastic mandible, glossoptosis, and small nasopharynx can lead to sleep apnoea.

Classification
Based on number of deformities present, and severity.

Investigation
Skeletal assessment: X-ray, CT (3D CT has now taken over predominantly in this regard). Particular note taken of the petrous temporal bone and middle/inner ear architecture. Early hearing aid placement if indicated will markedly improve communication skills and speech development.

Treatment
Should be structured, planned, and timed to fit with the physical and psychosocial growth of the child. Multidisciplinary team: plastic craniofacial surgeon, oral surgeon, orthodontist, occuloplastic surgeon, neurosurgeon, dietician, psychologist, social worker, speech and language therapist, ENT surgeon. Consider the various elements of the deformity. Reconstruct skeleton before the soft tissues. Multiple operations over many years are needed:

- **Early management** Airway—head-down crib may suffice. However, may require tracheostomy. Bilateral mandibular distraction may overcome glossoptotic airway difficulty, as genioglossus is short secondary to micrognathia. Treatment proceeds according to extent of defect/deformity.
- **Orbit** Deficient inferior lateral orbital floor, oval-shaped orbit, sloping supra-orbital ridge. Reconstruct lateral orbital floor defect and the supra-orbital ridge with calvarial, iliac crest, or rib bone graft. Rib resorbs rather more but is easier to work with.
- **Zygoma** Absent or hypoplastic. Reconstruct with bone graft.
- **Maxilla** Hypoplastic, flattened, narrow, and vertically short. Major deformities of the orbit, zygoma, and maxilla may require a bicoronal incision and use of vascularized split or full-thickness calvarial bone grafts on temporalis muscle. This option tends to leave a resultant temporal fossa hollow; can be corrected later with alloplastic material.
- **Mandible** Micrognathia and microgenia giving a retruded lower face and increased facial convexity. Mandible is advanced by sagittal split osteotomies of the mandibular ramus or distraction osteogenesis. Chin projection can be increased by advancement genioplasty or onlay bone graft. Further osteotomies may be needed to correct open bite deformities.
- **Eyelid** Anti-mongoloid slant to palpebral fissure, colobomas. These are repaired by a variety of flaps and techniques depending on the severity of the defects. Shortage of soft tissue is a problem. Principle is to resuspend the lateral canthus in addition to augmenting the lower lid tissues.
- **Prominent nose** This can be improved by rhinoplasty, principally to in-fracture, remove dorsal hump, and augment tip projection.
- **Ears** Varied degrees of hypoplasia through to absence (see ear reconstruction).

Reference
Jabs EW, Li X, Coss CA, et al. (1991). Genomics **11**, 193–8.

Pierre Robin sequence

A triad of micrognathia (small jaw), glossoptosis (falling back of the tongue), with airway obstruction and cleft palate. (Cleft palate was not a major feature in Pierre Robin's original description.)

Aetiology
- Unknown.
- Some may be familial.
- Developmental mandibular growth disturbance related. Possibly caused by failure to extend the head from the flexed position preventing the tongue from descending from between the palatal shelves causing (?) cleft palate and the other features.
- External intra-uterine pressure on the mandible which otherwise has normal growth potential.

Clinical presentation
Evident at birth:
- Micrognathia (hypoplasia of the mandible) and/or retrognathia (posterior position of the mandible). Because of the short posterior positioned chin the genioglossal muscles are short and cannot hold the tongue forward.
- Glossoptosis, whereby the tongue falls backwards and causes obstruction of the airway.
- Cleft palate—usually only type 1 or 2 (soft palate only or with posterior part hard palate).
- These produce a 'bird-like' facies with retruded chin and protruding tongue.
- Respiratory obstruction worse when the child relaxes or sleeps.
- Feeding difficulties. Small feeds, often regurgitated, with frequent aspiration leads to poor growth, exhaustion, and respiratory tract infections.

Management
- Early management is important to avoid death.
- Exclude other causes of obstruction such as choanal atresia by passing a catheter down each nostril. Also exclude tracheo-oesophageal fistula.
- Exclude other associations such as laryngomalacia, cervical spine anomalies, Stickler's syndrome (hereditary progressive arthro-ophthalmopathy).
- Lie in a face-down position, or intubate with nasopharyngeal or oropharyngeal tube.
- Retract the tongue and hold with a suture or clip safety pin. This is only temporary as the tongue will swell.
- Indications for surgery are failure to prevent obstruction with face-down position and monitoring, >7 days of obstructive episodes or infections, failure to gain weight, mandible >1 cm behind maxilla.
- Lip adhesion (Routledge procedure): the tongue is sutured forward to the lower lip and alveolus to prevent it falling back and obstructing the airway.

- Tongue transfixation with K wire: a K wire is placed through the protracted tongue and fixed to the mandible to prevent it falling back.
- Tracheostomy is only performed if the above procedures are ineffective.
- Palate repair when appropriate.

Prognosis

- Repeated episodes of hypoxia may lead to brain damage.
- Obstruction will cause death.
- If properly managed, the growth of the mandible depends on the underlying cause. Generally the mandible is small and later orthognathic surgery may be needed. Chin implants or a genioplasty may also be required.

Microtia

Definition
A congenital malformation of variable severity of the external and middle ear. A disorganized cartilage remnant and a lobule of varying size are often present.

Prevalence
- 1/4000–6000.
- Increased in the Navajo (1/1000).
- Male-to-female ratio 2:1.
- Ratio of right to left to bilateral is 5:3:1.

Aetiology
Syndromic causes include hemifacial microsomia and Treacher Collins syndrome. Vascular insults during development, rubella, and thalidomide have all been implicated, as has a genetic component.

Classification
Nagata classified microtia into five types:
- Lobule type—remnant lobule, without concha, acoustic meatus, or tragus.
- Concha type—remnant lobule, concha, acoustic meatus, tragus, and inter-tragal notch.
- Small concha type—remnant lobule with a small indentation representing the concha.
- Anotia.
- Atypical microtia—all other cases.

Timing
Nagata recommends waiting until age 10 for sufficient rib cartilage growth but other authors suggest that it is sufficient for framework construction from age 5 years. The normal ear is usually within 7 mm of normal height by this age, and body image concepts begin to form at age 4–5 years. Reconstructed auricles may grow in line with the other ear.

Middle ear surgery
Usually only recommended for bilateral microtia. It should take place after ear reconstruction to avoid scarring in the skin envelope region.

Technique
Basic steps to be achieved are:
- Cartilage framework construction.
- Dissection of pocket, removal of remnant cartilage, and placement of framework.
- Lobule transposition.
- Tragal and conchal construction.
- Projection of auricle.

Nagata two-stage reconstruction
The first stage involves framework construction from costal cartilages harvested from the ipsilateral side. A W-shaped skin incision is used to remove the cartilage remnant and develop a pocket for framework placement. The framework is sutured into place, and the lobule is transposed. Skin flaps are then sutured into place to cover the framework. In the second stage, the auricle is elevated from the scalp, and kept in position with a costal cartilage block placed posteriorly and covered with a temporoparietal fascia flap (TPFF) based on the superficial temporal artery. This is then covered with an 'ultra-delicate' split-thickness skin graft taken from the scalp. This graft is harvested so that the hair follicles are left at the donor site, thus avoiding hair growth on the ear and alopecia at the donor site.

Three-stage reconstruction
The first stage involves construction of the framework and placement in the pocket. The remnant cartilage is removed, and the lobule is transposed in the second stage. The third stage involves projection of the ear and construction of the tragus.

Branchial clefts

Nasal dermoid
- The tract can extend from the nasal midline to the crista gallae and cause meningitis, or be a blind-ended pit on the nasal midline.
- The first branchial arch relates to the trigeminal nerve and the second arch to the facial nerve.

Branchial clefts
- Type 1 arises between branchial pouches 1 and 2 and produces a pre-auricular pit with a tract *superficial* to the vessels.
- Type 2 arises between pouches 2 and 3. It lies at the junction of the upper two-thirds and lower third of the sternocleidomastoid and the tonsillar fossa and runs *between* the external and internal carotid arteries.
- Type 3 (rare) arises between pouches 3 and 4. The tract runs from the piriform sinus to the same point in the neck as type 2 but the tract passes *behind* the carotid vessels.

Cleft lip and palate: introduction

Cleft lip (CL)
Cleft lip is a congenital abnormality of the primary palate involving the lip, alveolus, and hard palate anterior to the incisive foramen. If extending posterior to the incisive foramen, it is termed cleft lip and palate (CLP).

Cleft palate (CP)
Cleft palate is aetiologically and embryologically distinct from CL and CLP, and represents a cleft of the secondary palate involving the hard palate (HP), posterior to the incisive foramen, and/or the soft palate (SP).

Submucous cleft palate
Submucous CP (Roux 1825) is a cleft of the secondary palate covered with mucosa. Cardinal signs include a bifid uvula, visible zona pellucida, and a palpable notch at the junction of the HP and the SP (Calnan 1954). A bifid uvula is present in 2% of the normal population. Adenoidectomy must be performed with caution as this may unmask previously undetectable velopharyngeal insufficiency. Surgical intervention is required in approximately 55% of patients.

Incidence
- General incidence of CL/CLP is ~1 in 700 live births. Considerable racial heterogeneity exists:
  - Caucasians: 1/1000.
  - Asians: 2/1000.
  - Africans: 0.5/1000.
- The non-syndromic CP rate is ~1/2000 and is relatively constant worldwide.
- CLP represents 45% of cases, isolated CP 30%, and isolated CL 20%.
- Ratio of unilateral left to unilateral right to bilateral CL deformity is 6:3:1.

Classification
General
- Unilateral or bilateral:
  - With respect to the palate, this is based on the whether the vomer is attached to one of the palatal shelves (i.e. unilateral CP) or neither of them (i.e. bilateral CP).
- Complete or incomplete.
- Based on supposed inheritance pattern:
  - Non-syndromic CL with or without CP.
  - Non-syndromic CP.
  - Syndromic CL with or without CP.
  - Syndromic CP.

Veau's classification (1931)
A   Incomplete cleft of secondary palate.
B   Complete cleft of secondary palate.
C   Complete unilateral cleft lip and palate.
D   Bilateral cleft lip and palate.

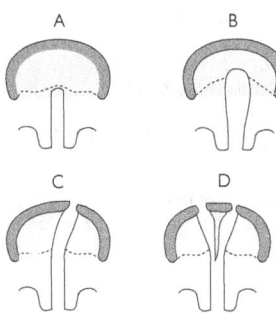

Fig. 5.1 Veau's classification of cleft palate.

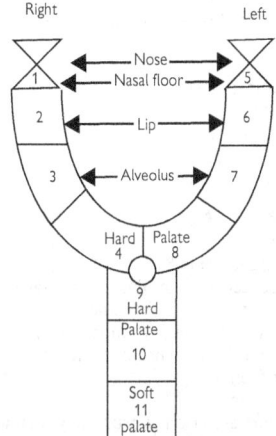

Fig. 5.2 Striped Y classification.

This classification has been criticized for ignoring isolated clefts of the primary palate and for being unable to differentiate incomplete and complete lip clefts.

Striped Y classification

First described by Kernahan and Stark (1958), and subsequently modified by Millard and Seider (1977), this classification provides a pictorial representation of the cleft lip and palate where an affected anatomical area is represented by stippling the relevant 'box(es)' on the Y. Cross-hatching represents an SMCP. Unfortunately, it does not allow isolated clefts of the secondary palate to be classified according to their side.

Unilateral cleft lip classification
- Microform (*forme fruste*):
  - Vertical groove or scar with notching of the vermilion and white roll, and variable shortening of the lip.
- Incomplete:
  - Characterized by complete lip separation but an intact nasal sill (Simonart's band).
- Complete:
  - Anatomical disruption of the nasal sill, lip, and alveolus.
  - If bilateral, associated with a cleft palate in 85% of cases.

Aetiology of CL and CLP
- Male-to female ratio 2:1.
- Infrequently associated with other congenital anomalies (syndromic in 14% of cases):
  - Trisomy 13 (Patau's syndrome) and trisomy 21.
  - Waardenburg's syndrome.
  - Van der Woude syndrome (associated with lip pits).
- Environmental factors:
  - Alcohol.
  - Anticonvulsants (e.g. phenytoin).
  - Folic acid deficiency.
  - 13-*cis*-retinoic acid.
  - Tobacco.
- Familial association: see Table 5.1.

Aetiology of isolated CP
- Male-to female ratio 1:2.
- Familial association: see Table 5.1.
- Syndromic or associated with another congenital anomaly in 60%:
  - Chromosomal (e.g. Down's syndrome).
  - Treacher Collins syndrome (chromosome 5).
  - Van de Woude syndrome (chromosome 1).
  - Klippel–Feil syndrome.
  - Pierre Robin sequence.
- Environmental factors are also important (e.g. vitamin A, riboflavin or folic acid deficiencies); also alcohol, tobacco, and anticonvulsants.

Embryology
CL results from failure of fusion of the medial and lateral nasal prominences (or processes) with the maxillary processes during week 5 of gestation. If associated with impaired palatal shelf fusion, CLP will result. The secondary palate develops by union of the two condensations of neural crest mesenchyme that arise from the medial aspects of the maxillary processes of the first branchial arch. The condensations undergo intramembranous ossification to form the palatal shelves, which are initially in a vertical orientation either side of the tongue and subsequently rotate to a horizontal plane dorsal to the tongue. The mechanisms responsible for palatal shelf adhesion are not entirely understood, but the transforming growth factor

Table 5.1 Familial association: risk of subsequent child with cleft lip or palate

Affected relative	Predicted recurrence (%)	
	CL or CLP	CP
No family history	0.1	0.04
Unaffected parents		
Single affected sibling	4	2
Two affected siblings	9	1
One parent affected		
No affected siblings	4	6
One affected sibling	17	15

beta gene family has been implicated. Fusion of the palatal shelves occurs between weeks 8 and 12 by apoptosis of the medial edge epithelial cells. CP results from partial or complete lack of fusion of the palatal shelves. It is believed that Pierre Robin sequence, a condition characterized by a wide U-shaped cleft palate, micrognathia, and glossoptosis, results from a disruption of this developmental cascade.

Prenatal diagnosis of CL or CLP

This is possible by ultrasound in the second trimester. It is not always possible to detect an isolated CP antenatally and most cases are diagnosed at birth.

Antenatal care

Early, preferably antenatal, referral to a specialist cleft centre is recommended. Parents may require genetic counselling; inheritance may be chromosomal (e.g. trisomy 13 or 21), Mendelian (e.g. Treacher Collins, Stickler, or Van der Woude syndromes), or sporadic. Cleft children will usually require expert multidisciplinary care until they have reached adulthood.

Multidisciplinary team

Comprises audiologist, clinical coordinator, ENT surgeon, geneticist, maxillofacial surgeon, orthodontist, paediatrician, plastic surgeon, psychologist, social worker, specialist nurse, and speech and language therapist. In the UK, the team is arranged in a 'hub and spoke' fashion.

Neonatal care

Airway obstruction

Especially in the case of Pierre Robin sequence in the presence of micrognathia. Nursing in prone position may prevent tongue from obstructing airway. An airway adjunct (nasopharyngeal tube) may be helpful. Do not divide tongue-ties initially (this could lead to the tongue occluding airway); indeed, a tongue stitch is sometimes used in severe cases.

Feeding
CP babies are unable to create a negative intra-oral pressure and thus are usually unable to breastfeed. Breastfeeding may be possible with unilateral CL. A modified teat is used for bottle feeding, preferably with expressed breastmilk (or milk formula). Lazarus et al. (1999) found that almost a third of cleft babies were underweight at the time of primary surgery (compared with approximately 14% of non-cleft controls); those children with a palatal cleft were most likely to be underweight. Following repair, average growth returns to normal compared with unaffected controls by the age of 4 years.

Risk of aspiration
Due to oro-nasal communication.

Genetic assessment
If indicated.

Surgical management
Treatment protocols vary considerably between different units and are usually individualized for the child's needs. The following is an approximate guide:
- Prenatal diagnosis (± genetic counselling).
- Birth: pre-surgical orthopaedics (if indicated).
- Age 6 weeks to 3 months: CL repair.
- Age 9–18 months: CP repair and ENT assessment ± grommets.
- Age 18 months to 5 years: revision surgery if indicated and cleft rhinoplasty.
- Age 6–10 years: orthodontic assessment and alveolar bone grafting.
- Age 11–20 years: orthodontic and restorative dental care. Possible skeletal surgery.
- Long-term issues include speech development (including velo-palatal insufficiency), orthodontic problems, and midfacial growth disturbance.

Hearing
Cleft palate deformity results in Eustachian tube dysfunction due to the misalignment of the normal palatal musculature. Tensor veli palatini and levator veli palatini both normally attach to the Eustachian tube and assist in tubal dilation, thus allowing the creation of a negative middle ear pressure during swallowing with subsequent drainage of any effusion. This mechanism is defective in the cleft child where the muscles attach directly into the rigid posterior element of the hard palate, thus negating any influence on tubal function.

The incidence of otitis media effusion can be 100% in cleft patients, with a significant risk of subsequent conductive hearing loss. This may pose particular problems for the child with abnormal speech development. Palatoplasty significantly reduces, but does not eliminate, the risk of permanent hearing loss. Thus all children require an ENT assessment and, if necessary, myringotomy with placement of grommets (ventilation tubes) if indicated. Adenoidectomy may also improve Eustachian tube patency.

The Clinical Standards Advisory Group (CSAG) Report on CL ± P (Clinical Standards Advisory Group 1998) identified wide disparity in quality of cleft care in UK. Too many units (n = 57) and too many surgeons performed too few operations (92 out of 99 surgeons performed <10 new primary repairs per annum). Thus it was recommended that the total number of cleft units should be reduced and that each surgeon should treat 40–50 new patients annually. Recommendations on the composition of the multi-disciplinary team were also made, with the use of a 'hub-and-spoke' network if necessary for geographical patient-access reasons.

References

Calnan J (1954). *Br J Plast Surg* **6**, 264–82.
Clinical Standards Advisory Group (1998). *Cleft lip and/or palate. Report of a CSAG Committee.* HMSO, London.
Kernahan DA, Stark RB (1958). *Plast Reconstr Surg Transplant Bull* **22**, 435–41.
Lazarus DD, Hudson DA, Fleming AN, Goddard EA, Fernandes DB (1999). *Plast Reconstr Surg* **103**, 1624–9.
Miller DR Jr, Seider HA (1977). *Br J Plast Surg* **30**, 300–5.

Cleft lip repair: unilateral

Aims of surgery
- Approximation of cleft edges with preservation of natural landmarks.
- Lengthening of the shortened lip on the cleft side.
- Functional reconstruction of orbicularis oris.

Historical perspectives
Cheiloplasty first reported in Chinese literature during the Chin Dynasty (c. 390AD). In 1949, LeMesurier was the first to recognize the importance of the Cupid's bow, although it was Tennison who preserved its anatomical position. Millard introduced his rotation–advancement method in 1957.

Relevant anatomy
The defect must be considered in terms of soft tissue, cartilage, and bony deficiencies. The normal lip comprises the central philtrum with adjacent philtral columns; the latter are created by the insertion of the pars peri pheralis, with the central dimple reflecting the absence of muscular insertion in the midline. The Cupid's bow, lying inferiorly, is created by the pull of the levator labii superioris inserting into the base of the ipsilateral philtral column. The white roll (of Gillies) is the musculocutaneous ridge created by the junction between the dry vermilion and the skin. The red vermilion has an associated midline tubercle (caused by the eversion of opposing pars marginalis fibres) and there is a distinct junction between the 'dry' and 'wet' vermilion.

The orbicularis oris is the highly complex primary muscle of the lip. It has deep internal fibres (the marginalis) running circumferentially between the two modioli which act in a purse-string manner to facilitate feeding and oral continence. The superficial external fibres (the pars peripheralis) fan out obliquely from the modioli to interdigitate with the other muscles of facial expression (including zygomaticus major superiorly and depressor labii inferioris inferiorly) and terminate within the dermis. Their role is primarily one of articulation and facial expression.

Clefting results in the abnormal attachment of the orbicularis oris into the nasal spine and the alar base respectively; the opposing forces result in splaying of the alar cartilages with broadening of the nasal tip and shortening of the columella. There is inherent instability of the dental arch segments, resulting in collapse of the lesser alveolar segment and lateral rotation of the greater segment, with the greatest deformity occurring with the most severe clefting. There is shortening of the philtrum and loss of the ipsilateral philtral column and a third of the Cupid's bow (and associated white roll) is absent.

The blood supply to the lip is from the superior and inferior labial branches of the facial artery, the mental and infra-orbital branches of the maxillary artery, and the transverse facial branch of the superficial temporal artery.

The nerve supply is from the facial nerve (buccal and mandibular branches).

Timing of surgery

Traditionally the 'rule of 10s' was applied: repair took place once the child weighed >10 lb, had Hb >10 g/dL, and was >10 weeks old. Because of anaesthetic concerns, most centres wait until the child is 3 months of age. Intra-uterine cleft lip repair is currently an experimental tool which has been performed with some success in animal studies. However, at present the perceived benefits (e.g. potentially scarless wound healing) do not outweigh the potential risks.

Pre-surgical alveolar moulding

Aims to narrow the cleft deformity and correct alveolar process malalignment. In its simplest form, it involves external taping (non-surgical lip adhesion) to allow moulding of the two halves of the maxilla and assist in approximating the cleft alveolus. This is often used in conjunction with a dental plate which prevents both the tongue from pressing into the cleft and collapse of the dental arch segments.

Pre-surgical orthopaedics

Introduced by McNeil and Burston in 1950. Aims to pre-operatively correct the skeletal deformities of the cleft maxilla such that the alveolar segments are sufficiently aligned so that the cleft of the alveolus and hard palate can be closed with a gingivoperiosteoplasty. Although narrowing of the alveolar cleft facilitates surgical repair, the long-term improvements on facial growth and secondary dentition remain unproven. May be passive (dental plate) or active (Latham's appliance, which is fixed to the maxilla and is activated by the child's parents by turning an integral coaxial screw, thus gradually aligning the alveolar segments). The use of these techniques is not universal, and is often reserved for severe deformities such as the wide bilateral cleft.

Operative technique

The key anatomical landmarks (Fig. 5.3) are marked prior to infiltration of local anaesthetic (with adrenaline).

A Vernier calliper is used to measure the distances involved accurately. The key to a successful aesthetic outcome is the final placement of the Cupid's bow and the final vertical length of the reconstructed philtral column. Point 2 is the peak of the Cupid's bow on the non-cleft side; the Vernier callipers are used to mark the exact desired location of the bow on the cleft side (based on a symmetrical relationship to the midpoint position 1). Point 4, the peak of the bow on the cleft side, can be difficult to determine precisely; measuring a distance from the commisure (point 11 to 4) and comparing it with the contralateral side (point 10 to 2) is inaccurate because of the asymmetrical tension created by the aberrant orbicularis oris insertion. However, point 4 is generally where the dry vermilion is widest and the white roll most prominent, with both features tapering off medially.

A primary cleft rhinoplasty is often performed concurrently and the child may require the simultaneous insertion of grommets.

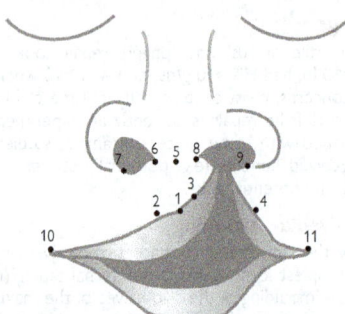

Fig. 5.3 Anatomical landmarks in cleft lip repair.

Tennison–Randall method
This method (Tennison 1952; modified by Randall 1959) avoids a straight-line scar by employing a triangular flap within a lower lip Z-plasty. However, it does cross the philtral column and flattens the philtral dimple.

Millard rotation advancement repair
This popular technique (Millard 1960) utilizes three flaps: the inferior rotation flap (R) of the medial lip element, the medial advancement flap (A) of the lateral lip element, and the columellar base flap (C) also arising from the medial lip element. The C-flap is used to recreate the nostril sill. The scars are within the philtral column and thus are well disguised. Furthermore, the lip length can be altered during surgery (the 'cut as you go technique'), which distinguishes it from the Tennison–Randall technique. The height of the new philtral column on the cleft side is governed by the length of the R-flap, and should, for symmetry, equal the length of the non-cleft philtral column. The nature of the flaps allows for secondary revision surgery. However, the technique is technically challenging and does leave a scar at the nasal base.

Post-operative management
Adequate wound toilet is required to prevent excessive crusting. The wound is often supported with Micropore tape, and topical antibiotic ointment is applied to the suture line on a regular basis. Children can resume feeding immediately. If non-dissolving sutures are used, removal is undertaken on the fifth post-operative day, often under sedation. Early wound massage is encouraged to minimize the risk of hypertrophic scar formation. Many surgeons use silicone nasal conformers for up to 6–12 months post-operatively, although success depends on parental cooperation.

Complications
Include wound infection and dehiscence and hypertrophic scarring. Although major revisions are unlikely, minor revisions may convert a good result to an excellent result; these include modifications to the Cupid's bow or white roll.

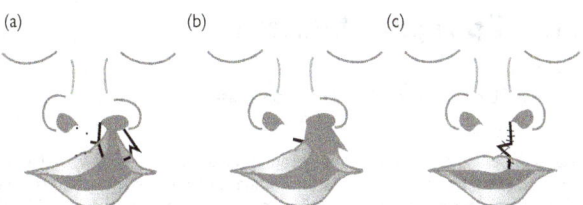

Fig. 5.4 Tennison–Randall cleft lip repair.

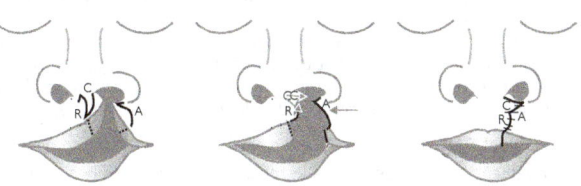

Fig. 5.5 Millard cleft lip repair.

References

Millard (1960). *Plast Reconstr Surg.* **25**: 595.
Randall (1959). *Plast Reconstr Surg.* **23**: 331.
Tennison (1952). *Plast Reconstr Surg.* **9**(2): 115.

Cleft lip repair: bilateral

Incidence
Bilateral CL represents ~15% of total cleft cases.

Anatomy
Bilateral clefting of the lip, alveolus, and anterior palate results in a characteristic central segment which is the remnant of the medial nasal process of the frontonasal prominence and comprises soft tissue (the prolabium) and bony elements (the premaxilla). Because of the combined effects of unrestrained cartilaginous growth and anterior pressure of the tongue, the premaxilla can be highly prominent, but becomes relatively hypoplastic as the child grows.

The nose is broad and flat with wide separation of the two crural domes which, if not corrected at the time of the primary repair, can result in severe secondary nasal deformity. The columellar is absent, and the prolabium is deficient in vermilion and white roll, and lacks muscle.

Historical perspectives
Management has changed radically over time. Traditionally the entire premaxilla was excised; however, this resulted in unacceptable nasal deformity and lip grossly deficient in its horizontal aspect. Attempts have been made to reset the premaxilla back with the vomer, although this has a detrimental effect on midfacial growth. It was then appreciated that the prolabium was an integral part of the upper central lip, which should be preserved in the surgical reconstruction.

Pre-surgical orthopaedics
Pre-surgical orthopaedics (e.g. Latham device) or naso-alveolar moulding (e.g. Grayson's device) are commonly used to narrow the cleft. Some advocate a simple lip adhesion (cheiloplasty) prior to formal repair at a later sitting. In very wide clefts, repair of each side may need to be staged. With adequate pre-surgical moulding resulting in anatomical alignment of the alveolar processes, subperiosteal repair of the alveolus (gingivoperiosteoplasty) is possible, but this remains controversial. Excessive undermining over the maxilla may hinder facial growth. However, advocates state that the technique significantly reduces the need for later alveolar bone grafting.

Principles of surgery
According to Mulliken (2000) these are:
- Maintain symmetry.
- Secure primary muscular union.
- Design the prolabial flap of correct size and configuration.
- Form the median tubercle and vermilion–cutaneous ridge from lateral labial tissue.
- Construct the nasal tip and columella by anatomical placement of the alar cartilages.

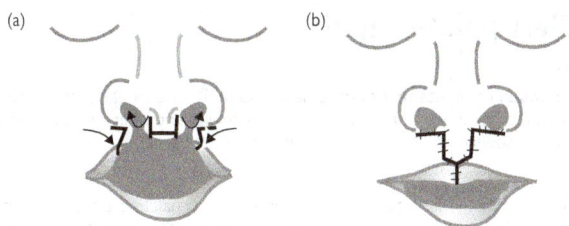

Fig. 5.6 Bilateral cleft lip repair.

Surgical repair

Techniques include straight-line repairs, Z-plasties (e.g. the Manchester upper lip Z-plasty), and the Millard two-stage repair (Millard 1971). The last of these has gained wide acceptance. A trapezoid-shaped prolabial flap is created by raising it off the premaxilla. The lateral elements of the prolabium are used to create superiorly based forked flaps which are banked by insetting end-on to the alar base flaps and are used for delayed lengthening of the columella. Orbicularis oris muscle from the lateral lip elements is dissected free, interdigitated in the midline, and sutured. The alar bases are set into place adjacent to the nasal spine, and the prolabial and lateral lip flaps are approximated. At a second stage the two fork flaps are used to lengthen the columellar in a V–Y manner

Further information

The Smile Train (http://www.smiletrain.org/) has excellent animations of both unilateral and bilateral cleft lip repair.

References

Millard DR Jr (1971). *Plast Reconstr Surg* **47**, 324–31.
Mulliken JB (2000). *Cleft Palate Craniofac J* **37**, 342–7.

Cleft palate repair

Aim
To obtain complete tension-free nasal and oral mucosal flap closure from the foremost point to the uvula with a technique and timing that produce optimal speech and minimize facial growth disturbances.

Anatomy
The hard secondary palate is composed of the palatine process of the maxilla anteriorly and the palatine bones posteriorly. The soft palate is a dynamic muscular sling and comprises five paired muscles (see Fig. 5.7):
- Tensor veli palatini (vents the Eustachian tube during swallowing).
- Levator veli palatini (comprises the 'sling' which elevates the soft palate).
- Palatoglossus.
- Palatopharyngeus.
- Muscularis uvulae.

The superior constrictor is a quadrangular muscle which originates from the medial pterygoid plate and sweeps around the upper pharynx to form its lateral and posterior walls. It acts in a sphincteric manner resulting in medial excursion of the lateral pharyngeal walls, thus assisting the seal between the velum and the posterior pharyngeal wall.

In cleft palate, the aponeurosis of the tensor veli palatini is attached along the bony margins of the cleft as opposed to the posterior border of the hard palate. Levator veli palatini is attached into the aponeurosis of tensor veli palatini and is cleft, thus interrupting its function as a muscular sling.

Blood supply
- Hard palate: greater palatine artery (branch of maxillary artery).
- Soft palate: lesser palatine artery, ascending palatine branch of the facial artery, and palatine branches of the ascending pharyngeal artery.

Nerve supply
- Sensory: maxillary division of the trigeminal nerve (CN V2). The greater palatine nerve enters through the greater palatine foramen to supply the hard palate and the lesser palatine nerve passes through the lesser palatine foramen to supply the soft palate.
- Motor: tensor veli palatine—internal pterygoid nerve (branch of the mandibular division of the trigeminal nerve (CN V3)). All other muscles are supplied by the pharyngeal plexus: the pharyngeal branch of the vagus nerve (CN X) and the glossopharyngeal nerve (CN XI).

Timing of repair
Timing is controversial. Whereas early surgery (<2 years) favours improved speech and hearing, delayed closure (>4 years) is associated with less retardation of midfacial growth. It is now generally accepted that early closure (<1 year) optimizes a favourable speech outcome and reduced hypernasality.

Late repair is associated with poor speech results and an increased palatal fistula rate. Cleft palate repair can assist only with speech production, not speech development. Thus it is reasonable to delay palatoplasty in syndromic children with severe developmental delay.

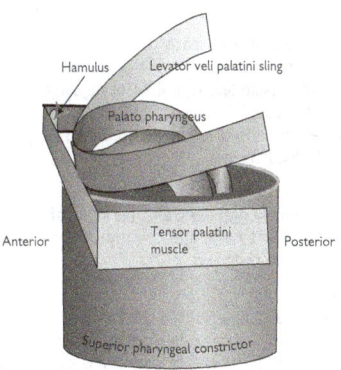

Fig. 5.7 Palate musculature anatomy.

Midfacial growth

In terms of the effect of surgery on midfacial growth, many authorities believe that the major deterrent to facial growth is not the timing of surgery *per se* but the surgical technique employed. Cephalometric analysis of adults with unrepaired clefts demonstrates normal maxillary growth (Ortiz-Monasterio *et al.* 1966). In some series, up to 20% of children with cleft palate may require a Le Fort I maxillary. The repairs which cause the greatest disturbance of palatal tissue architecture and thus palatal blood supply, such as the Veau–Wardill–Kilner pushback, are believed to have the most deleterious effect on midfacial growth. Ultimately it may be easier to correct a class III malocclusion with orthodontic treatment or orthognathic surgery rather than to establish normal speech in a older child after delayed cleft palate repair.

Surgical technique

Principles

The procedure is performed under GA using a feet-facing endotracheal tube and a Dingman gag to maintain intra-oral access. Throat packs are used and care must be taken to ensure that these are removed at the end of the procedure. The gag may cause tongue oedema post-operatively, particularly after prolonged surgery, and thus constant post-operative airway assessment is essential.

- After marking the planned surgical incisions, the palate is infiltrated with local anaesthesia and adrenaline (e.g. 0.5% lidocaine and 1:200 000 adrenaline).
- A small sandbag beneath the child's shoulders helps to extend the neck, and thus facilitate access.
- Many surgeons use a fibre-optic headlamp.
- Accidental damage to the greater palatine neurovascular bundle (NVB), as it emerges from the greater palatine foramen, must be avoided. Some surgeons advocate creating incisions with the contralateral hand, thus bevelling the incision away from the NVB.

- Aim for:
  - Two-layer closure of the palate.
  - Lengthening of the palate.
  - Restoration of muscle line of pull (muscle sling) across soft palate (intravelar veloplasty).
  - Minimal dissection and disturbance to blood supply to palate to avoid growth disturbance.

Straight line closure (or adhesion)

In children with extremely narrow clefts, paring of the medial palatal edges with elevation of sufficient nasal and oral mucosa to attain a two-layered closure is all that may be required.

von Langenbeck technique

The von Langenbeck technique (1861) can be used in children with slightly wider clefts. It combines a straight-line adhesion with lateral releasing incisions (lateral to the NVB) to create bipedicled oral mucoperiosteal flaps which allow closure of the oral layer. The raw lateral areas are normally packed with haemostat (e.g. Surgicel) and allowed to heal by secondary intention.

This procedure remains popular today, and it can be combined with an intravelar veloplasty in order to recreate the normal muscle sling of the soft palate. This approach produces a longitudinal midline scar which may be prone to contraction, and there is no facility to lengthen the soft palate, thus increasing the risk of subsequent speech disorder. The absence of anterior palatal incisions (cf. the 'pushback' technique) is thought to have benefits in terms of maxillary growth. Delaire described the creation of lateral releasing incisions which were medial to the NVB, thus reducing the deleterious effect on maxillary growth. However, the additional wound tension that resulted from the use of smaller flaps resulted in a higher post-operative fistula rate.

V–Y pushback technique (Veau–Wardill–Kilner repair)

This technique raises bilateral unipedicled mucoperiosteal flaps based on the greater palatine artery, repairing the nasal mucosal layer, performing an intravelar veloplasty, and then closing the oral mucosal flaps in a V–Y fashion. It is used for incomplete clefts or clefts of the secondary palate. The technique frequently leaves a sizeable area of the hard palate exposed, which subsequently granulates and heals by secondary intention. However, the 'push-back' has the advantage of lengthening the soft palate, but because of the adverse effects on anterior palatal fistula rate (due to the single layer of nasal mucosa anteriorly) and maxillary growth, this technique has been largely abandoned.

Double opposing Z-plasty

This technique (Furlow 1986) has gained wide acceptance as it addresses both the dynamic requirements of cleft palate repair by re-establishing the levator sling within a two-layered closure (thereby minimizing fistula formation) and concurrently lengthening the soft palate (without using tissue

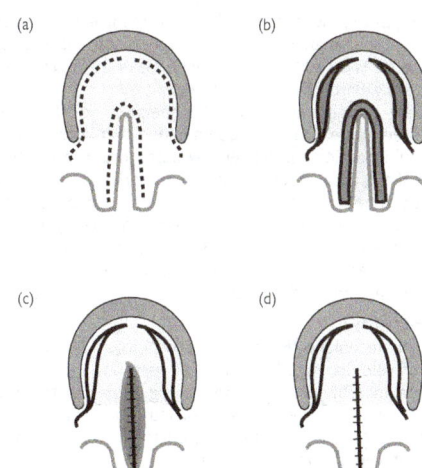

Fig. 5.8 The von Langenbeck palatal repair: (a) pre-operative markings; (b) bipedicled mucoperiosteal flaps raised with lateral releasing incisions; (c) closure of the nasal mucosa; (d) final appearance after closure of the oral mucosa.

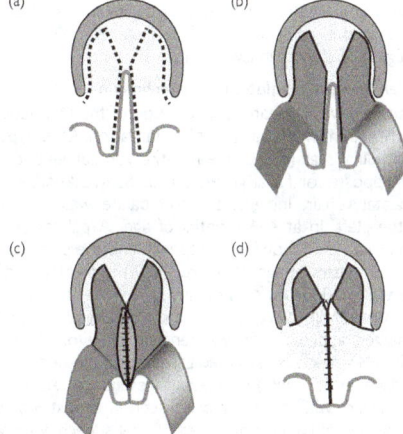

Fig. 5.9 V–Y pushback repair. (a) pre-operative markings; (b) posteriorly based mucoperiosteal flaps raised (NVB preserved within flap); (c) repair of the nasal layer and intravelar veloplasty; (d) flaps 'pushed back' to lengthen the soft palate and close the oral layer.

from the hard palate), thus theoretically reducing the risk of velopharyngeal incompetence. It is primarily intended to address soft palate closure; thus, with complete clefts an additional technique may be required to gain hard palate closure (e.g. Bardach's two-flap technique).

Anterior flaps contain mucosa only, but the posterior flaps also contain the levator mechanism. Furlow recommended that right-hand dominant surgeons should position the posteriorly based oral flap on the left side, as elevation of the nasal mucosa from the underlying muscle is the most challenging component of the operation. Without the need for lateral releasing incisions, there is less interference with maxillary growth. The technique has favourable long-term results in terms of speech and fistula rate when compared with other techniques. Fistulae tend to occur at the junction of the hard and soft palates.

Intravelar veloplasty
The aim of this technique (Braithwaite and Morris 1968; Kriens 1969) is restoration of velopharyngeal function by dissecting out the abnormally inserted palatal musculature and repositioning it in an anatomical manner. A prospective study of the influence of intravelar veloplasty on post-palatoplasty VPI (Marsh et al. 1989) failed to demonstrate a significant improvement in velopharyngeal function.

Two-flap technique
Bardach introduced the two-flap palatoplasty technique as a modification of the Langenbeck technique: the lateral releasing incisions are extended anteriorly to create two unipedicled mucoperiosteal flaps based on the NVB. These highly mobile flaps can be used to close anterior cleft defects securely, thus minimizing the risk of anterior palatal fistula. The procedure is normally performed in conjunction with an intravelar veloplasty prior to a standard straight-line closure in two layers.

Schweckendiek two-stage palatal repair technique
In the 1950's there was a greater appreciation of the link between palatal repair and subsequent midfacial growth retardation. One hypothesis was that the longitudinal scar (e.g. created by the von Langenbeck technique) impeded anteroposterior facial growth. Thus Schweckendiek proposed a two-stage palatal repair. Initially, the soft palate was repaired concurrently with the cleft lip at 4–6 months of age. A palatal obturator was then used to facilitate swallowing and speech and the palate subsequently repaired at 12–14 years of age. More recently the palatal repair has been brought forward to 18–24 months of age.

In 1978, Schweckendiek's son published the results of 25 years follow-up of the two-staged approach (Schweckendiek and Doz 1978). (A subsequent analysis of 45 randomly selected cases was published as the Marburg project (Bardach et al. 1984).) Excellent results in terms of maxillary growth were noted, with normal growth seen in almost 90% of patients, but less than a third of patients achieved normal speech, with VPI present in more than half of patients.

CLEFT PALATE REPAIR

1. Oral flaps designed

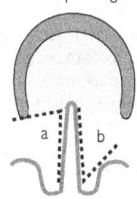

2. Oral flaps raised with muscle on patient's right (*) and mucosa only on left

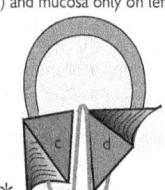

3. Nasal flaps designed with muscle on patient's left (*)

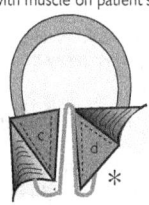

4. Nasal layer closed after flaps transposed

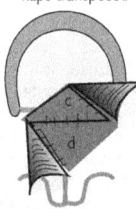

5. Oral layer closed

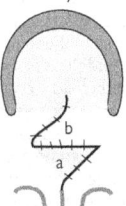

Fig. 5.10 Furlow double-opposing Z-plasty: (1) pre-operative markings; (2) elevation of oral mucosal flaps; (3) nasal flap design; (4) transposition and closure of nasal mucosal flaps; (5) final appearance after intravelar veloplasty closure of oral mucosa.

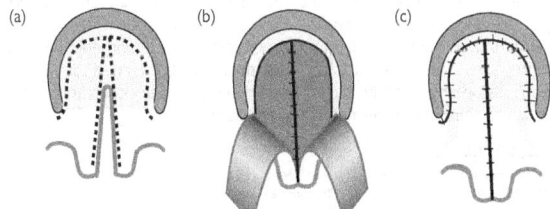

Fig. 5.11 Bardac two-flap palatoplasty: (a) pre-operative markings; (b) bilateral posteriorly based unipedicled flaps raised and closure of nasal layer; (c) closure of oral layer following intravelar veloplasty.

Vomerine flaps

These are used to assist in closure of the hard palate, particularly in wide unilateral or bilateral clefts. Wide superiorly based mucoperiosteal flaps are raised from the nasal mucosa overlying the vomer; both sides are utilized if closing a bilateral cleft. The flap is rotated laterally and sutured to small palatal mucoperiosteal flaps raised on the nasal (or oral) surface of the palatal shelf. Inferiorly based vomerine flaps were initially used, but these resulted in unacceptable maxillary growth retardation, presumably because of interference with the vomer–premaxillary suture.

Submucous cleft palate repair

A significant proportion of these children will be asymptomatic and therefore will not require surgery. Surgery is reserved for those who are symptomatic. A Furlow technique with intravelar veloplasty is normally favoured; alternatively, a pharyngoplasty may be used.

Post-operative recovery

The immediate post-operative issues are maintenance of a safe airway and adequate analgesia.

A nasopharyngeal airway adjunct is commonly used. Children with Pierre Robin sequence are at particular risk of airway obstruction and occasionally a tongue traction suture is used.

Peri-operative corticosteroid (dexamethasone) may reduce the risk of post-operative airway obstruction secondary to oedema. Excessive analgesia risks sedation and thus airway compromise.

Many surgeons use elbow splints in the immediate post-operative period to prevent the child from interfering with the delicate surgical repair. For similar reasons, spoons and other implements are avoided at feeding time to avoid accidental damage to the palate. Some surgeons insert a fine-bore nasogastric tube in theatre in order to augment fluid (or feed) intake post-operatively if needed. In the event of accidental removal, re-insertion must not be attempted because of the risk of palatal damage.

Oral hygiene is maintained by regular mouthwashes or gargling, and tooth brushing can normally be resumed after the first post-operative week.

Post-operative complications

Other than airway difficulties, haemorrhage is the prime concern. It normally arises from the raw area created by the lateral releasing incisions. If severe, digital pressure with an adrenaline-soaked swab is necessary and preparations should be made for the child to return to theatre immediately. Other complications include palatal fistula formation, speech disorders, and midfacial growth disturbance. Rarely, early wound dehiscence can occur; this warrants a return to theatre for attempted re-apposition.

References

Bardach J, Morris HL, Olin WH (1984). *Plast Reconstr Surg* **73**, 207–18.
Braithwaite F, Maurice DG (1968). *Br J Plast Surg* **21**, 60–2.
Furlow LT Jr (1986). *Plast Reconstr Surg* **78**, 724–38.
Kriens OB (1969). *Plast Reconstr Surg* **43**, 29–41.
Marsh JL, Grames LM, Holtman B (1989). *Cleft Palate J* **26**, 46–50.
Ortiz-Monasterio F, Serrano A, Barrera G, Rodriguez-Hoffman H, Vinageras E (1966). *Plast Reconstr Surg* **38**, 36–41.
Schweckendiek W, Doz P (1978). *Cleft Palate J* **15**, 268–74.

Cleft rhinoplasty

Cleft nose deformity
Associated with cleft lip deformity and thus may be considered as unilateral or bilateral. Correction is essential to achieving facial symmetry and a good aesthetic outcome.

Anatomy
The major defect of the unilateral cleft lip (UCL) nasal deformity is the wide alar base. Compared with the unaffected side, the alar lies inferolaterally, thus falsely lengthening the appearance of the nose. In more severe cases the alar cartilage is hypoplastic and convoluted, with a poorly projecting alar dome. The columella is both shortened and oblique, with its base directed away from the cleft side. The piriform aperture of the premaxilla is underdeveloped on the cleft side, thus exaggerating the alar deformity. Retarded growth of the nasal bones and the nasal process causes the nasal dorsum to tilt to the cleft side. The base of the nasal septum is deviated away from the cleft side because of the unopposed action of the normal musculature, and may be dislocated off the nasal spine. The bilateral cleft nasal deformity may be considered as a duplication of the UCL nasal deformity and comprises a significantly shortened columella as well as a broad depressed nasal tip.

Aims of nasal surgery
- Functional: to relieve soft tissue and skeletal occlusion of the cleft nasal airway.
- Aesthetic: to achieve bilateral symmetry of the nose with an improved nasolabial and nasofacial relationship with minimal surgical scarring.

Timing of surgery
Primary nasal surgery
Primary surgery is usually performed concurrently with the primary cleft lip repair (readily facilitated by Millard rotation–advancement procedure) or at 5–6 years of age. Primary nasal repair has not been demonstrated to adversely affect subsequent nasal growth.

Secondary nasal surgery
Secondary surgery is performed at preschool age if there is significant deformity (normally involving the lower lateral cartilage), or is delayed until nasal growth is complete (~16 years).

Interference with the vomer or nasal septum is best deferred until nasal growth is complete because of the deleterious effect on nasal growth. Likewise caution should be exercised when performing an primary open rhinoplasty in pre-school children because of reports of subsequent abnormal bulbous nasal growth during the adolescent growth spurt.

Secondary rhinoplasty may be deferred until adolescence or adulthood when definitive osteoplastic rhinoplasty may be safely undertaken. By the teenage years, the piriform aperture has been augmented post alveolar bone grafting and nasal growth is virtually complete.

By adulthood, maxillary growth is complete. Thus in the event of significant midfacial hypoplasia, Le Fort I advancement can safely proceed in order to improve maxillary projection before secondary rhinoplasty is undertaken.

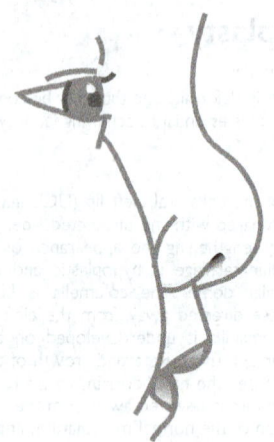

Fig. 5.12 Unaffected baby profile. Flattened nose and mid face in cleft lip and palate.

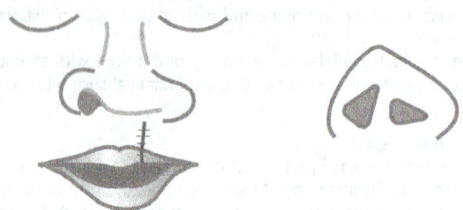

Fig. 5.13 Cleft nose deformity: anterior view and worm-eye view.

Unilateral cleft lip primary rhinoplasty

McComb technique
This technique (McComb 1975) is performed simultaneously with the UCL repair. Having mobilized the nasal skin free of the cartilaginous framework, the caudally rotated lower lateral cartilage is re-orientated and secured with percutaneous bolster sutures.

Tajima technique
An inverted-U incision is made within the nasal vestibule in order to reposition the alar cartilages (Tajima 1977).

Bilateral cleft lip primary rhinoplasty

Following a retrospective analysis of primary BCL repair using the Millard forked flap technique, McComb (1990) noted that, by puberty, the columella became too long with excessively large nostrils, there was downward drift of the lip–columella junction, and the nasal tip remained broad because of alar dome separation. Thus he avoids utilizing prolabium tissue for nasal reconstruction and advocates a two-stage nasal–lip repair.

Secondary rhinoplasty

This is normally performed using a standard open-tip technique adopting bilateral marginal or rim incisions with a stepped or V-shaped transcolumellar incision at either its base or midpoint. Numerous techniques exist for columella lengthening including V–Y advancement (Fig. 5.14, left) or the use of a rectangular columellar flap (Fig. 5.14, right).

The broad nasal bridge associated with a BCL may require medial and lateral osteotomies and infracture. Once nasal growth is complete, the septal deformity is usually corrected by submucous cartilaginous resection, repositioning of the caudal septum, and midline fixation.

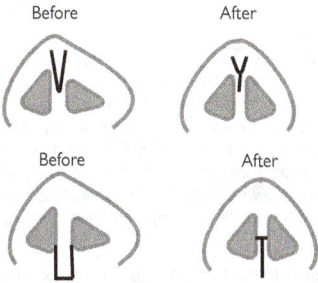

Fig. 5.14 Techniques for columella lengthening.

References

McComb H (1975). *Plast Reconstr Surg* **55**, 596–601.
McComb H (1990). *Plast Reconstr Surg* **86**, 882–93.
Tajima S, Maruyama M (1977). *Plast Reconstr Surg* **60**, 256–61.

Velopharyngeal incompetence

Definition
Velopharyngeal incompetence (or insufficiency) (VPI) is a generic term for the inability to completely occlude the velopharyngeal aperture during speech. Cleft palate affects speech. After primary palatoplasty, 80% of patients achieve satisfactory speech results, 15% are acceptable (with speech therapy), and 5% require secondary surgical management.

Aetiology
- Clefting of the secondary palate.
- Submucous cleft palate.
- Palatal fistula.
- Enlarged tonsils (thus obstructing velopharyngeal closure) or adenoid involution during puberty.
- Post-orthognathic surgery (e.g. for class III malocclusion correction).
- Neuromuscular dysfunction (e.g. CVA, myotonic dystrophy, MS, PD).
- Syndromic (e.g. velocardiofacial syndrome, trisomy 21).
- Behavioural/mislearning (phoneme-specific nasal emission).

Assessment
Speech and language
VPI has the characteristics of hypernasality (during vowel production) and nasal emission (or escape) (during consonant production). Many children attempt to compensate by speaking softly to minimize nasal airflow or use maladaptive articulation patterns (e.g. glottal stops). All phonemes in the English language are produced by oral airflow and thus require velopharyngeal closure. The exceptions are the nasal consonant phonemes M, N, and NG, which normally allow nasal escape. The articulation of plosives (P and B) and fricatives (F and S) requires a competent velopharynx.

Flexible nasoendoscopy
Can be performed in the outpatient setting on a conscious patient (topical anaesthetic nasal spray can be used) and allows direct visualization of the incompetent velopharynx to determine the relative contribution of poor velar excursion versus inadequate lateral pharyngeal wall mobility. Requires a cooperative child (~5 years or older).

Videofluoroscopy
Provides real-time visualization of the velopharynx by means of lateral soft-tissue fluoroscopy. Requires the use of a contrast medium (nasal barium). Exposes child to radiation.

Pressure-flow measurements
Provides quantitative information on the pressure-flow changes occurring during speech.

MRI
May be used to exclude velocardiofacial syndrome (Shprintzen's syndrome) in light of aberrant arterial vasculature.

Management
- Speech therapy is effective in minor cases of VPI, post-operative patients, and those with compensatory articulation techniques.
- Palatal obturators make suitable temporizing measures for those patients with palatal fistulae or a residual cleft. A palatal lift is used to elevate a soft palate that is of sufficient length but inadequate mobility, whereas a palatal bulb is used to augment a shortened palate.
- Surgery is indicated with VPI in the face of an adequately corrected cleft palate. It is normally undertaken after 5 years of age but before 12 (as the ability to train speech diminishes):
  - Tonsillectomy or adenoidectomy is often required before formal surgical correction. Adenoids can obstruct the insetting of pharyngoplasty flaps, whilst enlarged tonsils may hinder the raising of posterior tonsillar pillar flaps.
  - Pharyngoplasty.
  - Pharyngeal flap.
  - Palatal lengthening procedures (e.g. Furlow double opposing Z-plasty).
  - Posterior pharyngeal wall augmentation has been attempted with autogenous grafts (e.g. cartilage, fat, or fascia) or various alloplastic materials (e.g. Teflon and silicone). The technique has been abandoned because of the high infection, extrusion, and migration rates and is of historical interest only.

Velopharyngeal closure (VPC) pattern
It is essential to assess the pattern of velar and pharyngeal closure preoperatively with videofluoroscopy and/or naso-endoscopy to ensure that the appropriate surgical technique is used:
- Coronal (55%): the most common pattern, predominantly due to soft palate making contact with the posterior pharynx.
- Circular (20%): closure is obtained by contributions from both the soft palate and the lateral pharyngeal walls.
- Circular with the Passavant ridge (15%): as with circular but with a prominent Passavant ridge created by superior pharyngeal constrictor of the posterior pharyngeal wall.
- Sagittal (10%): this is most commonly seen post cleft palate repair. There is minimal soft palatal or superior constrictor contribution, and the majority of closure is via the lateral pharyngeal walls.

Sphincter pharyngoplasty
The aim is augment the pharyngeal wall in order to allow velopharyngeal closure in cases where there is deficient lateral pharyngeal wall movement. The best results appear to be in those flaps which are inset as high as possible on the posterior pharyngeal wall. Beware of abnormally medially placed internal carotid arteries in patients with velocardiofacial syndrome!

Hynes (1950, 1953) described raising bilateral superiorly based flaps consisting of the salpingopharyngeus muscle of the posterior tonsillar pillar and overlying mucosa. These were rotated through 90° and inset into the posterior pharyngeal wall at the level of Passavant's ridge such that the tips of the flaps were overlapping. Division of the soft palate was sometimes required to gain access to the posterior pharynx. He later used bulkier flaps also containing palatopharyngeus and part of the superior constrictor muscle. The procedure eliminates nasal escape in 95% of patients

Orticochea (1968) modified the placement of Hynes' flaps such that they were much lower in the posterior pharyngeal wall, thus obviating the need for soft palate division. Furthermore, the flaps were inset into an inferiorly based posterior pharyngeal flap to create a dynamic sphincter. Retrospective analysis demonstrates that the best results were in younger children and those where the flaps which were inset higher in the posterior pharynx, at the level of attempted velopharyngeal closure.

Jackson and Silverton (1977) again raised similar flaps to Hynes but inset them in the midline in a superiorly based posterior pharyngeal flap at the level of normal velopharyngeal closure closure (cf. Orticochea). Over 90% of patients experienced improved speech with this approach.

Posterior pharyngeal flap

The aim of this technique (Schoenborn 1875) is to obtain static closure of the velopharynx by means of a superiorly or inferiorly based flap which is elevated from the posterior pharyngeal wall (in the plane of the prevertebral fascia) and inset into the soft palate. It is most appropriate for those patients with adequate lateral pharyngeal wall motion but deficient velar function. Air passes around the flap (the 'lateral ports'). Although technically more demanding to perform, the superiorly based flap (raised to the level of C1) is preferred as it retracts the velum superiorly when cicatricial contracture occurs.

Outcome

Pharyngoplasty and posterior pharyngeal flaps have comparable success rates in excess of 80%. Hynes estimated that 20% of post-pharyngoplasty patients would require further surgery (e.g. palatal lengthening). Post-operative hyponasality occurs in approximately 15% of patients.

Complications

Excessive occlusion of the velopharynx (particularly with the posterior pharyngeal flap) can result in:
- Acute post-operative airway obstruction (necessitating immediate re-intubation).
- Hyponasality.
- Snoring and chronic obstructive sleep apnoea.
- Dehiscence of the 'bucket-handle' flap from the posterior pharynx.
- Bleeding.
- Infection.

Symptoms may settle as post-operative oedema resolves.

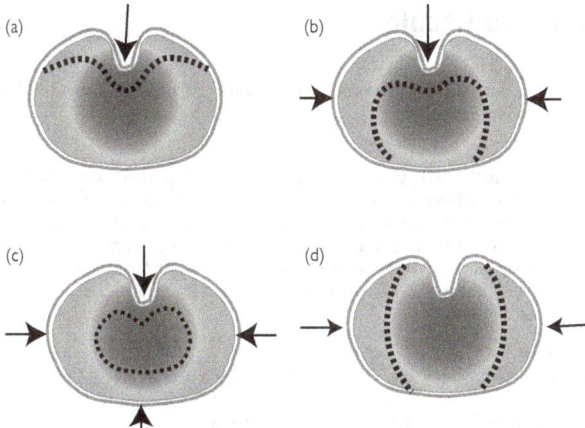

Fig. 5.15 Velopharyngeal closure patterns: (a) coronal; (b) circular; (c) circular with a Passavant ridge; (d) sagittal.

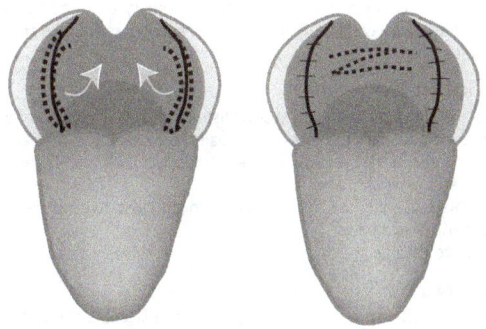

Fig. 5.16 Hynes pharyngoplasty.

References

Hynes W (1950). *Br J Plast Surg* **3**, 128–35.
Hynes W (1953). *Ann R Coll Surg Engl* **13**, 17–35.
Jackson IT, Silverton JS (1977). *Plast Reconstr Surg* **59**, 518–24.
Orticochea M (1968). *Plast Reconstr Surg* **41**, 323–7.
Schoenborn KWEJ (1875). *Verh Dtsch Ges Chir* **4**, 235–9.

Palatal fistula

Definition
An abnormal oro-nasal communication resulting from dehiscence of the primary cleft palate repair.

Incidence
Cohen et al. (1991) rated up to 23% in a retrospective series of 129 consecutive patients with non-syndromic cleft palate. Approximately half were ≤2 mm and were repaired in conjunction with lip or nasal revision surgery or alongside an alveolar bone graft; 14% were ≥5 mm and required early repair as they were symptomatic. The recurrent fistulation rate was 37%. 25% of patients were left with a permanent fistula at the end of their cleft management.

Risk factors
- Wide cleft palates (e.g. Pierre Robin sequence or Veau type 3 and 4 clefts).
- Surgical technique (e.g. pushback palatoplasty).
- Post-operative infection or haematoma.
- Mechanical (children's fingers!).

Prevention
Meticulous surgical technique at the time of primary palatoplasty including a tension-free two-layered closure of the oral and nasal layers and careful haemostasis.

Classification
- Naso-alveolar fistula: these anterior fistulae normally represent an unrepaired alveolar cleft; they are usually reconstructed with an alveolar bone graft just prior to the eruption of the canine teeth (8–10 years of age).
- Hard palate fistulae: the majority occur in the post-alveolar segment of the anterior hard palate.
- Soft palate fistulae.

Symptoms
Whereas tiny fistulae are often asymptomatic, a sizeable fistula can result in significant difficulties for the child, including oral fluid and food regurgitation into the nasal chamber and VPI. Food can become lodged in the fistula which may cause oral hygiene problems.

Management
Small asymptomatic fistulae do not require surgical closure. Larger symptomatic fistulae may be closed with local mucoperiosteal flaps.

It is crucial that, as with primary palatal surgery, a two-layer closure is achieved. Local turnover mucosal flaps may be used or, if hindered by excessive scarring, vomerine mucosal flaps can be utilized. Repair must be tension free with avoidance of overlapping oral and nasal layer suture lines to minimize the risk of recurrence if one of the layers dehisces.

In the event of recurrence, pharyngeal flaps may be useful, particularly for posterior fistulae in children with VPI. Alternatives include the pedicled dorsally based tongue flap, which requires delayed division at approximately 3 weeks. Occasionally inter-maxillary fixation (IMF) may be required to minimize the risk of flap avulsion from the recipient site.

Last-ditch options include free tissue transfer, where the radial forearm flap has been successfully used (Chen et al. 1992), or the use of submucoperiosteal tissue expanders (De Mey et al. 1990).

In recalcitrant cases, particularly where the patient has speech disturbance but is keen to avoid further (potentially complex) surgery, a palatal obturator prosthesis may be considered.

References

Cohen SR, Kalinowski J, LaRossa D, Randall P (1991). *Plast Reconstr Surg* **87**, 1041–7.
Chen HC, Ganos DL, Coessens BC, Kyutoku S, Noordhoff MS (1992). *Plast Reconstr Surg* **90**, 757–62.
De Mey A, Malevez C, Lejour M (1990). *Br J Plast Surg* **43**, 362–4.

Orthodontics

Definitions
- **Orthodontics** is a specialty of dentistry concerned with the study and treatment of malocclusions, which may be a result of tooth irregularity, disproportionate jaw relationships, or both.
- **Orthognathics** is the surgical manipulation of the elements of the facial skeleton to restore the proper anatomical and functional relationship in patients with dentofacial skeletal anomalies.

Multidisciplinary team
The orthodontist is a key member of the multidisciplinary cleft team and is involved throughout the patient care pathway.

Anatomy
The alveolar cleft normally occurs between the lateral incisor and the canine. Permanent lateral incisors are absent in up to 40% of patients.

Infancy
Many units use pre-surgical orthopaedics, particularly in wide clefts, in an attempt to improve alignment of the maxillary segments and the nasal cartilages prior to cleft lip repair. The prosthetic plate also acts as an obturator to assist feeding and allows the tongue to adopt a more physiological position (whilst also preventing it from forcing the maxillary segments to diverge). The device requires regular cleaning (1–3 times/day) to prevent fouling.

In UCL the plate may have a protruding nasal extension (an acrylic prong arising from the prosthesis) which helps to elevate the depressed nasal dome and straighten the columella. Post cleft lip repair, patients with severe nasal distortion are fitted with commercially available silastic stents which are kept *in situ* for up to 3 months following surgery by means of perforated facial taping.

The extremely protrusive premaxilla in BCL may be repositioned into a more favourable anatomical relationship with the maxillary segments by means of pre-surgical orthopaedics which utilize an intra-oral appliance with a means of strapping and thus retracting the premaxilla, with the aim of facilitating a more favourable surgical repair. This passive naso-alveolar moulding was introduced by Grayson *et al.* (1993). In addition to facilitating the lip repair, it assists in remodelling the nasal dome, tip, and hypoplastic columella. Active pre-surgical orthopaedic techniques include the use of the Latham device as described in the section on cleft lip repair.

Primary (deciduous) dentition (age 3–6 years)
The main themes of management are to correct severe dental cross-bites or to extract troublesome displaced deciduous teeth. Cross-bite correction is performed with transverse maxillary distraction (expansion) and anterior repositioning (protraction) using removable or fixed devices ('braces').

Transitional (mixed) dentition (age 7–11 years)

This period is critical as alveolar bone grafting (ABG) is conducted once 25–50% of the canine root is formed. Prior to bone grafting, anterior collapse of the maxillary arch is corrected with, for example, a quad helix device. This expands the collapsed arch to provide well-aligned maxillary segments and minimize the alveolar cleft. Prior to ABG, supernumerary teeth in the immediate vicinity of the cleft are extracted and all appliances/metalwork are removed to ensure that the gingiva is intact and healthy prior to surgery.

Permanent dentition (> 12 years)

The aim is for class 1 occlusion with ideal overjet (defined as the horizontal distance between the incisal edge of the maxillary incisor and the mandibular incisor) and overbite (defined as the vertical distance between the incisal edge of the maxillary incisor and the mandibular incisor). Replacement of an absent lateral incisor may be necessary (e.g. using an osseo-integrated prosthesis).

Angle's classification of occlusion (1899)

Based on the relationship of the maxillary first molar to the mandibular first molar (Fig. 5.17).

Orthognathic procedures

Cleft patients may have significant skeletal and dental discrepancies between the maxilla and mandible. Maxillary hypoplasia and a relative prognathism of the mandible (which is usually of normal size) result in the patient having an Angle class III malocclusion. Note that approximately 12% of American high school students have a class III malocclusion, and it may be even more prevalent in oriental populations.

Maxillary advancement

May be indicated in significant class III malocclusion. A pre-operative speech and language assessment is essential as such a procedure may precipitate VPI, which may necessitate a pharyngoplasty. Pre-operative cephalometric analysis is undertaken in order to evaluate the degree of surgical advancement necessary:

- *Le Fort I osteotomy*. Maxillary advancement for cleft-related maxillary hypoplasia is normally achieved by means of a Le Fort I osteotomy. The advanced lower maxilla is rigidly fixed in its new position with internal plates.
- *Distraction osteogenesis* In severe maxillary hypoplasia, or in younger children where there might be a risk of interfering with uninterrupted tooth buds, distraction osteogenesis may be employed. Based on the Ilizarov technique, distraction osteogenesis was first used in the craniofacial skeleton by McCarthy et al. (1992) who applied the technique to correction of the hypoplastic mandible. External devices with a rigid external frame secured using a cranial halo or internal devices (with a percutaneous port to facilitate distraction) may be employed. There are three phases of treatment:

- Post-operative latency period (typically 3–7 days).
- Distraction period: distraction occurs at a rate of 1 mm/day until the desired degree of distraction is obtained. Excessive distraction can lead to fibrous union.
- Consolidation period: the neo-position of the maxilla is allowed to consolidate for a minimum of 4 weeks at which point the external or internal distraction apparatus is removed.

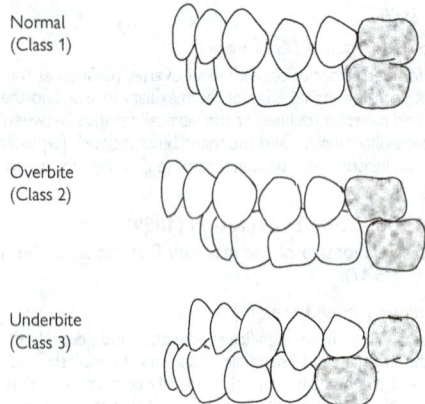

Fig. 5.17 Angle's classification of occlusion.

References

Grayson BH, Cutting C, Wood R (1993). *Plast Reconstr Surg* **92**, 1422–3.
McCarthy JG, Schreiber J, Karp N, Thorne CH, Grayson BH (1992). *Plast Reconstr Surg* **89**, 1–10.

Alveolar bone grafting

Alveolar bone grafting is an essential element of the contemporary surgical management of the cleft alveolus.

Aims

- Closure of the oro-nasal fistula.
- Stabilization of the maxillary arch.
- Provision of bony support for the eruption of permanent teeth adjacent to the cleft (usually the lateral incisor and canine).
- To allow prosthetic restoration of the missing lateral incisor by means of an osseo-integrated implant.
- Augment the piriform aperture, thus providing additional support to the alar base on the cleft side.

Gingivoperiosteoplasty

This was introduced by Skoog (1967) in order to primarily close the alveolar cleft using periosteal flaps, and has been used in conjunction with pre-surgical orthopaedics. Although decreasing the requirement for later alveolar bone grafting, it has generally fallen from favour on account of the adverse effect on facial growth (even though it does not directly interfere with the vomerine growth centres).

Timing

Historically this has proved somewhat controversial:
- Primary (<2 years, usually at the time of palatal repair).
- Early secondary (2–5 years).
- Secondary (>5 years) grafting (at eruption of canine).

Primary grafting was found to have a deleterious effect on maxillary growth. Furthermore, bone graft resorbs in the absence of an erupting tooth. Boyne and Sands (1972) demonstrated that the ideal timing for secondary grafting is prior to the eruption of the permanent canine, with excellent restoration of alveolar bone height. Thus close liaison with the orthodontic team is essential. Once grafted, the maxillary arch is stabilized; consequently any orthodontic movement of the maxillary segments must be performed before this time.

Bone graft harvest

Recognized sites for harvest include ileum (considered to be the 'gold standard'—iliac crest or posterior ileum), calvarium, tibia, rib, and mandibular symphysis. The ileum can be harvested by a traditional 'open' approach or by minimally invasive means.

Open iliac crest harvest

The patient is in the supine position, thus allowing concurrent preparation of the recipient site. Intravenous prophylactic antibiotics are administered at induction of anesthaesia. The area of the anterior superior iliac crest is infiltrated with local anaesthesia containing adrenaline. An incision is made parallel and approximately 1 cm inferior to the prominence of the iliac crest in order to ensure that the resulting scar does not lie directly over the crest. The aim is to harvest bone from where the ileum is thickest, namely between the iliac tubercle and the anterior superior iliac spine (ASIS). The immediate vicinity of the ASIS is avoided in order to prevent damage to the lateral femoral cutaneous nerve and the predominant growth centre of the bone. A distinct anatomical junction, corresponding to the cartilaginous cap of the ilium, exists between the insertion of the external oblique muscle fibres and the origin of gluteus medius muscle. This is readily breached with a scalpel, without the need for significant dissection, to form a medially based 'trapdoor' flap. The outermost layer of cancellous bone is discarded because of inevitable 'contamination' with chondrocytes. A block of cancellous bone is harvested by means of a narrow osteotome. If a further graft is required, then a gouge or Volkmann's spoon can be employed. Prior to trapdoor and wound closure, insert a paediatric feeding tube within the ileum in order to infuse bupivicaine post-operatively, thus providing excellent post-operative analgesia, aiding early mobilization.

Recipient site surgical technique

The cleft margins along the alveolus are incised and superiorly based mucoperiosteal flaps are elevated, with care taken not to interfere with the gingivodental junction. The lateral-most incision is extended into the vestibule lateral to the first two teeth, in order to expose the anterior maxilla and piriform aperture for additional grafting. A pocket is made within the cleft, bordered by either alveolar bone or gingival flap, and this potential space is packed with the cancellous autograft previously harvested from the iliac crest. The flaps are closed over the graft in a tension-free manner.

Post-operative management

Patients are kept on a strict fluid/soft food diet for the first 6 weeks. Meticulous oral hygiene is necessary and close parental supervision in this regard is beneficial. Orthodontic assessment of the quality of the graft is made radiologically with the aim to implant within 4–6 months.

Complications

Flap breakdown with bone graft exposure and subsequent infection and resorption of the graft are recognized complications (<2%). Long-bone fracture and pneumothorax have been reported for the tibial and rib donor sites, respectively.

References

Skoog T. (1967). *Scand J Plast Reconstr Surg* **1**, 113–30.
Boyne P, Sands N (1972). *J Oral Surg* **30**, 87–92.

Congenital upper limb anomalies

Incidence
- 1 in 506 live births.
- Male > female.
- 50% bilateral.
- 25% syndromic.

Aetiology
- Mainly unknown.
- Very varied causes may result in similar phenotype.
- Gene defects and embryological studies give us some idea for some conditions.

Classification (IFSSH–Swanson classification)
Failure of formation
- Transverse:
  - Description of level.
- Longitudinal:
  - Radial.
  - Central.
  - Ulnar.
  - Intercalated (phocomelia).

Failure of differentiation
- Soft tissue:
  - Syndactyly.
  - Trigger digit.
  - Camptodactyly.
  - Clasp thumb.
- Skeletal:
  - Clinodactyly.
- Tumerous.

Duplication
- Pre-axial.
- Central.
- Post-axial.

Undergrowth
- Brachydactyly.
- Symbrachydactyly.

Overgrowth
- Level of involvement of macrodactyly/gigantism.

Amniotic band syndrome/constriction ring

Generalized conditions
- Achondroplasia, dyschondroplasia.

Antenatal diagnosis
More obvious defects, such as failures of formation, are sometimes detected antenatally on ultrasound scans. The surgeon may be called upon to advise the parents on what to expect, prognosis, and possible future treatments.

Hand development:
- 0–3 months   ulnar-sided grasp.
- 3–6 months   palmar grasp.
- 6–9 months   extends wrist.
- 9–12 months   palmar pinch, uses thumb for adduction, pinch.

Timing of surgery
There is much discussion on timing of surgery, mostly based on personal preference with no good evidence other than the natural development of hand function. Generally, the earlier the reconstruction the better the integration of the reconstructed part, the more the part anatomically adapts; the growth potential is maximized and physical and psychological scarring is minimized.

Management
- Assess the child and their parents and siblings to detect mild inherited conditions.
- Take a family history.
- Observe the child's hand use and integration.
- Reassure the parents that they were not responsible for the anomaly and briefly explain hand embryology.
- Reassure the parents that even with the most severe anomalies children adapt amazingly.
- Psychological and genetic counselling can be helpful.
- For complex conditions it is wise to have several consultations to help decide the appropriate intervention and prepare the parents.

Indications for surgery
Ensure that treatment is designed to improve the child's function. Consider top and toe needs in bilateral cases. Opposing grasp, with sufficient stability and strength, would be ideal in cases lacking these functions. Always consider growth.

Radial dysplasia

Definition
Congenital failure of formation in longitudinal distribution affecting all pre-axial or radial structures but usually defined by the most obvious deficiency, that of the skeleton.

Incidence
- 1 in 30 000–100 000 live births.
- Half to two-thirds are bilateral, but not symmetrical.
- Type IV with absence > partial absence.
- Males > females.
- Right > left.
- Radial anomalies always associated with thumb anomaly except TAR.
- Thumb hypoplasia 50% associated with anomaly of radius.

Aetiology
- Sporadic, non-inherited.
- Syndromal.
- Teratogens:
  - Thalidomide.
  - Valproic acid.
  - Radiation.

Associated disorders
Frequently found. The most common are:
- VACTERL (VATER).
- Cardiac (septum and radius both form in week 5 of gestation).
- Holt–Oram syndrome (familial, with ASD).
- Gastrointestinal.
- Haemopoietic.
- Thrombocytopenia (thrombocytopenia absent radius (TAR) syndrome).
- Fanconi anaemia (with renal anomalies and pancytopenia).
- Skeletal:
  - Syndactyly.
  - Scoliosis.
  - Sprengel's deformity.
  - Knee deformity (tibia).

Classification (Bayne and Klug 1987)
Types of radial dysplasia:
I   short distal radius (second most common type).
II hypoplastic radius (rarest).
III partial absence.
IV complete absence (most common).

Note absent radius is usually associated with Blauth type 4 or 5 thumb except in TAR syndrome when the thumb is present.

Clinical presentation
At birth the hand and wrist are flexed, supinated, palmar subluxed, and radially displaced. This may be passively reducible. The thumb anomaly is obvious. Clinical severity correlates with radiological severity.

Skeletal
- Radius deficiency ranging from hypoplasia to absence. Distal radius worse affected.
- Fibrous anlage or mesenchymal 'scar' remnant in place of the radius thought to contribute to progressive deformity with growth by tethering.
- Curved ulna secondary to original cause or to tethering of growth.
- Humerus usually shorter then normal, and distal defects of coronoid, capitulum, and medial condyle, with reduced elbow flexion.
- Absent or hypoplastic radial carpal bones, especially scaphoid and trapezium.
- Thumb hypoplasia or absence.

Soft tissue
- Hypoplastic, fused, or absent radial wrist extensors (ECRL/B, BR, APL, EPL/B) and flexors (FPL, FCR), and in severe cases also FDS and EDC muscles and tendons.
- Stiff fingers progressively better as move from radial to ulnar digits.
- Absent radial artery.
- Absent superficial radial nerve and musculocutaneous nerve.
- Abnormal median nerve; may supply areas normally supplied by radial and musculocutaneous nerves.

The more severe the skeletal dysplasia, the more severe is the soft tissue deficiencies.

Management
Assess for associated anomalies.
Passive stretching regime and serial splintage as soon as born.
- Surgery, if indicated to stabilize wrist to improve:
  - Hand position.
  - More effective use of thumb (gets it out of the crotch of the elbow).
  - Flexion strength.
  - Aesthetics.
  - Ulnar epiphysis growth (possibly, by stimulation).
- Contraindications to surgery
  - Bilateral radial dysplasia
  - Lack of elbow flexion.
  - Very short forearm.
  - Severe systemic illness.
  - Adult who has adjusted to deformity.

Surgical principles are to correct
- Alignment of wrist.
- Stability of wrist.
- Tendon transfers to rebalance forces.
- Correct ulnar curvature/bowing.

Timing of surgery

Early (before 6–9 months)
- Type I: do nothing or lengthen radius.
- Type II: lengthen radius.
- Types III and IV: centralization/radialization with or without prior distraction.

Later (9–18 months)
- Pollicization or thumb reconstruction.

Late
- Scar revision.
- Revision of centralization or radialization.
- Distraction lengthening of ulna.
- Osteotomy of ulna.
- Opponensplasty.

Operative options

Distraction of soft tissues
- Indicated if passive reduction of wrist and hand are not possible, and not improved by serial splinting and stretches.
- Preliminary soft tissue distraction lengthening (apply at 6–9 months, distract at 0.5 mm/day for approximately 2 months, stabilize for 1 month, and then definitive operation. (Kessler 1989; Smith and Greene 1995; Tonkin and Nanchahal 1995).

Centralization
- Carpal slot (depth equal to width ulna head) created by excising lunate ± capitate.
- Skeletal shortening by trimming the ulna head but avoiding injury to the physis.
- Insertion of the ulna into the slot and temporary K-wire fixation.
- Ulnar capsulodesis, double-breasted if possible.
- Results in stiffer shorter limb.

Radialization
- Requires full passive correction pre-operatively.
- No carpal bones excised.
- Ulna is placed radial to carpus, overcorrecting the wrist.
- Temporary pin fixation.
- Maximizes lever arm for tendon transfers.
- Tendon transposition of radial deviators to ulnar side of wrist and hand.
- Results in better motion and possibly less disturbance to growth.

Ulnar osteotomy
- May be performed simultaneously or later.
- If performed simultaneously, there is a risk of devascularizing epiphysis.

Osseous support reconstruction
Replace missing radius with free fibula graft or flap (Albee), possibly including the epiphysis (Starr), second toe metatarsal, or index metacarpal.

Ulnocarpal arthrodesis
Usually a salvage procedure when skeletally mature.

Splintage until skeletal maturity is recommended after all procedures

Complications
- Recurrent deformity, especially carpal subluxation.
- Premature distal ulnar epiphyseal closure (maybe worse if operation performed over age 8).
- Wrist stiffness (usually limitation in extension to neutral, and ulnar deviation to neutral).

References
Bayne LG, Klug MS (1987). *J Hand Surg (Am)* **12**, 169–79.
Kessler I (1989). *J Hand Surg (Br)* **14**, 37–42.
Smith AA, Greene TL (1995). *J Hand Surg (Am)* **20**, 420–4.
Tonkin MA, Nanchahal J (1995). *Ann Acad Med Singapore* **24**(Suppl), 101–7.

Ulnar dysplasia

Definition
Defined as a congenital failure of formation of the ulnar portion of the hand and forearm.

Incidence
- 1 in 100 000 live births.
- Ratio of unilateral to bilateral 4:1.
- Males = females.
- Left > right.
- 50% associated with other musculoskeletal anomalies (fibular hemimelia, proximal femoral focal deficiency, phocomelia, scoliosis).
- Not associated with systemic anomalies.

Aetiology
- Sporadic.
- Not related to thalidomide.
- Some concerns raised about the role of hormonal therapy.
- Aetiology is thought be an injury to the zone of polarizing activity (ZPA). This leads to an absent ulnar but also a hand deformity as the ZPA codes for all digits.

Associated disorders
- Commonly found but not specifically related to ulnar dysplasia.
- Mainly skeletal.

Classification
- Use one for forearm and other for hand.
- Classified according to ulna and elbow (Bayne or Baur).

I	Hypoplastic ulna.
II	Partially absent ulna.
III	Absent ulna.
IV	Humeroradial synostosis.

Cole and Manske (1997) classification based on thumb and first web space

A	Normal.
B	Mild first web and thumb deficiency (narrow).
C	Moderate–severe (syndactyly thumb to index, thumb in palmar plane, lack of opposition, absent extension thumb, hypoplastic).
D	Absent thumb.

Clinical presentation
Presents with:
- Hypoplasia of whole upper limb.
- Elbow malformed and unstable with radial head dislocation or fused (radiohumeral synostosis).
- Ulna hypoplastic or absent.
- Radius bowed.
- Hypoplastic or absent digits in all.
- Syndactyly in 30%.
- 70% have some thumb or first web anomaly.
- Usually have less obvious deformity compared with radial dysplasia and good function.

Management
- Assess for associated anomalies.
- Splinting and stretches.
- Surgery.

Indications for surgery
- Syndactyly.
- Thumb hypoplasia.
- First web space deficiency.
- Marked internal rotation.
- Progressive curvature of radius.

Surgical principles are to correct
- Reconstruct thumb and digits to provide prehension.
- Widen and deepen first web space.
- Alignment of wrist and forearm.
- Stability of wrist.
- Tendon transfers to rebalance forces.

Operative options
- Release syndactyly.
- Thumb web procedures.
- Thumb reconstruction.
- Excision of fibrous ulnar anlage.
- Radius osteotomy.
- Radius or ulna lengthening.
- Rotational osteotomy of humerus.
- Rarely, conversion to one bone forearm.

Reference
Cole RJ, Manske PR (1997). *J Hand Surg (Am)* **22**, 479–88.

Cleft hand

Synonyms
Ectrodactyly, lobster claw hand, split hand, median hypoplasia.

Definition
Defined as a congenital failure of formation of the central portion of the hand and forearm. Very variable phenotype from the classic central cleft to single ulnar digit hand, probably related to great variety of pathogenesis.

Incidence
- Estimated at 1 in 30 000–100 000 live births.
- 50% bilateral and involve feet as well.
- Bilateral cases are familial; AD.

Aetiology of cleft hand
- Unknown, but AD relationship with greater then expected penetrance seen in familial types.
- Failure in formation of the interdigital spaces between gestational days 39 and 50. The mesodermal cells necrose between the digits and are replaced by migrating ectodermal cells from the apical ectodermal ridge. Failure of necrosis to occur results in osseous syndactyly; necrosis in the middle of a digit results in polydactyly; excess necrosis results in a cleft.

Associations
- Syndactyly.
- Polydactyly.
- Cross-bones and other bone fusions (proximal phalanx or metacarpals).
- Cleft feet.
- EEC syndrome (ectrodactyly, ectodermal dysplasia, and cleft lip and palate).
- Rarely, associated with deafness, ocular anomalies, Poland syndrome ventricular septal defect (VSD).

Classification
This category used to include typical and atypical cleft hands. Atypical cleft hands had U-shaped clefts with hypoplastic or absent index and middle fingers replaced by nubbins, which demonstrate some movement. Atypical cleft hands are now best classified with symbrachydactyly.

The Japanese classify cleft hands as failure of differentiation on the basis of the frequent association with syndactyly and call this 'syndactyly-cleft hand complex'.

Classified according to description and number of digits or on teratological sequence (with increasing severity of failure of formation) based on presumed aetiology:

- Type 1—central V-shaped cleft with absent middle finger.
- Type 2—central V-shaped cleft with absent middle and index fingers.
- Type 3—central V-shaped cleft with absent, middle, index, and ring fingers.
- Type 4—absent thumb, index, and middle fingers.
- Type 5—monodactylous–little finger only.
- Subtypes—s = syndactylized, p = polydactyly.

Manske's classification
Manske's classification (Table 5.2) is based on quality of thumb and first web as these are more important in hand function than the cleft.

Table 5.2 Manske's classification

Type	Web space	Treatment
1	Normal	Close cleft, excise extra bone, reconstruct transverse metacarpal ligament
2	Narrowed, mild	Close cleft + webplasty
2	Narrowed, severe	Close cleft + flap
3	Syndactylized	Close cleft, release syndactyly + flaps or excise index
4	Merged as missing index	No treatment, stabilize MCPJ
5	No thumb	Toe transfer

Clinical presentation
Presents with absence of the middle finger and to varying degrees the middle metacarpal. The adjacent digits may be absent or present. If present, they are often larger than the other side and frequently syndactylized. With increasing severity the radial side of the cleft becomes absent, leaving a single little finger or in worst cases no digits (peromelia). Cross-bones or fusions are often present in the palm. No carpal anomaly usually.

The intrinsic muscles and long tendons are present but insert anomalously either to the remaining digits or over the stumps.

Factors in management and prognosis
- Quality of thumb.
- Width of first web space.
- Number of digits.
- Movement and alignment of remaining digits.

Management and principles of surgery

Cleft hands are often described as having good function but poor aesthetics.
- Function can be improved by:
  - Increasing first web space.
  - Releasing any syndactyly.
  - Improving motion at MCPJs by excision or release of cross-bones.
  - Releasing PIPJ contractures by Z-plasty, and soft tissue release.
  - Osteotomies of metacarpals to align digits.
  - Improving abduction and opposition of the thumb, and providing opposition posts or digits when absent.
  - Occasionally a digit can be created by straightening and covering a cross-bone.
- Aesthetics are improved by closure of the cleft.

Indications for surgery

- Any deformity detected that may be improved by the above procedures.
- See Manske's classification (Table 5.2) and guide to surgery above.

Operative options for cleft closure

- Snow–Littler technique using a palmar-based flap from the cleft transposed to widen the first web space and simultaneously transposing the index finger at the metacarpal base onto the middle finger metacarpal base.
- Miura–Komada technique uses the same index transposition but with an incision along the web space and around the digit, and a dorsal extension for access to the metacarpal base, thus minimizing the risk of flap necrosis.
- Ueba technique uses the same digit transposition but the flaps lie transverse, with the dorsal flap from one side of the cleft and the palmar flap from the other side of the cleft.

Camptodactyly

Definition
Defined as a flexion deformity (bent over in dorsal/palmar plane) of the PIPJ of congenital origin. From *kampto* (Greek, bend over).

Incidence
- Common, 1% of population.
- Often unreported when mild.
- Most frequent in the little finger.
- Familial in some; AD.
- Two peaks of presentation at early childhood or adolescence, when it frequently presents after trauma. Possibly a female preponderance in the adolescent group.

Aetiology of camptodactyly
Results from a congenital imbalance of flexion and extension forces at the PIPJ.
- Abnormal intrinsics (especially anomalous lumbrical origin or insertion).
- Anomalous flexor digitorum superficialis (absent, shortened, or anomalous origin or insertion).
- Anomalous extensors.

Classification
Classified according to whether it is:
- Isolated deformity, multiple anomalies, or syndromic.
- Childhood or adolescent onset.
- Extensor lag, extensor block, or fixed flexion deformity.

Modified Adams classification
1. Flexion contracture of PIPJ.
2. Partially fixed.
3. Arthrographically fixed (a) without or (b) with changes on X-ray.
4. More than one digit involved.

Clinical presentation
- Presents with a flexion deformity at the PIPJ. Can usually obtain full flexion but full extension may need passive assistance or be impossible. Uncommonly, fixed deformity.
- Often presents with a history of preceding trauma, but this is unrelated.
- Check for other congenital limb anomalies.
- X-rays in adolescents show characteristic changes to the PIPJ:
    - Anvil (wedged) shaped proximal phalanx head.
    - Divot in the articular base of the middle phalanx.
    - Exaggerated subcondylar recess (Drucker's space).
    - PIPJ slopes off to ulnar aspect.
- Extension of the digit reveals the inclination of the joint to the ulnar side by abduction of the middle and distal phalanges.
- Always check function of the ulnar nerve, intrinsics, and the FDS.

Factors in management and prognosis
- Extensor lag, extensor block, or fixed flexion deformity.
- How bad is it?
- Is it symptomatic?
- Progressive?
- Secondary joint deformity present?
- Age of patient?
- Which finger is involved?
- Isolated/multiple?

Management
Splinting and stretches are recommended first.

Indications for surgery
- Contracture greater than 50°–70°.
- Symptoms.
- Failure of conservative therapy.
- Progressive contracture.
- Adams types 1 and 2 can be treated by exploration, release, splintage, and/or tendon transfer.
- Adams type 3(a) is best treated by TATA, and types 3(b) and 4 most successfully by osteotomy.

Principles of camptodactyly surgery
- Skin release.
- Soft tissue and joint release.
- Rebalance flexor and extensor forces.
- Stabilize.
- Reconstruct skin defect.

Operative options
- Exploration for anomaly, resection (and release), and then splintage.
- Tendon transfer to augment extension at central slip utilizing lumbrical, FDS, or EIP, or by extensor plication.
- FDS lasso procedure to increase MCP flexion.
- Total anterior teno-arthrolysis (TATA) (Saffar 1983). Involves a subperiosteal monobloc stripping of the flexor structures from the proximal and middle phalanx including the FDS insertion, palmar plate, and A2 pulley all in continuity, then releasing the PIPJ and subsequent pinning of the joint in extension which re-sets the balance of the flexors.
- Osteotomy to correct flexion and inclination (indicated in older patients with established PIPJ changes not amenable to soft tissue correction).
- Skin release is usually by FTSG or transposition flap from the side of the digit.

Reference
Saffar P (1983). *Ann Chir Main* **2**, 345–50.

Clinodactyly

Definition
Inclined (bent sideways) digit of congenital origin. Usually bent at middle phalanx level.

Incidence
- Common.
- Under-reported.
- Frequently familial (AD with incomplete penetrance).
- Usually little finger, angled towards ring finger at the middle phalanx.
- Usually bilateral.
- Occurs in other digits as part of brachydactyly and other conditions.

Aetiology
- Unknown.
- Deformity usually due to a longitudinal bracketed (C-shaped) epiphysis of the middle phalanx. Instead of a transverse physis at the proximal end of the phalanx, this abnormal physis extends as a C around the digit (usually with the open part of the C facing towards the ulna. The longitudinal portion of the physis prevents longitudinal growth on this side and encourages wedge-shaped growth of the phalanx.

Classification
Descriptive classification of degree of inclination and digit involved.

Clinical presentation
- Presents as a bent finger, appears angled sideways at the distal phalanx. May give a history of preceding trauma, which is unrelated.
- Check the opposite hand and parents.

Factors in management and prognosis
- How bad is it?
- Is it symptomatic?
- Progressive?
- Age of patient?
- Which finger is involved?
- Isolated anomaly or part of multiple anomalies?

Indications for surgery
- Inclination greater than 50°–70°.
- Symptoms (overlaps ring finger).
- Failure of conservative therapy.
- Progressive inclination.

Principles of clinodactyly surgery
- Skin release.
- Correct skeletal deformity.
- Reconstruct skin defect.

Operative management options
- Epiphyseolysis (Langenskiold described the destruction of the anomalous portion of the physis preventing further deformity and, if performed early enough, even allowing growth to correct the deformity).
- Closing wedge osteotomy.
- Opening wedge osteotomy.
- Exchange wedge osteotomy.

Reference
Langenskiold (1975). *JBJS* **57**(3): 325.

Clasp thumb

Definition
Thumb anomaly where it is flexed in the palm and not seen to extend. This is normal in babies under 6 weeks. Not to be confused with thumb-in-palm anomaly.

Incidence
- Variable.
- In some, due to hypoplasia of EPL.
- Association with digitotalar syndrome and Freeman–Sheldon syndrome ('whistling face syndrome').

Classification
Weckesser (Reed and Heiple) classification
1. Deficient extension.
2. Flexion contracture combined with deficient extension.
3. Hypoplasia of the thumb.
4. Others.

McCarroll classification
- Supple (absent EPL).
- Complex. (absent EPL and in addition a flexion contracture of the MCPJ, lax collateral ligaments, thenar hypoplasia, adduction of the CMCJ, and inadequate skin).

Clinical presentation
- Presents with parents noticing that the thumb is kept in the palm.
- May be first presentation of thumb hypoplasia or mild radial club hand.

Management
- Initially splint the thumb in extension; majority improve.
- Surgical management by tendon transfer using EDM, BR + PL graft (Flatt), ECU (Kelikan), or FDS (Crawford). Note that EI is also frequently absent.
- Complex thumbs may also need extensive palmar release, opponensplasty, and ulnar collateral ligament reconstruction.

Indications for surgery
- Failure of splinting, with failure of thumb extension.

References
Weckesser (1968). *J Bone Joint Surg (Am)* **50**: 1417–28.
McCarroll (1985). *Hand Clin* **1**: 567–75.

Trigger digit

Definition
Congenital discrepancy between the size of the pulley and the size of the flexor tendon leads to flexion contracture of the digit or less commonly the triggering one sees in adults.

Incidence
- Trigger thumb common.
- Trigger finger rare.

Aetiology
- Mostly sporadic and isolated.
- Note that it is common in complete obstetrical brachial plexus palsy children, indicating a growth cause.

Clinical presentation
- The child presents with a digit locked in flexion or extension. Most present in first year of age, but can present much later.
- A palpable nodule, called Notta's node, may be felt.

Classification
- Fixed.
- Mobile.

Management
- It is reported that one in three cases of trigger thumb self-resolve with stretches and splinting if mobile but triggering at presentation. However, the thumbs do not improve sufficiently to allow normal hyperextension.
- Operative release of the A1 pulley should be performed for full recovery.
- Finger triggering does not seem to resolve and should be treated operatively. Steroid injections are not indicated in children unless there is pathology such as diabetes or inflammatory arthritis.

Operation
Under GA incise transversely at the level of the MCPJ flexion crease, blunt dissect to expose the A1 pulley, and divide the pulley on its radial aspect (to avoid inadvertent injury to the oblique pulley). Suture the wound with absorbable mattress suture to ensure wound eversion in the flexion crease. Mobilize.

Outcome
Full recovery with a barely visible scar. Notta's node tends to resolve.

Syndactyly

Definition
Digits that are joined together are syndactylized. The term is usually used to describe congenital failure of separation, but can apply to post burn or trauma fusion of digits.

Incidence
- Most common hand anomaly or second most common hand anomaly after polydactyly.
- 1 in 650–2000 births.
- Males to female ratio 2:1.
- Highest incidence is second post-axial web space, i.e. second web in foot and third web in hand.
  - 50% third web space in hand.
  - 30% fourth web space.
  - 15% second web space.
  - 5% first web space.

Aetiology
- Unknown.
- Familial in 20% of cases.
- AD inheritance with incomplete penetration and variable expression.
- Failure of separation linked to steroids, fibroblast growth factor receptor deficiency.
- Some congenital cases are due to trauma and healing, as in amniotic band/constriction ring syndrome.

Associated disorders
- Apert's syndrome.
- Poland syndrome.
- Symbrachydactyly.
- Aarskog's syndrome.
- Acropectovertebral dysplasia.
- Many other syndromes and chromosomal anomalies.

Classification
Congenital syndactyly lies within the failure of differentiation category.

Syndactyly is classified according to whether it is
- Complete (extends to tips) or incomplete.
- Simple or complex (bone involved), or acrosyndactyly (digit tips fused but bases free).
- Single or multiple.
- Unilateral or bilateral.
- Hand, foot, or both,
- Isolated deformity, multiple anomalies, or syndromic.

Temtamy and McKusick (1956) classification
- Type I: second post axial web syndactyly.
- Type II: synpolydactyly (third web syndactyly and duplication finger 3 or 4.
- Type III: ring and little finger syndactyly.
- Type IV: complete syndactyly all fingers.
- Type V: syndactyly associated with metacarpal/tarsal synostosis.

Clinical presentation
- Presents at birth with joined fingers. Some mild incomplete cases may not be detected until later in life.
- Assess the web involved: whether the union is skin only or involves nails or bone.
- Assess the pattern of bone involvement and the differentiation of bone and joints, nailbed and nailfold, quality of skin and soft tissues, degree of syndactyly.
- Assess possible skin donor sites.

Timing of surgery
Some suggest results are poorer if done at less than 18 months of age; others say hand development occurs between 6–24 months and so it is important to perform surgery before then. Where digits involved are of different lengths it is important to separate before deformity occurs. Personally, I do the separation bilaterally before the child is 12 months of age.

Principles of syndactyly surgery
- Problems:
  - Skin shortage (circumference of two separate digits is greater than circumference of two fingers together (Flatt)).
  - Fascial connections running transverse between the digits.
  - Tendinous connections, (e.g. pollex abductus between EPL and FPL).
  - Neurovascular connections; distal division of nerve or vessel, Hartman loops (neural loop penetrations by digital arteries).
  - Bone, joined, inadequately formed, delta phalanges.
  - Joints, usually symphalangism.
- Principles:
  - Creating a web space sloping at 45° from dorsal to palmar with a free transverse distal edge.
  - An aesthetic slightly hour-glassed shape.
  - No scar contracture.
  - Minimally visible scars on dorsum.
  - No longitudinal scars on the digits.
  - Generally avoid separating a digit on both sides (in a three- or four-digit syndactyly) as there may be a risk to vascularity of the digit.

Operative options
- Digital separation is by a zig-zag design (Cronin 1956) creating interdigitating triangular skin flaps of varying width from the dorsum and palmar aspects of the digits to cover the sides of the same digits once separated. These flaps avoid creation of longitudinal scars along the digits which may cause flexion contracture. In digits with symphalangism (e.g. Apert's syndrome) longitudinal division is permissible as flexion contracture will not occur.
- Many more surgical options are described for web reconstruction. Most require skin grafts to fill in the lateral web/digital defect created by transposition of the dorsal web flap. Most use a modification of the Bauer (1956) design, which creates a dorsal rectangular flap to recreate the web space, or opposing palmar and dorsal triangles, or an omega and anchor design.
- There are techniques that avoid skin grafts by redistributing the dorsal digital skin (Niranjan, Giele).
- For complicated syndactyly some surgeons have attempted:
    - Using distraction of the digital skeleton laterally from the involved web.
    - Tissue expansion of the dorsal skin.
    - These techniques are not generally used because of the very high complication rate.
    - Reconstruction of the lateral nailfolds is by Buck-Gramcko triangular pulp flaps.
    - Skin cover by abdominal, groin, or thenar flaps have been described.

Complications
- Injury or inability to separate digital neurovascular bundles.
- Web creep (reconstructed web creeps to a more distal location due to digital scarring and growth). More common in complex syndactyly.
- Deformity of digit (flexion and lateral curvature due to scarring, growth disturbance due to length inequality between syndactylized digits).
- Hyperpigmentation of skin graft.
- Hair growth in skin graft.
- Skin graft loss or flap necrosis leading to delayed healing and scarring.

References
Bauer TB, Tondra JM, Trusler HM (1956). *Plast Reconstr Surg* **17**, 385–92.
Cronin TD (1956). *Plast Reconstr Surg* **18**, 460–8.
Niranjan N (2005). *BJPS* **58**: 15–21.
Temtamy SA, McKusick VA (1978). *Birth Defects* **14**, 1–619.

Polydactyly

Definition
Congenital formation of extra digit or part thereof.

Incidence
Most common congenital upper limb anomaly.

Aetiology
- Unknown.
- Can be hereditary (ususally autosomal recessive) especially if duplicated little finger.
- Associated with many syndromes such as Ellis–van Creveld syndrome, Lawrence–Moon–Bardet–Biedl syndrome, trisomy 13, Biemond syndrome.

Classification
Stelling classification for fingers:
A   Incomplete digit, soft tissue only, often attached by small pedicle.
B   Complete digit.
C   Complete digit and metacarpal.
Type A is the most common by far, and usually occurs on the ulnar border of the little finger at the level of the proximal phalanx.

Clinical presentation
Presents with extra digit noted at birth.

Management
- **Type A** Some midwives try strangulating the polydactyly by ligating it with silk. However, this is painful, and leaves a tender nodule on the contact ulnar border of the little finger due to the underlying neuroma. There is an apocryphal tale of a baby who bled to death after such a ligation! Excision is kindest. This can be done soon after childbirth under local anaesthesia, or under general anaesthesia at a later age. The principle of excision is to excise the stump with an ellipse ensuring adequate skin for tension-free closure, dissect out the neurovascular bundle with diathermy, and divide this sufficiently away from the skin so as to avoid a tender neuroma. Close with absorbable sutures.
- **Type B** Excision following the principles above. Beware that more skin is required than first appearances. If central polydactyly, may need to correct adjacent anomalies in bone or soft tissue.
- **Type C** Excision of the whole ray, closure of the space, and creation of the inter-metacarpal ligament. Try to excise a central rather than a border ray if there is no obvious choice.

Outcome
- In type A, a completely normal hand function, minimal scar.
- In type B, depending on the digit involved excision will leave a normally functioning hand. Occasionally a central polydactyly may cause adjacent growth or developmental anomaly inhibiting completely normal function.
- Type C leaves a normally functioning hand but there may be some widening of the interdigital space and scissoring if the central ray is excised.

Thumb duplication

Thumb duplication differs from other types of digital polydactyly in the complexity of the polydactyly and hence the reconstruction.

Classification
Wassel based his classification on the most proximal level of the duplication:
- Type 1 duplication   distal phalanx.
- Type 2 duplication   to IPJ.
- Type 3 duplication   proximal phalanx.
- Type 4 duplication   to MCPJ.
- Type 5 duplication   metacarpal.
- Type 6 duplication   to CMCJ.
- Type 7 duplication   triphalangeal thumb.

Note that even-numbered types are duplications to joint level. A Stelling A polydactyly type duplication of the thumb connected by a thin soft tissue pedicle (usually at the level of the metacarpophalangeal joint) is not covered adequately by this classification. It is sometimes described as a rudimentary thumb.

Incidence
One of the most common congenital hand anomalies. Most common type is type 4, next most common is type 2, then type 6.

Management
- Assess the level of duplication, development, and stability of the joints, and axial deviation of each element.
- Treatment does **not** consist of simple excision of the extra thumb.
- Excision of the most hypoplastic thumb if obvious, along with realignment of the skeletal axis by osteotomies, and reconstruction of the collateral ligaments. Osteotomies are needed to align the joint surfaces and the axis of the phalanges and to thin the widened metacarpal or phalangeal head. Realignment of the flexor and extensor tendon may also be needed.
- If 'balanced' thumbs with equal size, then options are to excise the radial most thumb preserving the thumb with the ulnar collateral ligaments and reconstructing the radial collateral ligaments, or to combine the two thumbs either equally as in the Bilhaut–Cloquet procedure or by using elements from one thumb to augment the retained thumb.
- Bilhaut–Cloquet procedure is the division of the two thumbs into two equal longitudinal halves, the outer elements of which are then joined together to create one thumb. The disadvantages are a frequently split nail and an incongruous and stiff IPJ.

Outcome
- In many cases the thumb is smaller and stiffer than the opposite thumb. This does not substantially effect function.
- Revision for zig-zag deformity is common if the osteotomies are not performed.

Congenital radial head dislocation

Definition
Defined as a congenital dislocation of the radial head. May occur as part of other anomaly such as ulnar dysplasia.

Incidence
- Most common elbow anomaly.
- Usually bilateral (60%).
- 40% AD.

Aetiology
- Hypoplastic capitellum.
- Hypoplastic forearm.
- Ulna may be short and have a negative variance.

Classification
- Posterior 65% (may restrict extension, head thin).
- Anterior 18% (may erode humerus and restrict flexion, head round).
- Lateral 17% (usually asymptomatic but more obvious).

Clinical presentation
- Presents at age 3–5 years; occasionally at birth with prominence or mass.
- Rarely causes pain or clicking; usually no loss of movement; no history of trauma; cannot reduce; pain may occur when older.
- Differentiate from pulled elbow, nurse maid's elbow, developmental radial head dislocation due to abnormal growth forces.
- Associated with numerous skeletal anomalies including Apert's syndrome.

Management
- Observation and reassurance.
- If surgery needed, results are better if treated early.

Indications for surgery
- Restriction of movement.
- Pain.
- Deformity.

Operative options
- Open reduction and reconstruction of annular ligament using triceps fascia.
- Shorten proximal radius.
- Lengthen biceps tendon to reduce deforming forces.
- Excise radial head at skeletal maturity (if done earlier the radius will migrate causing a wrist anomaly).
- Consider one bone forearm if very severe.

Radioulnar synostosis

Definition
Congenital fusion of radius and ulna. Failure of differentiation.

Incidence
- Rare.
- Bilateral in 60%.
- Female = male.

Aetiology
- Mostly sporadic.
- Some inherited AD with incomplete penetrance and variable expression.
- Associated with large range of limb and other congenital anomalies and some syndromes (mandibulofacial dysostosis, acrocephalopolysyndactyly, XXY, etc).

Clinical presentation
- The problem is loss of forearm rotation.
- Fixed pronation position but patients adapt through the radio carpal joint and there is little functional loss.
- Cleary and Omer (1985) found no association between the position of the forearm and level of synostosis, or between the position of the forearm and function.

Classification
- Depends on site: proximal, distal, or combined (latter two very rare).
- Or Cleary and Omer types.
  1. Fibrous union.
  2. Osseous synostosis.
  3. Osseous synostosis with hypoplastic posteriorly dislocated radial head.
  4. Osseous synostosis with anterior dislocated malformed radial head.

Management
- Do nothing, most patients adapt.
- There are some cultures where the forearm needs a certain position, e.g. full supination to hold a rice bowl in Asian cultures. Therefore intervention may be needed.
- Surgery may be indicated when there is fixed full pronation or pronation >60°.
- Best performed before the child is 6 years old.

Operative options
- De-rotation osteotomy to 10°–20° pronation position.
  - Proximal through fusion mass (Green and Mittal 1979).
  - Distal through each bone separately.
- Excision of synostosis and interposition of vascularized tissue.

Outcome
- Never improves as much as you would like.
- High complication rate of 20–30% including compartment syndrome, nerve and vascular injury, loss of movement, recurrence.

References
Cleary JE, Omer GE Jr (1985). *J Bone Joint Surg (Am)* **67**, 539–45.
Green and Mittal (1979). *J Bone Joint Surg (Am)* **61**: 738–43.

Thumb hypoplasia

Definition
Defined as a congenital hypoplasia or aplasia of the thumb. May fall in the failure of formation or in the hypoplasia category of the IFSSH classification.

Incidence
- Isolated.
- May occur as part of another condition such as radial dysplasia, cleft hand, symbrachydactyly.

Aetiology of isolated thumb hypoplasia
- Unknown.
- Fetal neurogenic injury.
- Thalidomide.
- Reduced oxygen tension.

Classification (Blauth 1967)
I   Smaller thumb, all structures present.
II   Hypoplastic thenar muscles; also hypoplasia of thumb metacarpal, phalanges, and radial carpal bones. There may be only one neurovascular bundle.
III   Absent thenar muscles, very reduced first web space, ulnar collateral ligament instability of the MCPJ. Varying degrees of partial aplasia of the proximal thumb metacarpal, and thumb extrinsic muscles (EPL, APL, EPB, FPL).
- IIIa With a CMCJ, hypoplastic extrinsic muscles.
- IIIb Without a CMCJ, thumb extrinsic extensors absent.

IV   Pouce flottant, (floating thumb or pendeldaumen). No metacarpal or musculotendinous structures.
V   Absent thumb.

This classification does not cover transverse absence of the thumb.

Clinical presentation
Presents with obvious thumb anomaly at birth. Assess the thumb looking for defects in the structures as listed in the classification. Mild thumb hypoplasia may be not noticed for years or ever!

Indications for surgery
- Type I may require no intervention.
- Types II and IIIa need to increase the first web space, stabilize the MCP joint, improve opposition, improve flexion and extension at the IPJ.
- Type IIIb is debatable: some attempt reconstruction and others excise.
- Types IV and V: pollicization of the index finger gives the best outcome.

Principles of surgery
- Increase function and appearance.
- Try to reconstruct all deficiencies in one operation.
- Try to do before 1 year old or preferably before 9 months as that is when full thumb function commences.

Operative options
- Increase the first web space width and depth:
  - Z-plasty.
  - Four-flap Z-plasty.
  - Flying man flap.
  - Dorsal rotational flap.
  - Transposing flap from index (Spinner).
  - Transposing flap from thumb (Strauch).
  - Pedicled groin flap.
  - Pedicled posterior interosseous artery flap.
  - Free groin flap.
  - Full thickness skin graft (from polydactylous digit if present).
- MCPJ stabilization (UCL reconstruction):
  - UCL plication.
  - Soft tissue gubbinsoplasty.
  - Ligament reconstruction with tendon graft (PL or EDM).
  - Ligament reconstruction with end of tendon used for opponensplasty. FDS ring finger tendon is used with one slip attached to radial side thumb MCPJ and used as opponensplasty and the other slip passed through metacarpal head to ulnar side and attached to the base of proximal phalanx.
  - Fusion.
- Opposition:
  - ADM (Huber–Nicolayson).
  - FDS ring finger.
- Extension and flexion:
  - EIP or EDM transfer.
  - Release pollex abductus tendon anomaly.
  - Flexor pulley reconstruction with FDS end, extensor hood.
  - FPL tendon reconstruction.
  - Fusion of IPJ.
- Pollicization.

Pollex abductus is the abduction of the thumb at the MCPJ when FPL contracts due to an anomalous insertion onto the extensor mechanism, the tight first web space, and the laxity of the UCL (Tupper).

Musculus lumbricalis pollicis is an anomalous muscle arising from the FPL passing across the first web space and attaching to the extensor hood of the index finger, perhaps contributing to the tight first web space (Lister).

Reference
Blauth W (1967). *Arch Orthop Unfallchir* **62**, 225–46.

Brachydactyly

Definition
Short fingers due to congenital anomaly.

Incidence
- Most common forms such as little finger clinodactyly are common, asymptomatic and often unnoticed.
- Inherited forms are uncommon.

Aetiology
- Mostly inherited AD.
- Sometimes syndromic (achondroplasia, hereditary multiple exostosis, Down's syndrome, Apert's syndrome, etc.).
- Can be part of systemic condition like pseudo-hypoparathyroidism (short metacarpals).

Clinical presentation
- The shortened digits may not be noticed until later in life.
- Other associated anamolies (syndactyly, symphalangism) may be more obvious.

Classification (Bell)
A Short middle phalanges:
 A1 Short middle phalanges (Farabee).
 A2 Delta middle phalanges: index finger and toe 2 (Mohr–Wriedt).
 A3 Delta middle phalanges: little finger (Bauer).
 A4 Short middle phalanges: index and little fingers (Temtamy).
 A5 No middle finger, small distal phalanges, tiny nails (Bass).
B Short distal phalanx, no nail (MacKinder).
C Short middle phalanges except ring finger, hyperphalangism of index and middle proximal phalanx (Drinkwater).
D Short distal phalanx thumb (Breitenbecher).
E Short metacarpals and metatarsals (Bell).
F Other (Pitt–Williams, Sugarman, smorgasbord (Meiselman et al. 1989)).

Management
- Good function means that little intervention is required.
- Longitudinally bracketed epiphyses may benefit from epiphyseolysis.
- Mature deformities causing functional problems may respond to osteotomies.
- Lengthening rarely indicated, but can be done acutely or by distraction.

Indications for surgery
- Treat associated conditions such as syndactyly.
- Functional problem (e.g. palpable painful short metacarpal head in palmar grip, piano playing with single short digit).
- Aesthetic loss of hand shape.
- Most patients do not need surgery.

Operative options
- Opening wedge osteotomy for angulated delta phalanges.
- Epiphysiolysis for angulated phalanges associated with longitudinally bracketed epiphysis.
- Immediate or single-stage lengthening, usually with interposition bone graft.
- Distraction lengthening.

Reference
Meiselman SA, Berkenstadt M, Ben-Ami T, Goodman RM (1989). *Clin Genet* **35**, 261–7.

Symbrachydactyly

Definition
Strictly translated as short fingers with stiff joints—a spectrum of digital failure of development, tending to preserve the thumb.

Incidence
One in 10 000.

Aetiology
- Mostly sporadic.
- Thought to be a mesodermal defect leaving ectodermal remnants such as skin and nails as nubbins.
- Sometimes associated with Poland syndrome.

Clinical presentation
- Symbrachydactyly has a spectrum of presentation.
- The best cases have all digits and all phalanges present but the fingers are slightly shorter and stiffer. This form can be indistinguishable from brachydactyly.
- The most extreme end of the spectrum has a transverse failure of formation which may be through the level of the forearm. This form can be indistinguishable from transverse failure of formation/reduction defect. Often there may be rudimentary digital remnants or 'nubbins' which suggests symbrachydactyly rather than reduction.
- Between these two extremes there are reducing patterns of digital loss (teratological sequence), starting with loss of the middle phalanges, then the distal phalanges, and then the metacarpals.
- The pattern with short/absent middle fingers preserving thumb and little finger was/is called atypical cleft hand.
- The pattern of loss tends to be more severe on the ulnar side, initially sparing the thumb.
- Compare with cleft hand when the tendency is to spare the ulnar side so that the extreme end of the spectrum has just a little finger.

Classification
Based on the teratological sequence and level of missing parts (Yamauchi):
- Triphalangia.
- Diphalangia.
- Monophalangia.
- Aphalangia.
- Ametacarpia.
- Acarpia.
- Forearm amputation.

Management
- In symbrachydactyly with short fingers no intervention is indicated as function is good.
- Where digits are absent (oligodactyly) the number of digits and their function determines treatment.

Operative options
- First web space release/deepening.
- Toe phalanx non-vascularized transfer.
- Toe transplant.
- On-top-plasty (parts of another digit transferred on-top of short digit).
- Distraction lengthening.

Macrodactyly

Definition
- Congenital overgrowth of digit.
- May be a component of other hypertrophic conditions or gigantism.
- Should be differentiated from secondary causes of a large digit but often is not.

Incidence
- Rare (2 per 100 000 live births).
- 1% of all congenital upper limb anomalies.
- Most common form is progressively growing lipofibromatous nerve overgrowth.
- 90% unilateral.
- 70% have more than one digit involved, usually adjacent.
- Index and middle digits most commonly affected than thumb.
- Distal elements usually worse affected than proximal elements.

Aetiology
- Unknown; probably different causes depending on type.
- ?Neural growth factor related.

Classification
- Primary or secondary.
- Static or progressive.

Primary
- Unknown cause.
- Congenital.
- Non-syndromic.
- Usually found to have generalized enlargement, particularly soft tissue enlargement of lipofibromatous tissue around the digital nerves.
- Often follows a nerve-like distribution and so can be seen to affect one side of a digit or frequently follows a median nerve distribution.
- Sometimes called *macrodystrophia lipoidotica* or *macrodactyly dystrophia lipomatosa progressiva*.

Secondary
- Related to other conditions or syndromes such as:
  - Neurofibromatosis.
  - Vascular malformations: both high-flow arterio-venous, and low-flow capillary-venous as in Klippel–Trenaunay–Weber syndrome or Maffucci's syndrome.
  - Enchondromatosis as in Ollier's disease.
  - Bone enlargement in Albright's polyostotic fibrous dysplasia or in acromegaly.
  - Congenital lymphoedema.
  - Proteus syndrome and others.

Pathology

Pathologically four types have been described:
1. Lipofibromatous.
2. Neurofibromatous.
3. Hyperostotic.
4. Hemi-hypertrophy or Proteus syndrome.

- Lipofibromatous is most common; primary and progressive. Apart from the proliferation of lipofibromatous tissue around the neurovascular bundles there is marked enlargement and fibrosis of the nerves and vessels similar to that found in median nerve lipomatosis or lipofibromatous hypertrophy of nerves. There is also periosteal fibrosis with foci of cartilage and bone formation. Enchondromatous metaplasia within diffuse periosteal fibromatosis has been described.
- Neurofibromatosis is secondary, progressive, and associated with the other signs of NF.
- Hyperostotic describes multiple osseous nodules that form soon after birth and grow. Note that bone growth also occurs in lipofibromatous and neurofibromatous types, but is a more regular expansion of the bone in the area affected.
- Proteus syndrome is characterized by hyperplasia of connective tissue including vessels and of bone. Often generalized gigantism of a limb or half a body.

Clinical presentation

- May be present at birth or may only be noticed after some years.
- Static or progressive growth:
  - Static form usually presents at birth and grows in proportion to other digits.
  - Progressive form may not be present at birth but appears in early childhood and grows rapidly and disproportionately to the other digits until puberty is complete.
- Skeletal involvement leads to stiffness and deformity, usually extended and inclined posture.
- Stiffness and deviation of the digits are common sequelae.

Management

Examination
Assess size difference, deviation or deformity, pattern of involvement. Look for secondary signs of other causes or syndromes. Look at other digits and measure the whole limb and compare. Look for movement, interference with the use of the other digits. Assess passive movement, vascularity. Palpate for masses.

X-ray
To assess the skeleton and joints. May see evidence of arthritis, osteophytes, hyperostotic masses, enlargement in width and length of bone, angulation, and inclination.

Indications for surgery
- Interference with function.
- Digit size approximates adult size.
- Large digit interfering with function, including social functioning.

Principles of surgery
- Create a relatively normal sized digit with some function.
- Do not interfere with function of the adjacent digits.

Operative options
- Amputation (only when all else fails and interferes with function; except for toes of course).
- Reduction (by combination of bone excision, osteotomies to correct angulation, and soft tissue excision, perhaps including the nerve);
- Epiphysiodesis (indicated where not severe and when at age 10 digit is already the size of the parents' digits. Usually is an epiphysiolysis rather then an epiphysiodesis. Secondary surgery may be needed to correct deformity. If done too early, can give very fat finger.)
- Excision of nerve to inhibit growth. (Believed by some to halt further growth but not proven!)

Reduction of macrodactyly (Hoshi–Ogino method)
Mid-lateral incision, particularly the convex side of the digit, extending in an L-shaped pattern at the pulp. Excise fat, the enlarged digital nerve, and the overlying skin. Perform a closing wedge osteotomy of the proximal phalanx and excise sufficient middle and distal phalanx to shorten the digit and fuse the DIPJ. Do a nail-plasty to reduce the length and width of the nail.

Alternative method (Barsky)
Bilateral mid-lateral incision with dorsal transverse joining incision at level mid-middle phalanx to create proximally based flap. Excise dorsal excess skin. Preserve nail on palmar flap, excise head middle phalanx and base distal phalanx, and fuse DIPJ. Later, excise dog-ear on pulp. The Tsuge method is similar but keeps nail on dorsal skin and excises palmar skin.

Outcome
- Generally poor, but better than no treatment.
- Often need secondary surgery.

Amniotic band syndrome

Also known as constriction ring syndrome. A congenital disorder mostly affecting the limbs but occasionally seen around the trunk and face.

Classification
Four types (Patterson):
- Circular groove.
- With distal oedema.
- With acrosyndactyly.
- Intra-uterine amputation.

Aetiology
- Intrinsic cause: band-like apoptosis.
- Extrinsic cause: amniotic band wound around extremities, possibly related to perforation of the sac.

Incidence
- Right = left.
- 50% of cases have another limb affected.
- Mostly distal parts affected.

Clinical findings
- Clinically, appearances are diagnostic, especially in types 1, 2, and 3. With amputation the diagnosis is more difficult, although there is tapering of the stumps and there are no nail remnants, unlike symbrachydactyly.
- X-rays show amputation occurring through bone or joint.
- What is left is not hypoplastic, and proximal structures are all present. This may influence reconstruction.
- There may be a temperature difference above and below the band even after it is treated.
- There may be major nerve involvement/division.

Treatment
- Release of acrosyndactyly if present before growth disturbance occurs.
- Z-plasty (multiple circumferential if required).
- Fat contouring (Upton has reported bunched up fat at each side of the band so that it is necessary to undermine the skin and redistribute the fat).
- Lengthening the thumb may be indicated; usually by toe transfer.
- On-top-plasty (extending the length of the thumb by moving the index on top) is rarely indicated.
- Early surgery if there is vascular compromise, severe lymphoedema, or acrosyndactyly affecting development.
- Urgent surgery rare.
- Treatment of distal lymphoedema may be needed.

Arthrogryposis

Definition
Arthrogryposis means curved joints (described by Rosenkrantz in 1905). Arthrogryposis is a term which groups together a heterogenous group of over 150 conditions. The key features are the presence of joint contractures at birth affecting at least two different areas, which are non-progressive and associated with muscle wasting.

Incidence
- One in 3000 live births has arthrogryposis multiplex congenita (AMC).
- Most common forms are amyoplasia ('classic arthrogryposis'), Freeman–Sheldon ('whistling face'), and distal forms.

Aetiology
- Unknown.
- Not inherited, sporadic.
- Considered failure of differentiation.
- Theories:
  - Obstruction to fetal movement.
  - Increased intra-uterine pressure, oligohydramnios.
  - Viral infection (Akabane virus in sheep).
  - Toxins such as chronic cyanide intoxication.
  - Aplasia of muscle due to embryonic failure of development.
  - Exposure of mother to paralyzing agents.
- Pathogenesis is *in utero* muscle fibre loss resulting in a fibrous fatty inelastic muscle belly. This occurs earlier and more severely in certain muscle groups, leading to muscle imbalance and joint contractures.

Classification
Classified according to whether it is myopathic or neuropathic but in practice impossible to distinguish.

Clinical presentation
- Presents with characteristic upper limb posture of shoulder internal rotation and adduction, elbow extension, forearm pronation, and wrist and finger flexion with the thumbs clasped in the palm.
- Lower limbs have hip dislocation, subluxed knees, and club feet.
- Lack of movement results in lack of flexion creases.
- Muscle atrophy results in fusiform joint appearance, although this is sometimes disguised by the subcutaneous fat.
- Disease is not progressive, although supple joints in the affected limbs at birth may contract due to lack of movement.
- Sensation is normal.
- Intellect is unaffected.
- Life expectancy is normal.

Associations
- Klippel–Feil syndrome.
- Sprengel's deformity.
- Hypoplastic mandible.
- Cleft palate.
- Dislocated radial head.
- Renal anomalies.
- Congenital heart disease.

Management
- Multidisciplinary.
- Stretches and splinting.
- Lower limb: aim for ambulation, stability.
- Upper limb: aim for hands to be able to be used at a desktop rather than one hand extended for toileting and the other flexed for feeding.
- Maintain movement.

Indications for surgery

Shoulder internal rotation contracture
- External de-rotation osteotomy of humerus.

Elbow extension contracture
- Triceps release and posterior capsulotomy.
- Active flexion by transfer:
  - Triceps to bicep.
  - Steindler flexorplasty.
  - Pectoralis major: unipolar or bipolar.
  - Latissimus dorsi.
  - ?Free gracilis innervated by intercostals.

Wrist flexion and pronation, and ulnar deviation
- Dorsal carpal closing wedge osteotomy (note carpal coalition).
- Proximal row or total carpectomy.
- Radius and ulnar decompression osteotomies.
- Flexor carpi ulnaris to extensor carpi radialis transfer in conjunction with any of above.

Finger flexion
- Osteotomies to correct flexion.
- Tendon transfers (FDS to extensor lateral bands).

Thumb in palm (flexion adduction contracture)
- Thenar muscle release.
- Thenar crease release with index transposition or Cadbury flap (four-flap Z-plasty).

Madelung's deformity

Madelung described this deformity in 1878 but credited Dupuytren.

Definition
Defined as a congenital 'dinner-fork' deformity of the distal radius and wrist.

Incidence
- Inheritable, AD, incomplete penetrance.
- Usually bilateral.
- Females > males.

Aetiology
- Anomaly of ulnar palmar aspect of the distal radial growth plate such that radial side grows but an abnormal bone bar on the ulnar side tethers growth.
- Early closure of ulnar aspect of distal radius physis.
- Abnormal radiolunate ligament.
- Associated with Leri–Weill mesomelic dwarfism, dyschondrostosis, and now with *SHOX* gene (short stature homeobox gene; if missing both, called Langer mesomelic dysplasia). This gene affects the mid-portion of the upper and lower limb, and so sitting height is close to normal.
- Also associated with achondroplasia, Turner's syndrome, and nail–patella syndrome.
- Related to reverse Madelung 'chevron carpus'.

Classification
- Ulno-dorsal (most common pattern).
- Ulno-palmar (causes more functional problems).

Clinical presentation
- Presents (usually at age 8–12 years) with spontaneous palmar subluxation of the wrist with increasing radio-palmar and ulnar tilt due to abnormal growth forces, producing a dinner-fork-like deformity.
- Short bowed radius (curve is dorsal and ulnar).
- Inclined (to palmar and ulnar) articular surface.
- Dorsally prominent ulna head.
- Triangular shape proximal carpus with lunate apparently retracted in between radius and ulna.
- Ulna carpal impingement.

Management
- Observation and reassurance as most have excellent function.
- Consider surgery.

Indications for surgery
- Pain secondary to impingement or degeneration.
- Deformity (be wary if this is the prime indication).

Operative options

- If before skeletal maturity (best at age 10–12 years), consider epiphysiolysis (Langenskiold, Vickers).
- If skeletally mature consider a volar approach, release pronator quadratus, expose distal radius, release ligament, do dome osteotomy radius, rotate distal radius.
- All achieve decreased pain, better appearance.
- Some recommend wedge osteotomy or excision of ulnar head or fusion, but none of these appear to have good results.
- Distraction has been described prior to surgery, but results are similar.
- Ulnar shortening for ulnar impaction.

Poland syndrome

Pectoral and hand anomalies described in 1841 by Alfred Poland, a medical student at Guy's Hospital.

Definition
Congenital pectoral muscle defect associated classically with symbrachydactyly but now extended to include any hand anomaly.

Incidence
- One in 20 000–30 000.
- Male = female.
- Right-to-left ratio 2:1.

Aetiology
- Mostly sporadic.
- Few families identified to date.
- One in 500 000 have Poland and Moebius syndromes (bilateral CN VI and VII palsy).
- Left-sided Poland syndrome also linked to leukaemia, non-Hodgkin's lymphoma, and dextrocardia.
- Currently vascular hypothesis for Poland syndrome and symbrachydactyly.
- Musculoskeletal malformations stem from hypoplastic subclavian artery in week 6 of gestation.
- As ribs grow forward and medially, the subclavian artery kinks and temporarily occludes, resulting in disruption of the blood supply.

Clinical presentation
- The hand anomaly is the most obvious defect:
  - Syndactyly.
  - Symbrachydactyly (symphalangism with syndactyly and hypoplasia/complete absence of middle phalanges).
- Upper limb girdle anomalies are less obvious:
  - Hypoplastic forearm or arm.
  - Absent sternal (and sometimes clavicular) head of pectoralis major.
  - Deficiency or absence pectoralis minor, latissimus dorsi, serratus anterior and other shoulder muscles.
- Chest:
  - Hypoplastic/aplastic ipsilateral breast and nipple areolar complex.
  - Abnormal ribs and costal cartilage.
  - Deficient subcutaneous fat and axillary hair.
  - Sternum rotates to involved side, causing contralateral carinate deformity.

Operative options

Hand
- Syndactyly correction.
- Brachydactyly can be improved by deepening webs to create illusion of longer fingers.
- First web often needs a flap to deepen and widen.

Rib cage
- Uncommonly requires intervention.
- Perform contralateral subperichondrial split rib resection and grafting with sternal osteotomy.

Axillary fold reconstruction
- Pectoralis major reconstruction using a latissimus dorsi transposition through limited scars to recreate the anterior axillary fold by detaching the origin and transferring it forward on the humerus (Hester and Bostwick).
- Contralateral latissimus dorsi free flap transfer.

Breast
- Males can be reconstructed using the latissimus dorsi and custom-made prostheses.
- Females need tissue expansion through puberty, followed by replacement with a permanent implant. Thin subcutaneous tissue will need simultaneous latissimus dorsi transfer. Alternatives are breast reconstruction using pedicled or free tissue transfer such as latissimus dorsi or TRAM flaps. Contralateral mastopexy may be useful.

Reference
Hester TR Jr, Bostwick J 3rd (1982). *Plast Reconstr Surg*, **69**, 226–33.

Toe phalanx non-vascularized transfer

Indication
Symbrachydactyly with loose digital soft tissue envelope and absent phalanges

Technique
- Longitudinal dorsal incision over third and fourth toes (avoid using the second in case it is needed for a second toe transfer).
- No growth if transferred subperiosteally (Carroll and Green 1975). Grows if transfer with periosteum and ligaments and restore function.
- Harvest extra-periosteally maintaining attachments of palmar plate and collateral ligaments.
- Repair the palmar plate and collateral ligament to any rudimentary tendon and soft tissue at recipient site, and K- wire for 3–4 weeks.
- Close donor site either by suturing flexor to extensor tendons or by bone graft from iliac crest.

Outcome
- Growth rate of 1.2 mm/year, achieves approximately 78% length of opposite toe phalanx, or 52% of opposite digital phalanx.
- Growth better if done before age 15 months.
- Donor site growth decreased in remaining middle and distal phalanx by 50%.
- Donor site usually ugly.

Reference
Carroll, Green (1975). *J Bone Joint Surg (Am)* **57**: 727.

Pollicization

Definition
Defined as creating a thumb by the transposition, stabilizing, and shortening of a finger ray (usually the index). The metacarpophalangeal joint becomes the basal joint of the new thumb, the proximal inter-phalangeal joint becomes the new metacarpophalangeal joint, and the distal inter-phalangeal joint becomes the new interphalangeal joint.

Indications for pollicization
- Congenital:
  - Thumb hypoplasia with absent CMCJ.
  - Thumb aplasia.
  - Five or more fingered hand.
- Acquired:
  - Traumatic total thumb loss.

Timing of surgery
Varies with surgeon but preferably before 2 years in congenital cases to maximize integration of the pollicized digit.

Principles of pollicization
- Design skin flaps according to preference or by planning in reverse.
- Elevate dorsal skin flaps preserving the dorsal veins which should be dissected to allow transposition.
- Dissect extensor tendon.
- Release lateral bands extensor mechanism for later attachment of intrinsics.
- Divide index metacarpal neck at level of the epiphysis.
- Destroy physis.
- Removal of second metacarpal shaft and base (index metacarpal head forms the trapezium), leaving intrinsics for later re-attachment.
- Elevate palmar flaps.
- Dissect neurovascular bundles to level of the proximal palm (this may need interfascicular neural dissection).
- Dissect flexor tendons and release A1 pulley.
- Hyperextension of MCPJ to stabilize new CMCJ and fix with longitudinal K-wire.
- Transpose digit.
- Axial rotation by 160° (pronation) to give good opposition.
- Angulation from palm by 40° to give good abduction.
- Place metacarpal head palmar to the base of the index metacarpal-carpal joint rather then in the same plane, adjust height of thumb so that it reaches the middle finger PIPJ, and fix with wire or suture.
- Shorten flexor and extensor tendons as required.
- If extensor indicis and EDC to index are present then preserve EI as EPL and use EDC as APL.
- Re-attach intrinsics to form new adductor and abductor.
- Close skin.

Outcome
Depends on the quality of the index finger and the presence of intrinsics and other musculotendinous structures.

Complications
- Overgrowth of the trapezium due to persistence of the physis.
- Stiffness.
- Instability; usually hyperextension of the new CMCJ.
- Lack of flexion or extension due to tendon imbalance.
- Poor opposition due to either inadequate rotation or poor intrinsics.
- Poor position of thumb.
- Marginal skin necrosis.

Chest wall deformity

Classification
- Congenital (pectus excavatum/carinatum, Poland syndrome).
- Post-traumatic.
- Following tumour resection.
- Post-radiation ulcers.
- Following chronic lung disease.

This section covers congenital chest wall deformities.

Congenital chest wall deformities
Congenital chest wall deformities may be primary or secondary to scoliosis or surgery. Primary is more common.

Pectus excavatum (funnel chest) and pectus carinatum (pigeon chest) are congenital anomalies resulting from costal cartilage overgrowth. This leads to either caving in of the sternum and associated ribs (excavatum), or a pigeon-chest-like protuberance (carinatum).

Treatment
- Camouflage.
- Osteotomies.

Treatment is categorized into either camouflage procedures using custom-shaped implants or injectable malleable implants to hide the sternal deformities, or corrective osteotomies. Parasternal osteotomies can be made and then supported by insertion of a substernal bar fixed to the lateral ribs (Ravitch's procedure), or the whole sternum can be excised and reversed to regain anatomical normality (Lexer's technique), or vascularized (Ishikawa 1988).

Chapter 6

Skin

Epidermolysis bullosa 234
Albinism 236
Pigmented melanocytic lesions 238
Skin tumours: classification 239
Melanocytic lesions 240
Epidermal lesions 240
Dermal lesions 241
Naevus cell lesions 242
Special naevi 243
Premalignant 245
Melanoma 246
Non-melanoma 250
Malignant 258

Benign skin lesions
Cysts 268
Fibrohistiocytic tumours 270
Epidermal tumours 272
Sweat gland tumours 274
Hair follicle tumours 276
Vascular tumours 277
Mast cell tumours 278
Port wine stain 279
Pyoderma gangrenosum 281

Epidermolysis bullosa

Definition
A group of inherited disorders in which the skin blisters in response to minor trauma, and which heal by scarring.

Incidence
Estimates vary; up to 50 per million live births.

Aetiology
Genetic.

Classification
- Epidermolysis bullosa simplex (EBS): intradermal skin separation. Usually mild and autosomal dominant (AD) inheritance; recessively inherited forms are more severe.
- Junctional epidermolysis bullosa (JEB): skin separates in lamina lucida or central basement membrane. Often fatal in early infancy. May be associated with pyloric atresia via common molecular pathway.
- Dystrophic epidermolysis bullosa (DEB): skin separates in the sublamina densa (deep basement membrane).
- (Hemidesmosomal epidermolysis bullosa: skin separates in the most superior part of the basement membrane—a new category).

Pathogenesis
The skin has a basement membrane to anchor the epidermis to the dermis. Keratin-containing filaments in the basal cells of the epidermis insert into hemidesmosomes, which are condensations of the basal cell membrane. Anchoring filaments extend deep from these hemidesmosomes and cross the lamina lucida to attach to the lamina densa. Fibrils containing type 7 collagen attach the lamina densa to the underlying dermis. Defects in the molecules responsible for basement membrane stability cause epidermolysis bullosa:
- EBS—abnormal keratin synthesis.
- JEB—mutations in genes encoding laminins or integrins.
- DEB—mutations in gene encoding type 7 collagen.

Clinical features
Usually noted at or soon after birth, except in very mild cases. Skin blisters are seen in response to minor trauma. Family history should be sought. Severity of disease is very variable. Blisters of oral, nasopharyngeal, ocular, genitourinary, or respiratory mucosae may also occur.

Complications
May include:
- Infection, which may be fatal.
- Mitten hand deformity—cocooning syndactyly due to recurrent blistering and atrophic scarring, which obliterates web spaces.
- Corneal ulceration.
- Tear duct obliteration.
- Cicatricial ectropion.
- Oesophageal strictures and malnutrition.
- SCC develops in non-sun-exposed skin between 15 and 35 years of age.

Investigations
Skin biopsy is analysed by electron microscopy to determine depth of blistering and immunoflorescence microscopy to help elucidate the mechanism. Genetic testing can identify the responsible mutation.

Management
Medical
- Wound care with semi-occlusive non-adherent dressings and topical antibiotics.
- Oral corticosteroids for oral mucosal disease.

Surgical
- Excision of SCCs.
- Reconstruction of syndactylous hand—high rate of recurrence.
- Split skin grafting to eyelids in cicatricial ectropion.
- Gastrostomy and tracheostomy.

Albinism

Definition
A group of genetic abnormalities of melanin synthesis with normal number and structure of melanocytes. Specific ocular changes must be present in order to diagnose albinism. Reduced melanin synthesis in skin, hair, or eyes is termed oculocutaneous albinism type 1, 2, or 3 (OCA1–3), respectively, whilst reduced synthesis limited to the eye is termed ocular albinism type 1 (OA1).

Prevalence
The overall worldwide prevalence is 1 in 10 000–20 000.

Classification and aetiology
- OCA1: autosomal recessive; caused by mutations in the tyrosinase gene (chromosome 11). Tyrosinase is the rate-limiting step in melanin synthesis. Most patients are compound heterozygotes. Different mutations cause different amounts of residual tyrosinase activity. No residual activity causes tyrosinase negative OCA1A; some residual tyrosinase activity leads to OCA1B.
- OCA2: autosomal recessive; caused by mutations in the *P* gene (chromosome 15).
- OCA3: autosomal recessive; caused by mutations in the *TYRP1* gene (chromosome 9). Only reported in African and African American individuals.
- OA: X-linked—caused by mutations in the *OA1* gene.

Clinical features
- **OCA1A** Classical albinism. Total absence of melanin in skin, hair, and eyes. Pigmentation does not develop as the patient matures. These patients never develop pigmented lesions in the skin, but amelanotic naevi may be present. Ophthalmological changes include lack of retinal and iris pigment, foveal hypoplasia, misrouting of the optic nerves, and nystagmus.
- **OCA1B** Broad variation in phenotype depending on the amount of residual tyrosinase activity. Pigment often develops in the first or second decade, leading to blond hair, blue eyes, and skin which tans upon sun exposure.
- **OCA2** Very light pigment is present in the hair and eyes at birth. Pigmented lesions (naevi, lentigines) may develop, particularly in sun-exposed areas.
- **OCA3** Described in African or African American individuals. Reddish-brown skin, red hair, and hazel or brown irises. The red colour results from accumulation of phaeomelanins. Ocular changes may be absent.
- **OA** Skin and hair are normal, irises are blue or brown, but retinal pigmentation is absent and the other ocular changes of albinism are present. Heterozygous females present with patchy retinal pigmentation and punctate iris translucency because of X-inactivation.

Pathogenesis
Simplified schematic pathway of melanin synthesis

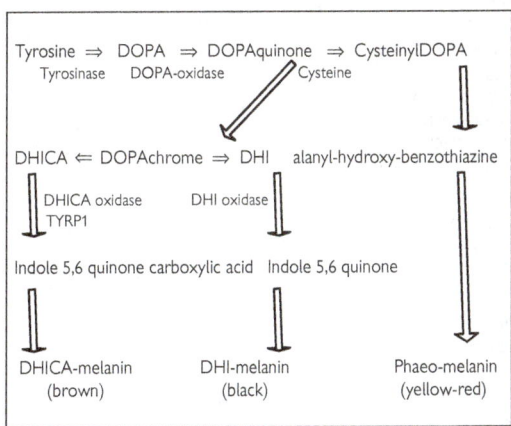

Investigations
Genetic counselling and genetic testing should be undertaken by a clinical geneticist experienced in dealing with hypopigmentation disorders.

Management
- **Skin care** Hypopigmentation mandates effective ultraviolet radiation protection. Physical methods including hats and long-sleeved/legged clothing are valuable, and a sunscreen with a high sun protection factor should be utilized.
- **Ophthalmological care** Regular ophthalmoligical follow-up to detect and treat hyperopia, myopia, and astigmatism.
- **Surgical** Any cutaneous tumours arising in individuals with albinism should be managed as described in the relevant chapter.

Pigmented melanocytic lesions

Benign
Melanocyte
Epidermal
- Ephelis.
- Lentigo simplex.
- Lentigo senilis.
- Becker's naevus.
- Albright's syndrome.

Dermal
- Mongolian blue spot.
- Naevus of Ito.
- Naevus of Ota.
- Blue naevus.

Naevus cell
- Junctional.
- Compound.
- Intradermal.
- Special:
  - Balloon.
  - Spindle.
  - Spitz.
  - Halo.
  - Congenital.

Malignant
- Melanoma:
  - Lentigo maligna melanoma.
  - Nodular.
  - Superficial spreading.
  - Acral lentiginous.
  - Arising in blue naevus.
  - Amelanotic.

Skin tumours: classification

This is best considered as part of a broad classification of pigmented lesions.

Non-melanocytic (melanin pigment)

Benign
- Epidermal naevi.
- Seborrhoeic keratosis.
- Actinic keratosis.
- Others, e.g. haemosiderin, vascular lesions.

Malignant
- Pigmented BCC.
- Pigmented SCC.

Melanocytic

Benign
Epidermal
- Ephelides.
- Lentigo simplex.
- Lentigo senilis.
- Becker's disease.
- Albright's syndrome.

Dermal
- Mongolian blue spot.
- Naevus of Ito.
- Naevus of Ota.
- Blue naevus.

Naevus cell
- Junctional.
- Compound.
- Intradermal.
- Special:
  - Balloon.
  - Spindle.
  - Spitz.
  - Halo.
  - Congenital.

Pre-malignant
- Dysplastic naevus.
- Lentigo maligna.
- Melanoma *in situ*.

Malignant
- Melanoma.

Melanocytic lesions

Embryology
Melanoblasts from the neural crest migrate to the basal epidermal layer and differentiate into melanocytes.

Physiology
Melanocytes are dendritic cells which produce melanin. Melanin when bound to protein is called a melanosome. Melanosomes are stored in other epidermal cells. The density of melanocytes varies around the body (e.g large amounts on the face) but does not differ between races. However, melanosome size does differ between races. On exposure to ultraviolet light, melanocytes produce melanin for protection. Melanocytic naevi are present at birth and become pigmented in response to circulating hormones in the first months after birth.

Epidermal lesions

Ephelides
Clinical features
Small <0.5 cm pale–dark brown smooth spots.

Pathology
Normal number of melanocytes. Increased pigment in response to sunlight.

Lentigo simplex
Clinical features
Develop in childhood; 1–2 mm in size: small brown and circumscribed. Not related to the sun.

Pathology
Increase in basal melanocytes and pigmentation.

Lentigo senilis
Clinical features
Sun-damaged skin in the middle-aged and elderly. Size ranges from very small to >1 cm. Light to dark brown in colour and generally uniform.

Pathology
Increased or normal number of melanocytes with increased pigmentation.

Becker's disease
Clinical features
Common, affecting 1/200; usually male (male-to-female ratio 5:1). Appear in adolescence, exaggerated by sunshine, generally on upper trunk and arms. Gradually spread in an irregular fashion and later usually becomes darker and hairy. Occasionally may develop acne-like lesions within it.

Pathology
Normal number of melanocytes with increased pigmentation. Epidermis thickened.

Treatment of epidermal naevi
Observation, unless biopsy is required for suspicious areas.

Dermal lesions

Mongolian blue spot
Clinical features
Slate blue discoloration over sacrum. <1% Caucasians. Usually fade and intervention is not required.

Pathology
Dermal melanocytes are due to failure of migration.

Naevi of Ito and Ota
Clinical features
Slate blue macular pigmentation of shoulder (Ito) or in the ophthalmic and maxillary distribution of the trigeminal nerve (Ota).

Pathology
Heavily pigmented dermal melanocytes. Epidermal melanocytes are sometimes involved.

Blue naevus
Clinical features
Blue black dome <1 cm in diameter. Common in the fourth decade and on the dorsum of hands and scalp. A cellular blue naevus is larger, slow growing, and may ulcerate with potential for malignant change.

Pathology
Melanocytes in deep reticular dermis and subcutaneous fat.

Treatment for dermal naevi
Observation, or excision if any diagnostic doubt.

Naevus cell lesions

Junctional
Clinical features
Flat pigmented area, variable size and colour between lesions but generally even pigmentation, occasionally darker in the centre. Usually a transient phase in children prior to becoming compound naevi. May remain junctional on the palms, soles and mucosae.

Pathology
Melanocytes present only at the epidermal–dermal junction.

Compound
Clinical features
Raised plaque to papillomatous lesions with variable colour. Increase in thickness during late childhood and adolescence and often cause concern at this stage. Associated with coarse terminal hairs.

Pathology
Central melanocytes push into dermis and peripheral melanocytes remain junctional.

Intra-dermal
Clinical features
Elevated as a dome, papilloma, or tag. Variable pigment. Rare in child.

Pathology
Melanocytes in dermis.

Treatment of naevus cell naevi
All naevi can be safely observed. If there is any doubt or significant change, treat with complete excision.

Special naevi

Balloon
Clinical features
Smooth dome-shaped red brown papule in people aged <30 years.

Pathology
Compound or intradermal melanocytes and balloon cells.

Spindle
Clinical features
5 mm–1 cm blue-black densely pigmented papilloma in females.

Pathology
Compound naevus with large amounts of melanin lying in the naevus cell and free.

Treatment
Both balloon and spindle can be observed but are generally excised because of the differential diagnosis of melanoma.

Spitz
Clinical features
Usually appear in early childhood as firm rounded red or brownish nodules. The colour is due to vascularity of tumour and associated pigment. The lesion may blanch with pressure. It grows rapidly over 3–6 months and the surface may be fragile and cause bleeding or crusting. Most common on the face, particularly the cheeks.

Pathology
Spindle-shaped cells in dermis and epidermis. Capillaries mixed with naevus cells. Kamino bodies.

Treatment
Usually the lesion is completely excised to confirm the diagnosis. Local recurrence is unusual.

Halo
Clinical features
Melanocytic naevus with a depigmented halo. Common, particularly in children and teenagers, and often the cause of concern to parents. Usually seen on the back and exaggerated by suntan. The pigmentation within the affected mole fades, becoming flesh coloured. In time the pigmentation returns to normal (may take years). Associated with vitiligo and thyroid disease.

Pathology
Compound naevus with lymphocytic infiltrate in the dermis.

Treatment
Manage conservatively.

Congenital

Clinical features
Present in 1–2% of newborns. Dark brown-black. May appear as pale macular lesions at birth and darken over the years. Develops hair as the lesion matures. Can become warty and develop nodules and be associated with underlying abnormalities such as meningeal involvement, spina bifida, or meningocoele.

Pathology
Melanocytes are junctional at birth and deepen to intradermal (in some cases even subcutaneous and fascial) in the first few months of life.

Classification
Giant (>2% BSA)
These can undergo malignant change with estimates of 1–40%. The real rate is probably 4–6%. Transformation can occur in the first year of life and over half the change occurs before puberty.
- Treatment:
  - Conservative: in some cases such as total scalp involvement excision is not cosmetically acceptable. After frank discussion with the parents close observation is an option.
  - Early: curettage and cautery or dermabrasion is an option in the first few months of life before the cells deepen.
  - Later:
    1. Surgical excision and direct closure.
    2. Serial excision.
    3. Deglove excision and FTSG or flap. Suture in enforced position (Chretien-Marquet *et al.* 1994); excise with no undermining; hyperextend wrist and fingers; excise and suture directly, splint in hyperextension and slowly reduce extension by changing splint weekly. The same principle can be applied at other joints.
    4. Serial tissue expansion for the very large.

Intermediate (1–2% BSA) and small (<1% BSA)
These have unproven malignant risk and management is as above.

Reference
Chrétien-Marquet B, Benaceur S, Cerceau M, Fernandez R, Saouma S, Murthy J (1994). *Plast Reconstr Surg* **93**, 337–44.

Premalignant

Dysplastic naevi

Clinical features
5–14 mm, irregular shape, varied colour (red, brown, black), 5–10% risk of malignant change. Dysplastic naevus syndrome (B–K mole): ≥75 naevi and a strong family history.

Pathology
Proliferation of atypical melanocytes disordered and discontinuous in basal layer of epidermis.

Treatment
Complete excision with 2 mm margin.

Melanoma *in situ*

Clinical features
Features in a spectrum similar to dysplastic naevi and melanoma.

Pathology
Proliferation of fully evolved cellular atypia continuous for sufficient breadth.

Treatment
Excision with 5 mm margin.

Lentigo maligna

Pathology
Non-nested atypical melanocytes in atrophic epidermis.

Clinical features
Variably sized and pigmented brown patch in sun-exposed areas (usually the face).

Treatment
Preferred management is excision with 5 mm margin. There is often a picture of field change with atypical melanocytes present at the resection margins once the pigmented area has been completely removed. This can be treated with imiquimod and observation. Observation with biopsy of changing areas in the very large lesion or infirm patient.

Melanoma

Definition
A malignant neoplasm of melanocytes.

Incidence
10–12/100 000 per year in UK; doubled over the last 20 years. Second-fastest growing cancer in USA. Lifetime risk around 1/70 for Caucasians. 4% of all skin cancers are melanoma, accounting for over 80% of skin cancer deaths. Rare under 20 years. Most common cancer in women aged 20–30 years.

Risk factors
- Type 1 skin, blond, red hair, blue eyes. Rare in dark-skinned people.
- UV exposure, both cumulative and childhood sunburn.
- Previous primary melanoma (8–10 times risk).
- Atypical naevus syndrome (8–10 times risk).
- Giant congenital pigmented hairy naevus (over 100 times risk).
- Family history of melanoma.
- Immunosuppression (4–5-times risk after organ transplant).
- Albinism, xeroderma pigmentosum.

Pathology
- Two phases described:
  - Radial growth phase with proliferation of neoplastic melanocytes within the epidermis.
  - Vertical growth phase where the neoplastic melanocytes extend into the papillary and reticular dermis.
- Breslow's thickness is measured from the stratum granulosum down to the maximum depth of the tumour.
- Other features that are important for prognosis are the presence of ulceration, neurovascular invasion, degree of mitotic activity, and Clarke's level in thin melanomas.

Clinical features
Appears as a change in a pre-existing naevus (congenital, acquired, or dysplastic) or as a new lesion. Assess lesion with particular attention to ABCDE (**A**symmetry; **B**order irregularity; **C**olour change or variegation; **D**iameter >6 mm; **E**xtra features (itch, bleeding or crusting, elevated area or palpable nodule)). This lesion may be in a site that has not been exposed to the sun. Lesions with any major feature or three minor features are suspicious for melanoma:
- Major features:
  - Change in size.
  - Irregular shape.
  - Irregular colour.

- Minor features:
  - Largest diameter ≥6 mm.
  - Inflammation.
  - Oozing
  - Change in sensation.

Record history, presence or absence of changes in size, colour, shape, and other symptoms (itching or bleeding). Examine site and size of lesion and describe it, including features above and ulceration. Examine all the skin and record other pigmented lesions. Examine for lymphadenopathy and hepatomegaly.

Extra-cutaneous sites for primary melanoma include eye, ear, gut, CNS, leptomeninges

Classification

By clinical-histopathologic subtypes.
- **Superficial spreading** Approximately 70% of melanomas; most common on trunk in men and legs in women. Typically a raised plaque with variegated pigmentation, irregular borders, >6 mm in diameter.
- **Nodular** 15–30%, mostly seen on legs and trunk. A dark nodule which may ulcerate and bleed.
- **Lentigo maligna melanoma** 4–15% melanomas. Typically on sun-exposed skin in older patients. Latent period of 5–20 years. Only about 5–8% of lentigo malignas develop to invasive melanoma.
- **Acral lentiginous melanoma** 2–8% melanomas in caucasians, but 29–72% of melanomas in dark-skinned people. On palms, soles, or under nailplate (subungual). Subungual melanoma presents as nail discoloration or a streak of pigment. Spread of pigment to a nailfold is Hutchinson's sign.
- Also desmoplastic melanoma, mucosal melanoma, malignant blue naevus, clear cell sarcoma, amelanotic melanoma.

Investigation

Stage 2B or over should have chest XR and liver ultrasound or ideally CT with contrast of chest, abdomen, ± pelvis, liver function tests, and FBC.

Treatment

- Melanoma is ideally managed in a multidisciplinary team.
- Excision biopsy of suspicious lesions with a 2–5 mm lateral margin of normal skin and to subcutaneous fat.
- Incision biopsy is occasionally indicated, e.g. within large suspected lentigo maligna on face. Subungual melanoma is biopsied by nail removal and sampling nail matrix.
- Excision margins for biopsy-proven melanoma is determined by Breslow thickness:
  - *in situ* lesions   2–5 mm margin
  - <1 mm thick   1 cm margin
  - 1–2 mm thick   1–2 cm
  - 2.1–4 mm thick   2–3 cm
  - >4 mm   2–3 cm

Staging for malignant melanoma

Table 6.1 TNM classification

Primary tumour	Breslow thickness
Tis	*In situ* tumour
T1	<1 mm (1b if Clark's >4)
T2	1.01–2 mm
T3	2.01–4 mm
T4	>4 mm
Ta	No ulcer
Tb	Ulcerated
Nodes	**Regional node involvement**
N0	No nodes
N1	One node
N2	Two or three nodes
N3	Four or more nodes/matted nodes/node plus in transit or satellite or ulcerated melanoma
Na	Micrometastases = not palpable, seen on SLNB
Nb	Macrometastases = palpable or extracapsular LNs
Nc	In transit metastases/satellites but no nodes
Metastases	
M0	No metastases
M1	Distant skin, subcutaneous or LNs
M2	Lung
M3	All other sites, or raised LDH with any metastases

Table 6.2 AJCC clinical staging (2001)

Stage	
0	Tis, N0, M0
1A	T1a, N0, M0
1B	T1b or T2a, N0, M0
2A	T2b or T3a, N0, M0
2B	T3b or T4a, N0, M0
2C	T4b, N0, M0
3A	Non-ulcerated any T, N1a–N2a, M0
3B	Ulcerated any T, N1a–N2a, M0
	Non-ulcerated T, N1b–N2b, M0
	Any T, N2c (intransit met and no nodes), M0
3C	Ulcerated T, N1b-N2b, M0
	Any T, N3, M0
4	Any T, Any N, Any M

Adjuvant therapy
There is currently no standard treatment in the UK. There are trials with interferon and vaccines in the UK. Patients with stage 2B disease should be referred to a cancer centre to consider entry into trials of adjuvant therapies.

Management of regional lymph nodes
- **Sentinel lymph node biopsy** A sensitive investigation and prognostic indicator. At present, there is no proven survival benefit for SLNB followed by elective lymph node dissection if micrometastases are found.
- **FNAC** For clinically or radiologically suspicious nodes.
- **Open biopsy** If FNAC is negative and suspicion remains.

Biopsy-proven lymph node metastases are treated by radical dissection after CT staging.

Local recurrence
Treatment is palliative by surgery, curettage or CO_2 laser. Isolated limb perfusion if multiple recurrences confined to one limb and no other disease.

Metastatic disease
Must be managed by a multidisciplinary team. Localized metastases may be excised (e.g. skin or solitary brain). Radiotherapy for symptom control in bone, skin, or brain metastases. Chemotherapy with dacarbazine or entry into a clinical trial; no survival benefit.

Follow-up
Patients should be taught self-examination. *In situ* melanoma, one postoperative visit. Invasive melanoma <1 mm, 3-monthly for 3 years plus 6-monthly for a further 2 years for lesions >1 mm thick.

Prognosis
Prognostic factors
Breslow thickness, ulceration, Clark's level, sentinel node positivity; age >70 years worse prognosis.

Table 6.3 Prognosis for malignant melanoma

Stage	Approximate 5 year survival
0	97%
I	90–95%
IIA	78%
IIB	63–70%
IIC	45%
IIIA	63–70%
IIIB	46–53%
IIIC	28%
IV	8–18%

Non-melanoma
(premalignant or *in situ* change)

Solar keratosis

Incidence
Very common in sun-exposed individuals with fair skin.

Aetiology
Usually associated with sun exposure.

Clinical presentation
Presents as a slow-growing adherent scale with an indistinct margin usually occurring on sun-exposed areas; often associated with surrounding inflammatory reaction; stinging or painful. May be pigmented.

Pathology
Pathologically characterized by:
- Atypia.
- Dysplasia of epidermis.
- Evidence of distorted maturation particularly:
  - Dyskeratosis.
  - Hyperkeratosis.
  - Parakeratosis.
  - Acanthosis.

Prognosis
3% develop into squamous cell carcinomas. Carcinomatous change is indicated by ulceration or induration.

Treatment
- 5-Fluorouracil.
- Cryotherapy.
- Curettage and cautery.
- Excision.

Bowen's disease

Definition
A skin lesion also known as psoriaform carcinoma. Considered squamous cell carcinoma in situ, or pre-malignant.

Incidence
Common in sun-exposed individuals with fair skin.

Aetiology
Usually associated with sun exposure. Arsenic exposure and HPV are other causes.

Clinical presentation
Presents as a slow-growing well-defined pink scaly plaque. It differs from a solar keratosis by having a well-defined border. Sometimes contains or is surrounded by telangectasia.

Pathology

Pathologically characterized by:
- Atypia.
- Dysplasia of epidermis.
- Mitoses.
- Pleomorphism.
- Evidence of distorted maturation particularly dyskeratosis.
- May be skip lesions or an extension down hair follicles.

Prognosis

8–10% develop into squamous cell carcinomas with an increased risk of metastases. Carcinomatous change is indicated by ulceration or induration.

Treatment

- Cryotherapy.
- Curettage and cautery.
- Excision.

Note that there are two types of Bowen's disease on the penis: erythroplasia of Queyrat and Bowenoid papulosis.

Keratoacanthoma (molluscum sebaceum)

A contentious tumour thought by some to be a self-resolving benign tumour of pilosebaceous origin but argued by others (particularly Ackerman) to be a variant of squamous cell carcinoma.

Incidence

Reasonably common (1/1000 population). Not as common as SCC but some cross-diagnosis. Twice as common in men. Increasing incidence with increasing age.

Aetiology

Unknown, but same factors as SCC. PRICTG mnemonic: **P**re-malignant, **R**adiation, **I**mmune deficiency/infection, **C**hronic wounds, **T**oxins, **G**enetic factors.

Clinical presentation

Rapidly growing proliferative polypoid lesion. Central ulceration and/or keratotic horn with raised epithelial edge and epithelial collarette. Lesion grows for weeks to 2 months; then remains static and may resolve within the next 3 months. Most common on sun-exposed face, hands, forearms.

Pathology

Well-differentiated squamous cells forming keratin, with only mild pleomorphism. Looks like a well-diffentiated SCC!

Treatment

Surgical excision is indicated despite possible self-resolution given difficulty in clinical and pathological separation from SCC. Margin of excision, 4 mm.

Prognosis

- At worst a low-grade malignancy, so prognosis is good.
- Increased risk of developing other skin cancers.

There are two multiple forms called keratoacanthoma of Grzybowski (do not resolve) and multiple Ferguson–Smith keratoacanthoma (do resolve).

Chondrodermatitis nodularis helicis

Clinical features
Scaly ulcerated lesions on the ear of elderly Caucasian males. Sharp pain when lying on the affected side.

Pathology
Actinic damage and destruction of underlying collagen, leading to cartilage exposure.

Management
A variety of methods from topical steroid to pressure relief (removing pressure from the affected area). However, excision biopsy, removing the affected cartilage, gives relief and gains pathological diagnosis. Malignant risk of SCC.

Porokeratosis

Clinical features
Many types:
- Atrophic centre with raised rim.
- Linear.
- Superficial—scaly 1 cm patches with typical raised thread-like rim.

Pathology
Coronoid lamella; plume of parakeratosis arising from one or two epidermal cells.

Management
Superficial cryotherapy or shave excision. Large lesions require excision. Malignant risk: 7% turn into BCC or SCC.

Cutaneous horn

Aetiology
These horns made of compacted keratin can be produced from any hyperplastic epidermal lesion, ranging from a wart (30%) to a solar keratosis (30%) to seborrhoeic keratosis to an SCC (20%).

Clinical features
Enlarged keratin growth protruding from the skin surface in a horn shape. More than 70% of horns are benign. Malignancy is suggested by tenderness, large size, and surrounding induration. Usually found in sun-exposed sites.

Treatment
Excision for diagnosis and to remove the horn which may cause problems because of its prominence and exposure to trauma.

Xeroderma pigmentosum

Genetics
Autosomal recessive.

Clinical
Equal incidence in males and females. Sunlight initially causes erythema, discomfort, and macular freckling. This progresses to patchy hyperpigmentation, depigmentation, and dryness. Eventually multiple cutaneous malignancies (melanoma 10%, others 90%). Eyes involved. Bird-like facies. Progressive decline in mental function.

Management
Prevention using sunscreen, clothing, and altered behaviour. Individual malignancy management.

Pinkus tumour (pre-malignant fibroepithelioma)
An unusual variant of BCC.

Aetiology
Caused by deletion or mutation of the *TP53* gene which codes for a tumour suppressor protein or mutation in the patched (*PTC*) gene which reduces an inhibitory signal for the hedgehog pathway which, if activated, can produce a BCC. Associated with previous radiotherapy.

Clinical features
Appears as a benign slowly growing pedunculated pink tumour with a warty surface. Pinkus tumours are most common on the trunk.

Pathology
Histologically differs from BCC by having long thin branching strands of basal cell carcinoma in a loose fibrovascular stroma. The basaloid cells show two populations: lighter cells in the strand and darker cells budding of the strands. They are malignant but with low metastatic potential.

Treatment
Treat as BCC.

Paget's disease of skin

Incidence
Rare.

Aetiology
Unknown.

Classification
Two types:
- Mammary.
- Extra-mammary.

Clinical presentation
- Mammary Paget's disease presents as an eczematous weeping scaly lesion, usually secondary to primary ductal carcinoma, extending into epidermis.
- Extra-mammary Paget's disease generally occurs in the pubis, perineum, thighs, or genitalia. It is usually related to underlying apocrine or eccrine sweat gland carcinoma, and rarely to secondary bowel or genitourinary cancer (note that the breast is an apocrine gland).

Investigation
- Biopsy.
- Look for primary.
- Stage tumour.

Pathology
Pathologically characterized by large cells with clear cytoplasm and oval nuclei within the epidermis. Lymphocytic reaction in the dermis and in some cases infiltration by malignant cells from the underlying tumour.

Treatment
- Referral to appropriate specialist to investigate for underlying tumour.
- Wide local excision and reconstruction. No data on margins; however, 2–5 mm should be sufficient.
- No medical management. Adjuvant therapy may be needed depending on cause. Radiotherapy and 5-FU ineffective.

Prognosis
High propensity for local recurrence. Outcome depends on type and treatment of underlying cause. Extra-mammary Paget's disease is related to sweat gland carcinoma and underlying malignancy, but often no underlying cause is found and therefore regular monitoring is required.

Linear epidermal (sebaceous) naevi (organoid naevi)

Definition
A benign proliferation of cells arising from embryonic ectoderm. As these ectodermal cells are pluripotential, an epidermal naevus is correctly termed a hamartoma because more than one of the normal components of the skin may be present. Present at birth. Sebaceous naevi have malignant potential.

Classification
Four main types:
- Linear epidermal naevus (LEN).
- Linear sebaceous naevus (LSN); also called Jadassohn naevus phacomatosis.
- Linear naevus comedonicus (LNC).
- Inflammatory linear verrucous epidermal naevus (ILVEN).

Incidence
- Uncommon (1:200). Approximately 60% of patients have LEN, 33% LSN, 6% ILVEN, and 1% LNC.
- ILVEN has a female-to-male ration of 4:21. The other types are distributed equally.

Aetiology
Unknown. It has been postulated that mosaicism (the presence of two genetically different populations of cells within the same individual) is responsible for the expression of the phenotype within specific groups of cells leading to the striking distribution of lesions.

The lesions are linear and often conform to the lines of Blashko. These are the lines of embryonic cell migration, and are linear on the limbs, S-shaped on the abdomen, and V-shaped on the chest and back, giving a 'fountain-like' appearance. These shapes are thought to be produced by the longitudinal growth and flexion of the embryo.

Clinical features
Lesions are present at birth, or develop within the first decade of life.
- LEN: plaques and nodules with a rough warty surface resembling seborrhoeic warts. Commonly found on the head, neck, and trunk.
- LSN: present at birth, but proliferate and reach full size at puberty. Respond to hormones. Raised hairless yellow or orange plaques surrounded by rounded elevations. Most common on face and scalp.
- LNC: numerous keratin-filled pits which resemble blackheads. Especially common on face, neck, trunk, and arms.
- ILVEN: linear, erythematous, and highly pruritic plaques on the long axis of a limb. These lesions may involve the nail.

Associated syndromes
Approximately a third of patients with an epidermal naevus have involvement of another organ system, most commonly the CNS, eyes and skeleton. Associated with Proteus syndrome, CHILD syndrome, McCune–Albright syndrome, and Klippel–Trenaunay syndrome.

Pathology
- LEN: variable pattern dependent on differentiated constituents. Commonly squamous papillomas with hyperkeratosis and acanthosis.
- LSN: combination of epidermal, apocrine, sebaceou, and follicular abnormalities. At puberty, enlarged mature sebaceous glands and papillomatous hyerplasia are present.
- LNC: cystically dilated hair follicles arise from an atrophic epidermis with open and closed comedones.
- ILVEN: inflammation and psoriform epidermal hyperplasia.

Complications
LSN may develop into benign or malignant neoplasms. The most common benign neoplasm is a syringocystadenoma papilliferum. BCC and SCC are the most common malignant tumours. The risk of malignant transformation is estimated at 10–20%. The tumours are usually low grade.

Management
Surgical removal of lesions may be requested for cosmetic reasons, and in LSN is indicated to prevent or treat malignant transformation.

Gorlin's syndrome

First described by Mikulicz in the nineteenth century. Also known as: Gorlin–Goltz syndrome, basal cell naevus syndrome, and naevoid basal cell syndrome.

Incidence
Rare. Prevalence 1/56 000. One in 200 who develop multiple BCCs have Gorlin's syndrome. Autosomal dominant inheritance.

Genetics
Abnormalities on chromosome 9q22–31. Chromosome 9: allelic loss in 9p13 and proximal part of 9q22–31 in 50%.
Hypothesis: caused by a mutation in a tumour suppressor gene on chromosome 9. Multiple genetic alterations are required for the transformation of completely normal to malignant cells, and in Gorlin's syndrome

the inactivation of the relevant gene on chromosome 9 always precedes other chromosomal loss.

The time interval between UV light exposure and the development of BCCs is about 6 months to 3 years, as opposed to 20–30 years.

Clinical features
Characterized by:
- Multiple BCCs.
- Palmar pits.
- Mandible cysts.
- Bifid or fused ribs.
- Calcification of falx cerebri.
- Cataracts.

Cutaneous
- Naevoid basal cell carcinomas:
  - Appear between 15 and 35 years of age.
  - Number of lesions varies from several to several thousand.
  - Most common on face and upper trunk.
  - Found in isolation or in groups.
  - Size 1–10 mm.
- Palmar and plantar pits–65%:
  - Rarely found in children and are age related.
  - Reports of BCC developing in the bases of such lesions.
- Other cutaneous manifestations:
  - Milia, epidermoid cysts, chalazia, comedones, and palmar and plantar calcinosis.

Head and neck
Odontogenic keratocysts: second most common feature (75–80%) Appear in first decade; peak incidence in second and third decades. Most common in the mandible > maxilla:
- Single or multiple.
- Unilateral or bilateral.
- Hallmark very high rate of recurrence due to satellite cysts.
- Calvarial thickening in a high percentage.
- Parietal and frontal bulging.
- Well developed supra-orbital ridges.
- Broad nasal bridge and mild hypertelorism.
- Congenital blindness secondary to cataracts, corneal opacities, and glaucoma.
- Strabismus and nystagmus.

CNS
- Calcification of the falx cerebri—CHX (85%).
- Also calcification of tentorium cerebelli, petroclinoid ligament, dura and pia mater, and choroid plexus.
- Medulloblastoma (20%).
- Meningiomas.
- Glioblastoma multiforme and astrocytoma.

Skeletal system
- Ribs: splayed, bifid and cervical (60%).
- Spina bifida occulta of cervical and thoracic vertebrae.
- Polydactyly of hands and feet.
- Sclerotic bone lesions of the pelvis and lumbar vertebrae.
- Sprengel's deformity.
- Shortened thumb metacarpals (cf. pseudo-hyperparathyroidism).

Other
- Ovarian and cardiac fibromas.
- Thoracic rhabdomyomas and bronchogenic cysts.

Malignant

Basal cell carcinoma

Definition
Malignant neoplasm of the basal cells of the epidermis. Colloquially called rodent ulcer.

Incidence
- Most common malignancy in humans with lifetime risk of 18–40% in Caucasians.
- Marked geographical variation.
- Age: rarely seen before 20 years; thereafter increases with age.
- Male-to-female ratio approximately 1.5:1.

Aetiology
- Pre-malignant (solar keratosis, Bowen's disease, organoid naevus of Jadassohn).
- Radiation (UV, X-ray, ionizing):
  - UV exposure, although relation with pattern of exposure unclear; childhood freckling or sunburn may be most important. Latency of over 20 years. Probably due to damage to *PTCH* tumour suppressor gene on chromosome 9q22.
  - PUVA treatment.
- Immune deficiency/infection (transplantation, HPV, HIV).
- Chronic wounds (Marjolin's ulcer).
- Toxins:
  - Arsenic, tar, coal.
  - Diet: high in fat, low in vitamins.
- Genetic predisposition:
  - Skin type 1 (always burns, never tans); red or blond hair; blue or green eyes.
  - Family history.
  - Albinism.
  - Gorlin's syndrome.
  - Xeroderma pigmentosa: rare, autosomal recessive. Failure of DNA repair.
  - Bazex's syndrome: follicular atrophoderma, BCCs, hipotrichosis, hypohidrosis.
  - Gardner's syndrome.
- Also fusion theory.

Classification
By histological morphology:
- Nodular.
- Cystic.
- Superficial.
- Morphoeic.
- Infiltrative.
- Micronodular.
- Pigmented.

MALIGNANT

Clinical features
Most are on head and neck; rarely seen on hands. They are slow growing and locally invasive; if neglected they can invade deep structures. Case reports of metastases from giant BCCs.

The appearance is very variable. Nodular type is most common, and appears as a raised, often pearly, nodule with a central dimple or ulcer and surface telangectasia. Superficial BCCs are scaly erythematous plaques which may ulcerate. Morphoeic BCCs often look like a flat slightly pale scar.

Microscopy
Basaloid blue-staining cells with large hyperchromatic oval nuclei with little cytoplasm. Aggregate in nests, and align peripherally in palisades. Usually connected to dermis (95%) or hair follicle (5%). Larger lobules of tumour degenerate to form cysts in cystic lesions.

Morphoeic and infiltrative types have thin strands of tumour. Morpheic forms show numerous fibroblasts with collagen often extending in subcutaneous areas, and chords with perineural invasion. Basi-squamous BCC has features of both BCC and SCC, and is more aggressive.

Treatment options
Excision, incision, or punch biopsy if unsure of the diagnosis and particularly if cosmetically sensitive site and resection will require flap or graft reconstruction. Essential if prior to radiotherapy or Mohs' micrographic surgery.

High-risk tumours: eyes, nose, lips, nasolabial folds, >2 cm diameter, ill-defined margins, recurrent, morphoeic, immunosuppressed patient.

Management
Excision: 4 mm margin if <2 cm diameter; 6 mm margin if >2 cm. Mohs' micrographic surgery. Radiotherapy if frail.

Low-risk tumours (others)
Management
Excision 3–4 mm. Curettage and cautery or cryotherapy if small and not on lower legs. Efudix or imiquimod for superficial BCCs; radiotherapy.

- Curettage and cautery: no pathological assessment of tumour and clearance margins.
- Excision and primary closure: 4 mm margins for primary lesions, and ≥6 mm for recurrences or ill-defined lesions.
- Mohs' micrographic surgery: in this technique microscopic control of the margins is achieved at the time of tumour removal. Closer margins are taken around the tumour and the base and margins are examined. Any positive margins are resected until clear of tumour. This is an expensive and time-consuming process. Indications include special sites such as eyelid where tissue preservation is important, ill-defined tumours on nose, recurrent tumours.
- Radiotherapy for patients in ill health unable to tolerate LA surgery. No pathology produced.
- Cryotherapy for dermatologists. No pathology produced.
- Imiquimod and efudix: used for superficial BCCs of trunk or limbs.

- Oral retinoids: used in Gorlin's syndrome. Appear to prevent or delay new BCCs and produce regression in existing lesions.
- Photodynamic therapy and interferon alpha have been used experimentally, but have substantial failure rates.

Incomplete excision
If incompletely excised as intra-lesional 33% recurrence rate; if within one high powered field 12% recurrence rate; if completely excised 1.2% recurrence rate.

Up to two-thirds of incompletely excised BCCs will not recur if left untreated. Primary BCCs which are incompletely excised on a lateral margin only, are of non-aggressive histological type, and are on non-critical anatomical sites may be observed. All others should be re-excised.

Prognosis
- 95% 5-year cure with excision.
- Mohs' surgery gives 99% 5-year cure for primary tumours, and 95% for recurrent BCCs.
- Radiotherapy has a 5-year cure rate of about 90%. Curettage and cautery, or cryotherapy of primary tumours, has a less successful outcome than the above.
- Metastasis is rare (0.0028–0.55%), but is usually fatal.

Prognostic factors
- Tumour size.
- Tumour site: lesions around eyes, nose, and ears appear to recur more frequently.
- Tumour type and definition of margins: basisquamous, micronodular, infiltrative, and morphoeic BCCs are all more likely to recur.
- Failed previous treatment.
- Having one BCC increases the risk of another by about 30%; risk increases with number of BCCs; about 80% occur within 5 years.
- Patients are also at increased risk of SCC and melanoma. Patients with BCC have an overall slightly increased risk of dying from cancer of all types. The reason is unknown.

Squamous cell carcinoma

Definition
A malignant neoplasm of keratinizing cells of the epidermis or its appendages.

Incidence
Affects about 0.1–0.2% Caucasians per year; rising. Varies geographically. Increasing incidence with increasing age. Male-to-female ratio 2:1.

Aetiology
- Pre-malignant (solar keratosis, Bowen's disease, erythroderma).
- Radiation (UV, X-ray, ionizing).
  - UV exposure; over 90% occur in sun-exposed skin. Probably due to inactivation of p53 tumour suppressor gene.
  - PUVA treatment.

- Immune deficiency/infection (transplantation, HPV infection, especially SCC of penis, vulva, and periungual; HPV type 16 has been implicated; HIV).
- Chronic wounds (Marjolin's ulcer).
- Toxins:
  - Arsenic, tar, coal, aromatic hydrocarbons, soot (historically, in chimney sweeps).
  - Diet: high in fat, low in vitamins.
- Genetic predisposition:
  - Skin type 1 (always burns, never tans); red or blond hair; blue or green eyes.
  - Family history.
  - Albinism.
  - Xeroderma pigmentosa: rare, autosomal recessive. Failure of DNA repair.

Classification
Thickness, Clark's level, histological morphology, stage, and grade are used.

Clinical features
The classical picture of raised rolled edges with a central ulcer is very variable. Frequently, it is an indurated nodular keratinizing tumour which may centrally ulcerate. It may also be a scaly erythematous patch which bleeds, or a flat granulating non-healing ulcer without rolled raised edges.

Pathology
Malignant epidermal cells invade deep to the epithelial basement membrane into the dermis. Nuclei are prominent, enlarged, and irregular, and often vesicular. Well-differentiated lesions have keratinized nuclei and extra-cellular keratin pearls. Poorly differentiated tumours do not show keratinization. Nuclei are large, with frequent dysplasia and mitoses. Pleomorphism, disturbance of normal maturation of the epidermis, and the presence of surrounding inflammation can also be seen.

Treatment
- Incision or excision biopsy if the diagnosis is uncertain.
- Surgical excision treatment of choice for most SCCs: 4 mm margin in tumours <2 cm in diameter, Broders' grade 1, and outside high-risk areas (ear, lip, scalp, eyelids, nose); otherwise, 6 mm margin.
- Mohs' micrographic surgery: best reported results, but has not been compared with excision in randomized controlled trial.
- Curettage and cautery: in <1 cm diameter, well-differentiated primary lesions on sun-exposed sites only. No pathology assessment of clearance.
- Cryotherapy: only for very superficial primary lesions in specialist centres.
- Radiotherapy: for non-resectable tumours.
- Lymph node dissection is used for clinically positive nodes, after FNA to confirm diagnosis. Parotidectomy and neck dissection for spread to parotid region.
- Distant metastases may be treated with radiotherapy and chemotherapy.

Staging for SCC

Table 6.4 TNM classification

Primary tumour (T)	
Tx	Cannot be assessed
T0	No evidence primary tumour
Tis	Carcinoma *in situ*
T1	<2 cm in greatest dimension
T2	2–5 cm
T3	>5 cm
T4	Invades deep structures
Regional nodes (N)	
Nx	Cannot be assessed
N0	No lymph node metastases
N1	Regional lymph node metastases
Distant metastases (M)	
Mx	Cannot be assessed
M0	No distant metastases
M1	Distant metastases

Table 6.5 AJCC staging for SCC

Stage 0	Tis, N0, M0
Stage 1	T1, N0, M0
Stage 2	T2 or 3, N0, M0
Stage 3	T4, N0, M0 or any T, N1, M0
Stage 4	Any T, any N, M1

Table 6.6 Broders' histological classification of differentiation in SCC

Grade 1	Differentiated: undifferentiated cell ratio 3:1
Grade 2	1:1
Grade 3	1:3
Grade 4	No differentiation

Prognosis

95% 5-year clearance with 4–6 mm excision margins. Recurrence and metastasis rates are not known precisely. 95% local recurrences or metastases are detected within 5 years.

Prognostic factors
- Site: metastatic potential increases in:
  - Lip, or other mucocutaneous site.
  - Ear.
  - Non-sun-exposed site (e.g. perineum, sacrum, penis).
  - Within area of radiation of thermal injury.
  - Chronic wound.
- Size:
  - Tumours with diameter >2 cm are twice as likely to recur and three times as likely to metastasize.
- Depth:
  - >4 mm or Clark level V are more likely to recur and metastasize.
- Differentiation:
  - Broders' grades 3 and 4 show more recurrence and metastasis.
  - Prognosis depends on the degree of differentiation/anaplasia, degree of acantholysis.
- Evidence of perineural spread:
  - Perineural involvement increases recurrence and metastasis.
- Evidence of lymphatic spread:
  - Lymphatic and vascular invasion at tumour site do not increase risk of recurrence or metastasis.
- Host immunosuppression is associated with poorer prognosis.
- Recurrent lesions are more likely to recur again.

Follow up

Tumours >2 mm in depth follow-up for 2 years.

Merkel cell carcinoma

A rare malignant tumour with a great propensity for local recurrence, skip lesions within compartments, and metastases. Treatment is very wide local excision and radiotherapy. Best prognosis from early detection and treatment.

Definition

A malignant tumour derived from Merkel cells. These cells are part of the amine precursor uptake and decarboxylase (APUD) lineage, which may be of neural crest origin. The Merkel cell is thought to be a touch receptor, and is ubiquitous but is particularly prevalent in the skin of the lip, hard palate, palms, and neck.

Incidence

Accounts for <1% of all skin cancer. In Rochester, MN, USA, the incidence is 2/1 000 000. Caucasians are affected more often than black people. Males and females are affected equally. Mean age at diagnosis is 75 years old.

Aetiology

Possible causative factors include UV radiation, immunosuppression, erythema ab igne, and congenital ectodermal dysplasia.

Pathogenesis
Cytogenetic abnormalities and loss of heterozygosity have been demonstrated at various loci, including chromosome 1p36 (a locus implicated in the pathogenesis of several neural crest derived tumours, including malignant melanoma) and encoding the tumour suppresser gene *P73*.

Clinical features
Merkel cell carcinoma presents as a painless subcutaneous nodule. It often has a slight red or purple hue. 50% of tumours occur on the head and neck, although any mucosal or cutaneous surface may be affected. It is locally aggressive and commonly metastasizes to the regional lymph nodes and distant sites. 30% present with lymphadenopathy of which 10–20% have no primary, which is a favourable prognostic sign. Examination includes the entire skin and regional lymph node groups. Differential diagnoses include SCC, BCC, amelanotic melanoma, cutaneous lymphoma, and metastatic small cell cancers.

Pathology
Immunohistochemistry distinguishes from differential diagnoses.

Investigations
Excision biopsy. Chest and abdomen CT is indicated to rule out metastasis from a small cell carcinoma of the lung as the cause of the lesion, and also to stage the disease.

Staging for Merkel cell carcinoma

Table 6.7 TNM classification

T_1 Tumour <2 cm in diameter	N_0 Regional lymph nodes not affected	M_0 No distant metastasis
T_2 Tumour >2 cm in diameter	N_1 Regional lymph nodes affected	M_1 Distant metastasis present

Table 6.8 AJCC staging

Stage		5-year survival
Stage IA	T1 N0 M0	64%
Stage IB	T2 N0 M0	
Stage II	Any T N1 M0	47%
Stage III	Any T Any N M1	0%. Median survival 9 months

Management and post-operative care
Owing to the rarity of Merkel cell carcinoma, no randomized controlled trials of treatment have been published. Treatment should be tailored for site of primary and fitness of patient.

Stage I
Wide local excision of the primary lesion. Margins should be at least 3 cm. Mohs' micrographic surgery is not recommended because tumour deposits may be microscopically non-contiguous. Often the site does not permit 3 cm excision; therefore complete excision with 1 cm margins and local flap cover to permit early post-operative radiotherapy. The risk of nodal relapse is 76%; therefore the nodal basin needs to be addressed. Options include radiotherapy and sentinel node biopsy with completion if positive and prophylactic dissection (generally reserved for the high-risk patient such as IB, x10 mitoses, lymph permeation).

Stage II
As above plus node dissection and post-operative radiotherapy or radiotherapy alone, depending on disease bulk and patient factors. Chemotherapy should be considered.

Stage III
Palliative care. Surgery for symptom control. In disseminated disease palliative chemotherapy.

Kaposi sarcoma

Definition
A skin lesion characterized by multicentric proliferation of vasoformative tissue.

Incidence
Rising due to association with AIDS. Nine males affected to one female.

Aetiology and classification
I   Classic occurring in elderly males of Mediterranean or eastern European Jewish descent.
II Endemic—central Africa.
III Immunosuppressed in organ transplant patients.
IV AIDS-related.

Clinical presentation
Slowly progressive presentation of red-purple patches progressing to papules and then nodules. In classic type they occur on the extremities and are associated with lymphoedema. AIDS-related type can occur anywhere but most commonly on the face.

Pathology
- Develops from the endothelial cells of the blood vessels and lymphatics.
- Vascular and spindle cell proliferation with endothelial atypia.
- Has a reactive picture but can undergo sarcomatous change.

Prognosis
High propensity for local recurrence.

Treatment
Classic form is radiosensitive. Isolated lesions excise or cryotherapy. Endemic is aggressive and is best treated with chemotherapy. Immunosuppressed patients should have a change of suppression and chemotherapy. AIDS-related type is complex and local excision, laser, cryotherapy all have a role for focal lesions. Generalized change requires retroviral agents.

Microcystic adnexal carcinoma
- Uncommon slow-growing tumour of eccrine glands.

Risk factors
- Previous radiotherapy (10%), sun damage.

Pathology
Superficially keratinocytes, deeper epithelial strands in sclerotic stroma. Low mitotic rate but perineural invasion.

Clinical features
Nondescript painful flesh-coloured papules on central face of Caucasians, especially periorbital and perioral. Associated with tingling and numbness. If left can infiltrate deeply to bone and cartilage.

Treatment
Mohs' resection as usually in cosmetically sensitive areas. Defect size can be up to four times the lesion size. Wide excision with at least 5 mm margin; repeat excision rate is higher than with Mohs' resection. Once clearance is achieved the recurrence rate is similar between both treatments. Metastatic rate is low: <1%.

Sebaceous carcinoma

Risk factors
Increase in females, Asian population? HPV association, arsenic ingestion, previous radiotherapy and associated with Muir Torre syndrome.

Pathology
Irregular lobules of basaloid cells with sebaceous differentiation. Many mitoses. Pagetoid spread.

Clinical features
75% on eyelid (upper 3x lower) Mainly on face especially around the eye. Slow growing painless, papule or nodule with yellow or orange hue.

Treatment
Ensure no Muir Torre, most likely associated with gastrointestinal or genitourinary cancer.

If orbit involved exenteration. If orbit not involved Mohs excision or excision with at least 5mm margin. 30% local recurrence if incompletely excised. Metastatic rate 14–25%.

Leiomyosarcoma

Classification
I Cutaneous from arrector pili muscle.
II Subcutaneous from smooth muscle in blood vessels.

Pathology
Spindle cells with cigar-shaped nuclei.

Clinical features
Lower extremities of older patients.

Treatment
Wide local excision with adjunctive radiotherapy for high-grade subcutaneous tumours. There is a high recurrence rate. The risk of metastases is low for grade I (1%) and high for grade II (30–60%).

Dermatomafibrosarcoma protruberans (DFSP)
Also known as storiform fibrous histiocytoma.

Definition
A dermal skin lesion that can be considered malignant. A very low grade fibrosarcoma arising from the dermis, locally recurrent, rarely metastatic.

Aetiology
Usually associated with sun exposure.

Clinical presentation
Clinically a DFSP develops as a slow-growing fibrous plaque or protruberant lesion from the dermis, usually on the trunk. It is red to brown in colour and slowly increases in size becoming multinodular. The margins are indistinct. It may cause discomfort or pain.

Pathology
Pathologically characterized by cartwheel or rush mat (storiform) arrangement of fibroblasts (spindle shape) within dermis and may extend subcutaneously.

Prognosis
High propensity for local recurrence.

Treatment
Mohs' excision with wide margin of 3–5 cm.

Cysts

Epidermoid cyst

Definition
Cutaneous or subcutaneous swelling derived from squamous epithelium.

Aetiology
Blocked gland, implantation of squamous epithelium. Increased incidence in smokers. Genetic (Gardner's syndrome, AD).

Clinical presentation
Varied from painless enlarging swelling in oily skin areas such as post-auricular, posterior neck, cheek, and back. History of infection, discharge of sebaceous (cheesy) material. Examination reveals a firm pea- to bean-sized swelling attached to skin, and often a visible punctum is seen.

Pathology
Wall is made of keratinizing stratified squamous epithelium.

Treatment
Complete excision of cyst and wall via skin crease incision. Otherwise, recurrence is likely. Infected cysts should be treated with antibiotics/drained and secondary surgery to remove residuum.

Tricholemmal cyst (pilar cyst)

Definition
Common benign cysts derived from outer root sheath of hair follicle.

Incidence
Very common; 5–10% population, of which 70% have more than one lesion. Most are on the scalp.

Aetiology
Rarely, may be familial (AD); otherwise unknown.

Clinical presentation
Slow-growing, smooth mobile subcutaneous scalp lesions, very much like sebaceous cyst but no punctum. Often multiple. Occasionally tender and may become infected.

Pathology
A cyst surrounded by a fibrous capsule with small dark cuboidal basal cells. May be calcification and cholesterol clefts. Differentiate from epidermoid cysts by the presence of a granular layer in the lining cells. If cyst has ruptured there will be inflammatory reaction and a foreign body giant cell reaction.

Treatment
Surgical excision.

Prognosis
Benign. Very rare malignant transformation.

Dermoid cyst

Definition
A cyst caused by the inclusion of embryonic epithelium at the sites of embryonic fusion.

Aetiology
As above.

Clinical
Classically at the outer third of the eyebrow in children. They are round and may be mobile or fixed to underlying periosteum. There is no punctum. Beware the midline location as this should be formally assessed with a CT scan to ensure no deeper connection.

Pathology
Squamous epithelium in the wall and virtually any form of contents, but usually adnexal structures.

Treatment
Complete excision.

Fibrohistiocytic tumours

Dermatofibroma

Sometimes called typical cutaneous fibrous histiocytoma. Probably not a true neoplasm but an inflammatory reaction secondary to trauma.

Definition
Common benign cutaneous nodule in the epidermis; usually asymptomatic.

Incidence
Common; four times more common in females. Any age but peak incidence in twenties.

Aetiology
Unknown, but patients frequently report a preceding insect bite or minor injury. Theories of origin include reactive or neoplastic. May be a differentiated matured histiocytoma where the histiocytes have left, leaving the fibroblasts.

Clinical presentation
Usually small (<1 cm) but can be larger (up to 10 cm in diameter). Can be painful and itchy. Usually solitary superficial skin-coloured hemispherical nodule that feels stuck on to the skin with no induration. Usually on the limbs; grows then remains static; occasionally painful, itchy, or may be traumatized. Can be erythematous and hyperpigmented.

Pathology
Histologically shows pseudo-epitheliomatous hyperplasia and basaloid proliferation within the dermis superficial to the papillary dermis. May have antibodies to factor XIIIa (marker of epidermal fibroblasts) and show dermal fibrohistiocytic infiltrate. Cellular variant has a 30% local recurrence rate after excision.

Treatment
Treatment is reassurance if the diagnosis is certain. However, simple excision may be required, especially if the diagnosis is uncertain or the lesion symptomatic or large.

Prognosis
Outcome is excellent if excised.

Juvenile xanthogranuloma (JXG)

Also known as naevoxanthoendothelioma.

Definition
Benign asymptomatic yellowish-reddish papules in children.

Aetiology
?Granulomatous reaction of histiocytes.

Clinical features
Tumour of infancy/early childhood mainly on upper body and trunk. Sudden appearance—usually single (81%), occasionally multiple, rarely in their hundreds. Less than ~1 cm in diameter, usually firm rubbery feel and

reddish-brown but occasionally bright yellow in colour. Tend to resolve spontaneously leaving atrophic scars, but may take months or years to do so. Multiple JXG is associated with neurofibromatosis type 1, juvenile myeloid leukemia, and café au lait spots.

Pathology
Histiocytic infiltate in dermis. Foam cells.

Treatment
Reassurance; if systemic or ocular lesions use steroids.

Prognosis
Visceral involvement in 10% with occasional eye involvement which can be mistaken for a malignant ocular tumour.

Epidermal tumours

Seborrhoeic keratosis
Also known as seborrhoeic warts, senile warts, basal cell papilloma.

Definition
A benign proliferation of epidermal cells producing characteristic lesions.

Incidence
Most common skin lesion in adults. Prevalence varies from 10% of under forties to 100% in over-75s especially in sunny areas. Most people have more than one seborrhoeic keratosis and an increasing number as they age, reportedly getting as many as a median of 69 lesions once over 75. No difference in sex distribution. There may be an AD inherited trait for multiple seborrhoeic keratoses.

Aetiology
Unknown. There is an increased rate of apoptosis. EGF or its receptor is implicated.

Clinical presentation
Well-defined lesions which look as if they are stuck on the skin, may feel soapy or greasy, often have a finely verrucous appearance with black heads, but may be flat. Colour can be pale to black. They often enlarge and bleed when traumatized. Parts may flake off, causing concern. The pigmentation may be variable. Most are on the trunk but can be anywhere except the palms and soles. Size is usually <1 cm but can be 5 cm in diameter. Largest recorded is 35 × 15 cm! Usually oval or round. If oval aligned along lines of tension. The colour is from haemosiderin and melanin. Lesions can become inflamed and secondarily infected if traumatized. Differential diagnoses include melanoma, naevus, BCC, SCC, verruca, solar keratosis, etc.

Pathology
Papillomatous epithelial (basal) proliferation. Horn cysts (intra-epidermal) filled with cornified skin cells including melanin. Verrucous architecture. 10% are reticulated or adenoid type with numerous thin tracts of branched interwoven basaloid epithelial cells.

Treatment
- Reassurance.
- Shave excision or curette and cautery.
- Ensure specimen or fragments are sent for pathology. One in 16 (6.4%) of specimens submitted as seborrhoeic keratosis were found to be a malignant tumour.

Prognosis
Rarely, maliganancy (Bowen's disease, SCC, or melanoma) can develop in pre-exisiting seborrhoeic keratoses. More frequently, lesions are misdiagnosed as seborrhoeic keratoses when in fact they are malignant tumours.

Acrochordon (fibro-epithelial polyps, skin tags)

Aetiology
Unknown. Theories include viral infection, hormone imbalances, and a localized paucity of elastic tissue. However, histologically this is not seen. Associated with obesity and non-insulin-dependent diabetes.

Clinical features
Small soft common pedunculated skin neoplasm, usually 2–5 mm, found in axilla or on neck. Very common; 46% of population have one.

Pathology
Keratinizing squamous epithelium overlying a fibrovascular centre.

Treatment
Reassurance; excision if symptomatic, such as when it is irritated by clothing.

Sweat gland tumours

Cylindroma (turban tumour)

Definition
Benign skin adnexal tumour usually apocrine in origin.

Aetiology
Unknown. Probably a primitive sweat gland tumour differentiating into eccrine and/or apocrine cells. Can be familial (AD) related to gene *CYLD* on 16q12–13.

Clinical presentation
Uncommon. Female-to-male ratio 6:1. Solitary or multiple. Usually on scalp, head, and neck. Slow-growing dermal nodules; pinkish red or bluish in colour. Multiple form resembles a bunch of grapes or tomatoes, or a turban if large. Occasionally will erode through skull!

Pathology
Small basophilic cells in dermis. Differs from spiradenomas as there are no lymphocytes.

Treatment
Surgical excision and reconstruction as required or serial excision.

Prognosis
Usually benign but rarely malignant transformation.

Syringoma (papillary eccrine adenoma)

Definition
Benign cyst of sweat ducts derived from cutaneous eccrine cells.

Aetiology
Unknown. Can be associated with diabetes and Down's syndrome.

Clinical presentation
Common; females slightly more than males; any age from puberty onwards. Skin-coloured yellowish rounded papules in the dermis, which can look translucent. Small: <3 mm in diameter. Usually on cheeks, axilla, chest, abdomen, genitals. Usually multiple. Differential diagnosis includes trichoepithelioma, milial cysts, xanthelasma, BCC, and microcystic adnexal carcinoma.

Pathology
Dermal tumour composed of numerous small ducts in a fibrotic background.

Treatment
Reassurance, surgical excision.

Apocrine hidrocystoma (cystadenoma)

Definition
A benign cystic growth from the apocrine glands.

Clinical features
Slow-growing lump around the eye in middle age. It is dome-shaped and cystic with telangiectasia. Often mistaken for BCC.

Pathology
Intradermal cyst lined with epithelium.

Treatment
Excision.

Hair follicle tumours

Calcifying epithelioma of Malherbe (pilomatrixoma)

Definition
A pilomatrixoma is a hamartoma of the hair matrix which often calcifies.

Incidence
Uncommon. Female-to-male ratio 1.5:1. Most common in childhood (5–15 years) with a second peak in incidence at age 50–65 years.

Pathogenesis
Pilomatrixomas stain strongly for Lef-1, a marker of hair cell differentiation. 75% of pilomatrixomas have somatic mutations in the gene *CTNNB1*. This suggests that dysregulation of the beta-catenin–Lef pathway contributes to tumorogenesis. They are also strongly positive for *bcl-2* (an anti-apoptotic factor) on immunohistochemistry, which suggests that decreased apoptosis also plays a role in pathogenesis.

Clinical features
Pilomatrixomas present as solitary nodules that have been growing slowly over several months or years. Initially soft, but as they mature become stony hard as they calcify. Calcification can be extruded from the skin They are often asymptomatic, but may cause pain during episodes of inflammation. Most lesions occur on the face and neck, and less commonly on the chest and upper limbs. They are associated with myotonic dystrophy.

On examination, they are a single firm stony hard nodules, 0.5–3 cm in diameter, which are the colour of normal skin. Rare giant lesions up to 15 cm in diameter are reported.

Tent sign: stretching the overlying skin reveals a lobulated appearance secondary to calcification within the lesion.

Pathology
Found in the lower dermis and subcutaneous fat. Sharply demarcated and encapsulated mass of epidermoid cells with basophilic cells merging into a zone of eosinophilic 'shadow' cells which have lost their nucleus. As the lesion ages, the number of basophilic cells decreases and the proportion of shadow cells increases. Calcium deposits are seen in 75% of lesions.

Treatment
Despite self-resolution, concern over aetiology, cosmesis, and continued growth often indicates surgery. Simple excision and closure; rarely, large lesions may require reconstruction. The lesions may be poorly delineated, and incomplete excision has been reported to be followed by local recurrence, but this is rare. Pilomatrix carcinoma is a rare tumour which may derive from a pilomatrixoma. It tends to occur in older patients, and is locally aggressive. Visceral metastasis and death have been reported.

Vascular tumours

Pyogenic granuloma (granuloma telangiectatum)

Definition
Benign skin tumour of vascular origin. Differential diagnosis is amelanotic melanoma or vascular malformation. In view of differential diagnosis must be sent for pathology.

Incidence
Common at any age, but more frequent in children. Sites include hands, face, and upper trunk, but similar lesions can occur on oral mucosa and genital skin.

Aetiology
Unknown. May arise *de novo* in an area of injury, especially if there is secondary infection or in association with a vascular naevus.

Clinical features
Exophytic polypoid lesion that grows rapidly in the early stages; later, size remains unchanged. Usually red or blue-black, partially compressible, haemorrhagic, and 5–10 mm in diameter (rarely, larger). Has an epithelial collarette. Central area either thinly epithelialized or ulcerated. If ulcerated sometimes has a fibrinous or scab cover. Frequently bleeds, requiring dressing. Sometimes called 'Band-Aid disease'. Surrounding skin may be secondarily infected.

Pathology
Resembles chronic vascular lesion with granulation tissue; vessels similar to vascular malformation.

Treatment
- Best option is surgical excision, very low recurrence rate with excision with 1 mm margin normal skin. Often vascular proliferation is deep and therefore narrow excision may be necessary to cure the lesion.
- Medical management with steroid creams, pressure dressings.
- Silver nitrate.
- Pulsed-dye laser.
- Radiotherapy.
- Curettage and cautery, although recurrence is frequent and the pathology is made more difficult.

Prognosis
High propensity for local recurrence with treatment other than surgery.

Senile haemangioma (Campbell de Morgan spot)

Aetiology
Unknown.

Clinical features
Multiple asymptomatic red macules or papules. Anywhere in the body.

Pathology
Capillary haemangioma.

Treatment
Nil, excision, laser or cautery.

Mast cell tumours

Mastocytoma

Definition
Mast cell proliferation in the skin.

Incidence
May be present from birth but can develop in early childhood. Only 25% of cases are in adults, usually at age 30–40.

Aetiology
Cause unknown but thought to be either over-reactive or neoplastic.

Clinical presentation
Initially starts as pruritic recurrent blistering papules with a persistent red/brown discoloration. The pigmentation is melanocytic caused by melanocyte stimulation generated by soluble mast cell growth factor. In time the patch becomes raised and may be ≥1 cm in diameter. If the patch is scratched or rubbed the lesion becomes palpable, edematous, and itchy with surrounding erythema (Darier sign). In the young, lesions may blister; in older patients lesion blistering is rare. Lesions may be nodular and are usually on the trunk. 50% of patients will show dermatographia (can draw on skin producing a wheal because of mast cell degranulation). When solitary are generally benign and resolve spontaneously. Rarely, mastocytomas are generalized (urticaria pigmentosa) and very rarely malignant. There may be systemic symptoms related to mast cell mediators such as headache, flushing, dizziness, tachycardia, syncope, nausea, diarrhoea, etc.

Pathology
Histologically see mast cell aggregates in dermis.

Treatment
Treatment is topical corticosteroids but a biopsy may be needed. Multiple lesions or systemic symptoms should be treated by a dermatologist with antihistamines and disodium cromoglycate (inhibits degranulation of mast cells).

Port wine stain

Definition
Port wine stains (PWSs) are a form of a low-flow venous capillary malformation. They are a congenital malformation present in 0.3–0.5% of newborns. They are best known to be in the distribution of the territory of the trigeminal nerve (CN V1), but may be present elsewhere.

Pathology
Capillary malformation of the venous type. Composed of small vessels (mean vessel size 0.46 mm). These vessels undergo progressive ectasia. Most PWSs are superficial.

Clinical behaviour
Initially present as a pink patch which is sharply delineated commonly involving the territories of the ophthalmic (CN V1) and maxillary (CN V2) nerves. These vessels become progressively ectatic, resulting in gradual darkening and thickening, and the development of nodularity or cobblestone appearance. This is accompanied by overgrowth of the local tissues in the form of macrochelia, macroglossia, macrotia, and macrognathia. These do not resolve spontaneously.

Complications
These may result from:
- Altered cosmesis.
- Local overgrowth.
- Involvement of other organ systems (eye, meninges, CNS).
- Rarely, malignancy.
- Cosmetic concerns are secondary to the vascular patch on the face, which may cover a large anatomical area and the overgrowth of local structures. This may also have a devastating psychological effect on the patient, especially in early life.
- The incidence of glaucoma is relatively high (45%) in patients having involvement of both the V1 and V2 territories of the trigeminal nerve.
- A well-known association of this condition is the Sturge–Weber syndrome, which comprises a PWS involving the V1 territory (ophthalmic), ipsilateral glaucoma, eyelid angiomas, choroidal haemangiomas (40%), calcification, and vascular anomalies of the brain with associated seizures and occasionally mental retardation.
- Skull radiographs often show tramline calcification.
- BCCs are known to develop on long-standing areas of nodularity on the PWS patches.

Treatment

- Laser therapy is the current mainstay of treatment of these lesions which in the past were subjected to a number of modalities including surgical excision with grafting, local flaps, dermabrasion, radium implants, radiotherapy, tattooing, sclerotherapy, and cosmetic camouflage. All the above had unpredictable results, often with devastating sequelae.
- Childhood PWSs respond well to flash-lamp pulsed dye (FLPD) lasers. Early treatment has many advantages which include quicker resolution, fewer episodes of treatment, lower laser pulse doses, and a decreased need for anaesthesia.
- PWSs in adults require longer treatment with FLPD lasers. There is usually an overall improvement in facial PWSs but those on extremities respond very poorly.
- Side effects of FLPD laser treatment, especially in adults, include hyper- and hypopigmentation, atrophic surface changes, punctate depressions, and occasionally scarring.
- Ultimately there is a 10% recurrence rate over 10 years.

Pyoderma gangrenosum

- An auto-immune mediated cutaneous ulcerative condition frequently misdiagnosed as infection, especially as may follow minor injury (pathergy).
- Skin is commonly involved but involves other systems:
  - Heart.
  - Lungs.
  - Liver.
- Produces sterile neutrophilic abcesses.

Incidence
- 1/100 000, equal sex distribution, any age including children but peaks at 30–40 years.
- 50% associated with other systemic immune mediated conditions including rheumatoid arthritis, ulcerative colitis, Crohn's disease, leukaemia, lymphomas, IgA gammopathies and myelomas, primary biliary cirrhosis, SLE, Sjögren's syndrome, and other arthritides.
- Has been reported to occur following plastic procedures!

Clinical presentation
- Initially a small wound or bite with a red papule that gradually ulcerates.
- Deep ulcer with violaceous overhanging border.
- May have areas of superficial ulceration that are very exudative.
- Pain.
- Arthralgia, myalgia.
- Differential diagnosis includes all causes of ulceration and Wegener granulomatosis, SCC, gumma, atypical mycobacterial and factitious ulceration.

Investigation
- Exclude other causes of ulceration.
- Biopsy.
- Culture: note that there may be secondary colonization with bacteria erroneously supporting an infective cause.
- FBC, U&E, ESR.
- Immune studies.
- Serum electrophoresis; bone marrow aspiration if blood malignancy suspected.
- Urinalysis.
- CXR.
- Colonoscopy?
- Doppler or venous studies.

Management
- Exclude other causes. Diagnosis of exclusion.
- Local dressings/wound care.
- Corticosteroids: topical or systemic.
- Immunosuppresants: cyclophosphamide, infliximab, azathioprine.
- Maintain mobility and range of motion.
- Surgery should be avoided except for biopsy as new lesions may occur at operation sites, e.g. SSG donor site (pathergy).
- Multidisciplinary management of these patients is recommended.

Outcome
- Prognosis is good once therapy is started.
- Recurrence possible.
- Scarring common.

Suspect pyoderma gangrenosum if condition becomes worse after an operation, especially if a remote donor site also becomes affected.

Chapter 7

Eyelid

Ectropion *284*
Entropion *288*
Blepharophimosis, ptosis, and epicanthus inversus syndrome (BPES) *290*
Anophthalmos and microphthalmia *291*
Hypertelorism, epicanthus, telecanthus, and hypotelorism *293*
Ptosis *295*
Eyelid reconstruction *297*
Eyelid reconstruction in facial nerve palsy *302*

Ectropion

Definition
Abnormal eversion or outward rotation of the (usually lower) eyelid from the globe.

Aetiology
- Congenital: rare; usually of lower lid; deficiency of anterior lamella.
- Cicatricial: facial burns; trauma; chronic dermatitis; skin excision or laser treatment; transcutaneous ORIF of fractures; radiotherapy.
  - Primary: deficiency of skin and muscle.
  - Secondary: inadequate SSG or scar contraction.
  - Complex: fusion of lid structures at level of orbital septum such as following organizing haematoma, oedema, severe trauma, and orbital floor explorations.
- Mechanical: large tumours (e.g. neurofibroma).
- Paralytic: paralysis of orbicularis occuli, such as after facial nerve injury, results in loss of support of lower lid so that involutional changes and gravity cause ectropion. Ectropion is usually not a feature of paralysis in the young.
- Involutional: horizontal laxity of anterior lamella and stretching or disinsertion of medial and lateral canthal tendons; disinsertion of capsulopalpebral fascia from inferior tarsal plate; laxity of retractors. Starts with lid sag and scleral show; then lid margin everts, exposing medial punctum which may become occluded in association with keratinization of the palpebral conjunctiva. Progresses to involve entire lower lid.

Clinical features
Symptoms include:
- Irritation, dryness, burning, itching.
- Red edematous lids.
- Tearing or epiphora.
- Long-term sequelae:
  - Corneal ulceration.
  - Visual loss.
  - Kertinization of palpebral conjunctiva and lid margin.
  - Punctal phimosis.

Classification
- Congenital.
- Acquired:
  - Involutional (senile).
  - Cicatricial.
  - Paralytic.
  - Mechanical.

Examination

- Examine cornea and conjunctiva.
- Check visual acuity and ocular movement;
- Assess lid laxity using:
  - Anterior distraction test in which the eyelid can normally only be pulled 6–8 mm from the globe.
  - Snap-back test in which the eyelid is pulled away from the globe, and normally snaps back immediately.
- Assess deficiency of the anterior lamella by superior displacement of the lower lid, which normally will lift >2 mm above its normal position.
- Assess integrity of medial canthal tendon by pulling lower lid laterally; it should move <5 mm.
- Lateral canthal tendon: lateral canthal angle should lie within 6 mm of orbital rim.
- Visible punctum suggests medial canthal laxity.
- In paralysis, look for corneal sensation, Bell's phenomenon, and lagophthalmos.

Management

Medical

- Lubrication and moisture shields (worn at night).
- Tape lateral canthal skin.
- Wipe eyes up and in.
- Massage and steroid injections to soften scars.
- External upper lid weights may reduce corneal exposure.

Surgical

- Congenital or cicatricial ectropion requires release and replacement of deficient tissues with grafts or local flaps, as utilized in eyelid reconstruction. These may be assisted by canthoplasty.
- Involutional or paralytic ectropion, usually involving the lower lid; the type of procedure used depends on the cause and degree of the ectropion.
  - Isolated punctual eversion. Excise horizontal diamond of tarsus and conjunctiva 4–8 mm wide with the apex 0.5–1 mm below and just lateral to punctum (use lacrimal probe to protect lacrimal duct).
  - Medial laxity with punctual eversion: Byron Smith 'lazy T' excision of conjunctiva and tarsus (Fig. 7.1) combined with pentagonal full-thickness excision of medial eyelid; shortens vertically and horizontally.
  - Horizontal lid laxity: excise full-thickness pentagon of eyelid. Kuhnt–Symanowsky procedure (Fig. 7.2) is pentagonal wedge excision of tarsus and conjunctiva from the lateral part of the lower lid via a blepharoplasty incision, with re-draping and excision of lower lid skin.
  - Medial canthal tendon laxity: the tendon is plicated, resected, and re-attached to Whitnall's tubercle, or the entire medial canthus is excised with the inferior canaliculus; the medial canthal tendon is then reattached to the posterior lacrimal crest, and the divided canaliculus is marsupialized to maintain its patency.

- Lateral canthal tendon laxity: lateral canthal plication or lateral canthal sling in which a strip of the lower limb is passed through a slit in the upper limb of the tendon (Tenzel); lateral tarsal strip involves excision of the lower part of the lateral canthal tendon and the skin over the lateral tarsus, and then suturing the tarsus to the orbital rim. Alternatively, Marsh–Edgerton periosteal pennant can be used for lateral canthal re-attachment.
- Recurrence in paralytic ectropion can be helped by fascial slings, dynamic temporalis muscle transfers, or tarsorrhaphy.

Lagophthalmos

Upper lid retraction due to unopposed action levator in orbicularis oculi paralysis can be corrected by insertion of upper lid margin gold lid weights or springs, by tarsorrhaphy, which aims to reduce the horizontal width of the palpebral aperture by creating adhesions between the lateral part of the upper and lower lids, or by levator recession.

ECTROPION 287

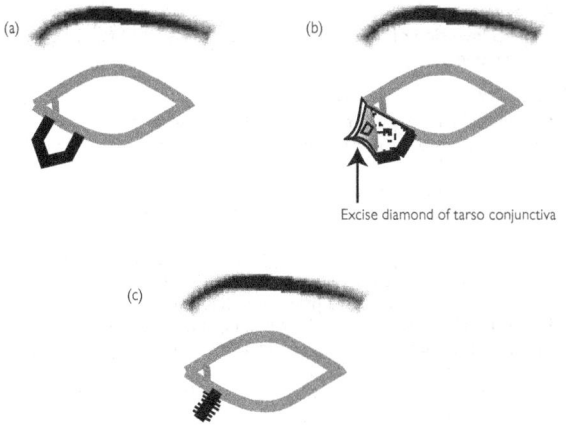

Excise diamond of tarso conjunctiva

Fig. 7.1 Lazy-T incision: (a) excise a full-thickness wedge medially at least 4 mm from the punctum; (b) reflect the medial remaining lower lid and excise a longitudinal diamond-shaped section of tarsoconjunctiva below the punctum, which inverts this part of the lid when sutured; (c) close the wedge.

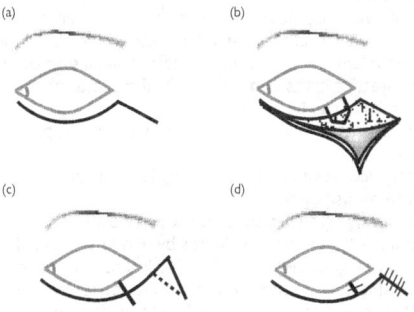

Fig. 7.2 Kuhnt–Zymanowsky procedure: (a) subciliary blepharoplasty incision; (b) elevate the skin flap and excise a lateral wedge of lower eyelid; (c) close the wedge and replace the skin, excising any excess laterally; (d) stitch.

Entropion

Definition
Abnormal inversion of the eyelid, causing the lashes to come into contact with the globe.

Aetiology
- **Congenital** Due to lack of the tarsal plate or hypertrophy of marginal pretarsal fibres of orbicularis occuli. May also be due to small or absent globe, or epiblepharon.
- **Cicatricial** Scarring of posterior lamella due to chemical injury, trachoma infection, Stevens–Johnson syndrome, ocular pemphigoid, or other inflammatory conditions.
- **Spastic** Overlapping of preseptal orbicularis fibres over pretarsal orbicularis causes the lower lid tarsal plate to rotate inwards. Usually young patients and a precursor to involutional entropion.
- **Involutional** ageing changes with a combination of disinsertion of the capsulopalpebral fascia, horizontal lid laxity, overlapping of preseptal orbicularis fibres over pretarsal orbicularis, and laxity of the lower lid retractors which causes the lower lid tarsal plate (which is thinner and buckles easily) to rotate inwards.

Clinical features
Symptoms are itching, burning, and grittiness due to eyelashes rubbing the globe and subsequent inflammation, which ultimately causes corneal ulceration. Signs include those of tight lid closure, lid inversion, scarring, and symblepharon (scarring or fusion of the bulbar and palpebral conjunctiva).

Management
- Congenital entropion due to hypertrophy of the pretarsal orbicularis can be treated by excision of infratarsal skin and pretarsal orbicularis with or without a lateral canthoplasty.
- Excision of overriding orbicularis muscle via transverse skin incision.
- Release of conjunctival scarring if this is causing vertical shortening of the posterior lamella, and pulling the tarsus and lashes onto the globe, and then insetting grafts of buccal or nasal mucosa, or conjunctiva. A localized band can be Z-plastied.
- Resection of anterior lamella and tarsus with sutures placed to evert lid margin.
- Transverse incision of tarsus (Weis, Fig. 7.3) may be transconjunctival, with suture repositioning.
- Conchal cartilage grafts to support lax tarsal plate.
- Horizontal lid-shortening procedures by mid-tarsal resection with a base-down triangular segment of conjuctival tarsus and lid retractors or by lateral tarsal resection, which can include lower lid suspension, tarsal rotation, and capsulopalpebral fascial tightening, or by canthal suspension.

Differential diagnoses
- **Epiblepharon** fold of redundant lower-lid skin which rolls over the lower lid margin, pushing the lashes onto the cornea. Sometimes called secondary entropion. Common in children, Chinese, and with swelling.
- **Trichiasis** Lashes only are turned in to touch cornea; lid margin in normal position.
- **Distichisis** Extra row of lashes on the inner margin of the lower lid abuts the cornea.
- **Symblepharon** Scarring or fusion of the bulbar and palpebral conjunctiva.

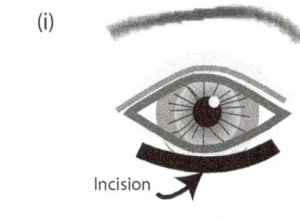

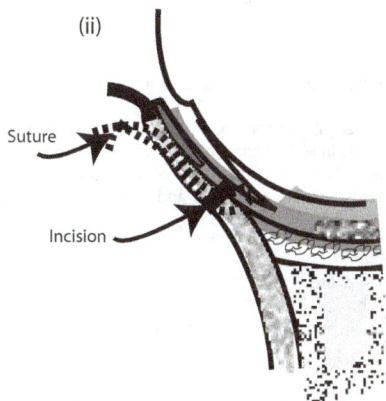

Fig. 7.3 Wies transverse tarsotomy and suture. A transverse incision completely through the lid to create a scar that prevents over riding of the pre-tarsal orbicularis, with a eversion suture to transfer pull of the lid retractors to the upper outer part of the tarsus.

Blepharophimosis, ptosis, and epicanthus inversus syndrome (BPES)

Definition
Constricted palpebral aperture and orbit.

Incidence
Rare.

Aetiology
- Autosomal dominant.
- Abnormalities located to 3q21–24.
- Mutation found in 50% of cases.

Classification
- Type I: associated with infertility due to ovarian failure; females only.
- Type II: no fertility problems; males and females affected.

Pathogenesis
Abnormalities in the *FOXL2* gene located on the long arm of chromosome 3 appear to cause developmental anomalies in eyelids and sometimes ovaries, possibly depending on the type of mutation.

Clinical features
- Ptosis.
- Epicanthal folds (epicanthus inversus, i.e. folds arise from lower lid).
- Telecanthus.

These cause reduced size of palpebral aperture. There may also be bony hypertelorism, microphthalmia, and abnormalities of the lacrimal apparatus. Extra-ocular manifestations which present variably include microcephaly, joint and limb anomalies, atrophy of uterus and ovaries, and growth and mental retardation.

Management
- Brow suspension for ptosis.
- Correction of epicanthic folds.
- Orbital remodelling by burring and bone grafts.

Anophthalmos and microphthalmia

Definition
Anophthalmos or anophthalmia is a complete absence of the globe within the orbital cavity. In microphthalmia the size of the globe is reduced, although it is still present.

Incidence
Estimated anophthalmia: 1/100 000.
Microphthalmia: 1/10 000.

Aetiology
Several genes have been identified in the formation of the globe and may be abnormal in anophthalmia and microphthalmia. Environmental factors, including radiation, toxins, drugs, and viruses, have also been implicated. The majority of cases are sporadic, or part of a recognized syndrome of congenital anomaly. Autosomal recessive, single-gene inherited anophthalmia has also been described.

Classification
- Primary anophthalmos: no evagination of optic vesicle occurs.
- Secondary anophthalmos: diffuse failure of forebrain development including eye.
- Degenerative anophthalmos: optic vesicle develops and then regresses.

Pathogenesis
The eye is formed in the embryo from a combination of neurectoderm of the forebrain (forming retina), neural crest mesenchyme (fibrous coats of globe), and surface ectoderm (lens and cornea). At day 22 of gestation the optic sulcus is visible on the forebrain. This projects laterally towards the surface ectoderm, forming the optic vesicle. The surface ectoderm overlying it thickens by day 28 into a lens placode, which invaginates into the vesicle at day 32–33 to form a lens vesicle. The surface ectoderm re-forms over the optic vesicle to create the cornea. Reciprocal interactions between the optic vesicle and lens placode are necessary for successful globe formation. The lacrimal apparatus, conjunctiva, and eyelids are of ectodermal origin. The eyelids unite over the cornea during the third month, and remain fused until the end of the sixth month. The globe is necessary for normal development of the orbital cavity.

Clinical features
Unilateral or bilateral anomaly. In microphthalmos the eye is reduced in size (axis <21 mm in adult, <19 mm in child) along a spectrum to complete absence of the eye. In anophthalmos eyelids are small and concave and when opened reveal a small empty conjunctival sac. Lacrimal apparatus is present and may function. Size of orbital cavity depends on size of globe, if any. Muscles of orbit are present.

Management

The aim is to create an adequate pocket for a prosthesis, and to match the contralateral eye if present. Tissue expansion is ideally started neonatally and continues over years. The following may also be required:
- Tissue expansion by implants.
- Bony resurfacing or osteotomies to enlarge the orbital cavity.
- Mucosal grafts to the enlarged cavity.
- Skin grafts or local flaps to eyelid skin.
- Tarsorrhaphy.
- Cartilage grafts or fascia lata sling to augment and support the lower lid.
- Upper lid surgery for ptosis.

Related conditions
- Fraser's syndrome consists of anophthalmia, abnormal genitalia, mental deficiency, renal agenesis, and abnormal ears.
- Coloboma: failure of fusion of optic fissure leading to a gap in some or all of the structures of the eye. May represent less severe form of the anophthalmia–microphthalmia spectrum of anomaly.

Acquired anophthalmos (i.e. secondary to surgery)
- Evisceration: the contents of the globe are removed and replaced with an acrylic spacer.
- Enucleation: the globe is removed from the orbit, leaving the other contents intact. An implant may be sutured to the orbital muscles to provide synergistic movement with the other eye.
- Exenteration removes the entire contents of the orbit, including the periosteum, and the eyelids. It can be reconstructed with a combination of bone graft, flaps, and grafts, or heal by secondary intention, which takes up to 3 months.

Hypertelorism, epicanthus, telecanthus, and hypotelorism

Hypertelorism

Increased distance between medial orbital walls. Normal distance is 23–28 mm.

Classification (Tessier)
- Type 1: 30–34 mm.
- Type 2: 35–39 mm.
- Type 3: >40 mm.

Cause
Usually congenital.

Treatment
Intracranial (more predictable) or subcranial osteotomies.

Epicanthus

A fold of skin from the nasal bridge that overhangs and obscures the medial canthus. It occurs commonly in oriental races. The fold arises from the upper lid (epicanthus palpebralis), the skin over the tarsus (epicanthus tarsalis), or the eyebrow (superciliaris). Epicanthus inversus is a variant where the fold arises from the lower lid.

Treatment
By variations of Z-plasty, jumping man flaps (Fig. 7.4).

Telecanthus

Increased distance between medial canthal edges.

Cause
Can be traumatic, congenital, or rarely tumour.

Treatment
Medial canthopexy either to each other (trans-ethmoidal) or to medial orbital wall.

Hypotelorism

Reduced distance between medial orbital walls (<23 mm).

Cause
Includes trigonocephaly, arrhinea (0–14 cleft), Binder's syndrome.

Treatment
Treat the cause; intracranial osteotomies.

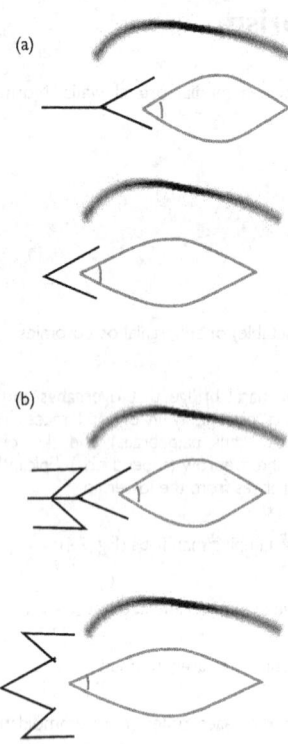

Fig. 7.4 Epicanthus and telecanthus procedures: (a) Y–V; (b) Mustardé double Z-plasty ('flying man').

Ptosis

Definition
Abnormally low level of upper eyelid (during straight ahead gaze).

Clinical presentation
- Obscures vision.
- Aesthetic concerns.

Classification
Congenital
- 85% congenital dystrophic (dystrophy of levator).
- 15% congenital aponeurotic or nerve palsy (non-dystrophic).

Acquired
- Neurogenic:
    - Oculomotor.
    - Sympathetic (Horner's syndrome).
- Myogenic:
    - Myasthenia gravis.
    - Chronic external ophthalmoplegia.
- Aponeurotic:
    - Trauma.
    - Senile/involutional.
- Mechanical:
    - Senile/involutional (excess eyelid).
    - Tumours.

Assessment
A detailed history may help to determine the cause.

Examination
- Degree of ptosis: measure distance from upper eyelid margin to reflected light reflex (corresponds to patient's visual axis).
- Position of lid in relation to cornea: measure extent that lid covers limbus (usually lid extends 1–2 mm below limbus).
- Levator function (normal 12–15 mm).
- Position of upper lid fold: if high, indicates levator aponeurotic dehiscence as levator is still attached to skin, but not distally.
- Bell's phenomenon.
- Lid lag (on downward gaze) suggests congenital origin.
- Quality of lid skin.
- Rate of return to inversion after manual eversion.
- Does ptosis increase on downward gaze?
- Hering's law: enhanced ptosis in myasthenia gravis, and brow ptosis.
- Visual acuity.
- Range of eye movement, especially superior rectus.
- Jaw winking.
- Corneal sensation.

Treatment

Generally, over-correct when levator function is bad and under-correct if levator function is good.

Treatment depends on levator function

- If levator lifts the lid ≥10 mm consider the degree of ptosis present. If the degree of ptosis is <2 mm do a Fasanella–Servat procedure; if 2–3 mm do a levator plication; if the degree of ptosis is >3 mm try aponeurosis surgery.
- If levator lifts the lid <10 mm and the degree of ptosis is >4 mm do a levator resection procedure, but if the degree of ptosis is <4 mm a brow suspension or occipitofrontal suspension is needed.

Fasanella-Servat procedure (Fig. 7.5)

Essentially a trans-conjunctival Müllerectomy. There are many modifications (Beard, Smith, Iliff).

Levator plication or resection

Transcutaneous or trans-conjunctival. The levator aponeurosis is plicated or resected and advanced directly onto the tarsus.

Aponeurosis surgery

- Can comprise levator aponeurosis resection, advancement, or repair; used when levator function is good.
- Conjunctival approach is good when levator function is adequate.
- Cutaneous approach is better when levator function is poor or fair.

Frontalis muscle suspension

Done using a variety of suspension materials (usually strips of fascia lata) and suspension patterns (usually Crawford's pattern: an M with an inverted V roof on top). It is difficult to achieve symmetry.

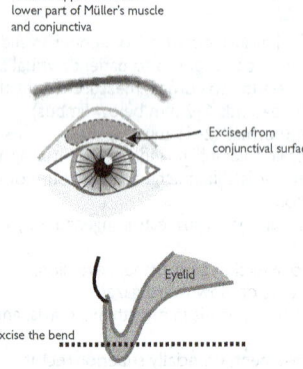

Fig. 7.5 Fasanella–Servat upper border tarsectomy and Müllerectomy via conjunctival approach. (a) Anterior view showing the area of excision from the conjunctival surface; (b) Lateral view: evert the lid and excise an ellipse of conjunctiva, upper pole tarsus, and lower insertion of Müller's muscle.

Eyelid reconstruction

Eyelid injuries are common, as are eyelid tumours requiring excision and reconstruction. Careful repair or reconstruction can restore function and aesthetics.

Repair of eyelid injuries

Debridement
Do not excise tissue. Most losses are apparent rather than real (due to retraction).

Repair
- Re-appropriate all tissues accurately.
- Do not need to suture orbital septum if in line with orbicularis fibres.
- Repair any muscles/aponeuroses.
- Repair or intubate lower canniculus but not upper canniculus. Leave tube in for 6 months.
- If common cannaliculus and/or lacrimal sac are injured may need dacryocystorhinostomy.
- If medial canthal tendon is divided, giving traumatic telecanthus, repair across nasal bridge with transnasal wire/suture.

Orbital fractures
- Assess:
  - If fractured.
  - If muscle trapped.
  - Enophthalmos.
  - Diplopia—mostly due to haemorrhage/traction on septa/muscle rather than entrapped muscle. Allow to settle.
- If there is a large fracture or if it is depressed, or causing muscle herniation or entrapment, consider operative reduction and fixation.
- Approaches to orbital floor:
  - Trans-conjunctival plus lateral canthoplasty.
  - Subciliary blepharoplasty—variations on plane, superficial or deep to orbicularis or both, i.e. superficial to pre-tarsal and deep to preseptal muscle.

Eyelid reconstruction
- Depends on size, position, and composition of defect.
- Excise tumour with 4–6 mm margin peripherally and on the deep surface to 1 mm clear surgical plane (therefore if fixed to tarsus do full-thickness excision of tarsus).
- Consider function of that portion of lid, i.e. mid-upper: corneal contact, very mobile. If outer lower eyelid: more structural, static.
- Beware ectropion/corneal abrasion.
- Consider whether defect will include margin. If not, much easier reconstruction as usual partial-thickness or full-thickness skin graft or flap.

Defect size

If it does include the margin, consider the size of the defect.

Lower lid
- Less than a third: direct closure plus cantholysis.
- Less than half: semicircular flap or cheek rotation flap (Mustardé) (Fig. 7.6).
- More than half: cheek rotation flap.
- Unless defect is lid margin only, i.e. vertical defect<5 mm from lid margin, then tarso-conjunctival flap and full-thickness skin graft (Hughes) (Fig. 7.7).

Upper lid
- Less than a third: direct closure plus cantholysis.
- More than a third: semicircular flap (Tenzel).
- More than a half: lower lid bridge flap (Cutler–Beard) (Fig. 7.8).
- If vertical defect <5 mm consider tarsal graft and local skin mobilization.

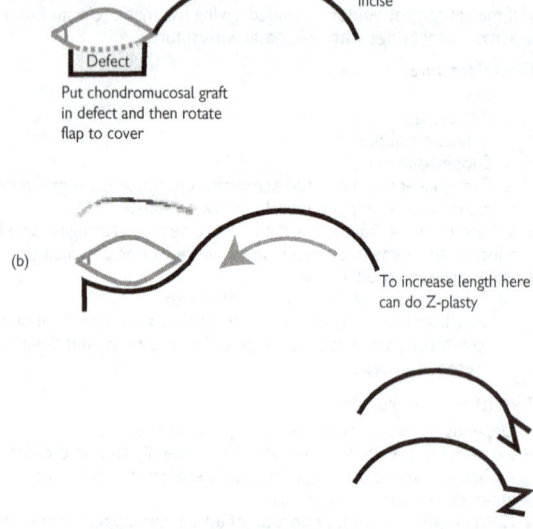

Fig. 7.6 Mustardé cheek rotation flap and chondro-mucosal graft. (a) Large defect of lower lid reconstructed with a cheek rotation flap with support given by a septal chondro-mucosal graft. (b) The cheek flap advanced. Greater length can be achieved by incorporating a Z-plasty at the distal end of the flap.

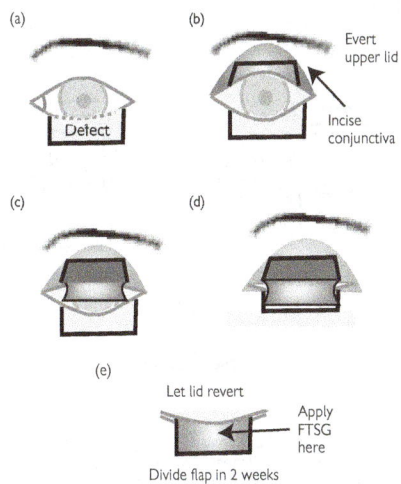

Fig. 7.7 Hughes tarso-conjunctival flap and skin graft eyelid reconstruction: (a) large lower lid defect; (b) upper eyelid everted and a conjunctival flap raised; (c) flap advanced into the defect; (d) flap sutured into defect, and upper lid allowed to revert; (e) FTSG applied on top of flap.

Direct closure
- Lower lid: beware ectropion. Therefore always try to close vertically but beware secondary scar contracture causing ectropion. If the scar is long do a vertical scar Z-plasty.
- Upper lid: place scar in skin crease (similar to blepharoplasty).

Skin graft
- Almost always full thickness.
- Almost always similar skin, i.e. thin 'blush skin' from clavicles and post-auricular groove or contralateral upper eyelid.

Wedge excision (full thickness) (Fig. 7.9)
- Do not excise as a wedge as this leads to notch in eyelid margin.
- Ensure the excision is at right angles to lid margin and then complete the wedge with an ellipse or angles, creating a pentagon.
- Close lid margin first at grey line with 6/0 silk to align it correctly (leave long ends to avoid eye irritation). With slight traction then suture the tarsal plate with the suture buried in the tarsus or anterior to the tarsus and conjunctiva.
- Suture conjunctiva with an inverting suture with absorbable 6/0 vicryl. Then suture orbicularis.
- Suture skin, catching long ends of suture closest to eyelid margin.
- Removal of stitches 5–7/7, leave margin sutures 10–14/7.

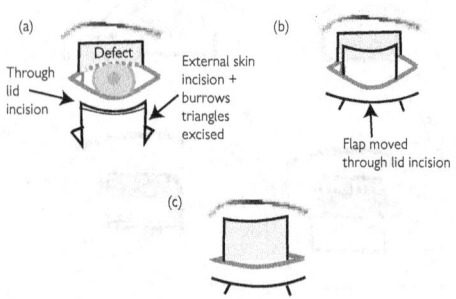

Fig. 7.8 Cutler-Beard lower lid bridge flap. (a) Large upper eyelid defect. A skin flap is raised from the lower eyelid/cheek skin and advanced under a full-thickness lower lid incision 4–6 mm below lid margin. (b) The flap is pulled through and inset into the upper eyelid defect. (c) Inset; divided later to restore vision.

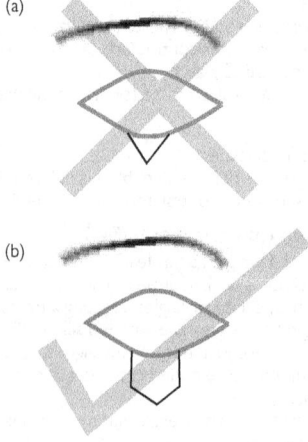

Fig. 7.9 Wedge excision of eyelid: (a) should not be a wedge; (b) should be a pentagon.

Lateral cantholysis

Release of appropriate limb of lateral canthal tendon, i.e superior for upper eyelid and inferior for lower eyelid.

Technique (Fig. 7.10)

- Horizontal incision in line with palpebral fissure.
- Scissor dissection to isolate appropriate limb.
- Divide under tension; leave other limb intact.
- Move divided limb towards midline.
- The conjunctiva from the fornix advances across to reconstruct the eyelid.
- May need to close this conjunctiva to skin.

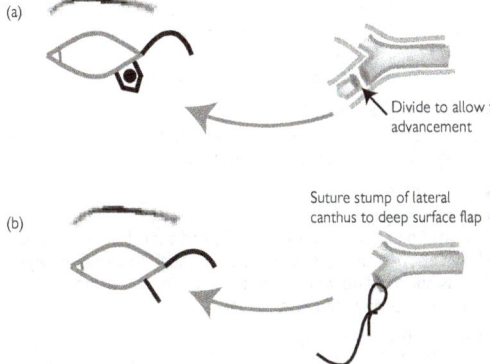

Fig. 7.10 Tenzel semicircular flap and lateral cantholysis: (a) wedge excision of lesion, design of the semicircular flap, release of the lower limb of the lateral tendon to allow advancement of the flap and conjunctiva; (b) suture and fixation of the lateral canthal stump to prevent retraction.

Eyelid reconstruction in facial nerve palsy

- Lid tightening procedures.
- Lateral canthus shortening.
- Fascial sling.

Tarsorrhaphy

Indicated for corneal protection (McLaughlin).

Temporary (Fig. 7.11)
- Do not excise much if any eyelid tissue, so that when it is reversed, it looks normal.
- Excise only a rim of margin of conjunctiva posterior to the grey line of both the upper and lower eyelids for the required distance.
- Suture together with another suture to bolster, leave 4–6/52.

Permanent (Fig. 7.12)
- Lower eyelid is split at grey line and anterior tissues excised. The superior eyelid has a corresponding area excised, posterior to the grey line and partial thickness of tarsus.
- The two areas are overlapped and sutured.

Encirclement (file d'Arion)
A central tarsorrhaphy with sling indicated if there is corneal exposure following a facial nerve palsy and lower eyelid ectropion.

Lagophthalmos
Upper eyelid weights:
- Use gold place deep to orbicularis, and superficial to tarsus.
- Heavy enough to close lid but light enough to allow the eye to open.
- Assess appropriate weight by taping on in first instance.

Upper eyelid springs can also be used.

See also Ectropion surgery.

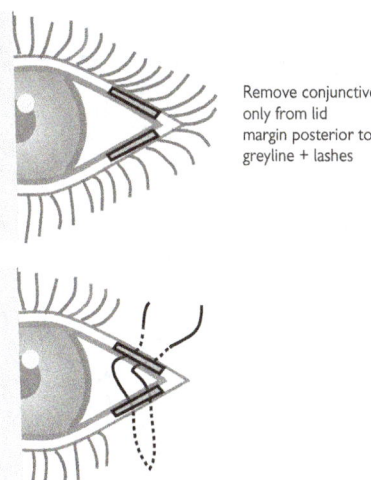

Fig. 7.11 Temporary tarsorrhaphy: Remove a rim of posterior conjunctiva only from both lids.

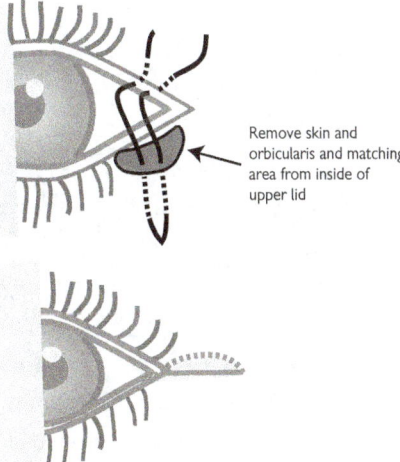

Fig. 7.12 Permanent tarsorrhaphy. Remove anterior tissues on the lower lid and posterior tissues on the upper lid and suture with bolster sutures.

Chapter 8

Nose, ear, face, mouth

Nasal reconstruction 306
Rhinophyma 314
Ear reconstruction 315
Facial nerve palsy 318
Cheek reconstruction 323
Drooling 327
Lip reconstruction 329
Swallowing 336

Nasal reconstruction

Historical perspectives
The first recorded nasal reconstruction was with cheek (not forehead) flap skin as described in the *Hindu Book of Revelation* by Sushruta Samhita in 600BC. In the sixteenth century, Gaspare Tagliacozzi, Professor of Anatomy at the University of Bologna, used a distally based medial arm flap to reconstruct the nasal tip. The pedicle was divided at 3 weeks (and, curiously, at 2 weeks in damp weather).

Aetiology
- Malignancy (particularly BCC and to a lesser extent SCC).
- Trauma.
- Congenital.

Anatomy
The nose is a complex structure involving the nasal skeleton, an internal mucosal lining, and an external skin covering. The mucosal lining is tightly adherent to the underlying deep surfaces of the nasal skeleton, thus limiting primary closure of mucosal defects to those <5 mm in diameter. The skin becomes progressively less distensible from the glabella to the nasal tip, with greatest pliability over the nasal dorsum and lateral walls. The skin is highly sebaceous, particularly at the tip, but it heals well with minimal scarring. The nose can be considered in terms of a number of aesthetic units:

The nasal skeleton may be considered in thirds:
- Upper—nasal bones and ascending processes of the maxilla.
- Middle—the paired upper lateral cartilages.
- Lower—the paired lower lateral (alar) cartilages.

These unite in the midline as the dome (the medial crura) in a tripod formation, thus suspending the nasal tip. The medial crura also support the columella. The lateral crura attach to the piriform aperture.

Aims of reconstruction
These are both aesthetic and functional (i.e. patent airway). The principles were described by Burget (1985):
- Restoration of 'normal' in terms of colour, texture, contour.
- Replacement of missing parts with tissue that is like in both quality and quantity. Flaps are generally preferred to grafts because of their superior aesthetic qualities, ability to cover the nasal skeleton, and resistance to contracture.
- A template (suture packet foil) is helpful to reconstruct 3D defects accurately.
- Recreate the aesthetic subunit, not just fill the defect. Thus a defect of ≥50% in an aesthetic unit necessitates reconstruction of the entire unit.
- Place surgical scars in the borders between aesthetic units for optimal results (Fig. 8.1).

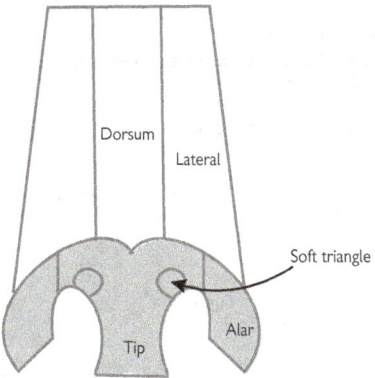

Fig. 8.1 Nasal aesthetic subunits.

Reconstructive techniques

The 'reconstructive ladder' approach is commonly used for cutaneous defects of the nose, but is not always appropriate.

Healing by secondary intention
May be appropriate for partial-thickness defects <10 mm in diameter.

Primary closure
Only suitable for the smallest lesions, particularly in the lower third, because of the immobility of the nasal skin. Better in dorsal skin.

Split skin graft
Prone to cicatricial contracture, although may be useful as a temporary measure until, for example, formal histology is available prior to embarking on a major nasal reconstruction post tumour excison.

Full-thickness skin graft
As with SSG, should aim to replace the entire cosmetic unit. Pre-auricular skin makes a satisfactory match for the upper part of the nose. Post-auricular or supraclavicular skin may also be used, but the colour match is less satisfactory.

Composite grafts
Useful for reconstructing full-thickness defects of the alar rim. A well-vascularized bed is essential. Limited to a maximum size of 1 cm from vascularized border or overall size <2 cm width. Graft 'take' can be made more reliable by increasing the area of inset by turning down para-defect skin for lining, thus making the skin defect larger but reducing the proportion of the defect that is full thickness.
- Helical rim.
- Root of helix.

Donor site is closed directly. Can notch at the scar line, especially if inset is not stepped. Central necrosis can occur, also producing a notch.

Local flaps
- Bilobed flap (Esser 1918).
- Nasolabial flap (Dieffenbach, nineteenth century).
- Banner flap (Elliott 1969).
- Nasalis flap.
- Dorsal nasal flap (Rieger, Marchac).
- Horn flap.
- V–Y advancement flap from the cheek.
- Alar advancement rotation flap (like Antia–Buch on helical rim but advancing the alar and closing the secondary defect on the nostril sill and base by V–Y closure.)

Distant flaps
- Forehead flap ('Indian technique').
- Scalping flaps (Washio, Converse).

Free tissue transfer
- Radial forearm flap ± bone.
- Dorsalis pedis flap.
- Postauricular flap.
- Auriculo-temporal flap.

Reconstruction of the nasal lining

Lining is often neglected, but inadequate nasal lining is a common cause of aesthetic and functional failure in nasal reconstruction. An adequately vascularized lining is essential for the successful placement of primary cartilage grafts. To line the entire nose anterior to the maxilla requires a piece of skin of dimensions 8 × 9 cm. Options include:
- Turn-down flaps of adjacent skin (Fig. 8.2).
- Mucosal grafts from the septum or intra-oral mucosa.
- Skin or composite grafts.
- Intra-nasal mucosal flaps.
- Intra-nasal chondromucosal flaps.
- Intra-oral mucosa buccinator flap.
- Cutaneous flaps.

Millard (1974) described a nasolabial lining flap. However, it tended to be bulky and thus capable of occluding the airway in bilateral cases.

The ipsilateral septal pivot flap (Burget and Menick 1972) is an anteriorly based septal mucoperichondrial flap based on the septal branch of the superior labial artery. It can adequately cover the internal aspect of the nasal tip.

Millard (1967) described a bipedicled mucosal advancement flap (subsequently modified by Burget and Menick (1986)) based medially on the remaining septum and laterally on the piriform aperture. It can be used to support defects of the distal half of the nose including auricular cartilage used to support a reconstructed alar rim. The dimensions of the defect are marked out on the septum using a template. The flap is dissected free in a submucoperichondrial plane, maintaining a base diameter. of at least 15 mm. A back-cut is made in the distal flap to allow transposition into the defect. The resulting exposed septal cartilage will re-epithelialize provided that the contralateral mucosal lining is left undisturbed.

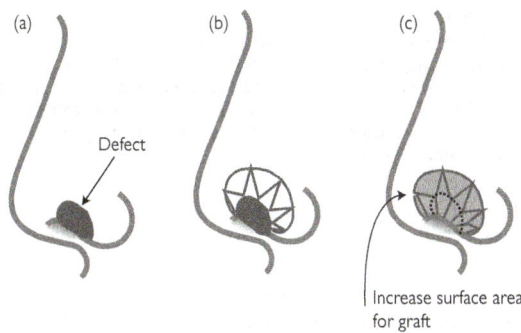

Fig. 8.2 Turn-down flaps to reconstruct nasal lining: (a) the defect; (b) a larger defect is outlined at least the radius of the original defect in width; (c) the skin from this outlined area is raised in the subcutaneous plane and turned down to provide lining and covered with a further flap or graft for external cover.

Skeletal support

This is a critical component of any nasal reconstruction. Much like limb reconstruction, skeletal stability and reconstruction is the essential step. Anatomically, the skeletal support of the nose can be considered in terms of a rigid central scaffold which maintains projection of the nose and tip elevation with lateral alar cartilages which tent the vestibule, thus permitting adequate air flow.

Options are prosthetic implants, cartilage, and osteochondral or osseous grafts or flaps. It goes without saying that any such grafts require a well-vascularized bed to minimize the risk of delayed resorption, distortion, extrusion or infection.

Septal support

L-strut (Gillies 1920) utilizes bone (e.g. olecranon) or cartilage (e.g. costochondral) to bridge the nose from the nasal radix to the tip, where it angulates in order to rest on the anterior nasal spine. It has a tendency to be unstable in a lateral plane and to produce an excessively wide columella.

The hinged septal flap is not dissimilar to the L-strut, except that the strut is made from a carved flap of septum which is hinged superiorly to augment the nasal angle.

The cantilever bone graft is secured at the nasal radix and extends to the nasal tip where it sits unsupported by an additional strut. Stability relies entirely on the fixation to the radix. Donor sites include split calvarium, ileum, rib, and tibia.

Lateral support
Free cartilage grafts are used. Donor sites include septal cartilage (in limited supply), conchal cartilage (curved and thus ideally suited to alar reconstruction), costal cartilage (plentiful and strong, and thus able to afford projection, although prone to warping in patients aged <35 years), and costochondral cartilage (less prone to warping compared with pure costal cartilage).

Tip grafts
Cartilage grafts, usually conchal or septal, are used. Conchal already has a nice curve or dome shape. Can be layered to produce the required contour.

Determinants of reconstructive choice
Choice of reconstruction depends on the site, size, and complexity of the defect, the patient (age, health, other scars, requirements), and the surgeon (experience, knowledge, preference). In general there are some techniques that are more suitable for some areas and size defects than others. FTSGs are a safe fall-back position but do not provide the best aesthetic result. Consider reconstruction in the following sites.

Nasal dorsum
Skin-only defects
- Glabella advancement rotation V–Y flaps.
- Direct closure.

Nasal sides
Skin-only defects
- Small:
  - V–Y advancement flaps from the cheek (parallel to nasolabial fold).
  - Banner flap.
  - Bilobed flap.
- Long or large:
  - Cheek advancement flap.
- Junction with alar:
  - Nasolabial flap.
  - Bilobed flap.
  - Nasalis flap.
  - Horn flap.

Nasal tip

Skin-only defects

- Small:
  - <0.5 cm and not near rim or soft triangle. Leave to heal, bilobed flap, banner flap, horn flap, nasalis flap, FTSG, direct closure in longitudinal direction if in midline. Near rim or soft triangle:
    —Dorsal nasal flap.
    —Bilobed flap.
- Large (whole tip or hemi-tip and alar):
  - Dorsal nasal flap.
  - Forehead flap.
  - Free auriculo-temporal flap.

Skin and cartilage defect

- Chondral graft (conchal) and flap as above.
- Composite graft.
- Forehead flap and conchal cartilage graft.
- Free auriculo-temporal flap.

Nasal alar

Skin only defects

- Small:
  - <0.25 cm and not near rim. Leave to heal, direct closure in longitudinal direction.
  - >0.25 cm. Bilobed flap, banner flap, horn flap, nasalis flap, dorsal nasal flap, FTSG.
  - Near rim or includes rim:
    —Bilobed flap.
    —Dorsal nasal flap.
    —Nasolabial flap.
    —Composite graft.
    —Direct closure—will narrow nostril.
  - Rim defect (small):
    —Alar advancement rotation flap (like Antia–Buch on helical rim but advancing the alar, closing the secondary defect on the nostril sill and base by V–Y closure) (Fig. 8.3).
    —Composite graft.
- Large (whole alar or hemi-alar):
  - Composite graft.
  - Nasolabial flap.
  - Forehead flap.
  - Free auriculo-temporal flap.

Skin and cartilage defect

- Chondral graft (conchal) and flap of choice as above.
- Composite graft.
- Forehead flap and conchal cartilage graft.
- Free auriculo-temporal flap.

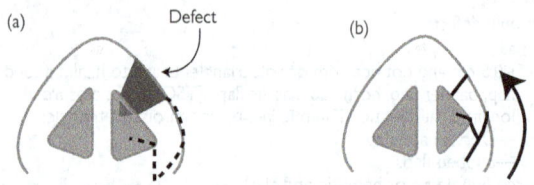

Fig. 8.3 Alar advancement flap to close alar rim defect.

Columella
- Advancement flaps: V–Y or rectangular with nasal base advancement (see cleft nose section).
- Composite graft.

Hemi-nasal
Skin only defects
- Mix of techniques to reconstruct each aesthetic unit. Therefore cheek advancement flap for side of nose, and composite graft, forehead flap, or auriculo-temporal flap for tip and alar.
- Forehead flap.

Skin and cartilage defect
- As above but with cartilage graft, or increased emphasis on composite tissue transfer.

Total nasal
- Lining by nasolabial flaps, septal mucosa, oral mucosa, buccinator flaps.
- Skeleton reconstructed by cantilever of L-strut bone or costochondral graft.
- Tip and alar by cartilage graft (conchal).
- Skin by forehead flap.
- Alternatively prefabricated nose in forearm pocket and free radial forearm flap.

Prosthetic reconstruction
In patients either unwilling or unfit to undergo major nasal reconstruction, a Bränemark osseo-integrated prosthesis or external spectacle-mounted prosthesis may be an appropriate management option.

Tips
- Big flaps are beautiful.
- Big flaps are harder for the eye to focus on and hence are better disguised, especially when the margins are on aesthetic boundaries. Big flaps are also less likely to trapdoor, suffer scar contracture, or cause nostril notching.

- See the flap sections for details on the various flaps. Specific tips for nasal application of the following flaps are:
  - Bilobed flap: try to keep the flaps on one side of the nose rather than cross the nasal midline as this disturbs aesthetic boundaries, and as the scar crosses a convex surface it is liable to contract and result in a contour deformity. As the skin is quite stiff in this region, wide undermining in a submuscular plane (just above perichondrium and periosteum) aids success.
  - Nasolabial flap: beware obliterating important boundaries such as the alar groove. Second procedure may be required to recreate the normal alar crease, but it is easier not to harm it in the first place. Techniques include island flap on a subcutaneous pedicle, exteriorize the pedicle, and do in two stages. Design as high as possible on the nose cheek margin.

References

Burget GC (1985). *Clin Plast Surg* **12**, 463–80.
Burget GC, Menick FJ (1972). *Plast Reconstr Surg* **50**, 580–7.
Burget GC, Menick FJ (1986). *Plast Reconstr Surg* **78**, 145–57.
Millard DR, Jr (1967). *Plast Reconstr Surg* **40**, 337–42.
Millard DR, Jr (1974). *Plast Reconstr Surg* **53**, 133–9.

Rhinophyma

Definition
A phyma is a localized swelling of facial soft tissue due to a combination of fibrosis, sebaceous hyperplasia, and lymphoedema. A rhinophyma is such a swelling on the nose.

Epidemiology
Phymas may also occur on the ears, forehead, or chin. They are more common in men than women.

Aetiology
Frequently associated with end-stage rosacea. Not related to alcohol.

Clinical appearance
Usually starts on the nasal tip and progresses to alae and columella. Colour varies from normal to deep red and purple. Forms a bulbous irregular swelling with a pitted surface.

Microscopic
Sebaceous hyperplasia with fibrosis.

Management
Physical ablation by paring off the excess tissue, sculpting the soft tissues to the contour of the nose, and allowing healing by re-epitheliazation is the optimal treatment. This can be achieved by shave excision, dermabrasion, electrosurgery, or carbon dioxide laser. Alginate dressings can help with haemostasis and will wash off within days.

Complications
- Recurrence.
- Delayed healing.

Ear reconstruction

An intimate knowledge of ear anatomy, relationships to facial structures, and proportions is required to reconstruct the ear. This section focuses on reconstruction of acquired defects. An earlier section covers ear reconstruction of congenital defects.

Functions of the external ear
- Cosmetic.
- Establishing the directional source of sound.
- Supporting spectacles.

Aetiology of external ear defects
Congenital
- Microtia (syndromic or non-syndromic).
- Cryptocia.
- Prominent ear.

Acquired
- Neoplasia (SCC, BCC, melanoma):
  - 10% of all cutaneous malignancies affect the ear.
  - Age 50 or above.
  - Male-to-female ratio 9:1. May be related to occupational hazards (e.g. construction industry) and hairstyle differences.
  - 60% SCC, 35% BCC, 5% MM.
  - 60% affect the helical rim.
- Trauma:
  - Laceration.
  - Abrasion.
  - Avulsion.
  - Haematoma.
- Thermal injury:
  - Frostbite—ears are an exposed extremity susceptible to frostbite.
  - Burns—ears are involved in 90% of facial burns.

Treatment
Frostbite
Rapid rewarming with towels soaked in sterile water at 30°C. Dress with Sulfamylon ointment which has good cartilage penetration. No debridement until clear demarcation has occurred.

Burns
Initial conservative management with cleansing of the burn and application of Sulfamylon ointment. Avoid pressure injury (e.g. from an endotracheal tube), and aggressively treat bacterial chondritis with debridement and intravenous and topical antibiotics. Reconstruction is delayed.

Haematoma
Blood accumulates between cartilage and perichondrium. Prompt drainage and irrigation followed by a pressure dressing to obliterate the dead-space prevents re-accumulation of haematoma, which can subsequently act as a nidus for new cartilage formation, leading to a 'cauliflower ear'.

Laceration/abrasion
In principle, thoroughly cleanse with minimal debridement. Marginally viable tissue can be excised at a later stage if it becomes necrotic. Anatomical landmarks should be meticulously aligned.

Avulsion/amputation
The ear is more commonly subject to avulsion than sharp amputation, making microvascular replantation difficult. The vessels within the pinna are frequently 0.3–0.7 mm in diameter, and differentiating arteries from veins may be difficult. Use of the superficial temporal vessels for end-to-end anastomosis will result in the loss of the temporo-parietal fascia flap (TPFF) which may be required for salvage if the replantation fails. Despite these drawbacks, successful replantation has been reported, and gives the most favourable long-term results.

Many methods of salvage of the cartilage framework have been described, including banking the cartilage in a subcutaneous pocket, removing the posterior skin and fenestrating the cartilage before placing in an auricular pocket, and covering denuded cartilage with a TPFF. All methods lead to relatively poor long-term results as the delicate auricular cartilage cannot effectively counteract the contractile forces of wound healing.

Cutaneous defects
Random pattern flaps from auriculo-cephalic sulcus or mastoid area. Hairless skin can easily be provided by random pattern flaps from the retro-auricular or mastoid area for coverage of lateral skin defects. Flaps can be passed through a cartilage window. Donor defects can be closed by advancing local tissue or by SSG.

Helical defects
Wedge excision, FTSG, Antia–Buch chondro-cutaneous flap, tunnel procedure, and tubed pedicle flap.

Less than 15 mm
Can be closed directly by extending the defect centrally as a wedge or using the star modification to avoid buckling of the cartilage.

Less than 30 mm
The Antia–Buch flap utilizes an anterior incision through skin and cartilage in the scaphoid fossa on one or both sides of the defect. Posteriorly, the skin of the auricle is elevated from the perichondrium medially, leaving a helical flap based on the skin of the posterior auricle.

More than 30 mm
In the tunnel procedure the helical defect is sutured to the retro-auricular skin, with a strut of costal cartilage sculpted to reconstruct the defect placed in a pocket of retro-auricular skin. In the second stage, the reconstructed ear is elevated with a covering of retro-auricular skin. The tubed pedicled flap can be used for large defects. Two tubes of retro-auricular skin are constructed with a common base and divergent free ends. These ends are sutured to the edges of the helical defect. At the second stage, the common base is elevated and inset into the centre of the defect.

Upper third defects
Antia–Buch chondro-cutaneous flap, pre-auricular banner flap, random pattern flaps from auriculo-cephalic sulcus, contralateral conchal graft, ipsilateral chondro-cutaneous conchal flap, costal cartilage framework construction, and TPFF.

Small defects
Can be closed using a pre-auricular banner flap, or Antia–Buch flap.

Intermediate defects
Require random pattern flaps from auriculo-cephalic sulcus.

Large defects
If the skin bed is favourable, contralateral conchal grafting may be appropriate, although this is seldom the case. An ipsilateral chondro-cutaneous flap of the whole concha based at the crus helix is useful to restore the silhouette of the ear, but lacks an antihelical fold. Costal cartilage framework construction with TPFF and skin grafting as described for microtia repair, may be the most appropriate technique.

Middle third defects
Small defects
Antia–Buch chondro-cutaneous flap.

Large defects
Tunnel procedure.

Lower third defects
Auriculomastoid flap, Pardue flap for cleft lobe. The auriculomastoid flap is a retro-auricular flap with a mastoid extension, shaped like an inverted Y. The limbs of the Y are sutured together to construct the lobe and the stem attaches to the auricle.

Cleft lobe
Traumatic clefts from pulled earrings are common. Many repair techniques have been described, but Pardue maintained an epithelialized hole in the lobe for continued jewellery wear by rolling a flap of tissue from the adjacent lobe into the apex of the defect and then closing the remaining defect primarily.

Total ear defects
Prosthesis, total ear reconstruction These defects require cartilage reconstruction as described for microtia repair. However, the costal cartilage in an adult is firmer because of calcification and ossification, rendering framework sculpture more difficult. Skin coverage is more limited because of scarring or cutaneous loss, and the lack of spare skin from excision of the cartilage remnant. Tissue expansion or the use of the TPFF in the first stage may be necessary, with subsequent use of a deep temporal fascia and a periosteum flap at the second stage.

Prosthetic ears may be considered if the patient does not wish to undertake reconstruction. Problems include inadequate colour match and insecure fixation. This can be overcome with the use of osseo-integrated implants.

Facial nerve palsy

Facial nerve palsy is a diagnostic and management challenge. There are an enormous number of aetiologies, all creating massive functional and psychological disturbance of such intricacy and balance that, despite the best attempts at reconstruction using all the tools in our armentarium, total reconstruction remains currently impossible. However, it is an excellent model for all the reconstructive options, and for the multidisciplinary working that forms the basis of our speciality.

Aetiology of facial paralysis

Facial nerve injury: partial, total. Level of injury detected by pattern of motor loss.

Central
- Vascular abnormalities.
- CNS degenerative diseases.
- Tumours.
- Trauma.
- Congenital (Mobius syndrome).

Temporal
- Bacterial/viral infections.
- Cholesteatoma.
- Trauma.
- Tumours.
- Iatrogenic.

Parotid
- Tumours (parotid).
- Trauma.
- Primary tumour of facial nerve.
- Malignant tumours of mandible/pterygoid.
- Iatrogenic.
- Idiopathic
- Intraneural tumour spread.

Facial palsy problems

- Ear:
  - Hyperacusis (nerve to stapedius).
- Brow:
  - Failure to elevate.
  - Ptosis.
  - Lacrimal gland ptosis.
- Eyes:
  - Failure to close.
  - Lagophthalmos.
  - Loss of corneal reflex.
  - Corneal ulceration.
  - Loss of tearing.
  - Epiphora.
  - Ectropion.

- Nose alar:
  - Collapse.
  - Ptosis.
- Upper lip:
  - Failure to elevate.
  - Failure to purse, retract, or kiss.
  - Ptosis.
  - Food entrapment in buccal sulcus.
  - Bite inside of lip in buccal sulcus.
  - Lip enlarges.
- Lower lip:
  - Ectropion.
  - Failure to purse, depress.
  - Dribbles, drools.
  - Incontinence.
- Tongue:
  - Loss of taste (may see loss of taste papillae).
- Normal side of face contracts the affected side, producing facial scoliosis.

Diagnosis and examination

Try to identify cause on history and examination.
- Observe for facial posture at rest:
  - Brow ptosis.
  - Eyelid ptosis, ectropion, epiphora.
  - Degree of eye protection by Bell's phenomenon (upward rotation of eyeball to protect cornea).
  - Loss of malar prominence.
  - Nasal alar ptosis.
  - Cheek ptosis.
  - Upper lip ptosis.
  - Lower lip ptosis, ectropion, incontinence.
- Head and neck examination including all facial muscles by assessing:
  - Brow elevation.
  - Eye closure.
  - Smiling.
  - Lip depressing.
  - Blowing/whistling.
  - Neck tensing.
- Hearing.
- Stapes reflex.
- Schirmer tearing test.
- Submandibular flow.
- Taste.

Investigations

- Neurophysiology.
- X-ray.
- MRI/CT for imaging internal structure.

Goals of reconstruction

- Normal appearance at rest.

- Symmetry with voluntary motion.
- Restoration of sphincter control.
- Symmetry with involuntary motion/expression of emotion.

Management
Repair divided into three stages:
- Immediate (0–3 weeks).
- Delayed (3 weeks–2 years).
- Late (>2 years).

Cell body, proximal nerve segment, and muscles capable of regeneration for up to 2 years. However, given rate of nerve regeneration, this is effectively reduced to 18 months. This is further reduced in the over forties.

Acute facial nerve injury
Two elements required—healthy nerve and healthy muscle:
- Direct repair.
- Nerve grafting.
- Myoneurotization.
- Cross-facial nerve grafting.
- Nerve transfer.

Chronic facial nerve injury
Need to find healthy nerve and transfer healthy muscle:
- Cross-facial nerve grafting to innervated functional free muscle transfer.

Both
As above plus muscle tendinous transfers/ transposition:
- Masseter.
- Temporalis.
- Sternocleidomastoid/platysma.

Static procedures
- Forehead:
  - Brow lift.
- Eye:
  - Artificial tears/ointment.
  - Taping.
  - Tarsorraphy.
  - Wedge excision.
  - Lateral canthopexy or canthoplasty.
  - Eyelid closure devices—magnets, weights, palpebral springs.
  - Partial temporalis transfer.
- Nose:
  - Alar lift.
  - Static support of nasa ala—fascia lata graft to periosteum, temporalis fascia.
- Upper lip and cheek:
  - Facelift.
- Lower lip:
  - Wedge excision.

- Plication orbicularis oris.
- Orbicularis advancement flap.
- Reconstruction nasolabial fold.
- Fascial slings.
- Depressor anguli oris procedure.
- Opposite face:
  - Selective balancing neurectomy.
  - Selective balancing myectomy.

Direct nerve repair
- Rarely possible because of tension in remaining segments.
- Intra-temporal facial nerve is not very fibrous and is very difficult to stitch.

Interposition nerve graft
- Donor nerve from sural, great auricular, cervical plexus (C3,4), lateral femoral cutaneous, ansa hypoglossi, or cutaneous nerves of forearm.
- Connect facial nerve stump to zygomatic and/or buccal branches.
- Recovery takes 6 months to 2 years for recovery of movement.
- Tone then movement in middle face. Forehead and lower lip movement only return in 15% of patients.
- Recovery is never completely normal. There is always mass movement (all muscles function together rather than independently so there is loss of facial emotion), dyskinesia (muscle movement disturbed), synkinesis. (mass movement or unintentional movement of a muscle when voluntarily moving another, usually winking the eye when smiling). These abnormal movements can be improved by therapy, exercises, and judicious use of botulinum toxin.
- Recovered muscle also shows increased fatiguability.
- Recovery takes place even in the presence of post repair radiotherapy.
- If no distal nerve, try direct muscle implantation.

Myoneurotization
Neuromuscular pedicle grafts (myoneurotization) in which a motor nerve and its motor endplate (with a small amount of muscle) are transplanted into the denervated muscle. Unfortunately, this only produces tone in the clinical setting. An alternative is suturing a denervated to an innervated muscle to obtain cross-innervation and hopefully mass action.

Cross-facial nerve graft
Used when there is no proximal stump to repair. The principle is to cross innervate from the normal side, using a buccal branch, using a two-stage procedure:
- **Stage 1** Pass a nerve graft from one buccal branch on the good side across the upper lip at the base of the nose to the tragus on the affected side. Await nerve regeneration, assessing by Tinel testing. Takes 6–9 months.
- **Stage 2** Harvest functional muscle for free microneurovascular transfer to the affected side and re-innervate it with the cross-facial nerve graft.

Nerve transfer
A nerve (usually spinal accessory, phrenic, or hypoglossal) is transferred to the distal facial nerve to restore some neural innervation to the facial

muscles. Outcome is no spontaneous facial expression, as facial movement depends on voluntarily or involuntarily moving the donor muscle. Thus in hypoglossal transfer there is synkinesis with tongue movement. Along with this poor recovery there is donor deficit, e.g. in hypoglossal transfer may be difficulties with swallowing and speech because of atrophy and paralysis of the tongue, requiring later dorsal Z-plasty of tongue.

Cross-facial nerve grafting to functional free muscle transfer
- Gracilis.
- Extensor digitorum brevis.
- Latissimus dorsi.
- Pectoralis minor.

The muscle is fixed to the zygomatic arch and the distal end is split to insert to the upper lip, lower lip, and modiolus. Sometimes slips are passed around the eye with fascial extensions to aid eye closure.

Dynamic muscle transposition
- Temporalis:
  - Fold-over—the temporal portion of temporalis with superficial temporal fascia used to extend length is reflected down over the zygomatic arch and sutured to the upper and lower lips, and the oral commissure. Modifications include excising a segment of the arch to increase the length and using strips to go around the eye for eye closure. Can be used for eye closure only.
  - Direct—the coronoid attachment of the temporalis is elevated and elongated by fascial strips and sutured to the mouth.
- Masseter (may cause trouble with speech and mastication):
  - Split anterior half of the masseter and transpose to modiolus. Beware the intramuscular nerve travelling obliquely across the muscle fibre split.
  - Total masseter transfer.
- Sternomastoid:
  - Can be detached from the clavicle and transposed to attach to the mouth.
- Platysma:
  - Weak flimsy transfer; attached to lip but depresses.
- Anterior belly of digastric:
  - To reconstruct depressor labii function.

Static support procedures
- Suspension of superficial musculo-aponeurotic system (SMAS).
- Plicate SMAS to buccinator external surface to stiffen it and hold it out.
- Buccinator plication.
- Supraciliary brow lift.
- Z-plasty of oral commisure.
- Wedge resection of lateral lower lip/eyelid.
- Conservative nasolabial fold resection.
- Face lift.
- Fascia lata grafts.
- Intra-oral redundant mucosa excision.

Cheek reconstruction

Anatomy
The lower lid skin abuts the cheek at the superior border of the sub-orbital cheek at the lid–cheek margin. The skin thickens and deep to the skin the lip elevators commence and the orbicularis oculi terminates. Deep to this the masseter originates from the lateral maxillary buttress, superficial to which the facial nerve runs anteriorly. The SMAS lies superficial to the facial muscles.

Blood supply
- Facial artery (from the external carotid artery) which enters the cheek approximately 2–3 cm anterior to the angle of the mandible and transverses obliquely to terminate as the angular artery.
- The superficial temporal artery (also arising from the external carotid artery) provides the transverse facial artery.
- The ophthalmic artery (a terminal branch of the internal carotid artery) provides the dorsal nasal artery.
- Venous drainage is predominantly via the anterior facial vein which drains into the internal jugular vein. Substantial communications exist with the cavernous sinus via the ophthalmic, infra-orbital, and deep facial veins. This is clinically relevant because it is a potential avenue for the spread of sepsis with the risk of cavernous sinus thrombosis.

Nerve supply
- Sensory—trigeminal nerve (CN V):
  - Second division (maxillary)—infra-orbital, zygomatico-facial, and zygomatico-temporal branches.
  - Third division (mandibular)—mental, buccal, and auriculo-temporal branches.
- Motor—facial nerve (CN VII) to the muscles of facial expression. It branches within the substance of the parotid gland into upper (zygomatico-facial) and lower (cervico-facial) divisions. The branches of CN VII lie deep to the SMAS which overlies the muscles of facial expression:
  - Upper division—temporal and zygomatic branches.
  - Lower division—buccal, marginal mandibular, and cervical branches.

Classification
Three aesthetic units, with some overlap (Gonzalez Ulloa et al. 1954):
- Suborbital.
- Pre-auricular.
- Bucco-mandibular.

In additional to the anatomical unit affected, the defect can be considered in terms of the depth: superficial, full-thickness, or through-and-through.

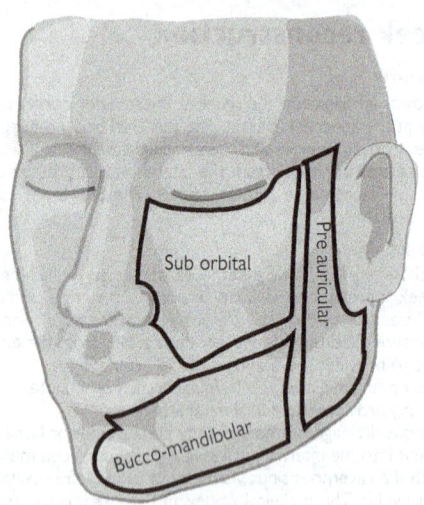

Fig. 8.4 Aesthetic subunits of cheek.

Aetiology of cheek defects
- Congenital:
  - Romberg's hemifacial atrophy.
  - Hemifacial microsomia.
  - Giant hairy naevus.
- Acquired:
  - Trauma.
  - Neoplasia.
  - Scleroderma.
  - Lipodystrophy (increasing incidence because of increasing use of anti-retroviral medication).

Aims and principles
- Repair of facial nerve and parotid duct.
- Reconstruction of convex contour of cheek and nasolabial fold.
- Reconstruction of skin cover with like skin.
- Respect aesthetic boundaries.
- Prevention of contracture or disturbance of anatomical features (lips, nose, eyelids, ears, and nasolabial fold).
- Beware causing ectropion and disturbing anatomical boundaries, facial nerve, and parotid duct.

Options

- Suborbital:
  - Direct closure vertically to avoid ectropion.
  - Cheek advancement flap (if para-nasal defect) (Fig. 8.5).
  - Mustardé rotation flap.
  - Cervico-facial flap anteriorly and inferiorly based rotation advancement flap (face lift type incision extending along crow's feet and then under lower eyelid).
  - Cervico-facial flap posteriorly based rotation advancement flap or inferio-laterally based, moving superior medially along the nasolabial fold (incision along nasolabial fold, paranasal, then under lower eyelid).
  - Limberg rhomboid flap.
  - Transposition flap.
  - V–Y advancement flap.
  - FTSG (often looks patch-like).
- Pre-auricular:
  - FTSG.
  - Limberg.
  - Transposition.
  - Cervico-facial flap anteriorly and inferiorly based rotation advancement flap but extending much further down the neck.
  - Cervico-pectoral flap—a variant of the above but extending onto the chest over pectoralis major in the deltopectoral flap zone.
  - Deltopectoral flap.
  - Pectoralis major myocutaneous flap.
  - Trapezius myocutaneous flap.
  - Free cutaneous flap.
- Bucco-mandibular:
  - As above
  - Lining reconstruction with:
    - Tongue.
    - Nasolabial flap.
    - Turnover flaps
    - Split flaps (i.e. split the cutaneous elements of the above flaps using one for lining and the other for cover).
- Contour defects:
  - Injection of fillers (silicon, collagen, fat).
  - Dermal or dermal fat grafts.
  - De-epithelialized free cutaneous flap (sutured dermis side down).
  - Omentum free transfer (but difficult to contour, and will change size as patient gains or loses weight).

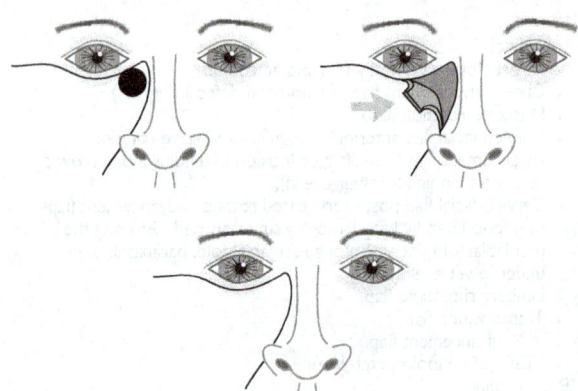

Fig. 8.5 Cheek advancement flaps (beware causing an ectropion).

Selection

- Size of the defect.
- Thickness of defect.
  - Does mucosal lining need to be reconstructed?
- Complexity of defect:
  - Facial nerve.
  - Parotid duct.
- Site of defect.
- Hairiness of proposed flap advancement (more of a problem in men in the beard area and the pre-auricular zone).
- Wherever possible try to reconstruct with adjacent tissue which has the best colour, contour, and mobility match.

Controversies

Purse-string deforming closure in children where the defect is pursestringed and closed as much as possible even if it deforms sensitive structures. As the wound settles the structures return to their usual position with minimal long-lasting deformity!

Reference

Gonzalez-Ulloa M, Castillo A, Stevens E, et al. (1954). *Plast Reconstr Surg* **13**, 151–61.

Drooling

Also known as salivation, sialismus, sialorrhoea, sialism, ptyalism.

Definition
Loss of control of saliva so that it drips out of the mouth.

Incidence
Unknown. Normal in babies up to 18 months; not usually considered pathological under 4 years. Up to 37% of patients with cerebral palsy experience drooling.

Aetiology
- Occurs normally during light sleep, when excited, nervous, or when eating certain foods (sialogogues).
- Neuromuscular: cerebral palsy, mental retardation, stroke, Parkinson's disease, Alzheimer's disease, epilepsy, facial nerve palsy.
- Abnormal shape of mouth or jaw.
- Large tongue or abnormal tongue movements.
- Mouth breathers, e.g. due to adenoid hypertrophy.
- Gingivitis and dental caries increase drooling.
- Drugs may cause hypersecretion of saliva, e.g. haloperidol, clozapine.

Classification
There are many classifications, based on amount of salivation:
- Mild: only onto lips.
- Moderate: reaches chin.
- Severe: drips off chin and onto clothes.
- Profuse: runs off the body onto surroundings.

Pathogenesis
1.5 L of saliva are produced per day: 70% from submandibular glands, 20% from parotid glands, and 10% from sublingual and minor salivary glands. Secretion is increased by parasympathetic stimulation of muscarinic cholinergic receptors. Nerves reach the parotid gland from the inferior salivary nucleus via the glossopharyngeal nerve, tympanic plexus, otic ganglion, and auriculo-temporal nerve. The submandibular and sublingual nerves are supplied by the superior salivary nucleus via the facial nerve and chorda tympani. Deglutition relies on coordinated movement of the peri-oral muscles, tongue, pharynx, and oesophagus, and intact intra-oral sensation and gag reflex. It is initiated under voluntary control. Reduced function at any stage, or lack of coordination, will cause drooling. Hypersecretion is a rare cause of drooling.

Clinical features
- Social embarrassment.
- Soiled clothing or surroundings.
- Skin maceration and infection.

Investigations
- Barium swallow may reveal oesophageal dysmotility.
- Nasopharyngoscopy may be used to assess the adenoids.
- Audiometry prior to surgery to chorda tympani.

Management
Medical
- Dental appliance moulded for individual patient to keep tongue and lips in place.
- Speech therapy to strengthen oral muscles and learn to improve control of saliva.
- Neck supports to stop head drooping forward.
- Skin care, e.g. with bibs or oral suction.
- Anticholinergic drugs, e.g. glycopyrrolate, atropine, scopolamine patches. Side effects include blurred vision, dry mouth, reduced sweating, constipation, urinary retention.

Surgical
- Adenoidectomy.
- Wilkie procedure: excise both submandibular glands and re-route parotid ducts to open into tonsillar fossa.
- Bilateral submandibular gland excision with unilateral parotid duct ligation.
- Henderson procedure: bilateral transposition of submandibular ducts to the tonsillar fossa with unilateral parotid duct ligation.
- Transtympanic neurectomy aims to transect the tympanic plexus and chorda tympani. May grow back over 6 months, leading to recurrence. Taste to anterior two-thirds of tongue is inevitably sacrificed. May also lose hearing.

Post-operative care
- Intravenous fluids until adequate oral intake.
- May need to keep intubated for 24–48 hours post-operatively until swelling resolves, e.g. in parotid or submandibular duct re-routing.

Complications
- Damage to hypoglossal, lingual, and marginal mandibular nerves during excision of submandibular glands. This may worsen control of saliva.
- Swelling, ranula cyst formation, or sialadenitis after salivary duct surgery.
- Salivary duct re-routing procedures may risk aspiration if oesophageal motility is impaired.
- Under- or over-correction of salivation.
- Dry mouth with malodorous thick saliva due to reduced volume.
- Dental caries due to loss of protective effect of saliva.

Future developments
Botox to parotid and submandibular glands reduces salivation safely and reversibly, but must be repeated every 3–6 months. Optimal administration under investigation.

Lip reconstruction

Anatomy (Fig. 8.6)
- Upper lip: between the nasolabial folds, below the nose, across the vermilion to the gingivolabial sulcus.
- Lower lip: from the labiomental fold to the gingivolabial sulcus.
- Muscles: orbicularis oris maintains oral competence; levator labii superioris, zygomaticus major, and levator anguli oris elevate the upper lip; depressor anguli oris and depressor labii inferioris depress the lower lip; and mentalis elevates and protrudes the central lower lip.
- The modiolus is the confluence of the cheek and lip muscles at the corner of the mouth.
- Nerve supply:
    - Motor—buccal and marginal mandibular nerves (CN VII).
    - Sensory—inferior alveolar nerve (CN Vb) and mental nerve (CN Vc).
- Blood supply: superior and inferior labial arteries (from the facial arteries) travel in the vermilion border.
- Lymphatic drainage via the submental and submandibular nodes.

Function of the lips
- Oral competence.
- Facial expression.
- Speech.
- Kissing.
- Eating and drinking.
- Aesthetic role.

Aetiology of lip defects
- Congenital:
    - Clefts.
    - Haemangiomata.
    - Naevi.
- Acquired:
    - Neoplasia (SCC, BCC, melanoma).
    - Trauma (bites, gunshot wounds), infection.

Aims
To reconstruct and provide the following elements.
- Skin: thin, supple, and appropriately coloured.
- Mucosa: thin, supple, and sensate.
- Vermilion: sensate and appropriately coloured.
- Commissure: well defined for expressive function.
- Stomal diameter: adequate for eating, oral hygiene, and denture insertion.
- Oral sphincter: competent to retain gases, solids, and liquids.
- Labial sulcus, upper and lower: to prevent spillage, drooling.

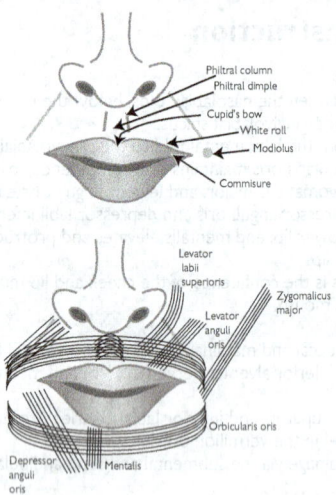

Fig. 8.6 Lip features and nomenclature; muscles of the lip.

Options

Upper lip
- <25%: primary closure using V-shaped wedge resection. Can be >25% in the elderly. The wedge can be stepped or modified to maintain/respect anatomical boundaries.
- 25–65%: Abbé flap, upside-down Karapandzic flap, unilateral modified upside-down Webster–Bernard flap.
- >65%: up side down Webster-Bernard (Zisser-Maddern) technique, advancement cheek flaps, bilateral nasolabial flaps, combination flaps, free flaps.

Lower lip (Fig. 8.7)
- <10%: simple wedge.
- <25%: primary closure using W-wedge, flared W, or single- or double-barrel wedge technique.
- 25–65%: Abbé flap, Abbé–Estlander flap, Gillies fan flap, McGregor–Nakajima flap, Karapandzic technique.
- >65%: double Abbé flaps, Webster–Bernard technique, Karapandzic technique, nasolabial flaps, combination flaps, free flaps.

Vermilion
- Total vermilionectomy by 'shave' excision and closure, or closure by bipedicled mucosal flap, or by V–Y musculomucosal flap.
- Total vermilion reconstruction by tongue flap or sensate musculomucosal flaps.
- Partial vermilion defect can be closed by advancing adjacent vermilion (and labial artery) or vermilion switch flaps.

Selection

Primary closure

- Simple wedge excision. Ensure that it traverses the vermilion and white roll at right angles, and ensure that it does not cross anatomical boundaries such as the labiomental or nasolabial folds.
- W-wedge (fish-tail wedge) for larger defects to truncate the length of the wedge so that it does not cross anatomical boundaries such as the labiomental or nasolabial folds. Modifications of this include curving the tails of the W into a barrel shape or into discrete steps (staircase method). Treatment of choice if feasible, because function and aesthetic outcome is optimal. Exception is resection of the philtrum, where an Abbé flap should be used to avoid ablation of this important landmark.

Abbé flap (Fig. 8.8a)

- Lip switch flap based on the labial artery which is maintained in a vermilion pedicle.
- Usually designed as a wedge, but may be tailored to suit the needs of the defect.
- The width of the Abbé flap is designed to be half the width of the defect, so that the loss of lip tissue is evenly distributed between upper and lower lip. The pedicle /pivot point is designed such that it sits at the midpoint of the opposing lip defect.
- Before raising the flap, place ink marks on the white roll on either side of the proposed incision. The inner marks will facilitate inset of the flap, and the outer marks will facilitate donor site closure.
- May be based on either a medial or a lateral pedicle.
- Observe the position of the labial artery when incising the non-pedicled side of the flap to facilitate identification of the labial artery in the pedicle.
- The flap is rotated through 180° and inset. The donor site is closed directly.
- Two weeks after the initial operation, the pedicle is divided and the final inset performed.

Abbé–Estlander flap (Fig. 8.7f)

Lip switch flap based on the labial artery, and specifically designed for commisure defects. The design is similar to an Abbé flap, but the pedicle is always medial to enable a commisure to be reconstructed. The final commisure may be indistinct and require later revision.

Gillies fan flap (Fig. 8.8b)

A fan-shaped rotational advancement flap based on the superior labial vessels. The flap is designed lateral to the base of the defect and carried into the nasolabial fold. A 1 cm back-cut is made superiorly to allow rotational advancement. The flap distorts the oral commisure, changes the direction of pull of the orbicularis oris fibres, and denervates the muscle, skin, and mucosa. The oral stoma is also reduced.

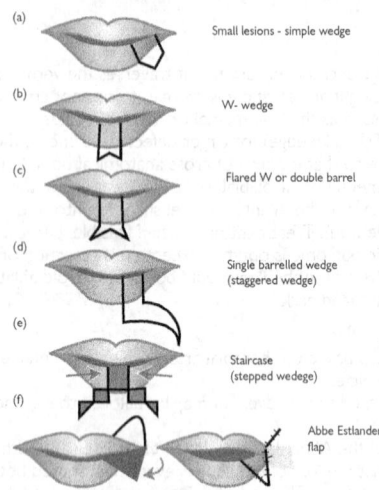

Fig. 8.7 Lip reconstruction by primary closure techniques: (a) simple wedge; (b) W-wedge; (c) flared W or barrel; (d) single-barrelled; (e) staircase or stepped wedge: (f) Abbé–Estlander flap.

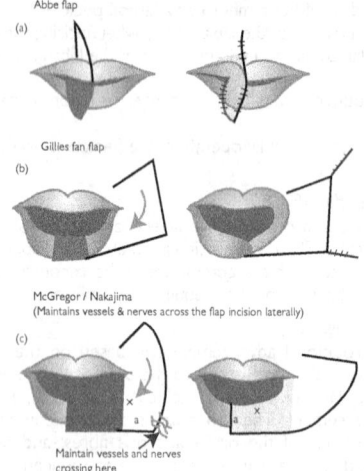

Fig. 8.8 Lip reconstruction by flap techniques: (a) Abbé flap; (b) Gillies fan flap; (c) McGregor–Nakajima flap.

McGregor-Nakajima flap (Fig. 8.8c)
- A modification of the Gillies flap to reduce the distortion at the commissure and also to replace all the vermilion.
- The pivot point is the oral commisure, so less distortion results. The size of the oral stoma is maintained. However, as the flap pivots through 90° rather then advances/rotates, the vertical incision becomes the new vermilion border.
- Vermilion must be replaced by either mucosal advancement or a tongue flap. Again, in the McGregor flap, the muscle, skin, and mucosa are denervated.
- The Nakajima method maintains the facial vessels and nerves supplying the flap.

Karapandzic technique (Fig. 8.9a)
- An innervated orbicularis oris flap.
- The flap is designed using semicircular incisions from the base of the defect to the nasal ala bilaterally. These incisions overlie the lateral border of the orbicularis oris muscle.
- Careful lateral dissection preserves the branches of the trigeminal and facial nerve, and superior and inferior labial arteries.
- The mucosa is incised and the flap rotated medially into place.
- This technique maintains the correct orientation of muscle fibres and provides a sensate lip, preserving lower lip function.
- Microstomia is a common complication; secondary revision or prosthetic stretching may be needed.

Webster–Bernard technique (Fig. 8.9b)
Allows for reconstruction of total lip defects. The initial resection is fashioned as a rectangle. Bilateral full-thickness cheek advancement flaps are created, and medially advanced into place. Burrow's triangles are resected in the nasolabial folds, but composed of skin and subcutaneous tissue only to preserve the deep neuromuscular structures. Mucosal advancement flaps from the transverse flap limbs are used to provide the vermilion. Z-plasties are used to close vertical suture lines to prevent notching with the inevitable scar contracture which accompanies wound healing.

Free flaps
- Used when local flaps are unavailable.
- Compromise functional and aesthetic outcomes.
- Free radial forearm flap may be designed to include palmaris longus tendon which can be sutured into the modiolus to provide some passive support.

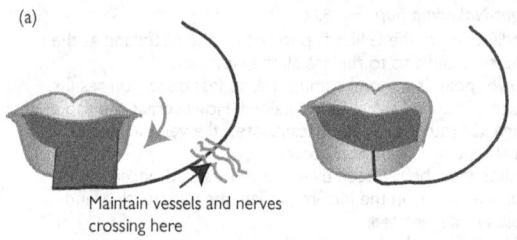
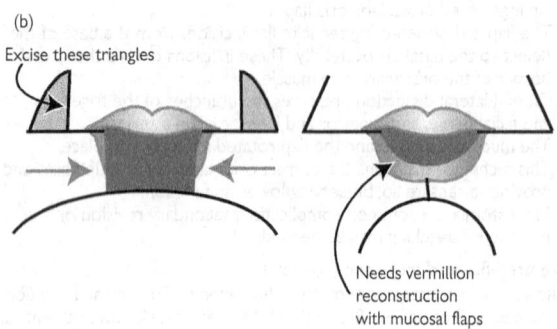

Fig. 8.9 Lip reconstruction by flap techniques: (a) Karapandzic; (b) Webster–Bernard.

(a) Nasolabial flaps—Fujimori gate flaps

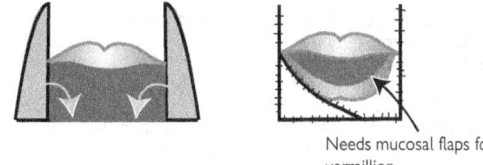

Needs mucosal flaps for vermillion

(b) Commisure lesions
Zisser method

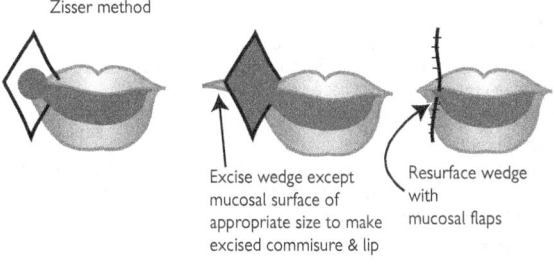

Excise wedge except mucosal surface of appropriate size to make excised commisure & lip

Resurface wedge with mucosal flaps

(c) Upper lip wedge modifications along anatomical boundaries

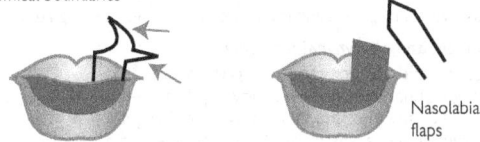

Nasolabial flaps

Fig. 8.10 Lip reconstruction by flap techniques: (a) nasolabial Fujimori gate flaps (b) Commisure reconstruction: Zisser method. (c) Variations of wedges to follow anatomical boundaries.

Swallowing

A complicated coordinated movement involving:
- Stage 1—food in mouth.
- Stage 2—food in pharynx.

Stage 1
- Voluntary stage: pass bolus through oropharyngeal isthmus.
- Intrinsic muscles of tongue alter its shape.
- Extrinsic muscles stabilize its position and by contraction alter its position.

Tongue
- Essential point is that the volume of the tongue remains constant.
- Contraction of the vertical intrinsic muscle makes a longitudinal groove in the dorsum to capture liquid.
- Heaped-up tip and edges contact hard palate and teeth.

Floor of mouth
- Contraction of the mylohyoid muscle raises the floor of the mouth.
- Vertical intrinsic muscle relaxes from anterior to posterior.
- Contraction of the mylohoid forces the bolus posteriorly.

Soft palate
- Flap-like valve can shut off oropharynx from the mouth (e.g. during chewing) or can close off the oropharynx from the nasopharynx.
- During swallowing soft palate is elevated against the projecting shelf of Passavant's ridge, sealing the nasopharynx and opening auditory tubes.

Laryngeal and pharyngeal movement
1. Larynx and pharynx move up to the hyoid.
2. Larynx, pharynx, and hyoid move up together.
3. Larynx , pharynx, and hyoid move down together.
4. Larynx and pharynx move down from the hyoid.

Swallowing
- Protection of the inlet.
- Sphincteric action of the aryepiglottic muscles.
- Rima of the glottis.
- Larynx hauled up beneath the posteriorly bulging tongue.
- Epiglottis tilted backwards and inferiorly by the passing bolus and acts as a lid over the laryngeal inlet.

Size of bolus
- Large bolus: epiglottis is separated from the posterior pharyngeal wall by the bolus.
- Smaller bolus: epiglottis touches posterior wall, producing lateral food channels.

Stage 2 (pharyngeal)
- Nose and pharynx seal off; bolus has to enter the pharynx.
- Entry of bolus into pharynx is accelerated by ascent of pharynx; wave of peristaltic contraction passes behind it down the pharyngeal contractors.

Oesophagus
- Peristaltic wave continues at 3–5 cm/sec.
- No change in velocity on change from skeletal to visceral muscle.
- Once clear of threat of aspiration, laryngeal inlet reopens to resume respiration.

Chapter 9

Head and neck

Tumours of the nasal cavity, sinuses, and nasopharynx *340*
Tumours of the oral cavity, oropharynx, and hypopharynx *344*
Head and neck cancer reconstruction *351*
Salivary gland tumours *354*
Superficial parotidectomy *357*
Neck dissection *359*

Tumours of the nasal cavity, sinuses, and nasopharynx

Nasal cavity and paranasal sinuses

Epidemiology
- 0.2–0.8% of all cancers; 3% of head and neck malignancies.
- 60% maxillary sinus, 25% nasal cavity, 14% ethmoid, 1% sphenoid and frontal.
- More frequent in men and in the fifth decade.
- Presentation is late with T3/4 disease.
- Increased incidence in the Far East.

Risk factors
- Cigarette smoke and alcohol (especially in combination).
- Occupational agents such as wood dust, nickel, and chromium, which seem to exert a synergistic effect.
- Organic chemicals (e.g. benzene), ionizing radiation, oncocytic papilloma, and possibly HPV may play a role.

Classification
By anatomical site or pathology.

Pathology
- Benign tumours include osteoma and fibroma.
- Malignant tumours can be subdivided as follows:
  - Epithelial—SCC (75–90% generally well or moderately differentiated), adenocarcinoma (accounts for 45% of carcinoma with occupational causes), malignant melanoma, undifferentiated carcinoma, small cell carcinoma, adenoid cystic carcinoma.
  - Osseous—osteogenic sarcoma, Ewing's sarcoma.
  - Connective tissue—chondrosarcoma, fibrosarcoma.

Diagnosis
History and examination, scrapings, incisional biopsy or excisional biopsy if small, and FNA of any palpable node will all aid diagnosis.

Investigations
Baseline blood investigations to look for malnutrition, anaemia, and liver metastases; FBC, U&E, LFT, thyroid function tests, clotting, cross-match (pre-operative 4–6 U). CXR, OPG (if tumour may be invading mandible), CT/MRI (to detect the extent and infiltration of the tumour and any nodes >1.5 cm or spherical with central necrosis), and chest CT scan for staging purposes. Comprehensive examination under anaesthetic should include palpation and panendoscopy.

Management
This requires a multidisciplinary team including an oncological surgeon, reconstructive surgeon, specialist nurse, speech therapist, dietician, oral hygienist, dentist, prosthodontist, psychologist, social worker, administrative and audit support, and an ex-patient.

Supportive management

Assessment by the above team and ensure suitable pre- and post-operative support as appropriate. Pre-operative feeding via an NG tube, PEG tube, or jejunostomy. Blood transfusion or tracheostomy may be required. Dental evaluation prior to radiotherapy. Helping the patient to stop smoking is important, as radiotherapy is less effective in patients who continue to smoke.

Maxillary carcinoma

Clinical features

- Nasal symptoms such as epistaxis, rhinorrhea, obstruction, swelling, and pain.
- Oral symptoms including loosening of teeth, referred molar pain, ulceration, or fistula of the hard palate.
- Ocular problems such as proptosis, swelling of the eyelids, and excessive tearing.
- Facial signs of swelling and asymmetric cheeks.
- Neurological evidence of involvement of the infra-orbital nerve.

Differential diagnosis

Sinusitis, polyps, papilloma.

TNM classification

- TX, T0, Tis: as for oral cavity tumours.
- T1: tumour in maxillary sinus mucosa.
- T2: tumour into bone but not posterior wall.
- T3: tumour invading any of posterior wall, subcutaneous tissues, orbital floor or medial wall, infra-temporal fossa, pterygoid plates, ethmoid sinus.
- T4: tumour into orbital contents beyond floor or medial wall, dura, brain, or nasopharynx.
- N and M as oral cavity.

Staging

- Stage 1: T1, N0, M0.
- Stage 2: T2, N0, M0.
- Stage 3: T3, N0, M0 or T1–3, N1, M0.
- Stage 4: T4, N0–1, M0 or T1–4, N2–3, M0–1, any T, any N, M1.

Treatment

Multidisciplinary team approach

Surgery and radiotherapy for all stages if the disease is resectable, including skull base resection for more advanced disease. Orbital exenteration should be performed if there is evidence of ocular involvement. If the tumour is in the orbital floor alone the eye can be saved, but if the orbital floor is resected and post-operative radiotherapy is planned many experts recommend eye removal anyway because of post-radiotherapy morbidity.

Reconstruction

- If the skin and orbit are preserved no reconstruction is needed.
- If the hard palate alone is involved a palatal prosthesis will suffice.

- With orbit and skin loss a fasciocutaneous flap is used (radial forearm flap).
- With loss of orbit, skin, and hard palate, a myocutaneous flap should be placed to fill the space (VRAM) using a double-skin paddle to reconstruct skin and hard palate mucosa.

Prognosis
- Local recurrence in 45%, mostly in the first year.
- Nodal disease in 22% and distant metastases in 18%.
- Five year survival is ~42%.
- >75% chance of mortality if patient presents with orbital, palatal, or infra-orbital nerve involvement.
- Tumours anterior and inferior to Ohngren's line (medial canthus to angle of the mandible) have a better prognosis.

Nasal cavity tumours
Clinical features
- Epistaxis.
- Congestion.
- Rhinorrhea.
- Obstruction.
- Swelling.

Differential diagnosis
Rhinitis, nasal polyp.

Treatment
Surgery/radiotherapy/both. Frequently radiotherapy alone is used because of cosmetic concerns.

Prognosis
If there is local recurrence, it is usually within the first year. 15% of patients get a second primary (40% in the head and neck, 60% elsewhere.)

Nasopharyngeal carcinoma
Anatomy
The nasopharynx continues from the nasal cavity anteriorly, including the post-nasal space. It ends inferiorly at an imaginary line between the upper surface of the soft palate and the posterior pharyngeal wall. Inferior to this is the oropharynx.

Epidemiology
0.25% of all carcinomas in Caucasians. Mainly occurs in the fifth decade. Common in southern China and in sub-Saharan and North Africa.

Pathology
Virtually all SCC (keratinizing or non keratinizing).

Risk factors
- Race.
- EBV.
- Genetic HLA link.
- Nitrosamines and nasal balms.
- Alcohol and smoking do not appear to be linked.

TNM classification
- Tx, Tis, T0, as for oral cavity tumours.
- T1: tumour confined to the nasopharynx.
- T2: tumour extends to the soft tissues in oropharynx, nasal cavity, or parapharynx.
- T3: tumour into bone or paranasal sinuses.
- T4: tumour with intracranial extension or to hypopharynx orbit or cranial nerves.
- NX, N0: as oral cavity.
- N1: unilateral node <6 cm above supraclavicular fossa.
- N2: bilateral nodes <6 cm above supraclavicular fossa.
- N3: lymph node metastases >6 cm or in supraclavicular fossa.
- MX, M0, M1: as above.

Staging
- Stage 1: T1, N0, M0.
- Stage 2: T1, N1, M0 or T2, N0–1, M0.
- Stage 3: T1-2, N2, M0 or T3, N0–2, M0.
- Stage 4: T4, N0-2, M0, or any T, N3, M0, or any T, any N, M1.

Clinical features
Nasal obstruction, epistaxis, otitis media, and asymptomatic upper jugular neck mass. The most common site is the lateral wall near the Eustachian tube. At presentation, lymph nodes are involved in 70% of cases (bilateral in 35%), the skull base is involved in 30%, and the cranial nerves may also be involved. Distant metastases are rare (<5%).

Investigation
As for nasal cavity tumours.

Management
As for nasal cavity tumours.

Treatment
- Stage 1: radiotherapy to primary and neck.
- Stages 2–4: either radiotherapy alone or chemo-radiotherapy.
- Surgical management is reserved for persistent or recurrent lymphadenopathy of the N2 neck. In selected cases it may be used for recurrent disease.

Prognosis
- 20–60% of patients develop distant disease.
- There is a greater chance with larger or lower neck nodes.
- There is no increased incidence of second neoplasia occurring in the head and neck.

Complications
In addition to the complications covered in this chapter, there is a significant rate of hypothyroidism post-radiation.

Tumours of the oral cavity, oropharynx, and hypopharynx

Anatomy
The oral cavity is defined as the area from the start of the lip vermilion to the junction of the hard and soft palates above to the line of the circumvallate papillae below. The oropharynx extends from there back to the tip of the epiglottis, which is at the level of the hyoid. The hypopharynx extends from the lower point of the oropharynx above to the plane of the inferior border of the cricoid cartilage below.

Epidemiology
These comprise 3% of all tumours in men and 2% in women. In India they comprise 40% of all cancers. Most common in sixth and seventh decades.

Classification
By anatomical site.

Pathology
Over 90% are squamous cell carcinomas. Other tumours include accessory salivary gland tumours, lymphoma, bone tumours, secondary deposits, spindle cell carcinoma, verrucous carcinoma, malignant melanoma, and sarcoma.

Risk factors
- The long-term use of tobacco and alcohol is related to 75% of cases.
- Spices, betel quid chewing, and smoking of *bidis* in India.
- Other risk factors are malnutrition, chronic irritation from dentures or poor dentition, chronic infection, marijuana, occupational agents such as nickel and formaldehyde, immunosuppression, previous tumour, and premalignant lesions.
- Viral aetiology such as HPV is being increasingly implicated as is EBV in tonsillar tumours.

Premalignant lesions
Leukoplakia (white patch) is reported to undergo dysplastic change in 15% of cases and malignant change in 5% (some authorities believe that it is a benign lesion). Differential diagnosis includes candida and lichen planus (these can be scraped off; leukoplakia cannot). Erythroplakia (red patch) converts to SCC in 55% of cases. Differential diagnosis includes infection and iron deficiency anaemia. Diagnosis is by biopsy. Treatment is by excision, carbon dioxide laser ablation, or retinoids. Regular follow-up and cessation of risk factors is recommended.

Clinical features
Symptoms include pain, discharge, haemorrhage, swelling or mass, speech and swallowing difficulties, and bad breath. Site-specific symptoms include referred pain such as otalgia, trismus, hoarseness of voice, or stridor. Signs include a visible ulcer or palpable mass and palpable lymphadenopathy.

Diagnosis

History and examination, scrapings, incisional biopsy, or excisional biopsy if small. FNA of any palpable node. In patients who present with palpable lymphadenopathy and no obvious primary, blind biopsies of common occult tumour sites such as tongue base and tonsillar fossa at time of panendoscopy is indicated.

Investigations

Baseline blood investigations to look for malnutrition, anaemia, and liver metastases; FBC, U&E, LFT, thyroid function tests; clotting, cross-matching (pre-operative 4–6 U); CXR, OPG (if tumour may be invading mandible), CT/MRI (to detect the extent and infiltration of the tumour and any nodes >1.5 cm or spherical with central necrosis) including chest for staging. Comprehensive examination under anaesthetic should include palpation and panendoscopy (synchronous tumour is picked up in 1–6%).

TNM definitions for oral cavity and oropharynx

- TX: cannot assess primary tumour.
- T0: no evidence of primary tumour.
- Tis: carcinoma *in situ*.
- T1: tumour ≤2 cm.
- T2: tumour 2–4 cm.
- T3: tumour >4 cm.
- T4: tumour invades adjacent structures.
- T4 oral cavity invades (a) extrinsic muscles of the tongue, through cortical bone and into skin and maxillary sinus, and (b) pterygoid plates, masticator space, and skull base, and encases carotid artery.
- T4 oropharynx invades (a) larynx, extrinsic muscles of the tongue, medial pterygoid, hard palate, and mandible, and (b) lateral pterygoid, pterygoid plates, lateral nasopharynx, and skull base, or encases carotid artery.
- NX: nodes cannot be assessed.
- N0: no nodal metastases.
- N1: single ipsilateral node ≤3 cm.
- N2a: nodal metastases in ipsilateral nodes <6 cm.
- N2b: nodal metastases in multiple ipsilateral nodes <6 cm.
- N2c: nodal metastases in bilateral or contralateral nodes <6 cm.
- N3: nodal metastases >6 cm.
- MX: distant metastases cannot be assessed.
- M0: no distant metastases.
- M1: distant metastases.

TMN definitions for hypopharynx

- TX, T0, Tis: as oral cavity.
- T1: tumour ≤2 cm in one subsite of hypopharynx.
- T2: tumour size 2–4 cm; invades from one subsite but no fixation of the hemilarynx.
- T3: tumour >4 cm or with fixation of the hemilarynx.
- T4: invasion of tumour from hypopharynx into local structures.

Staging (AJCC 2002)
- Stage 0: Tis, N0, M0.
- Stage 1: T1, N0, M0.
- Stage 2: T2, N0, M0.
- Stage 3: T1–2, N1, M0 or T3, N0–1, M0.
- Stage 4: T1–3, N2–3, M0 or T4, N0–3, M0 or any T, any N, M1.

Management
This requires a multidisciplinary team including an oncological surgeon, reconstructive surgeon, specialist nurse, speech therapist, dietician, oral hygienist, dentist, prosthodontist, psychologist, social worker, administrative and audit support, and an ex-patient.

Supportive management
Assessment by the above team and ensure suitable pre- and post-operative support as appropriate. Pre-operative feeding via an NG tube, PEG tube, or jejunostomy. Blood transfusion or tracheostomy may be required. Effective pain control. Dental evaluation prior to radiotherapy. Help to stop smoking is important, as radiotherapy is less effective in patients who continue to smoke.

Treatment principles of primary tumours
T1 and mobile T2 tumours (stages 1 and 2) can be treated by either surgery or radiotherapy (external beam or brachytherapy). If, following surgery, these tumours are >5 mm deep or are incompletely excised, post-operative radiotherapy is indicated.

Larger or fixed tumours (stages 3 and 4) are generally treated with a combination of surgery, reconstruction, and post-operative radiotherapy. However, the treatment options must be adjusted on an individual patient basis, which is why the multidisciplinary approach is vital. It is important to take the general health and the preference of the patient, and the local expertise, into account. Radical radiotherapy and chemoradiotherapy are alternatives in stage 3 and 4 disease at certain sites (e.g. tonsillar fossa and tongue base), where they are the preferred options in the infirm patient who will do poorly with the duration and stress of surgery required for major resection and reconstruction.

Excision margins
This should include the tumour and any *in situ* changes around it. Clearly defined tumour blocks are ideally excised with a 1 cm margin, and infiltrative or post-radiation recurrence with a 2 cm margin. Use frozen section analysis if any doubt exists.

Surgical approach
Accessible T1 and some T2 tumours can be excised via an intra-oral approach. Larger and more distant tumours will require a lip split and mandibular osteotomy.

Indications for primary radiotherapy
- T1 or T2 lesions.
- Indistinct margins.
- Synchronous primaries.

- Generalized field change.
- Patient choice.
- Infirm patient.
- No invasion of the mandible.

Treatment principles of neck nodes

In the N0 neck, node dissection is generally not performed for T1 tumours, but is performed for T3 and T4 tumours, including bilateral dissections where the tumour crosses the midline. The debate lies over T2 tumours. For sites where there is a high risk of occult metastases (e.g. the tongue and floor of mouth) or where the neck is opened for access (e.g. the oropharynx), a neck dissection should be performed (some authorities argue that this principle should also be applied to T1 tumours). Also consider performing a neck dissection when follow-up or monitoring of the neck may be difficult. Sentinel lymph node biopsy may have a future role in these patients.

Neck dissection should be performed on an N-positive neck. Surgeons can tailor the extent of the neck dissection depending on the N stage, the primary tumour site, and the proximity of the involved nodes to vital structures that should be preserved. For the N0 or N1 (<2 cm) neck, primary radiotherapy is an option with equivalent results.

Indications for post-operative radiotherapy
- Incomplete excision.
- Close excision (<5 mm).
- Extracapsular lymph node spread.
- N2 and N3 disease (some say any N-positive neck).

Poor prognostic factors
- High TNM stage.
- Thickness of tumour (>0.5 cm).
- Invasion of perineurium, lymph and blood vessels.
- Irregular pattern of invasion.
- Poorly differentiated tumour.
- Carotid adherence.
- Extracapsular spread from lymph nodes.
- Tumour recurrence.

Tumour recurrence

This is likely if excision is incomplete, margins are close (<0.5 cm), or margins contain *in situ* change. Note that 8.8% of 'clear' resections have positive margins.

Survival (5-year)
- Overall: <50%.
- Stage 1: 85%.
- Stage 2: 66%.
- Stage 3: 41%.
- Stage 4: 9%.

However, there are large variations depending on site.

Chemotherapy
Chemotherapy is generally used as part of a controlled trial or as part of the palliative regime in advanced or recurrent disease. Neoadjuvant chemotherapy (given prior to other modalities) has been used to shrink tumours to allow surgical treatment. Trials that demonstrate survival benefit are awaited.

Post-operative care
Intensive post-operative care as for free flaps. Test swallow 8–10 days post–operatively. Continuing supportive management as described above.

Follow-up
Close follow-up initially monthly after treatment to exclude recurrence and detect new primaries.

Recurrent disease
This requires careful pre-operative decision-making and counselling with the patient and the multidisciplinary team. If there is a curative intent this usually will require surgery and reconstruction in a previously operated or irradiated field which is associated with higher morbidity and mortality. If there is no curative possibility, palliative chemo- or radiotherapy (if not previously used), together with supportive and palliative care, will be needed.

Oral cavity

Lip
Incidence
30% of all oral carcinomas; 90% occur on lower lip.

Differential diagnosis
All forms of skin pathology, especially SCC, BCC. and melanoma.

Risk factors
Long-term sun exposure and all skin malignancy risk factors.

Nodal spread
There is an increased risk of nodal spread depending on size of tumour (T1, <5%; T2, 5–35%; T3/4, 20–100%), depth of tumour (>6 mm, 15%), poor differentiation, perineural invasion (50%).

Treatment
T1 tumours can be treated with surgery or radiotherapy. Radiotherapy leaves better cosmesis and function, especially at the commissure, but surgery provides staging details, margin assessment, and is more rapid. Both achieve 90% local control. Excision margins for lesions smaller than 1 cm can be 0.5 cm, but anything larger should have a 1 cm margin. Mohs' surgery can be considered. A T2 tumour with N0 neck should be considered for prophylactic neck dissection. Field change of the vermilion is amenable to radiotherapy or vermilionectomy and mucosal advancement.

Reconstruction
Defects of <30% of the lip will close directly, with a W or barrel excision. Between 30% and 60% lip defect consider Abbé, Estlander, Johansen's

step or Karapandzic flaps. Larger defects will require a Bernard–Webster, Gillies fan, or MacGregor flap. For total defects free tissue transfer is considered.

Prognosis

The main determinants are tumour stage and perineural involvement. Minor factors include histological grade and patient age (worse if <40 or >80 years).

Buccal mucosa

Most tumours occur on or inferior to the plane of occlusion; 60% present having extended beyond the cheek mucosa. Advanced disease may necessitate parotidectomy and mandibular resection. An N0 neck has occult metastases in <10%. Depth of tumour is the most significant prognostic factor, as patients with tumours <6 mm have a >98% 5-year survival. Radiotherapy is the preferred option for small tumours around the commissure.

Gingiva and alveolar mucosa

This is often misdiagnosed, as it is similar to benign conditions such as gingivitis. It is most common in the molar area and invades the bone early. There is a high incidence of nodal metastases (T1, 25%). Small tumours are best treated with surgery with or without rim resection rather than radiotherapy. Deeper tumours require mandibulectomy. The N0 neck should be dissected.

Retromolar trigone

80% of these tumours occur in men. They present early and often with nodal disease (27–60%).

Floor of mouth

70% occur anteriorly near the lingual frenulum and the lymph drainage may be bilateral. T1 tumours can be treated by surgery or radiotherapy. T2 tumours encroaching on the mandible are better treated with surgery. Mandibular invasion occurs in 15–30%, and 30% of patients have positive nodes at presentation.

Mandible

Rim excision is performed in non-irradiated patients if the tumour is on the occlusal surface or has reached the alveolus but there are no clinical or radiological signs of involvement. Any doubt or definite involvement requires segmental resection. In irradiated mandibles, if the tumour is in close proximity to bone, segmental excision is carried out. If the mandible is edentulous and involved with tumour, segmental excision is the only option because of the poor bone stock.

Hard palate

This is the rarest site for a tumour and systemic metastases are rare.

Anterior two-thirds of tongue

This most commonly presents as a painless indurated ulcer on the lateral tongue (75%). Some units are treat all stages with brachytherapy with equal survival but significant side effects. 80% of patients who die from this tumour do so because of locoregional disease.

Oropharynx

This site is associated with a high incidence of synchronous primaries. The tumour spreads into the nasopharynx and hypopharynx submucosally and often invades the prevertebral fascia.

Tongue base

The extent of tumour infiltration can be appreciated by palpation and ability to protrude the tongue (paralysis of CN XII). There are no pain fibres in the tongue base; hence these tumours are often painless until they have infiltrated further. When considering surgical treatment, management of the larynx is important. If the larynx is involved or the entire base of tongue and hypoglossal nerves need to be resected, laryngectomy should be considered. Nodal spread to ipsilateral nodes in 70% and bilateral in 30%.

Soft palate

These tumours are detected early because of early symptoms and ease of visualization.

Tonsils

There is a suggested link to EBV in primary tumours. 1% of tumours are secondary deposits. The internal carotid artery lies only 2.5 cm posteriolateral to the tonsillar fossa and advanced tumours are often continuous with the neck nodes. Over 50% patients have positive nodes at presentation and dissection of the N0 neck is indicated.

Pharyngeal wall

Tend to present late with spread past the midline; hence bilateral nodal metastases are common.

Hypopharynx

Tumours in this area tend to spread submucosally, leaving an intact epithelium, and produce skip lesions. As a consequence the tumour is rarely localized to one subsite and tends to present with stage 3 or 4 disease in approximately 80% of patients. Up to 17% of patients may also have distant metastases.

Piriform sinus

Approximately 70% of hypopharyngeal tumours originate here.

Posterior pharyngeal wall

20% of tumours.

Postcricoid

10% of tumours.

Treatment

Laryngopharyngectomy, reconstruction, and post-operative radiation are the mainstay treatment for all stages of tumour. In the rare finding of a T1 tumour (1–2%), radiation alone may be used. Trials using chemoradiotherapy without surgery have had some success but this should not be considered standard treatment.

Head and neck cancer reconstruction

Reconstructive principles
Allow remaining normal anatomy to return to place and function. Match type, volume, surface area, elasticity, and function of tissues removed.

Reconstructive aims
- Restore function of oral continence, speech, and swallowing.
- Cover vital structures and promote rapid healing to permit early adjunctive radiotherapy and prolong disease-free period.
- Restore external appearance.
- Resection and reconstruction is only the preferred alternative when it is done well with low morbidity.

Reconstructive options

Direct closure and secondary intention
Small tumours, T1, and some T2 can be excised with a laser or knife and left to mucosalize. This is best in areas where contraction of the wound will not distort function (e.g. tongue).

Skin grafts
These can be fenestrated and plicated in place for small intra-oral tumours. Their success rate is variable and often the wound mucosalizes when the graft disappears.

Local flaps
Intra-oral flaps have their place in selected cases but cause further distortion of local anatomy and the pedicle can limit the inset. They are also using oral mucosa which can be prone to further malignant change. The most commonly used is the buccinator flap, which requires an intact facial artery which may not be present after neck dissection. The nasolabial flap, based inferiorly and tunnelled through the cheek to lie intra-orally, is suitable for small inferior alveolar or floor of mouth tumours. Others that should be considered are submental and forehead flaps.

Distant flaps
Predominantly the pectoralis major but also the deltopectoral flap for salvage cases.

Free flaps
The main soft tissue flaps are the radial forearm, anterior lateral thigh, and vertical rectus abdominus myocutaneous. The latissimus dorsi and the lateral arm (short pedicle) are used less frequently. The fibula and DCIA (iliac crest) are most commonly used for bone reconstruction.

Reconstructive selection
This takes various factors into account.

Patient factors
The general health of the patient, their ability to withstand a major procedure, and the likelihood of post-operative problems must be considered. It may be necessary to compromise on the quality of the reconstruction if the risks are too great. For example, sometimes the pedicled flap may be indicated before the free flap.

Resection site
The size, site, three-dimensionality of the defect, and availability of a nerve for flap innervation may influence the reconstruction. Consider what is removed in terms of tissue bulk, content, and function (e.g. bone) to guide what may need to be replaced. Smaller defects that require pliable flaps in three dimensions, such as the oropharynx, will be better with a radial forearm flap, larger defects will be better with an anterior lateral thigh flap, and volume is provided by a VRAM. The vessels remaining in the neck, and hence the length of pedicle required, will also influence flap selection.

Donor site
Consider which donors are available and the morbidity associated with using them. The anterior lateral thigh defect, if directly closed, is a very low morbidity donor site. However, if it cannot be closed, it is a poor donor site.

The radial forearm flap and the anterior lateral thigh flaps are the workhorse flaps for mucosal replacement in the oral cavity and oropharynx. Taking the tongue as a whole organ, if up to 75% is removed the ideal construct is with an innervated radial forearm flap. If the total tongue is removed, more bulk is required to initiate swallowing and a VRAM or anterior lateral thigh flap is the best choice. In the hypopharynx, pharyngeal mucosa can be replaced by a radial forearm flap, anterior lateral thigh flap, or pectoralis major skin, tubed or as a patch as needed. Free jejunum may also be used, either opened for partial defects or as a tube. The choice depends on the factors outlined above and the level of expertise available. Occasional practitioners of jejunal flaps have higher complication rates and would be better served with tubing skin if they are more familiar with this technique.

Mandibular reconstruction
For small defects (<6 cm) a bone graft wrapped in well-vascularized tissue is sometimes used. However, failure rates of over 30% have been reported. Vascularized bone is the optimum reconstruction. The free fibula is the most often used because of the large amount of bone available, the ability to contour the bone, cortical thickness for implantation, and minimal donor site complication. Other options include the DCIA or the radial forearm flap with bone. Not performing a mandibular reconstruction in the elderly is an option for defects lateral to the parasymphyseal region when the TMJ has been removed. In these cases soft tissue reconstruction alone is used.

General consensus dictates that if a patient receives post-operative radiotherapy, osseo-integrated implants are not considered.

More than one flap may be required for large or composite defects. The fibula with skin can be used for bone and mucosal replacement. However, failure rates of up to 10% in the skin paddle are reported, and some surgeons advocate using two free flaps in this situation.

Peri-operative care
Prophylactic antibiotics, thromboprophylaxis, nutrition, oral hygiene, tracheostomy care, and flap observation will all be needed.

Complications

- Complications relating to excision:
  - Haemorrhage, haematoma.
  - Unintended damage to neurovascular structures.
  - Incomplete excision.
  - Recurrence.
- Complications relating to soft tissue reconstruction:
  - Flap donor site complications.
  - Flap necrosis.
  - Incomplete healing with fistula formation.
  - Infection.
  - Insensate reconstruction.
  - Chewing flap.
  - Hair in mouth.
  - Impaired swallowing of food.
  - Drooling.
  - Pooling of food.
  - Impaired speech.
  - Trismus.
  - Psychological and psychosexual problems.
  - Scarring and contour defects.
- Complications relating to bone reconstruction:
  - Loosening, infection, or exposure of the osteotomy fixation.
  - Bone necrosis.
  - Bone resorption.
  - Non-union or malunion.
- Complications relating to neck dissection:
  - Lymph leak.
  - Infection.
  - Skin flap necrosis.
- Radiation complications especially:
  - Xerostomia.
  - Osteoradionecrosis.

Salivary gland tumours

Incidence
- 3% of head and neck tumours.
- 80% are in the parotid, and 80% of parotid masses are benign.
- 50% of submandibular, 50% of sublingual, and only 25% of accessory gland tumours are benign.

WHO classification
- Adenoma:
  - Pleomorphic (60%).
  - Adenolymphoma (Warthin's tumour, 8%).
  - Oncocytoma.
- Carcinoma:
  - Muco-epidermoid (9%).
  - Malignant mixed tumour (arising in pleomorphic adenoma, 5%).
  - Acinic cell.
  - Adenocarcinoma.
  - Adenoid cystic carcinoma (4%).
  - Squamous carcinoma.
- Non-epithelial tumours:
  - Soft tissue.
  - Mesenchymal.
- Malignant lymphomas.
- Secondary tumours:
  - Melanoma.
  - SCC.
  - Breast.
  - Thyroid.
- Unclassified tumours.
- Tumour-like lesions.
  - Sialadenosis.
  - Oncocytosis.
  - Cysts.
  - Infection.
  - Granulomatous disease.

Pleomorphic adenoma
Pleomorphic adenoma is a mixed tumour combining components of the duct epithelium, myoepithelium, and stroma. It is more common in women, and 2–10% undergo malignant change. It presents as a slow-growing lump that is firm and slightly irregular. Macroscopically it appears encapsulated, but often has invisible extensions (bosselations).

Warthin's tumour
Warthin's tumour is a lympho-epithelial tumour. It is five times more common in men, particularly smokers in their fifties. It is multicentric and bilateral (10%), and has a high recurrence rate.

Muco-epidermoid carcinoma
There are three grades. Well-differentiated tumours have a large number of mucous cells, limited local invasiveness, and rarely metastasize. Intermediate tumours behave in a similar fashion to a well-differentiated SCC. Poorly differentiated tumours are aggressive tumours that invade locally and metastasize regionally.

Adenoid cystic carcinoma
Adenoid cystic carcinoma exhibits unusual behaviour. It is prone to perineural and vascular invasion, skip lesions are common, and it excites very little host response. As a consequence it tends to be painless and can silently invade bone. There are three grades (Szanto):
- Grade 1 —cibrose (no solidity, good prognosis).
- Grade 2 —tubular (<30% solid).
- Grade 3 —solid (poor prognosis).

It can recur very late (after 25 years) and usually presents as lung metastases.

Clinical features of malignant salivary gland tumours
- Painful and hard lump arising in the body of the gland.
- Duct obstruction and infection.
- Bleeding from the duct.
- Invasion of local structures and fixation.
- In the parotid:
  - Paralysis of CN VII.
  - Ear problems.
  - Trismus.
  - Dysphagia with deep lobe involvement.
- Examination should be bilateral (exclude Sjögren's syndrome) and include intra-oral examination, bimanual palpation, and cranial nerve examination.

TNM classification
- TX, T0, Tis: as for oral cavity tumours.
- T1: tumour ≤2 cm with no clinical extraparenchymal extension.
- T2: tumour 2–4 cm without clinical extraparenchymal extension.
- T3: tumour >4 cm or having clinical extraparanchymal extension.
- T4: tumour into one of skin, mandible, ear canal, facial nerve, skull base, or around carotid.

Staging
- Stage 1: T1, N0, M0.
- Stage 2: T2, N0, M0.
- Stage 3: T3, N0, M0 or T1–3, N1, M0.
- Stage 4: T4, N0, M0 or T1–4 N 2–3 M0 or any T, any N, M1.

Investigations
- CT/MRI with gadolinium contrast of head neck and chest.
- Sialography.
- FNA or US-guided biopsy of tumour.

Treatment of parotid lumps
- Limited superficial parotidectomy, removing the tumour and a cuff of normal tissue, is performed for benign disease.
- Formal superficial parotidectomy is carried out for malignancy confined to this area.
- Total parotidectomy is performed if the tumour is large (T3) or in the deep lobe, preserving the facial nerve if it is not involved (this may involve splitting the tumour).
- Post-operative radiotherapy is indicated for malignant tumours and for benign tumours if excision is incomplete or the capsule is breached.
- A node-positive neck requires neck dissection.
- Some adjunctive chemotherapeutic regimens can be effective.
- If the pathology is uncertain, it is appropriate to perform a superficial parotidectomy with frozen section and proceed to total parotidectomy only if this is positive.

Prognosis
Poor in high-grade tumours in the elderly that present with pain, nerve involvement, and local invasion.

Superficial parotidectomy

Parotid anatomy
Bilateral gland found anterior and inferior to ear. Wraps around the posterior ramus of the mandible. Extends anteriorly over masseter. 75% of the gland is the superficial lobe lying anterior to the facial nerve. The posterior lobe has a retromandibular portion. The facial nerve enters the posterior aspect of the gland and separates the lobes. The connection between the lobes is called the isthmus.

The parotid duct (Stensen's duct) is 5–6 cm long and traverses the cheek in a line from the inter-tragal notch to the midpoint between the upper lip and the alar base, from the parotid to empty into the oral cavity through an orifice opposite the second upper molar. The parotid fascia attaches to the zygoma, masseter, and sternomastoid.

The parotid gland is supplied by parasympathetic branches that hitch a ride on the glossopharyngeal nerve after the otic ganglion from the inferior salivary nucleus.

Indications
Benign and low-grade malignant disease of the parotid gland superficial to the facial nerve. Removal of the lymph nodes within the parotid, usually as part of a neck dissection.

Aims
Removal of the superficial parotid gland with preservation of the facial and great auricular nerves.

Planning
Head up, shoulder pillow, head ring, LA with adrenaline, GA with no muscle relaxant, nerve stimulator, fine suction, and bipolar diathermy.

Incision
Modified Blair incision. Start at the upper border of the ear and continue down in the pre-auricular crease, curving in towards the pinna above the tragus and then out into the pre-auricular crease again. The incision loops under the ear lobe arches over the mastoid tip and turns anteriorly to run two fingerbreadths below the mandible, arching towards the hyoid bone.

Exposure
The skin incision is deepened through the SMAS–platysma layer and elevated in this plane off the parotid fascia. Posteriorly over the mastoid tip the skin flap is elevated off the SCM, taking care not to damage the great auricular nerve (as it courses obliquely across the upper third of the SCM) and the EJV.

Procedure
Start posteriorly by incising the investing fascia and elevating the posterior tip of the parotid gland off the mastoid tip and the anterior border of the SCM, taking great care not to cut the posterior facial vein (ligation causes congestion). Dissection should now proceed using mosquito forceps and bipolar cautery to free the gland from the ear canal and the zygomatic root. The next step is to identify the tragal pointer at the deep extent of

the cartilaginous canal. The previous manoeuvres have ensured that this is done with greater access. The facial nerve lies 1 cm deep to this pointer. Suction, bipolar diathermy, and good retraction on the gland aid this search. The parotid is dissected off the bony canal and then in a plane parallel to the facial nerve. Connective tissue bands may look similar to the facial nerve; the use of a nerve stimulator facilitates identification of the nerve and is recommended.

Dissection progresses by placing the tips of the mosquito forceps in the perineural space lateral to the nerve. Tissue is cut down to the tips as they are lifted away from the nerve. The cut edges are clamped and diathermied. In a true superficial parotidectomy this is continued from the first branch off the main trunk to the termination of the gland. Sometimes, because of the placement of the tumour, it is necessary to perform retrograde dissection of the nerve. The options are to find the cervical branch as it runs with the retromandibular vein, the marginal branch superficial to the facial artery, or the buccal branch by cannulating Stensen's duct.

Closure
5/0 or 6/0 nylon sutures and a suction drain.

Complications
- Facial nerve division is the most significant complication. Primary repair or grafting where necessary should be carried out at the time.
- Frey's syndrome (gustatory sweating), which is caused when regenerating parasympathetic fibres from the facial nerve enter the skin. On response to stimuli the impulse errantly passes to these new connections, causing sweating. Skin flap re-elevation, with or without interposition of dermofat grafts or alloderm between nerve and skin at closure, has been recommended to treat this condition.

Neck dissection

Radical neck dissection (ND) is an operative procedure for the removal of the lymphatic field of the neck from the mandible above to the clavicle below, and from the midline to the anterior border of the trapezius. It is attributed to Crile (1906), who is said to have performed it in 45 minutes!

Anatomy

- The submandibular triangle is bounded by the anterior and posterior bellies of the diagastric muscle and the inferior border of the mandible.
- The submental triangle is bounded by the bilateral anterior bellies of digastric and the mandible.
- The upper jugular nodes are in the area from the skull base to the level of the hyoid. The anterior border is the sternohyoid and the posterior is the posterior border of the SCM (as for levels 3 and 4).
- Middle jugular nodes lie between the hyoid and the omohyoid muscle or cricothyroid membrane.
- Lower jugular nodes lie from the lower border of omohyoid to the clavicle.
- The posterior triangle is formed by the clavicle below and the posterior border of SCM and anterior border of trapezius muscle.
- Subclavicular and mediastinal nodes may also be involved and can be resected in a extended neck dissection.

Memorial Sloane–Kettering Cancer Center Classification

The cervical lymph nodes are described in terms of seven levels:

I   Submental and submandibular triangles.
II Nodes around upper third of IJV and medial to SCM; above the level of the hyoid bone.
III Nodes around middle third of IJV and medial to SCM; above the level where the omohyoid crosses the IJV.
IV Lower jugular, scalene, and supraclavicular nodes deep to the lower third of SCM.
V   Posterior triangle nodes.
VI Anterior.
VII Superior mediastinum.

The classification takes into account primarily the lymph node levels cleared, and secondarily the anatomical structures preserved. There are essentially three anatomical types of ND.

Extended

- Any of the other types are extended to include either a lymph node group not usually removed (such as paratracheal) or structures not routinely removed (such as carotid artery).
- Extended radical ND includes levels 1–5 plus levels 6 and 7, and parotidectomy.

Comprehensive
- Radical ND includes clearance of levels 1–5 plus accessory nerve, SCM, and IJV.
- Three types of modified radical ND or functional ND:
  - Type 1 preserves the accessory nerve.
  - Type 2 preserves the accessory nerve and the SCM.
  - Type 3 preserves the accessory nerve the SCM and the IJV (sometimes the term functional ND is reserved for this type).

Selective
Clearance of only some levels with preservation of IJV, accessory nerve, and SCM:
- Supra-omohyoid (levels 1, 2, 3).
- Antero-lateral (levels 2, 3, 4).
- Anterior (levels 2, 3, 4, and 6—those around the trachea).
- Posterior (levels 2, 3, 4, 5 with sub-occipital and retro-auricular nodes).

Indications
- Neck lymph node metastases.
- Prophylactic neck dissection when size or site of tumour predicts likely lymph node spread.

Contraindications

Contraindications to functional ND
- Fixed nodes.
- Nodes >3 cm with impaired mobility.
- Fixed nodes which become mobile after radiotherapy.
- Recurrent nodes post surgery/radiotherapy.

Contraindications to radical ND
- Fixation to vertebral column.
- Fixation to brachial plexus.

Planning
Head up and tilted away from the operative side, with a sandbag under the shoulders. The upper chest, neck, and hemi-face should be prepared and draped.

Incision
There are many to choose from. The tri-radiate is the most commonly used. The upper incision lies in a cervical skin crease three fingerbreadths below the mandible, running from the mastoid to below the chin. The vertical limb lies at the junction of the posterior third and anterior two-thirds, to afford some protection to the great vessels in the event of a wound breakdown.

Exposure
The incisions are deepened through the platysma and flaps are raised in the subplatysmal plane. Caution should be exercised posteriorly where the SCM is close to the skin, and the flaps should be raised subcutaneously and superiorly where the marginal mandibular branch lies in the subplatysmal plane.

Procedure

The lymphatic contents are excised *en bloc*, commencing at the anterior border of the trapezius muscle. Incise down to the deep cervical fascia and peel the contents off this fascia as you move anteriorly. The omohyoid muscle is divided and taken with the specimen. Contents of the posterior triangle include the accessory and lesser occipital nerves and the transverse cervical vessels. The nerves from the cervical plexus are divided and direct you to the phrenic nerve lying on the scalenius anterior muscle. Take care not to go under the clavicle. Inferiorly the tissue is clipped and tied, including the external jugular vein. The SCM is divided and the IJV is tied, being cautious of the thoracic duct (on the left). The specimen is dissected superiorly off the vagus nerve and carotid artery. At the mastoid the SCM is divided and the top of the IJV is tied. Moving anteriorly, the submandibular fascia is incised and the facial vessels are tied, creating a superior flap which protects the marginal mandibular nerve. In the anterior corner of the dissection the lingual and hypoglossal nerves are located and Wharton's duct is tied. The gland is dissected of the mylohyoid muscle and the specimen cleared off the strap muscles to finish the dissection. The wound is washed out with sterile water.

Closure

3/0 absorbable to platysma–dermal layer and 4/0 absorbable to the skin. Two large suction drains.

Post-operative care

Wake the patient gently and sit them up. Keep the drains in for 5 days.

Complications

This procedure carries a mortality of ~1%.

Intra-operative

- Nerve injury.
- Carotid problems (bradycardia and emboli).
- IJV bleeding or air emboli.
- Lung problems (pneumothorax).
- Chyle leak.

Early

- Skin flap necrosis.
- Carotid blow-out.
- Haematoma.
- Pain.
- Respiratory difficulty.

Intermediate

- Infection.
- Deep vein thrombosis
- Pulmonary embolism.
- Pneumonia.
- Continuing wound problems (5–10%).

Late
- Seroma.
- Horner's syndrome.
- Poor cosmetic appearance.
- Shoulder pain syndrome.
- Accessory nerve damage.
- Neuroma.
- Recurrent tumour.
- Scar contracture.
- Fistula.
- Facial oedema.
- Cerebral oedema.

Carotid artery protection is essential in any patient whose skin wound is liable to break down (irradiated, poorly nourished, diabetic). A levator scapulae flap, dermal graft, or free flap may be used.

Chapter 10

Chest

Breast cancer *364*
Breast reconstruction *367*
Nipple–areolar complex reconstruction *373*
Chest wall reconstruction *375*
Sternum reconstruction *378*

Breast cancer

Epidemiology
- Incidence: 1/9 women in USA; 1/12 women in UK.
- 30% of all cancer in women is of the breast; 1% of male cancers.

Risk factors
- Hormonal: increased duration of uninterrupted oestrogen exposure due to menarche <12 years, menopause >55 years, and nulliparous or first child at over 30 years. HRT long duration of the contraceptive pill, and diethylstilboestrol use have also been implicated.
- Genetic predisposition: a family history (especially first-degree relative <40 years with breast cancer) can increase the risk threefold; *BRCA1*, AD inheritance, linked with ovarian cancer, *BRCA2*.
- Previous breast carcinoma (up to 30%), previous *in situ* change (tenfold) and previous cellular atypia (fivefold).
- Radiation exposure.
- Geography: higher incidence in West compared with East. Related to lifestyle: ?higher dietary fat, affluence.

Classification
By pathological type:
- Invasive ductal (65–80%).
- Tubular (variant of ductal) (2–18%).
- Mucinous (1–4%).
- Medullary (<5%).
- Others such as invasive lobular and inflammatory.

Pathophysiology
The breast can undergo various changes, but these do not necessarily lead on to the next stage:
- Normal hyperplasia.
- Hyperplasia with atypia.
- Carcinoma *in situ* (invasive carcinoma). There are two forms of *in situ* disease:
  - Lobular carcinoma *in situ* (LCIS) occurs commonly in both breasts and only leads to malignancy in 14% of cases.
  - Ductal carcinoma *in situ* (DCIS) is often multifocal, is less likely to be bilateral than lobular, and has ~43% risk of becoming invasive disease.

Clinical features
- Lump in the breast or axilla.
- Recent history of distortion or inversion of the nipple.
- Nipple discharge that is blood-stained, bilateral, or in >50 years.
- Skin changes such as ulceration, eczema, distortion, or *peau d'orange*.

Diagnosis
Triple assessment, i.e. examination, imaging (usually mammography but also ultrasound or MRI), and FNA or core biopsy. If all are positive or negative the result is 99% accurate.

Management

As part of a multidisciplinary team.

Prophylactic mastectomy

This is a contentious issue and various guidelines have been drawn up in different areas. This should be considered if the risk is greater than one in four.

- Bilateral mastectomy: *BRCA* positive; strong family history (two first-degree relatives aged <40 years with cancer) and LCIS/DCIS; bilateral LCIS/DCIS.
- Unilateral mastectomy (remaining breast): DCIS/LCIS; one first-degree relative.
- Nipple conservation is possible but ~4% risk of cancer in remnant; patient choice.

LCIS

Three options:
- Observation with regular examination and yearly mammogram.
- Bilateral prophylactic mastectomy (very aggressive considering only 14% risk of malignant change).
- Tamoxifen.

DCIS

- Excision alone if small area (<2.5 cm), margins clear by >10 mm, and well differentiated.
- Lumpectomy and radiotherapy, although some controversy as ~57% do not go on to cancer.
- Mastectomy has a local recurrence rate of 1.4% and long-term survival of 98%.

Invasive carcinoma

- Breast conservation via wide local excision and radiotherapy may be used if the disease is not multifocal and the ratio of tumour size to breast size is not too high. The overall survival and distant-disease-free survival is the same as mastectomy, but the local recurrence rate may be higher (Milan 20 year study 8.8% vs. 2.3% with mastectomy).
- Modified radical mastectomy ± radiotherapy to prevent local recurrence in large tumours.
- Axilla: with non-palpable disease this should be assessed by sampling (>four level I nodes) or sentinel node biopsy. If positive or macroscopic disease the axilla should be treated with either dissection or radiotherapy.
- Chemotherapy increases survival and decreases recurrence rate, especially in younger women.
- Hormonal therapy with tamoxifen increases survival in patients <50 years who are oestrogen receptor positive and the over-fifties. Can also use aromatase inhibitors.
- Biological therapy with herceptin if herceptin receptor positive.

Table 10.1 TNM classification of breast cancer

T0, Tx, Tis	
T1	<2 cm
T2	2–5 cm
T3	>5 cm
T4	Attached to skin/chest wall
N0, Nx	
N1	Mobile ipsilateral nodes
N2	Fixed ipsilateral nodes
N3	Ipsilateral internal mammary nodes
M0, Mx	
M1	Distant metastases

Table 10.2 Breast cancer staging and survival (M0 unless specified)

Stage	TNM	5-year survival
0	Tis N0	Stage 0—95%
I	T1 N0	Stage I—88%
IIA	T0 N1, T1 N1, T2 N0	Stage II—66%
IIB	T2 N1, T3 N0	
IIIA	T3 N1, T0–3 N2	
IIIB	T4 N0–2	Stage III—36%
IIIC	Any T N3	
IV	Any T Any N M1	Stage IV—7%

Breast reconstruction

Principles
Restoration of aesthetic breast form using autologous and/or prosthetic material.

Aims
- Replacement of skin.
- Replacement of volume.
- Achieve bilateral breast symmetry.
- Reconstruction of nipple.

History
- **Tumour factors** Surgery, chemotherapy, radiotherapy stage, and survival. How long since original treatment and any recurrence? Family history of breast cancer. Discussion re risks to other breast and possibility of contralateral mastectomy.
- **Patient wishes** Has the patient decided on autologous or expander-based reconstruction? Does she wish symmetry within or outwith a bra? What is her attitude to scarring, length of surgery, and recovery time? Does she have any preconceptions or firm ideas?
- **Contralateral breast** What is her current bra size? Does she like her remaining breast? Does she want it to be larger, smaller, uplifted, or matched?
- **Donor site** Specific questioning re potential donor sites. Does the patient have a preference? Has there been any surgery or trauma to exclude any donor site?
- **Patient factors** Full medical and surgical history. Smoking, allergies, and scarring history.

Examination
BMI and general examination.

Breast examination
Ensure that there are no masses, lumps, or recurrence. Assess suitability of contralateral breast for procedures if requested.

Skin and soft tissue
Assess radiation damage. If serious, check back skin for damage. Look for laxity, thickness, and general quality of the skin. Measure the amount of skin required to symmetrize. This is best done by measuring clavicle to infra-mammary fold on the breast meridian and subtracting the mastectomy side measurement from the contralateral measurement to give X. In some autologous reconstructions the skin from the scar to the infra-mammary fold should be removed and so this distance should be measured and added on to X to give a final measurement of the amount of skin required. In the event of reduction or mastopexy on the normal side, the measurement of the contralateral breast will have to be adjusted accordingly. Assess how much infill (tissue under the superior mastectomy flap which gives the superior pole of the breast) is required. Measure breast width and nipple distance from the sternal notch as this will be important in expander choice.

Muscle

Check for pectoralis and anterior axillary fold preservation. Check for function of latissimus dorsi (if the nerve is working, thoracodorsal vessels are probably preserved).

Donor sites

Check donor sites for scarring, hernias, and defects. Measure maximum skin dimensions that can be taken, allowing closure.

Investigations
- Recent contralateral mammogram.
- Restaging before reconstruction should be considered and discussed with the oncologist.
- CXR, FBC, U&E, LFT, clotting, and cross-match.

Timing of reconstruction

Immediate

This preserves skin and infra-mammary fold and the scar can be designed in the most aesthetically pleasing direction. This produces the optimal breast reconstruction. Mastectomy and reconstruction are performed at one sitting and therefore this is a cheaper and more efficient use of resources. There is reduced anxiety for the patient over loss of the breast. It is possible to irradiate the reconstructed breast (autologous is more resistant then prosthetic) but there is increased risk of capsular contracture and fat necrosis. Recent studies report inferior results, even of TRAMs, after radiotherapy. In breast-conserving treatment, reconstruction of partial defects is best done immediately, thus reducing the incidence of fat necrosis and skin loss.

Delayed

Surgery is delayed until after chemotherapy and radiotherapy, usually for 6 months but longer if irradiation change is severe. This reduces the risk of capsular contracture and fat necrosis. It is logistically easier to organize as only one surgical team is required. Psychologically allows the patient to adjust to her mastectomy and more time to decide if and what reconstruction she wishes.

Reconstructive options after wide local excision/ quadrantectomy

Autologous

Reshape by undermining the breast to redistribute the tissue and suturing in layers. Use pedicles for larger defects: lower pedicle for upper defects, and upper pedicle for lower defects. As part of reduction mammaplasty. The nipple pedicle can be adjusted depending on the cancer site. Latissimus dorsi flap.

Non-autologous: implant
- Indications: as part of breast-conserving treatment.
- Complications: breast tissue necrosis; requires complete tumour excision as breast is distorted after procedure; risk of nipple necrosis.

- Disadvantages: in larger defects the use of the latissimus dorsi means the loss of a reconstructive option in the event of mastectomy; may need contralateral symmetrizing surgery; significant increase in complications after radiotherapy.
- Advantages: much improved aesthetic result over wide local excision or quadrantectomy alone.

Reconstructive options after mastectomy

Autologous with or without expander

- Pedicled: latissimus dorsi, unilateral TRAM, bilateral TRAM (with or without delay in the case of the TRAM flaps).
- Free: TRAM, muscle-sparing TRAM, DIEP, others (superficial inferior epigastric artery, superior gluteal, inferior gluteal, Rubens/peri-iliac, anterolateral thigh, gracilis).
- Latissimus dorsi (pedicled TRAM) with expander.
- Indications: ulcerated tumour; thin poor quality skin; skin discrepancy >6 cm; loss of pectoralis major and the anterior axillary fold; ptotic breast the patient wishes to be matched; failed prosthesis; patient preference; surgeon preference.
- Donor vessel: in a free flap the internal mammary, thoracodorsal, or circumflex scapular vessels are used.
- Complications: problems due to longer procedures (e.g. DVT, PE, chest infection); complete or partial flap failure; fat necrosis; prolonged wound healing at donor or recipient site; seroma; haematoma; abscess; abdominal bulge or hernia (TRAM). See individual flaps.
- Disadvantages: longer operation and recovery; more scarring.
- Advantages of autologous alone: gold standard result that gives a more natural appearance and changes as the body changes.

Non-autologous

- Expander or implant: silicone, saline, or mixed; anatomical (silicone or mixed) or round.
- Indications: good-quality skin (usually no radiotherapy); enough skin to cover the prosthesis and a discrepancy <6 cm; opposite breast 350 mL or less (when reduced); non-ptotic or patient wishes it augmented; pectoralis major intact; patient preference; surgeon preference.
- Placement: usually submuscular, either partial (subpectoral) or complete (subpectoral and serratus); subcutaneous in the obese.
- Complications: see under breast augmentation. The capsular contracture rate is ~20% in non-irradiated and 50% in irradiated. The risks of haematoma, seroma, and infection are all higher than in immediate reconstruction than in delayed.
- Disadvantages: frequent visits for expansion; less natural shape; difficulty with ptosis and re-creation of the infra-mammary fold; long-term consequences of implants requiring further surgery and disruption of life.
- Advantages: shorter operation and recovery, no additional scarring or donor site problems.

Reconstructive choice

The main factors contributing to the choice are patient preference, surgeon preference, patient factors, contralateral breast dimensions, mastectomy site features, and donor site availability. A broad algorithm can be proposed.

- No radiotherapy; contralateral breast small to medium; no ptosis (or after reduction and mastopexy); 50–60% lower abdomen required:
  - Autologous: DIEP, autologous latissimus dorsi, muscle-sparing TRAM, TRAM, unilateral pedicled TRAM.
  - Non-autologous: Tissue expander (especially if contralateral augmentation).
- Radiotherapy, contralateral breast small to medium, no ptosis (or after reduction and mastopexy):
  - Autologous: DIEP, TRAM, muscle-sparing TRAM, autologous latissimus dorsi.
  - Autologous with expander: latissimus dorsi and expander.
- Contralateral breast large or ptotic and requires to be matched; ≥75% lower abdomen required:
  - Autologous: muscle-sparing TRAM; TRAM; bilateral pedicled TRAM; DIEP with two or three perforators; delayed unilateral pedicled TRAM (tie off the deep inferior epigastric system 2 weeks before).
  - Autologous with expander: latissimus dorsi and expander can match the size but not the ptosis.

TRAM vs. DIEP

A TRAM flap takes the entire rectus muscle and fascia. As a consequence donor site morbidity is higher, with more hernias and bulges (up to 20%) and objectively (not subjectively) greater abdominal wall morbidity. However, the rates of fat necrosis and partial flap failure are lower in a TRAM flap. Muscle- and fascia-sparing TRAMs may reduce the more overt complications whilst retaining the vascular advantages. Refinements of DIEP such as taking more perforators with larger flaps or limiting it to reconstructions involving 60–70% of the abdominal wall may further reduce complications.

Abdominal flap inset

Skin

Orientate the skin paddle to best replace the skin and infill the superior pole. This may be vertical, oblique, or horizontal depending on the nature of the defect and the chest wall dimensions.

Pedicle

Pedicled flaps can be transferred on an ipsilateral or contralateral pedicle. Ensure that the tunnel is not tight and the muscle is not kinked. Free flaps can be anastomosed to axilla or internal mammary vessels. Temporarily secure the flap on the chest wall, do the anastomoses, sit the patient up, and inset. Fix the muscle to the chest wall to prevent tension or kinking on the anastomoses. Then shape the breast and suture the skin, leaving it larger to allow for shrinkage.

Latissimus dorsi inset

Skin
The flap is usually rotated through 180° so that the inferior tissue is placed on top of the pectoralis major and becomes the infill. The axilla is closed off by suturing the latissimus muscle to the chest wall.

Pedicle
The pedicle is visualized via the back. The insertion can be divided or left attached to the humerus.

Expander
Superiorly this is placed underneath the pectoralis muscle and inferiorly and laterally is sub-latissimus.

Secondary surgery
The reconstructed breast should be assessed 3–6 months post surgery. This is the ideal time to adjust the reconstruction and do any surgery to the contralateral breast.

- Volume: too much volume in autologous reconstruction can be removed with liposuction; too little can be treated with lipofilling. Expanders can be exchanged for implants or the ports removed if required.
- Contour: flap or implant adjustment may be required. Contour defects can be filled with fat injection.
- Infra-mammary fold: this may need to be adjusted via either an external or an internal approach.
- Scar revision.
- Nipple reconstruction.

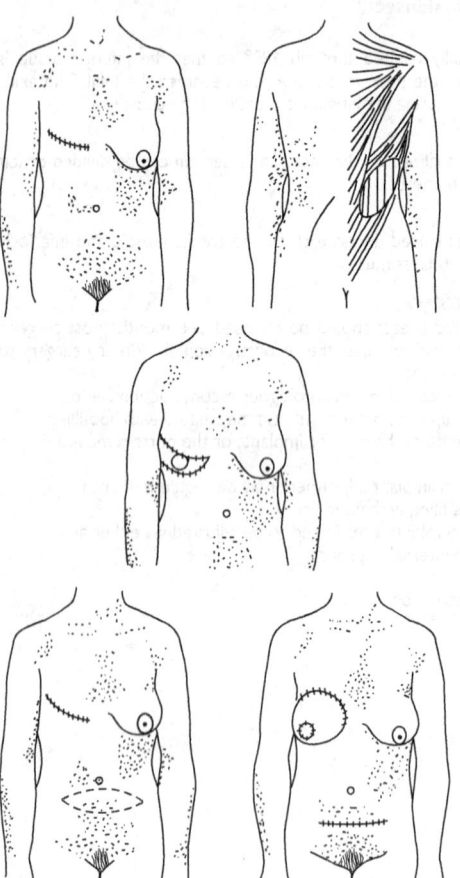

Fig. 10.1 Methods of reconstruction of the breast after mastectomy.

Nipple–areolar complex reconstruction

Nipple-areolar complex (NAC) reconstruction is performed in patients who have undergone breast reconstruction after mastectomy. After a breast reconstruction, tissue swelling takes time to settle and the effect of gravity affects the ultimate position of the breast. Therefore NAC reconstruction is normally performed at least 3 months after breast reconstruction to allow accurate symmetrical NAC placement. Nipple and areolar reconstruction can be performed at the same time and under local anaesthetic.

Nipple reconstruction
Nipple sharing procedures
Part of the opposite nipple is used as a composite graft. Not ideal in that the normal breast is affected. Either the lower half of the opposite nipple or its most prominent half is used.

Local flaps
- Skate flap: resembles the skate fish; requires FTSG.
- Modified skate flap: direct closure of donor site; avoids FTSG.
- Quadripod flap: four flaps elevated and drawn centrally to form the sides of the nipple; post-operative retraction a problem.
- Double opposing tab flap.
- C–V flap.

Design new nipple height to be twice that of the opposite side, immediately after operation, as significant loss of projection is to be expected.

Areolar complex reconstruction
Skin graft
- FTSG as part of skate flap procedure.
  - Donor sites:
  - Opposite areola: not ideal in that the normal breast is affected; ideal if breast reduction being done.
  - Groin, upper inner thigh, labia: graft pigments with time, but colour may then fade.
  - Axilla: not so pigmented.
  - Resected areola if not involved in disease.

Tattooing
Often performed at the time of nipple reconstruction. Some delay tattooing to allow new nipple to heal. Colour at time of procedure is darkened by haemosidirin pigment which will fade. Also ink colour fades in time. Therefore aim for the new nipple to be slightly darker than the the opposite nipple.

Quadrapod flap

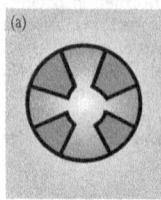 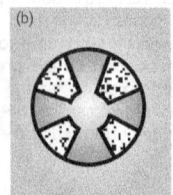 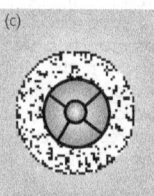

Skate

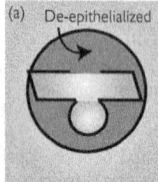 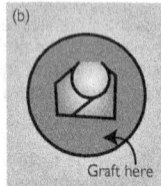

Fig. 10.2 Quadrapod flap: (a) design; (b) de-epithelialize between the spokes; (c) pull up the central hub and suture spokes together, and FTSG the surrounding neo-areolar. Skate flap (modified): (a) design and de-epithelialize the grey area; (b) elevate the head and arms of the flap, leaving it attached to the chest, wrap the arms around to support the head, and FTSG the surround.

Chest wall reconstruction

Anatomy
- Bony composition
  - Thoracic vertebrae, ribs, costal cartilages, sternum.
  - Major muscular attachments: latissimus dorsi, serratus anterior, pectoralis major and minor, external, internal, and innermost intercostals, rectus abdominus, and external oblique.
- Vascular supply
  - Intercostal arteries, internal thoracic artery, subscapular artery giving off the thoracodorsal artery and serratus branch, and thoraco-acromial artery.

Functions of the chest wall
- Protection of chest and upper abdominal viscera.
- Attachment for muscles of respiration.
- Overall integrity of chest wall is vital to prevent paradoxical movements during respiration and provide normal respiratory function.
- Contribution to movements of the shoulder and arm.
- Respiration.

Aetiology of chest wall defects
- Congenital:
  - Poland's syndrome.
  - Pectus excavatum.
  - Pectus carinatum.
  - Scoliosis.
- Acquired:
  - Infection (necrotizing fasciitis, infected mesh, chronic empyema).
  - Neoplasia, (lung tumour involving wall, or primary wall tumour including breast).
  - Iatrogenic (rib excision, radiotherapy).
  - Trauma (gunshot wounds, RTA).

Problems with chest wall defects
- Loss of respiratory support and respiratory difficulties.
- Flail segment.
- Loss of ability to raise abdominal pressure for defecation, urination, coughing.
- Discomfort.
- Deformity.

Aims
- Restore the integrity of the chest wall.
- Provide stable soft tissue coverage.
- Remove deformity.

Options for acquired chest wall defects
- Prosthetic mesh in a methyl methacrylate cement sandwich: to restore the integrity of the chest wall in stable non-infected wounds. Temporary measure in grossly contaminated wounds. Needed where flail segment likely to compromise respiratory function, which varies according to respiratory status of patient. Can be very large: five or six rib segments in young fit adult or much smaller (three or four rib segments) in respiratory cripple. Site of the defect is also critical. A posterior para vertebral defect causes less paradoxical respiration than an equivalent defect in the more mobile anterior–lateral area.
- Skin grafts: temporary method of wound closure in massive chest trauma. Secondary removal and definitive wound cover is required when the patient is fit.
- Tissue expansion can provide sufficient expansion of adjacent tissue to enable closure by advancement or flap cover. Easier than on the abdomen as has a firm base against which to expand.
- Topical negative pressure: provides a *temporary* wound dressing which decontaminates the wound and promotes granulation tissue formation. Good for very productive exudative wounds.
- Flaps: provide skin, subcutaneous tissue, fascia, and muscle.
- Local flaps and regional flaps
  - Skin only—delto-pectoral, scapular, parascapular, superior abdominoplasty.
  - Muscle and fascia—latissimus dorsi, pectoralis major, rectus abdominus, serratus anterior.
  - Skin, muscle, and fascia—rectus abdominus musculocutaneous flap, latissimus dorsi musculocutaneous flap, pectoralis major musculocutaneous flap.
  - Omental transposition flap.
- Free tissue transfer—tensor fascia lata flap, anterior lateral thigh.

Selection
- General considerations.
- Aetiology and timing: immediate repair in the case of non-infected wounds caused iatrogenically or by neoplasia excision, delayed if the wound is contaminated or infected. Prefer muscle flap to close infected defects to optimize dead-space filling, blood and antibiotic therapy, and better antibacterial properties.
- Depth and complexity of defect:
  - Bronchopleural fistula will need well-conforming flap of omentum or muscle to seal.
  - Chronic empyema defect with deep dead-space due to fibrosis will need good conforming tissue to close dead-space such as muscle or omentum.

- Chest wall layers involved:
  - Ribs only with adequate soft tissue are repaired with nothing, suturing ribs together, synthetic patch with mesh alone, mesh cement sandwich, or autologous fascial or muscle layer patch.
  - Skin only with ribs intact is repaired with wide undermining and direct closure, or local or regional flaps. Tissue expansion with secondary closure is also used when the soft tissue deficit is large.
  - Ribs and skin: use single composite tissue reconstruction (eg. TFL with iliotibial tract) or two separate techniques for each defect (eg. mesh for rib defect and Latissimus dorsi myocutaneous flap for skin).
- Site:
  - Posterior chest wall:
    — Trapezius.
    — Latissimus dorsi flap.
  - Anterior lateral chest wall:
    — Superiorly based rectus abdominus muscle or myocutaneous flap.
    — Latissimus dorsi flap.
    — Pectoralis major (medial or superiorly based).
    — Serratus anterior.
    — Tensor fascia lata flap.
    — Omentum.
- Options appraisal:
  - Other wounds, drains, scars.
  - Note that previous thoracotomy will have divided the latissimus dorsi and serratus!
  - Vascularity and nerve supply to remaining muscles and skin/fat.
  - Age, health, and requirements of patient.
  - Ability of patient to tolerate raised thoracic pressures once wound is closed.

Sternum reconstruction

Most commonly performed for post-sternotomy dehiscence and infection.

Anatomy
- Bony composition: manubrium, sternum body, xiphoid process.
- Bony attachments: clavicle, first to seventh costal cartilages.
- Major muscular attachments: pectoralis major, sternocleidomastoid, sternohyoid, sternothyroid, innermost intercostals, rectus abdominus, and external oblique.
- Vascular supply: intercostal arteries, internal thoracic artery.

Functions of the sternum
- Protection of chest and upper abdominal viscera.
- Attachment for muscles of respiration.
- Overall integrity of chest wall is vital to prevent paradoxical movements during respiration and provide normal respiratory function.
- Contribution to movements of the shoulder and arm.
- Respiration.

Aetiology of sternal defects
- Congenital:
  - Clefts.
  - Pectus excavatum.
  - Pectus carinatum.
  - Scoliosis.
- Acquired:
  - Infection (infected sternotomy, chronic mediastinitis, necrotizing fasciitis).
  - Neoplasia, (lung tumour involving wall, or primary wall tumour including breast).
  - Iatrogenic (sternotomy, radiotherapy).
  - Trauma (gunshot wounds, RTA).

Problems with sternal defects
- Loss of respiratory support and respiratory difficulties.
- Flail central segment.
- Loss of protection for heart and mediastinum.
- Discomfort.
- Deformity.

Aims
- Excise the cause.
- Obliterate dead-space.
- Restore the integrity of the sternum and chest wall.
- Provide stable soft tissue coverage.
- Remove deformity.

Post-sternotomy infection

- Most common indication for reconstruction.
- Reported in up to 5% of median sternotomies.
- Infection may involve the mediastinum, prosthetic valves, prosthetic aorta, and suture lines.
- Mortality ranges from 5% to 50%.
- Incidence increases when either internal thoracic artery is used for coronary artery bypass.
- Incidence increases further when both internal thoracic arteries are used.

Classification

Pairolero classified into three types:

- Type 1: within 3 days of operation. Serosanguinous drainage; no cellulitis, costochondritis or osteomyelitis; negative cultures.
- Type 2: 2–3 weeks post-sternotomy. Purulent discharge, cellulitis, costochondritis, and/or osteomyelitis; positive cultures.
- Type 3: Months to years post-sternotomy. Draining sinus tract with underlying costochondritis or osteomyelitis.

Options for acquired sternal defects

- Tissue expansion can provide sufficient expansion of adjacent tissue to enable closure by advancement or flap cover. Easier than on the abdomen as has a firm base against which to expand. Very rarely used given adjacent infection.
- Topical negative pressure (TNP): provides a *temporary* wound dressing which decontaminates the wound and promotes granulation tissue formation. Good for very productive exudative wounds. Presence of collapsed foam in wound cavity splints the sternum and helps optimize pulmonary function. In high-risk patients unfit to undergo reconstructive surgery, TNP has been reported to lead to fibrous union of the sternum, providing adequate respiratory function.
- Flaps: provide skin, subcutaneous tissue fascia, and muscle.
- Local flaps and regional flaps.
  - Skin only—advancement flap of anterior chest wall skin (overlying pec major).
  - Muscle—latissimus dorsi, pectoralis major (medially based and cannot be used if IMA has been harvested! Or superiorly based, on thoraco-acromial pedicle), or rectus abdominus (less reliable if IMA has been harvested but can survive on intercostal anastomoses from intercostal 8 to SEA).
  - Skin and muscle—rectus abdominus musculocutaneous flap, latissimus dorsi musculocutaneous flap, pectoralis major musculocutaneous flap.
  - Omental transposition flap.
- Free tissue transfer–latissimus dorsi, omentum, tensor fascia lata flap.

Selection
- General Considerations.
- Aetiology and timing: immediate repair in the case of non-infected wounds caused iatrogenically or by neoplasia excision, delayed if the wound is contaminated or infected. Prefer muscle flap to close infected defects to optimize dead space filling, blood and antibiotic therapy, and better antibacterial properties.
- Depth and complexity of defect.
  - A deep wound will need well conforming flap of omentum or muscle to seal.
- Sternal layers involved.
  - Skin only with sternum intact is repaired with wide undermining and direct closure, or local or regional flaps. Tissue expansion with secondary closure is also used when the soft tissue deficit is large, or tissue expansion of the flap prior to transfer.
  - Sternum and skin: use single composite tissue reconstruction (eg. Rectus abdominus myocutaneous flap) or 2 separate techniques for each defect (eg. Pectoralis major for sternal defect and chest wall advancement flap for skin).
- Site.
- Superior sternum.
  - Pectoralis major muscle in hole and then advance chest wall skin to close.
- Middle sternum.
  - Pectoralis major (medial—not if IMA has been harvested!—or superiorly based) for sternal hole and contralateral pectoralis major muscle superiorly based and left attached to humerus to double breast over other pec major in hole to provide sternal splinting and then advance chest wall skin to close.
  - Rectus abdominus muscle in hole, and pec major for splinting and then advance chest wall skin to close.
  - Omentum in hole then SSG over omentum. Note does not provide any chest wall and sternal splinting.
- Lower sternum—less common but more of a problem because of the reduced ability to advance the lateral skin, especially in the area of convergence of the inferior mammary folds!
  - Rectus abdominus muscle in hole, and pec major for splinting and then advance chest wall skin to close.
  - Rectus abdominus myocutaneous flap—less reliable when IMA is gone.
  - Rectus abdominus ± pec major for splinting and SSG.
  - Rectus abdominus and breast flap (beware the lower medial quadrant of breast is also devascularized when IMA is gone).
  - Omentum in hole; then SSG over omentum. Note that this does not provide any chest wall and sternal splinting.
- Whole sternum:
  - Combine middle and lower techniques.
  - Free latissimus dorsi and SSG.

- Options appraisal:
  - Other wounds, drains, scars.
  - Note that IMA harvest has significant impact on reconstructive options.
  - Vascularity and nerve supply to remaining muscles and skin/fat.
  - Age, health, and requirements of patient.
  - Ability of patient to tolerate raised thoracic pressures once closed.

Note

Respiratory function can be severely disturbed by an absent sternum and this is considerably restored by reconstructing the sternum by a method that splints it in respiratory effort. Hence the neurotized functioning superiorly based pectoralis major flap across the defect (and a hole filling one in the defect if required) provides the best restoration of pulmonary function.

Chapter 11

Abdomen and trunk

Abdominal wall reconstruction *384*
Spinal closure *387*

Abdominal wall reconstruction

Anatomy
- Layers: skin, Camper's fascia, Scarpa's fascia, musculo-aponeurotic layer, transversalis fascia, pre-peritoneal fat, peritoneum.
- Muscles: laterally—external oblique, internal oblique, transversus abdominus. Midline—rectus abdominus surrounded by the rectus sheath.
- Vascular supply: Superior epigastric, intercostal, deep and superficial inferior epigastric, deep and superficial circumflex iliac arteries.

Functions of the abdominal wall
- Protection of abdominal viscera.
- Locomotion.
- Increasing intra-abdominal pressure.
- Respiration.

Aetiology of abdominal wall defects
- Congenital:
  - Omphalocele.
  - Gastroschisis.
- Acquired:
  - Infection (necrotizing fasciitis, infected mesh).
  - Neoplasia (intra-abdominal involving wall, or primary wall tumour).
  - Iatrogenic (incisional hernia, radiotherapy).
  - Trauma (gunshot wounds, RTA).

Problems with abdominal wall defects
- Hernia.
- Loss of respiratory support.
- Loss of ability to raise abdominal pressure for defecation, urination, coughing.
- Discomfort.
- Deformity.
- Fragility of skin leading to ulceration.

Aims
- Restore the integrity of the abdominal wall.
- Provide soft tissue coverage.

Options
- Prosthetic mesh: to restore the integrity of the abdominal wall in stable wounds. Temporary measure in grossly contaminated wounds.
- Skin grafts: temporary method of wound closure in massive abdominal trauma. Secondary removal and definitive wound cover is required when the patient is fit.
- Tissue expansion can provide sufficient expansion of adjacent tissue to enable closure by advancement or flap cover.

- Topical negative pressure: provides a *temporary* wound dressing which decontaminates the wound and promotes granulation tissue formation. May also have a role in the management of enterocutaneous fistulae, allowing healing by removal of irritant enteric secretions.
- Flaps: provide skin, subcutaneous tissue, and fascia.
- Local flaps:
  - Skin only: groin flap, superficial epigastric, abdominoplasty.
  - Muscle and fascia: external oblique turnover flap, components separation technique.
  - Skin, muscle and fascia: rectus abdominus musculo-cutaneous flap, external oblique musculo-cutaneous flap.
- Regional flaps:
  - Skin, muscle, and fascia: tensor fascia lata, rectus femoris, or extended latissimus dorsi flap.
- Free tissue transfer: tensor fascia lata flap.

Selection

- General considerations.
- Aetiology and timing: immediate repair in the case of non-infected wounds caused iatrogenically or by neoplasia; delayed repair if wound is contaminated or infected.
- Abdominal wall layers involved:
  - Fascia only with adequate soft tissue is repaired with mesh or component separation technique.
  - Skin only with fascia intact is repaired with wide undermining and direct closure or local flaps. Tissue expansion with secondary closure is also used when the soft tissue deficit is large.
  - Fascia and skin: use single composite tissue reconstruction (e.g. TFL with iliotibial tract) or two separate techniques for each defect (e.g. mesh for fascial defect and abdominoplasty advancement for skin).
- Site.
- Upper abdominal wall:
  - Superiorly based rectus abdominus musculo-cutaneous flap.
  - External oblique muscle and aponeurosis.
  - Extended latissimus dorsi flap.
- Lower abdominal wall:
  - Tensor fascia lata flap.
  - Rectus femoris flap: may include a fascial extension (the 'mutton chop' flap) to enable reach to the epigastrium.
  - Inferiorly based rectus abdominus musculo-cutaneous flap.
  - External oblique muscle and aponeurosis.
  - Groin flap.
- Options appraisal:
  - Other wounds, stoma, scars.
  - Vascularity and nerve supply to remaining muscles and skin/fat.
  - Age, health, and requirements of patient.
  - Ability of patient to tolerate raised intra-abdominal pressure, and hence raised thoracic pressures. once abdomen closed.

Component separation (Ramirez et al. 1990)

Separation of the components of the abdominal wall allows mobilization of each unit over a greater distance than would be possible if they were moved *en bloc*. The external oblique is separated by an incision over the linea semilunaris. The rectus abdominus is separated from the medial two-thirds of the posterior rectus sheath by an incision just lateral to the linea alba. These incisions preserve the neurovascular supply to the rectus between the internal oblique and transversus abdominus layers. Each rectus can be advanced 10 cm, and the anterior sheath is sutured to the opposite anterior sheath. This provides dynamic abdominal wall support.

Reference

Ramirez OM, Ruas E, Dellon AL (1990). *Plast Reconstr Surg* **86**, 519–26.

Spinal closure

Indications
- Spina bifida.
- Post-operative spinal surgery.
- Pressure sores.
- Burns.

Classification
- High, middle, low.

or
- Cervical.
- Thoracic.
- Lumbar.
- Sacral.

Options
- Any level:
    - Paravertebral muscles.
    - Flap plus direct closure skin.
    - Tissue expansion, (except cervical).
- Cervical:
    - Trapezius.
    - Latissimus dorsi.
    - Releasing incision mid-lateral line.
- Thoracic:
    - Trapezius.
    - Latissimus dorsi.
    - Latissimus–gluteus combined flap.
    - Releasing incision mid-lateral line.
- Lumbar:
    - V–Y based on paravertebral perforators.
    - Latissimus dorsi.
    - Latissimus-gluteus combined flap.
- Sacral:
    - Gluteus.
    - Tensor fascia lata flap, extended.

Principles
- Excisional debridement.
- Close dead space with muscle; may need one flap for dead space and another for skin closure.
- Try to avoid midline scar.
- Try to have a double-breasted closure.
- Beware tension-free closure whilst patient is prone. May be under tension when the patient is supine, sitting, or flexed.

Special flaps

For others see flap section.

Latissimus dorsi-gluteus combined flap

When the latissimus dorsi is raised, based on its thoracodorsal pedicle, the inferior third of the muscle has a much reduced blood supply and so consequently does the overlying skin if raised as a myocutaneous flap. The skin around the posterior lateral iliac crest is a watershed area for blood supply. The inferior crest skin is supplied by perforators from the gluteus. For long spinal defects, including the thoracic, lumbar, and sacral regions or just lower thoracic to upper sacral levels, the latissimus dorsi and the gluteus can both be raised on their thoracodorsal and superior gluteal arteries, respectively, through a midlateral skin incision. Keep the skin overlying these muscles in continuity, creating a massive flap from axilla to greater trochanter. This myocutaneous flap can be advanced medially. The advancing edge can have the muscle and skin separated for a short distance to allow the muscle to fill the dead space and the skin to close in a double-breasted manner. The mid-lateral skin incision can be partly closed directly and the remainder split-skin grafted.

Latissimus flap designs

These can be based on thoracodorsal artery and just the muscle origin elevated and the flap transposed medially. This remains innervated and functional, but the reach of this pedicle means that it is suitable for thoracic and upper lumbar defects only.

Defects lower than this can be based on the lumbar perforators, but with denervation of the muscle. If distally based, the skin component can be the V–Y pattern or transposition utilizing the skin laxity in the flanks. The V–Y pattern can be designed transversely or obliquely, moving from axilla to lumbo-sacral junction.

Chapter 12

Upper limb

Anatomy of extensor mechanism of the fingers *390*
Digital extensor mechanism defects and assessment *392*
Hand infections *394*
Dystonia *400*
Hand tumours *401*
Soft tissue tumours *405*
Vascular tumours *409*
Bone tumours *412*
Metastatic tumours *417*
Upper limb amputations *418*
Ray amputation *420*
Upper limb proximal amputations *421*
Prostheses *422*
Arthrodesis: digital *423*
Examination of the wrist *425*

Anatomy of extensor mechanism of the fingers

Knowledge of the intricacies of the extensor mechanism is important to understand the pattern of deformity and disability produced by injury/disease of the various elements of the system, and consequently to treat these injuries/diseases appropriately.

Extension is produced by an intricate combination of extensor and intrinsic muscle action. The extensor mechanism of the middle finger can be classified into extrinsic extensors and intrinsic extensors, and a retinacular system.

Extrinsic extension is produced by the EDC. The EDC tendon inserts into the dorsal hood overlying the MCPJ, and is the principle extensor of this joint. There may be attachments deep to the tendon adhering it to articular margins and the base of the proximal phalanx. However, most of the tendon passes freely over the joint distally and flattens out into the dorsal hood. Over the proximal phalanx it divides into three parts, one central and two lateral. The two lateral bands diverge around the central slip (as it attaches to the base of the middle phalanx) and then converge over the distal half of the middle phalanx, being brought together by the triangular ligament, and eventually coalesce and insert at the base of the distal phalanx. The central slip attaches to the base of the middle phalanx, and is the prime extensor of the PIPJ (Fig. 12.1).

Intrinsic finger extension includes the action of the interossei and lumbricals. These produce interphalangeal extension of the fingers. The interosseii originate from the adjacent metacarpals and the lumbrical from the flexor digitorum profundus tendon.

The interossei insert proximally into the lateral aspects of the dorsal hood separated from the EDC tendon by the sagittal bands. The sagittal bands are the transverse and vertically orientated fibres of the dorsal hood that surround the MCPJ. They serve to centralize and stabilize the EDC tendon on the dorsum of the MCPJ. The interossei form the majority of the lateral bands; the rest are formed by divergent fibres from the EDC tendon and are reinforced more distally on the radial side of the digit by the insertion of the lumbrical. Distally, the lateral bands are further reinforced by the contribution from the lateral slips of the trifurcation of the central slip. In exchange the lateral bands contribute to the central slip and assist PIPJ extension.

The retinacular system described by Landsmeer (1963) stabilizes the above tendon system and is comprised of the transverse and oblique retinacular (ligament) fibres.

The transverse fibres arising from the proximal phalanx and flexor tendon sheath pass through a window in Cleland's ligament volar to the axis of the PIPJ and insert on the lateral bands dorsal to the axis, and on the triangular ligament that separates the lateral bands at this level. They can be compared in function to the sagittal bands at the MCPJ.

ANATOMY OF EXTENSOR MECHANISM OF THE FINGERS

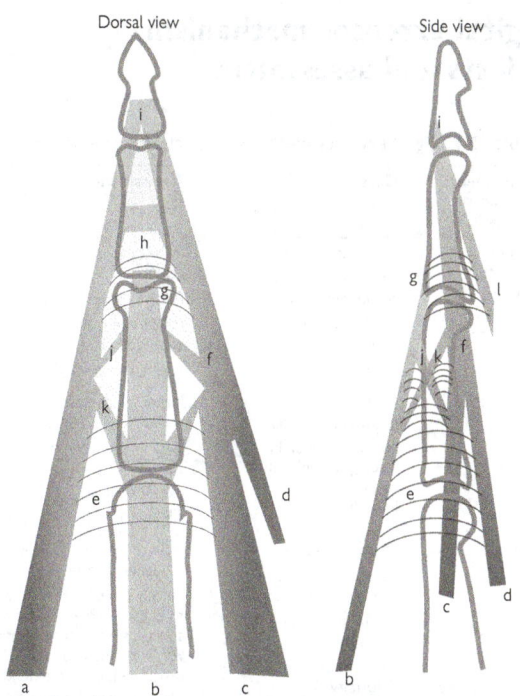

Fig. 12.1 The extensor mechanism of the left ring finger: (a) lateral band (dorsal interosseous); (b) extensor tendon; (c) lateral band (palmar interosseous); (d) lumbrical; (e) sagittal bands; (f) lateral band; (g) transverse retinacular fibres; (h) bare area; (i) triangular fibres and distal extensor tendon; (j) divergent fibres from lateral bands to central slip; (k) divergent fibres from extensor tendon to lateral bands; (l) oblique retinacular fibres (Landsmeer).

The oblique fibres (oblique retinacular ligament (ORL) of Landsmeer) are deeper and more tendinous, originate from the proximal phalanx and flexor sheath of the proximal phalanx, and have a broad insertion on the side of the lateral bands from the PIPJ to the distal third of the middle phalanx. The axis passes volar to the PIPJ and dorsal to the DIPJ as the ORL passes to insert on the lateral bands to extend the DIPJ.

Flexion of the PIPJ slackens the ORL and allows flexion of the DIPJ, whereas extension of the PIPJ tightens the ORL and extends the DIPJ. This produces coordinated movement between the interphalangeal joints.

Reference

Landsmeer JM (1963). *J Bone Joint Surg Am* **45**, 1654–62.

Digital extensor mechanism defects and assessment

Table 12.1 Digital extensor mechanism defects and assessment

Component of extensor mechanis	Cause	Assessment
Extrinsic extensor tendon	Sharp laceration Attritional rupture on bone/metal Attritional rupture ▶ synovitis (Vaughan–Jackson lesion)	Inability to extend digit actively Passive extension possible Inability to maintain passively extended digit Ability to extend IPJs retained
Sagittal band	Closed trauma Rupture of usually radial sagittal band leading to subluxation of extensor into ulnar gutter	Inability to extend digit actively Passive extension possible Ability to maintain passively extended digit Ability to extend IPJs retained
Central slip	Sharp laceration Closed traumatic rupture or avulsion Attritional rupture ▶ synovitis Leads to Boutonnière deformity	Able to extend MCPJ; shows tendency to hyper-extend Initially (first few weeks) able to extend PIPJ, but in doing so against resistance forms a 90° flexed position (Elson's test); the DIPJ also extends Later ability to extend PIPJ is lost: initially active loss only but progresses to passive loss as well, and later to DIPJ hyper-extension
Lateral band	Unilateral laceration poses no deficit Bilateral laceration rare Most problems relate to contracted intrinsics/lateral bands	Difficulty or inability to extend MCPJ Difficulty in flexing PIPJ when MCPJ extended (Finochietto–Bunnell test)
Transverse retinacular ligaments	Rarely injured in isolation Deficiency or laxity in these allows the lateral bands to sublux palmarwards until palmar to the axis of rotation, where they become a PIPJ flexor instead of an extensor	Development of Boutonnière deformity, with loss of passive extension of PIPJ Hyper-extension of DIPJ Reduced ability to flex DIPJ when PIPJ extended (Haines–Zancolli test)

Table 12.1 (Contd.)

Oblique retinacular ligaments	Rarely injured in isolation Deficiency of these contributes to swan-neck deformity Contracture of these leads to Boutonnière deformity	Loss of coordination of extension and flexion of the IPJs Flexed DIPJ even with extension of PIPJ
Distal extensor tendon	Sharp laceration Attritional over bony spur Stretched in osteoarthritis, synovitis, nodes	Inability to extend DIPJ actively (Mallet deformity)

Other conditions affecting extensor mechanism

Intrinsic tightness	Post-traumatic (Watson's syndrome) Postural after prolonged MCPJ flexion	Difficulty or inability to extend MCPJ Inability or difficulty in flexing PIPJ when MCPJ extended. (Finochietto–Bunnell test)
Lumbrical plus	Post division of flexor tendon distal to origin of lumbrical	Flexion of MCPJ and contrary extension of PIPJ on attempted flexion of digit

Other conditions that may mimic extensor mechanism defects

Locked MCPJ	Snagging of palmar plate of the MCPJ on an osteophyte	Inability to extend MCPJ passively or actively Can flex further and extend to the blocking point IPJ flexion and extension normal
Trigger digit	Stenosing tenovaginits of the flexor tendons at the A1 pulley	If severe, inability to fully extend MCPJ and PIPJ passively or actively Flexion may also be reduced in range Crepitus or Notta's node may be palpable

Hand infections

Aetiology
- There is usually a history of penetrating injury, although infections around the nail may be due to maceration of the skin in people who work with their hands immersed in water, or suck their fingers.
- The traumatic incident may have been very minor and not remembered by the patient.
- Haematogenous infection of bone or the flexor sheath is rare.
- *Staphylococcus aureus* is the most common organism in cultures; streptococci, Gram-negative bacteria, and anaerobes are also encountered. Fungi infect the nailfolds.

Clinical features
- Heat, redness, pain, swelling, and loss of function are typical.
- Progress from cellulitis to abscess.
- The four cardinal signs of flexor sheath infection (first three described by Kanavel, and the fourth added later) are:
  - Pain on passive extension of the finger.
  - Tenderness over the flexor sheath.
  - Symmetrical fusiform swelling of the whole finger; prompt surgical drainage is required.
  - Flexed finger posture.
- Some of these signs may be apparent in subcutaneous collections.
- Joint infections show signs of flexion posture, pain on movement of involved joint, fusiform swelling, and tenderness around and on the joint. However, adjacent joints will move without pain or tenderness indicating pain-free movement of the flexor tendons.
- Cellulitis will show redness, swelling, heat, and tenderness but there will not be increased pain on joint or tendon movement within restricted range caused by the swelling. If no collection or foreign body present, antibiotics can be tried. If in doubt, operate.
- Differentiating between infection and inflammatory conditions (such as gout, acute rheumatoid arthritis) is sometimes extremely difficult. Careful consideration of the history, patient, and examination findings can help in most cases but in the immunosuppressed (rheumatoid arthritis) it can be very difficult. If in doubt, treat as infection and get operative samples.

Investigations
- FBC, ESR, CRP if the patient is septic; uric acid if you suspect gout (closed joint infection).
- X-ray looking for foreign body (organic matter may be radiolucent), osteomyelitis, and gas in soft tissues.
- Culture of pus, preferably before antibiotics are commenced.

Management: medical
- Elevation.
- Splint to relieve pain.
- Exercises to maintain mobility, rest in between.

- In very early infections (24–48 hr) high-dose intravenous antibiotics may treat the infection.
- Surgery is required if there is a collection of pus or if conservative management has not resolved the infection within 2 days.
- The patient must be observed closely.

Management: surgical

General principles
- Tourniquet control.
- Extensile incisions.
- Release of pus and infective material.
- Specimens sent for microbiological and histopathological examination.
- Debridement excision of necrotic tissue.
- Wash-out.
- Loose closure allowing mobilization.
- Administration of intravenous antibiotics.
- Consider return to theatre in 24–48 hr to re-debride, wash out, and close.

Post-operative care
- Wounds are packed lightly with dressing changes and soaks in iodine or saline twice daily.
- Mobilize the hand in the soak.
- Continuous or intermittent irrigation with normal saline is an alternative, particularly for flexor sheath or palmar space infections.
- Elevate the hand.
- Splint the hand for 24–48 hr for pain relief.
- Start physiotherapy when pain and swelling are resolving (24–48 hr).

Complications
If hand infections are not treated promptly, tendon adhesions, necrosis and even rupture, stiffness, and permanent loss of function will ensue. Hand infections are a surgical emergency.

Cellulitis

Usually a very minor skin break, with infection by streptococci or staphylococci. Produces redness, tenderness, and mild swelling. May see ascending lymphangitis in beta-haemolytic streptococcal infection. No collection formation and responds to antibiotics (penicillin, flucloxacillin, cephalosporin) within 24 hr.

Felon

Closed-space subcutaneous infection of the pulp due to a minor puncture wound or rarely a flexor tendon sheath infection spreading distally. The pulp spaces are formed by the firm fascial connections between the pulp skin and the distal phalanx which create the loculations of fat to pad the pulp. Felons usually 'point' towards the mid-pulp and should be incised and drained through most superficial pointing area. *Staphyloccocus aureus* is the most common pathogen. If not treated, felons lead to pressure necrosis of the pulp, osteomyelitis of the distal phalanx, and rarely flexor tendon sheath infection.

Management

Incise longitudinally and drain over the pointing area, usually the mid-pulp, avoiding the digital nerves. If not obviously pointing, do a midlateral pulp incision and extend the incision through the pulp in the plane of the nail, dividing all the involved vertical septa near the palmar aspect of the distal phalanx. An alternative approach is a fish-mouth incision around the base of the hyponychium (Fig. 12.2), but this leaves an apical scar that may be tender.

Paronychia

Most common infection in the hand. An infection of the perionychium (the soft tissue fold around the nail) usually due to a hangnail laceration or avulsion usually by using one's teeth (hence organisms reflect oral flora, staphylococci, streptococci) which becomes infected. Pus then tracks around the perionychium in a horse-shoe shape producing a 'run around'. Pressure necrosis can lead to death of the nailfold. The area is hot, swollen, and tender. Pus can also track under the nailplate and collect subungually where it can also necrose the nailbed. It may also track into the pulp.

Management

- If non-operative management fails, do operation under ring block. Incise over the fold where the pus is pointing (do *not* incise parallel to the fold through out its length as this will necrose the distal strip), or longitudinally along the lateral nailfold, or perpendicular to and through the nailfold, or at the junction of the nailbed and the nailfold in the crease. May need to elevate and remove the nailplate.
- Occasionally pus can be released by merely lifting the nailfold off the nail.
- Pack the wound with a small wick.
- Change the dressing daily or on alternate days and soak the wound in Betadine.
- Antibiotics.

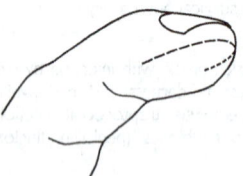

Fig. 12.2 Fish-mouth incision of finger pulp.

Herpetic whitlow

This is caused by herpes simplex virus type 1 infection and should not be treated by surgery, unless there is a secondary bacterial infection. It is common in children, perhaps related to maceration from finger sucking. Typically, the finger tip (nailfold or pulp) or whole finger becomes throbbing, painful, red and swollen. Small vesicles coalesce to form bullae; become haemorrhagic, crust, desquamate, and then heal. Each crop of vesicles lasts 10–12 days. Vesicle fluid can be cultured. The infection resolves spontaneously within a month. Can be treated using acyclovir 400 mg four times daily for 10 days if serious infection in immuno-compromised patient.

Flexor sheath infection

This is a surgical emergency as the pressure and pus in the tendon sheath causes ischaemic necrosis of the tendon, leading to rupture. In lesser states, the tendon rapidly adheres to its sheath, resulting in permanent stiffness. The cause is usually a penetrating injury of the flexor surface at the level of the DIPJ or PIPJ. The injury may not be noticed by the patient, although most recall one. It is important to know the penetrating instrument and whether it was all retrieved. For example, a needle-stick injury usually does not leave any foreign body behind; however, a thorn may well break or shed, leaving foreign material in the flexor sheath.

Management
If foreign body retention is suspected, arrange an urgent US scan to see if it can be localized. Once in the sheath, any foreign body can move some way from the entry site. There are two principle operative techniques for draining a flexor tendon sheath infection—open or closed.

Open
A midlateral incision along the digit from the DIPJ with a transverse or oblique incision from the web space over the A1 pulley can be used to expose the whole tendon sheath. A Bruner type incision can be used, especially if it needs to incorporate a palmar wound over the PIPJ of phalanges, or preferably it can be a midlateral incision which swaps sides incorporating the entry site. The advantage of the mid-lateral wound is that it is less painful to mobilize, gives the flexor tendon more support, and in the event of wound problems does not lead to exposure of the flexor tendons. In addition it is the preferred incision if later tendon grafting is likely. The cruciate and flimsy portions of the sheath are then excised (leaving the annular pulleys intact). Look for any foreign body. Excise thickened synovium. Remove insipated fibrinous material and pus. Irrigate the wound. Closure is delayed for 48 hr, after a second look and wash-out or the wound heals secondarily. Intensive physiotherapy is essential to regain full range of movement.

Closed
Two incisions are made to access the flexor sheath—one transverse or zig-zag just proximal to the distal palmar crease over the A1 pulley, and the other over the DIPJ either transverse or mid-lateral. The sheath is entered and a catheter passed down it for a short distance. Saline injected through the catheter drains the infection and irrigates the sheath, exiting through the distal hole. The catheter is left *in situ* for continuous or intermittent irrigation of the flexor sheath with normal saline over 24–48 hr.

This technique does not explore or allow removal of any foreign material or inspissated pus or fibrinous material or any synovial thickening, nor does it allow for debridement of the entry wound. Hence it should be reserved for very early presentations of flexor sheath infections where the penetrating object is known to have been removed entirely and ther is no possibility of remnant being left in the sheath. The open technique should be used for all other flexor tendon sheath infections.

Joint infections

The joint is hot, swollen, and tender, and range of motion is reduced. There is pain in the joint on motion. The digit assumes a flexed posture similar to a tendon sheath infection but the swelling may be more localized to a joint. The cause is usually a penetrating injury from the dorsum of the joint into a very flexed joint. Commonly the MCPJ is infected due to a human bite or, rather, the patient has punched someone in the mouth causing them to involuntarily 'bite' them. The penetrating injury passes directly through the various tissue planes into the joint, but when the joint moves back into a position of rest the planes move differently, occluding the entry into the joint and making the infection a closed one.

Management
This is a surgical emergency to avoid destruction of the articular cartilage.

Metacarpophalangeal joints
Approach the joint dorsally through a longitudinal or zig-zag incision, incorporating the wound in the transverse limb. Split the extensor tendon centrally, incorporating the tendon injury/laceration, or incise along the ulnar side of the central extensor tendon through the sagittal band. Retracting the tendon, incise the joint capsule and expose the joint. Irrigate, debride any thickened synovium, leave open with a wick, or close the skin loosely. Wash hand, mobilizing it within a Betadine (povidine iodine) soak.

Proximal interphalangeal joints
Approach the joint from a midlateral incision. Divide the accessory collateral ligaments as they attach to the palmar plate to access the joint. If needed, the accessory collaterals can be excised, creating a triangular defect which allows more effective joint irrigation. Maintain the true collateral ligaments. In severe infections approach the joint from bilateral midlateral incisions. This enables through-and-through wash-out. Leave the wounds open and wash twice daily in Betadine baths.

Distal interphalangeal joints
These can be washed out through either midlateral incisions or dorsal incisions of longitudinal Mercedes (or Y) transverse with lateral extensions (H). The extensor is retracted or split to expose the joint and wash it out.

Web space infections

Web space or collar-stud (collar-button) abscesses occur in the web space subcutaneous tissue between the metacarpal heads and around the inter-metacarpal ligaments. They usually start palmar, but may track dorsal from palmar in the web space. They cause abduction of the fingers from the affected web, unlike a dorsal subcutaneous infection, extending down to the level of the web. Because of the palmar and dorsal extent, these abscesses may need combined dorsal and palmar drainage. Dorsal drainage is through a longitudinal incision, and palmar drainage is via a longitudinal or zig-zag incision.

Palmar space infections

Palmar spaces are described by Kanavel as the mid-palmar (deep palmar ulnar) space and the thenar (adductor) space (Kaplan's alternative nomenclature in parentheses). The mid-palmar space is a central space which is a continuation of the carpal tunnel lying deep to the palmar aponeurosis and superficial to the deep palmar interosseous and adductor fascia. The mid-palmar space has multiple septa distally which divide the space to direct the flexor tendons to their digits, and canals for the lumbricals and their accompanying neurovascular bundles. The thenar space overlies the adductor and is bounded ulnarly by the insertion of the adductor on the third metacarpal. Pus here can track dorsally around the adductor or between the two heads of the adductor to collect in the space between the adductor and the first dorsal interosseous. Both spaces are traversed by the flexor tendons and nerves but pus usually collects deep to these structures.

Mid-palmar space infections cause dorsal swelling, with loss of the cup of the palm, palmar tenderness, and pain on moving the ring and middle fingers. Although the dorsum is swollen, the incision should be palmar longitudinal in line with the fourth ray, distally to or including the carpal tunnel.

Thenar space infections cause swelling with abduction of the thumb. They can be drained via dorsal or palmar incisions following the thenar crease. Be sure to explore the space between the adductor and the FDI.

The space of Parona is the space on the palmar aspect of the wrist deep to the flexor tendons, superficial to the pronator quadratus, and bounded radially by the FCR and ulnarly by the FCU. It connects distally with the radial and ulna bursa, thus acting as a passage by which pus can spread from one side of the hand to the other, producing a horseshoe abscess. This is decompressed by an extended carpal tunnel incision, extended by a zig-zag incision with the transverse limb lying along the distal wrist flexion crease, allowing nerve protection even in the event of swelling.

Dystonia

Definition
Dystonia is defined as a painless movement disorder. It is often isolated and associated with a single task (often a complex motor task).

Incidence
- 100 per million.
- Higher in muscians.
- ?Prevalence 0.2%.

Classification
Classified according to:
- Age: early (<26 years) and late?
- Site: focal, segmental, and multifocal.
- Aetiology: primary or secondary.

Clinical presentation
Dystonia usually presents in 30–50-year-olds secondary to complex motor tasks such as writing or playing musical instruments. Patients complain of a slow clumsy movement without pain, although cramp may be present. Posture may become bizarre. Other hand activities are normal. Differential diagnosis includes carpal tunnel syndrome, tendonitis, and arthritis.

Investigations
- Nerve conduction studies.
- X-rays and other imaging.

Treatment
- Adaptive (change tools, technique, avoid tasks).
- Therapy (splints, retraining).
- Interventional (acupuncture, botulinum toxin).

Indications for surgery
- None for dystonia.

Prognosis
Prognosis is poor. For example, most sufferers from writer's cramp change hands to write.

Hand tumours

Definition
Hand tumours are very common. Occasionally, they appear following trauma (10%), but most present incidentally. The vast majority are soft tissue and benign. Management comprises diagnosis and reassurance in many cases, but some tumours require excision. Skin cancers are common on the hand; these are discussed elsewhere. Sarcomas are also discussed elsewhere.

Classification
- Skin, soft tissue, or bone.
- Solid or cystic.
- Benign or malignant.
- Component cells or origin of tumour.

Diagnosis
Based on history, examination, and investigations.

History
- Onset.
- Duration.
- Progression/regression/course.
- Symptoms.
- Any associated conditions—gout, rheumatoid arthritis, neurofibromatosis, malignancies, previous masses.

Examination
- Site.
- Size.
- Shape.
- Surface.
- Solidity/consistency.
- Symptoms, especially tenderness or pain.
- Secondary effects:
  - Pathological fracture.
  - Deformity.
  - Stiffness.
  - Laxity.
  - Compression nerves/vessels/bone/nail.

Investigations
- X-ray: essential for assessment of secondary effects, potential sites of origin (such as arthritic joint in ganglia), and bone tumours; helpful for all other tumours as may show calcification, chondromatous elements, and other pathology.
- Ultrasound: excellent in soft tissue tumours for determining solid from cystic tumours, and can show origin or associations of the tumour with surrounding structures.

- MRI and CT scans may be required for more precise delineation of site, extent, and associations of both bone and soft tissue tumours prior to excision, and can be diagnostic in bone tumours.
- Biopsy may extend from simple needle aspiration of cystic contents to incisional biopsies of suspected malignancies. The latter should be performed through a longitudinal incision, with consideration of the eventual wide excision (which should include the biopsy tract) and reconstruction, and preferably by the eventual treating cancer centre. The most common biopsy method is large-bore FNA, which is useful for most tumours, but there are difficulties in the pathological diagnosis of neural and lipid tumours using this technique.
- Microbiology: infection can mimic tumour and tumour may mimic infection.

Treatment
- If benign, reassurance may be all that is necessary. Warn the patient to re-attend if significant change or symptoms appear.
- Tumours causing symptoms should be treated.
- Treatment is guided by the Enneking staging system of soft tissue and bone sarcomas (Table 12.2) and the AJCC staging system (Table 12.3) together with the site, extent, and behaviour of the tumour.

Excision margins (Table 12.4)
- Intralesional: resection cuts across the primary lesion (macroscopic tumour left), 'curettage'.
- Marginal: tumour mass removed from normal tissue within the reactive zone (microscopic tumour left), 'shelling out'.
- Wide: Significant cuff of normal tissue taken around the tissue.
- Radical: entire compartment containing the tumour is excised; most radical is amputation.

Note that some benign tumours, such as aggressive fibromatosis, have a locally aggressive clinical behaviour pattern necessitating wide local excision for cure.

Reconstruction
Avoid reconstructing with local or pedicled flaps because of the risk of metastatic spread along the contiguous operative site and pedicle.

Table 12.2 Enneking (Musculoskeletal Tumour Society) staging system for bone and soft tissue tumours

Stage	Surgical grade (G)	Anatomical location (T)	Metastases (M)
0	Benign (G0)	Any (T1 or T2)	None (M0)
IA	Low (G1)	Intra-compartmental (T1)	None (M0)
IB	Low (G1)	Extra-compartmental (T2)	None (M0)
IIA	High (G2)	Intra-compartmental (T1)	None (M0)
IIB	High (G2)	Extra-compartmental (T2)	None (M0)
III	Any grade	Any (T1 or T2)	Mets (M1)

Table 12.3 AJCC staging system for soft tissue sarcomas

Stage	Grade	Size	Relation to fascia
IA	Low	<5 cm	Any
IB	Low	>5 cm	Superficial
IIA	Low	>5 cm	Deep
IIB	High	<5 cm	Any
IIC	High	>5 cm	Superficial
III	High	>5 cm	Deep
IV	Any metastases		

Table 12.4 Excision margins related to surgical grade of tumour

Grade	Behaviour	Histology	Excision
G0	Benign		Intralesional or marginal excision
G1	Low	<5 mitoses/HPF, more differentiated, more stroma and fewer cells, less necrosis	Marginal or wide
G2	High	>10 mitoses/HPF, less differentiated, less stroma and more cells, more necrosis	Wide or radical

HPF, high-power field.

Table 12.5 Grading of hand tumours

Benign (G0)	Low grade (G1)	High grade (G2)
Skin		
Pyogenic granuloma	Keratoacanthoma	Melanoma
Epidermal cyst	SCC	Merkel cell
Keratoses	BCC	Sweat gland
		Sebaceous gland SCC
Soft tissue		
Ganglion	Desmoid	Synovial sarcoma
Giant cell tumour (tendon sheath)	Liposarcoma (LG)	Malignant fibrous histiocytoma (MFH)
Lipoma	Fibrosarcoma (LG)	Liposarcoma (HG)
Neurilemmoma	Kaposi's sarcoma	Rhabdomyosarcoma
Neurofibroma		Epitheliod sarcoma
Chondromatosis		Clear cell sarcoma
Glomus tumour		Angiosarcoma
Dermatofibroma		Haemangiopericytoma
Vascular malformation		Malignant peripheral nerve sheath
		Kaposi's sarcoma (HIV)
Bone/cartilage		
Enchondroma	Giant cell tumour	Osteosarcoma
Osteochondroma	Desmoplastic fibroma	Ewing's tumour
Fibrous dysplasia	Chondrosarcoma (LG)	Lymphoma
Osteoid osteoma	Parosteal osteosarcoma	Chondrosarcoma
Bone cysts		Myeloma
Osteoblastoma		

Based on Mankin (1987).

Reference
Mankin HJ (1987). *Hand Clin* **3**,185–95.

Soft tissue tumours

Ganglia
Soft to hard mucin-filled cysts attached to tendon sheath or joint capsule.

Incidence
- Very common; comprise 50–80% of hand lumps. Dorsal wrist most common at 70%, palmar wrist 10–20%, DIPJ ganglion 10–20%, flexor sheath 10%. Can occur in relation to any joint or tendon.
- Female > male.
- All ages but most common in twenties to forties. Different sites have differing age of peak incidence: dorsal wrist, twenties; palmar wrist, forties; DIPJ, fifties and sixties.
- 60% of dorsal wrist ganglia persist over 6 years.

Aetiology
Unknown: three theories:
- Aperture in joint capsule with ball valve effect—high pressure in the joint forces out synovial fluid and lower pressure externally cannot force it back. The cause of the aperture may be trauma, degeneration, or congenital. Support for the theory is identification of a tract and aperture on many occasions.
- Mucoid degeneration of the joint capsule. Support for the theory is based on the pathological finding of tiny mucoid cysts within the substance of the joint capsule adjacent to the ganglion.
- Embryonic rest of synovial tissue left behind in the subcutaneous tissues.

Ganglia are not a herniation of synovium.

Clinical features
- May appear gradually or suddenly as a lump.
- May follow trauma.
- Can be symptomatic, causing aches or pains possibly secondary to expansion or mechanically blocking movement.
- Be wary of the very painful ganglion; the pain may arise from elsewhere and will remain even when the ganglion has gone.
- Exclude underlying pathology such as ligamentous injury, stenosing vaginitides, arthritis with bone spurs.

Classification
- Dorsal wrist ganglia arise from the scapholunate ligament or from the carpometacarpal joint in association with a metacarpal boss.
- Palmar wrist ganglia arise from the flexor carpi radialis sheath, the trapeziometacarpal joint, the radio-scaphoid, or the scapho-trapezial joint.
- Palmar digital ganglia arise from the flexor tendon sheath at metacarpal joint level.
- Distal interphalangeal joint ganglia arise from the DIPJ in association with degenerative arthritis and Heberden's nodes.

Macroscopic
The ganglion wall is neither synovium nor epithelium, but is compressed collagen fibres. It may be multiloculated. There may be a duct leading to the joint.

Microscopic
The ganglion contains mucin, a viscous jelly comprising glucosamine, hyaluronic acid, and other mucopolysaccharides.

Investigations
- X-rays: may show underlying degenerative arthritis or osteophytes.
- US or MRI scanning: shows the cystic structure and perhaps the duct.

Treatment
- Rupture (classically with the Bible).
- Reassure.
- Aspirate.
- Inject with steroids, sclerosants, fibrin glue.

Surgery
Excise ganglion and its duct down to the origin.

Prognosis
- Doing nothing results in 60% persistence beyond 5 years.
- Aspiration results in 60% recurrence.
- Excision results in 40% recurrence, especially if incompletely excised, and 9% complications.

Complications
- Pain or persistence of pain.
- Stiffness.
- Recurrence.
- Scar.
- Collateral injury to nerve, vessel, tendon, or ligament.

Pigmented villa nodular synovitis/synovioma

Also known as giant cell tumour of tendon sheath, fibrous xanthoma, localized nodular synovitis.

Incidence
- Second most common soft tissue tumour in the hand (7–12%), mainly found in the palm and fingers, especially around the DIPJ of the thumb, index, and middle fingers. Benign but can infiltrate and invade bone, or involve tendon sheath and joint, making it difficult to excise fully.
- Males = females.

Aetiology
Unknown.

Clinical features
- Slowly increasing size, asymptomatic mass.
- Firm.
- Multinodular.
- May have a yellow-brown appearance at surgery because of haemosiderin accumulation.

Investigations
X-ray: may show pressure effect on bone.

Treatment
Treated by marginal excision, attempting to clear to achieve complete excision.

Prognosis
Significant recurrence rate (30%), especially if arising from joint or if excision incomplete. Rate of recurrence said by some to be related to gene *nm-23-H1* expression, others disagree.

Implantation dermoid
Also known as epidermal or inclusion cysts.
- Epithelial cysts, soft to hard, lie subdermal or subcutaneous.
- May have a history of penetrating trauma, especially a thorn, or other puncture wound, or may follow more severe trauma such as abrading or crush injuries or surgery.

Incidence
- Third most common soft tissue tumour of the hand (5–9%).
- Comprise 10–20% of hand lumps.
- Male > female.
- All ages, but most common in twenties to forties.
- Most common on fingertips, especially pulp or web spaces (in barbers).

Aetiology
Implantation of epithelial cells which enucleate and continue to produce squamous epithelium and sebaceous products which accumulate within the cyst. Slowly growing they can become pea or hazelnut sized, and symptomatic due to their hardness and position.

Clinical features
- Subcutaneous firm cyst.
- Spherical.
- Non-tender.
- History of trauma.
- Situated on pulp or flexor surface, web space.

Investigations
X-rays: may show indentation in adjacent bone due to pressure effect.

Treatment
Surgery: excision of the cyst is generally curative.

Prognosis
Excellent; recurrence rate is very low.

Schwannoma (neurllemmoma)
Peripheral nerve tumours arising from Schwann cells, firm to hard, attached to nerve, and so move from side to side but not longitudinally.

Incidence
- Isolated.
- 10% multiple (multiple schwannomatosis); can be multiple in neurofibromatosis.

- Found along the course of nerves.
- Grow from a fascicle, but displace surrounding fascicles allowing easy extirpation, preserving the nerve.

Aetiology
Unknown.

Clinical features
- Slowly increasing size.
- Some are tender or transmit shooting neural pain when percussed.
- Often asymptomatic.
- Clinically difficult to differentiate from neurofibroma or MPNST.

Classification
Simple or ancient: Antoni A cells and B cells pathologically.

Investigations
MRI scanning can usually determine neural nature of tumour, but ultrasound is better at showing the tumour's relationship to the nerve.

Treatment
- Reassurance if asymptomatic and small.
- Surgical excision if symptomatic (or open biopsy if not easily extirpated or if excision will lead to neural deficit).
- 'Schwannomas shell out; neurofibromas never do.'

Prognosis
- Recurrence rates are low.
- Usually excised with no neural deficit.
- Risk of malignant transformation is low.

Lipoma

Benign tumours of fat that tend to occur along neurovascular bundles in the hand, or less commonly subcutaneously on the hand.

Incidence
Fifth or sixth most common soft tissue tumour in the hand—lower rank than elsewhere in the body where they are the most common subcutaneous tumour.

Clinical features
- Often asymptomatic soft mass, with mobile edges.
- Slow growing.
- May cause compression symptoms particularly in carpal tunnel, or Guyon's canal.
- Rarely tender unless angiolipoma or Dercum's disease

Treatment
Excision, if symptomatic. Marginal excision is usually easy.

Prognosis
Recurrence rates are low.

Vascular tumours

A wide range of pathologies fall into this category, some of which are not real tumours (e.g. venous malformations). The most common in the hand are vascular malformations and glomus tumours.

Vascular malformations

Vascular malformations in the hand are usually venous. They may be isolated or, rarely, occur in syndromes such as Maffucci's syndrome. They may be asymptomatic if small, but with increasing size can cause symptoms of hypertrophy, interference with function due to size or swelling, and aching pain and discomfort. Phleboliths may form within the venous channels, creating palpable hard masses. The vascular malformation can involve all structures, making it difficult to excise fully. Recurrence rate is high following surgery.

Incidence
- May be apparent only as a minor lesion at birth or in childhood, and develop with age.
- Minor lesions are very common; major malformations are rare.

Aetiology
Unknown.

Clinical features
- May be asymptomatic, or painful.
- May cause symptoms due to secondary compression or erosion, including bleeding, pathological fracture, neuropathy, or due to increased blood flow such as hypertrophy.
- Soft compressible blue-black irregular mass.

Investigations
- X-ray: may show phleboliths, erosion of bone by expanding vascular channels.
- MRI or US: demonstrates extent and nature of lesion. Vascular, so will be high signal on T1 and T2 images.

Treatment
- Supportive therapy such as compressive garments, elevation, and reduced activity can help symptoms.
- Surgical excision is indicated in symptomatic lesions, especially those causing pain, reduced function, hypertrophy, bleeding, or disability.

Prognosis
- Moderate (long-term recurrence rate 20–100%).
- If completely excised, recurrence is rare. However, complete excision is frequently impossible due to the infiltrating and invisible nature of the extent of the vascular malformation. In these circumstances the recurrence rate is almost 100%.
- Malignant transformation is rare (Maffucci's syndrome has a high risk of developing soft tissue sarcomas and other malignancies).

Glomus tumours

Tumours of the glomus bodies, which are arteriovenous shunts which regulate blood flow through the peripheries and skin. When the body or hand is cold the glomus system dilates shunting blood; when the body is warm it constricts, causing blood to flow through the capillary network.

Incidence
- Most common at dorsal fingertip, periungual.
- Any age and sex.
- Commonly a delayed diagnosis.

Aetiology
Unknown.

Clinical features
- Exquisitely tender area.
- With or without a palpable mass.
- Symptoms exaggerated by cold.
- Cherry-red mass may be visible on trans-illumination of the pulp.
- Love's sign: pinpoint tenderness.
- Hildreth's sign: tenderness diminishes on exsanguination.

Investigations
- X-ray: may show an indentation of the dorsum of the distal phalanx.
- MRI or US: demonstrates lesion.

Treatment
Surgical excision. Avoid exsanguinating the limb otherwise the glomus tumour can be difficult to find, or allow a brief deflation of the tourniquet to expose the tumour. The tumours are frequently found along the vessels supplying the nailbed and hence an intimate knowledge of their anatomy is essential pre-operatively. Nailbed tumours are best excised by fish-mouth hyponychial incisions and elevating the nailbed, approaching the tumour from the deep more visible surface. This also diminishes the risk of nail injury.

Prognosis
Good (recurrence rate <10%) if completely excised. However, frequently the tumour is hard to find and is not excised.

Granuloma

Foreign body granulomas or reactions are pseudo-tumours of inflammatory masses which form in response to the implantation and retention of a foreign body. The size and intensity of the granuloma depends on the nature of the foreign body and the immune response of the patient. Generally, organic materials are more provocative.

Incidence
- Very common.
- Male > female.
- All ages.

Clinical features
- History of penetrating injury.
- Growing response which stabilizes.
- Spontaneous ejection of material.

Investigations
- X-ray: may show radio-opaque bodies.
- US: the best method for detecting foreign bodies.

Treatment
Surgical excision of the mass and removal of the foreign body. Some say removal of the foreign body is sufficient, as without it the granuloma resolves.

Prognosis
Excellent.

Bone tumours

- Bone tumours in the hand are relatively rare.
- The majority are benign. The difficulty lies in accurate confident diagnosis, enabling reassurance if the tumour is benign, but timely excision of the suspicious ones.

Classification

According to component:
- Cartilage.
- Bone and cartilage.
- Bone.
- Tumour-like lesions:
  - Inclusion cysts.
  - Intraosseous ganglion.
  - Bone island (very common, eccentrically placed sclerotic lesions).
  - Brown tumour (hyperparathyroidism, look for radiological evidence of subperiosteal erosions pathognomic of hyperparathyroidism; also known as von Recklinghausen's disease of bone).
  - Fibrous dysplasia.
  - Carpal boss (bony spur at second or third carpo-metacarpal joint, often with overlying ganglion; common in young women twenties and thirties; treatment is excision ± fusion of joint; beware excision causing avulsion of ECRL/B).

Principles of management

- Identify lesion: this is usually a clinical diagnosis based on behaviour, swelling pain, pathological fracture, site, with the help of radiology, rarely CT scan, bone scan, and biopsy.
- Treatment if required:
  - External lesion—excise.
  - Internal lesion—curette, excise, ± bone graft or other reconstruction, rarely amputation.

Enchondroma

Benign tumour of cartilage within bone. Most common primary tumour of bone in the hand (90%).

Incidence
- Common in the hand especially the proximal phalanx of the little finger.
- Usually incidental and solitary, but occasionally syndromic and multiple (Ollier's and Mafucci's syndromes—in these syndromes there is an up to 60% risk of malignant change).
- Age 10–60 years.

Aetiology
- Unknown.

Clinical features
- Often presents as a pathological fracture.
- Occasionally presents as swelling or deformity.
- Not usually painful.
- May be found incidentally.

Investigations
- X-ray: stippled calcification within a well-defined expansile eccentric defect within the bone with a thinned cortex: there may be a cortical hole, but no soft tissue involvement.

Treatment
- Reassure, unless symptomatic or causing deformity.

Surgery
- Curette through cortical bone window; bone grafts are not necessary.
- Pathological fractures through enchondromas should be reduced, stabilized (splint or K-wires) and left to heal.

Prognosis
- Good: recurrence rate <5% after curette.
- Small risk of malignant transformation; higher in polyostotic varieties, such as Ollier's multiple enchondromatosis.

Eccondroma
Uncommon chondroid tumour (benign) external to the bone cortex; commonly at the base of the phalanges in young adults.

Treatment
- Excise.

Osteochondroma
Common benign bone tumour with a hyaline cartilage cap, growing near the physis or tendon insertions. The thickness of the cap (if thick) is prognostic/diagnostic of malignant change.

Incidence
- Common.
- Usually isolated.
- Multiple in patients with multiple hereditary exostoses.
- Most common at distal end of proximal phalanx.
- Age 10–30 years.

Aetiology
- Unknown.

Clinical features
- Hard mass.
- May cause stiffness, deformity, growth deviation.
- Can be confused with exostoses which may have a fibrocartilaginous cap.

Investigations
- X-ray: characteristic appearance of exophytic bone lesion near the end of a bone; stuck onto cortex, perhaps with adjacent bone deformity.

Treatment
- Excise if causing symptoms, deformity, or required for diagnosis.
- Correct deformity as required.

Prognosis
- Recurrence is rare. Excision will not correct any established deformity.

Exostosis
- Benign bone tumour that grows from the superficial bone surface, often subungually, possibly in response to trauma. Can grow rapidly and be destructive to the overlying nail and nailbed.
- May be covered by a fibrocartilaginous cap, confusing it with an osteochondroma.

Incidence
- Common, especially on distal phalanx.

Clinical features
- Mass; aymptomatic or tender due to external pressure on mass.
- If subungual causes nail deformity.

Investigations
- X-ray: bony mass with thin cartilaginous cap.

Treatment
- Excision.

Prognosis
- Recurrence rate is low.

Osteoid osteoma
Benign painful bone lesion that provokes an inflammatory response. Often difficult to diagnose, and confused with inflammatory and infective conditions.

Incidence
- Relatively common in the hand and wrist (5–15% of osteoid osteomas).
- Age 20–50 years.
- Most common in proximal phalanx (head and neck) and carpus.

Aetiology
Unknown.

Clinical features
- Pain (often worse at night), tenderness over lesion.
- Inflammation.
- Relieved by aspirin or NSAIDs.
- May have associated swelling, stiffness, and disability.

Investigations
- X-ray: especially on CT—lucent nidus surrounded by a sclerotic ring and surrounding bone inflammation/reaction.
- Bone scan will show hot spot.

Treatment
- Some suggest that osteoid osteomas may be self-limiting, but because of difficulty of diagnosis many hand cases have already had symptoms for more than a year.
- Radiologically guided radiofrequency ablation and CT guided core biopsy excision have been attempted and are successful, but depend on site, size, and expertise.
- Surgery: *en bloc* excision or curettage must excise the nidus or the tumour will recur. The tumour can be difficult to localize and excise.

Prognosis
- Recurrence rates are low if the tumour is completely excised, but re-operation is frequent because of failure to excise or incomplete excision.

Aneurysmal bone cyst

Locally destructive, very expansile bone cyst with fluid levels.

Incidence
- Reasonably common once enchondromas are accounted for.
- Tends to occur in metacarpals.
- Young adults.

Aetiology
- Unknown.

Clinical features
- Incidental finding or pathological fracture.
- Swelling.

Investigations
- X-ray: expansile cystic lesion similar to giant cell tumour, well demarcated by sclerotic margin.

Treatment
- Curette ± graft/cement.

Prognosis
- Recurrence rate 14%.

Unicameral bone cyst

Benign asymptomatic bone cysts; more common in the femur and humerus.

Incidence
- Rare.

Aetiology
- Unknown.

Clinical features
- Present incidentally or on pathological fracture.
- Differential is enchondroma.

Investigations
- X-ray: well-defined septated cyst in metaphysis with fluid level.

Treatment
- Aspiration and injection steroid.
- Curette.

Prognosis
- Good.

Giant cell tumour of bone

Benign but locally aggressive tumours of bone that invade, destroy, and may even metastasize.

Incidence
- Very uncommon in the hand, relatively common in distal radius.
- Middle-aged.

Clinical features
- Swelling.
- Pain.
- Incidental finding or pathological fracture.

Investigations
- X-ray: expansile lytic eccentric epiphyseal or metaphyseal lesion with indistinct borders; no sclerotic margins. May extend into the soft tissues.
- MRI scanning: helpful in diagnosis and surgical planning.
- Biopsy for diagnosis.
- CXR or CT scan staging for metastases.

Treatment
- Curette ± graft/cement.
- Excision and reconstruction.

Prognosis
Radial giant cell tumour has greater than average risk of recurrence (50%) with curette methods, so wide excision and reconstruction is advised.

Metastatic tumours

Bone and soft tissue metastases to the hand are rare. When they do occur, they tend to indicate widespread disseminated metastases.

Incidence
- Rare.
- Lung cancer most common, followed by renal, breast, colonic, melanoma.

Clinical features
- Increasing mass.
- Usually expansile lytic lesion in phalanges, except prostrate (sclerotic) may produce symptoms of pain, swelling, inflammation.

Investigations
- X-ray and MRI scanning will help diagnosis and assessment of extent of lesion.
- Biopsy is needed to confirm histology.
- Search for primary if unknown.
- Staging studies.

Treatment
- Excision if indicated for symptom control, or if solitary lesion.
- Radiotherapy.

Upper limb amputations

Definition and aims
Procedure that aims to remove an affected part or tidy a damaged part and produce an aesthetic stump which must be pain free, sensate, and not interfere with the function of the remaining parts.

Incidence and aetiology
- Very common procedure, particularly for hand injuries.
- Other upper limb trauma.
- Peripheral vascular disease, especially renal transplants with associated arteriovenous shunting (steal syndrome).
- Infection.
- Malignancy.

Classification
Traumatic hand amputation
Beasley classification:
- Transverse (the more proximal the greater the loss of function).
- Radial (loss of thumb is unique).
- Ulnar (leads to loss of power grip.
- Central (ugly and can lead to palmar incontinence; loss of middle finger also causes loss of three-point fixation).

Other amputations
Classified according to level:
- Above elbow.
- Below elbow.
- Through *specified* joint.
- Through *specified* bone.

Surgical principles
- Preserve length.
- Prevent neuroma (trim nerves back so that they lie in well-padded uninjured tissue and not in areas of function).
- Management of bone:
  - Smooth edges.
  - Taper the stump.
  - Can leave the articular cartilage if through joint.
- Management of soft tissue:
  - Good tension free closure.
  - Design flaps so that scars lie in non-contact areas and maximum sensation is preserved in contact or functional areas.
  - Avoid contractures by incision and scar design.
  - Achieve primary closure/healing.
- Prevent complications:
  - Complete excision of nail germinal matrix where indicated will prevent nail spikes.
  - Early mobilization will prevent stiffness.
  - Desensitization will prevent hyperpathia.
  - Do not suture tendon ends over the stump (to avoid quadriga effect).

Quadriga is the tethering of a flexor digitorum profundus, preventing the other FDP tendons from their full excursion. For example, if you hold one of your fingers extended at the DIPJ (other than your index finger which has an independent FDP), you cannot fully flex the DIPJs of your other digits!

Complications

- Early:
  - Wound dehiscence.
  - Bone exposure.
  - Infection (usually secondary to inadequate debridement or closure under tension).
- Late:
  - Neuroma.
  - Bone spurs.
  - Nail spikes.
  - Pain.
  - Fragile tight skin.
  - Overly loose unstable tip.
  - Ugly bulky tip.
  - Cold intolerance.
  - Quadriga.
  - Hypersensitivity.
  - Loss of function.
  - Gapping if central digit.

Post-operative care

- Light dressing reduced early.
- Early mobilization.
- Desensitization programme.
- Stump moulding.

Ray amputation

Definition
Technique to amputate the whole ray of a digit (includes metacarpal/tarsal) rather than the digit alone.

Aims/indications
- Required for clearance of disease.
- Aesthetic improvement.
- To reduce palmar gap (incontinence).

Contraindications
Ray amputation will reduce the width of the palm and reduce grip torque whilst straight-line grip strength remains the same.

Method of ray amputation

Index finger
- Remove the index finger metacarpal but re-attach the interossei and other intrinsics to the middle finger metacarpal to maintain pinch power/abduction (Chase).

Middle or ring finger
- Amputate the digit through the base of the metacarpal and then transpose the index or little finger across to the remaining middle (ring) finger metacarpals and excise the base of index/ or little finger metacarpal. This will reduce scissoring and improve a radial splay.
- Alternatively, excise the middle (ring) finger ray but include a bow-shaped wedge resection of the capitate (hamate) to obtain closure of the ray rather than leave a basal metacarpal gap which, with closure distally, leads to scissoring (Le Viet).

Little finger
- As with index finger, remove the ray and re-attach the abductor digiti minimi to the ring finger.

Upper limb proximal amputations

Through carpus
Worth preserving any possible wrist motion.

Wrist disarticulation
Worth preserving distal DRUJ to allow pro-supination.

Forearm
- Preserve maximum length, as any pronation and supination is useful proximally.
- A minimum of 8 cm is required for stump fitting. If there is any less than 8 cm the biceps insertion becomes obstructive and may need to be proximalized.

Through elbow
This is better than above elbow as it allows transmission of humeral rotation to prostheses, but prosthesis fitting is difficult because of the bulge at the stump end.

Above elbow
- Preserve all possible length.
- Functional prostheses are heavy and require greater lever arm and thus stump length.
- Length is measured from the axilla, so apparent length can be gained by deepening the axilla.

Prostheses

Aim
To assist function and aesthetics or both.

Classification
- Static: silicone mimic.
- Dynamic (e.g. hook, claw, or pinch):
  - Mechanical.
  - Myoelectric.

Even a static prosthesis can confer functional benefit as a support or restraining hand, or by closing a gap.

Fitting
Depends on a tapered well-padded sensate stump. Most fitting depends on a silicone liner and suction cup with a terminal bracket onto which the prosthesis locks. This can be reinforced by straps if the stump is short or the suction fit is inadequate.

Osseo-integrated prosthesis (Branemark prosthesis)
A recent innovation is the osseo-integrated bracket onto which the prosthesis can be locked or mounted. This requires good bone stock with thin stable adherent skin overlying the bone. The first procedure fits the osseo-integrated socket into the bone. Once integrated, an opening is made in the overlying epithelium and the post is mounted into the socket. A prosthesis is then mounted onto the post. Meticulous care must be taken over the hygiene of the post-epithelium interface. This technique has proved most useful for facial prostheses as they are light and have relatively little load and shear passing through them. However, the technique is being trialled in digital and larger limb prosthesis.

Arthrodesis: digital

Definition
Surgical fusion of a digital joint.

Aim
The prime requisite is painless stable union in the shortest possible time, which allows good function.

Indications
- Unsalvageable joint.
  - Degenerative arthritis.
  - Inflammatory arthritis.
  - Traumatic joint loss.
- Pain causing loss of function.
- Stiffness causing loss of function due to malposition.
- Failure of conservative treatment—splinting, change of use, exercises, steroids, NSAIDS.
- Alternative strategies (osteotomy, arthroplasty–excision or replacement, denervation) have failed or are inappropriate.

Classification
According to joint to be fused.

Options

Fixation
- K-wire.
- Tension band wire.
- Screw.
- Plate and screws.
- Intra-medullary pin (Harrison peg).

K-wire
No compression and only relative stability, but is sufficient for easy fusers such as rheumatoids.

Tension band
Converts tension into compression force. It requires an eccentric load and a stable structure on the opposite side against which forces can compress. Tension band wire needs to be pre-stressed and strong enough to resist the tension force.

Tension band K-wires
Can be intramedullary or into the palmar cortex. The latter have less loosening of the wires. Can use screw intramedullary instead of wires. These wires or screws act to neutralize slipping/translational forces.

Lag screw
Gives stability by compression. Compressive forces create friction which resists shear, giving stable fixation. Screws can only fuse DIPJs in an extended neutral position. Easiest to use cannulated lag screws such as the Herbert screw.

Plates and screws
These are bulky and require good-fitting bone surfaces and precise plate application skills with pre-bending and compression to achieve good stability.

Intramedullary pins
These are only relatively stable but are adequate for good fusers.

Our personal preference is to use a 2.4 mm cannulated screw for DIPJ, tension band wires or a screw for PIPJ, tension band wires or a plate for MCPJ, and a plate for CMCJ.

Bone preparation
- None (only suitable for rheumatoids).
- Nibble articular surface.
- Saw cut.
- Cup and cone.

Parallel or concentric surfaces
- Concentric surface gives greater surface area and better variability in setting the angle in all three dimensions, but is harder to cut unless use special cup-and-cone instruments are used. These need to be used with care as they can remove a great deal of bone!
- Parallel surface is easier to perform and fix but there is less variability in altering the position once cut. Start with a 90° cut in the distal bit and then cut the proximal surface at the angle required (Tip: use an intramedullary pin to help alignment of cuts).

Position
The aim is to achieve thumb tip pulp to finger tip pulp opposition. The exact angle depends on the degree of bone shortening. If there is more bone shortening, less flexion is required to reach the thumb tip. If there is no bone shortening and fusion occurs in an extended position, you may cause quadriga.

Table 12.6 Fusion angles for finger joints

	Index	Middle	Ring	Little
DIPJ	5°	10°	15°	20°
PIPJ	25°	30°	35°	40°
MCPJ	45°	50°	55°	60°

Results
Good fusion rates with all techniques.

Examination of the wrist

Diagnosis is helped immeasurably by detailed knowledge of the anatomy and biomechanics of the wrist and of course some inkling of the pathology. Obviously examination of the wrist is preceded by a thorough history.

Look
- Search for bruising, swelling, erythema, deformity, abnormalities of posture, scars, or wounds.
- Observe the range of motion possible by asking the patient to show the range of flexion, extension, radial and ulnar deviation, and rotation, comparing both sides.
- Note any limitations, difficulties, or symptoms provoked by the demonstration

Feel
- Start away from the symptomatic or painful areas.
- Slightly flex and ulnar deviate the wrist.
- Palpate the radial styloid, dorsal distal edge of the radius, Lister's tubercle, and the dorsum of the DRUJ.
- Return and palpate the snuff box, feeling the APL, EPB, and EPL tendons individually before feeling the scaphoid. Compare this with the opposite side as it is normally tender.
- Continue heading ulnarwards on the dorsum feeling the proximal pole of the scaphoid, the scapho-lunate joint just distal to Lister's tubercle, and then the lunate itself. Note any tenderness.
- Move the wrist into radial deviation causing the triquetrum to flex and become palpable from the dorsum. Palpate this and the lunotriquetral joint.
- Palpate the pisiform and rub it onto the triquetrum, noting pain or crepitus.
- Feel the head of the ulnar and the DRUJ.
- Palpate along the course of the flexor and extensor carpi ulnaris.
- Move distally and feel the dorsum of the hamate and capitate including their joints. To feel the trapezoid and trapezium requires the wrist to move into ulnar deviation and flexion.
- Turn the wrist over, and palpate the scaphoid tubercle and the trapezial ridge on the radial aspect, and on the ulnar aspect the pisiform and the hook of the hamate lying a centimeter distal and radial.
- Compress the lunate between your fingers dorsally and palmarly.

Move
- Move the wrist passively into flexion and extension, feeling the smoothness of the motion and the range of motion.
- Move the wrist from radial to ulnar deviation and back again, noting the same properties.
- Check the range of motion of pronation and supination, noting any change in position of the ulnar head.

Provocative tests

Watson scaphoid shift test (examines scapholunate dissociation)
Place the olecranon on the table and flex the elbow. Ulnar deviate the wrist. Pinch the scaphoid between your thumb and index finger. Place your thumb pulp perpendicular to the distal dorsal edge of the radius covering Lister's tubercle, such that the tip of the thumb touches the proximal pole of the scaphoid. The index lies distally and palmar, pushing on the scaphoid tubercle. The object is to try to resist scaphoid flexion as the wrist moves into radial deviation. Normally it is impossible to prevent the scaphoid from flexing. However, in scapholunate dissociation, your index prevents the scaphoid from flexing. To accommodate the reducing space, the scaphoid tries to shift dorsally, increasing the prominence of the proximal pole, until such time as the bony contact of the rest of the flexing carpus forces the scaphoid to flex with a painful clunk.

Lunotriquetral ballotement (assesses lunotriquetral instability)
The lunate is pinched in one hand and the triquetrum (and pisiform) are held in the other, and they are moved in opposite directions. Positive if excess movement, pain, and crepitus. Lunotriquetral instability can also be tested by the Shuck test, whereby whist holding the lunate one moves the wrist through its range of motion eliciting pain at the joint.

Manual stress test or midcarpal shift test
Grasp the hand with one hand and the distal forearm with the other and passively assess the range of motion and instability of the carpus. Apply an axial load to the hand onto the forearm in a slight palmar direction. A clunk occurs as the lunate flips from a flexed to an extended position.

Midcarpal clunk
Passively move the wrist from ulnar to radial deviation and back again, with and without compressive load. Midcarpal instability will be evident as a stepped jerky movement rather than a smooth arc of progression, accompanied by a mid-motion clunk which may or may not be painful.

Ulna carpal stress test or TFCC load test (examines the DRUJ)
Ulnar deviate the wrist and rotate the forearm, with and without axial load. Postive if painful, clicky, or reduced range. Positive test indicates ulnocarpal area pathology (TFCC tear or perforation, ulna abutment, DRUJ pathology).

Piano key test (examines stability of ulnar head, ulnocarpal ligaments)
With forearm pronated, push down on ulnar head. It should depress and then return to position, as does a piano key. Positive test if fails or is painful, indicating instability or ulnocarpal pathology.

DRUJ instability test
Pinch the ulnar head in one hand and the radius in the other and move in opposite directions, assessing the stability of the radioulnar ligaments. By doing the test in pronation, supination, and mid-position it may be possible to differentiate whether the palmar or dorsal ligament is affected. Grind the ulnar head against the radius sigmoid notch to elicit pain or crepitus.

Common differential diagnoses

Radial sided wrist pain
- Trapezio-metacarpal (thumb basal) joint arthritis.
- Scapho-trapezial-trapezoid (STT) arthritis.
- Scaphoid pathology (Preiser's avascular scaphoid, non-union, fracture).
- De Quervain's stenosing tenovaginitis.
- Flexor carpi radialis tendonitis.
- Radio-carpal joint arthritis.
- Wartenberg's syndrome (radial neuritis).
- Intersection syndrome.

Ulnar sided wrist pain
- Extensor carpi ulnaris tendonitis.
- Pisi-triquetral arthritis.
- TFCC pathology (tear, detachment, perforation, loose body).
- DRUJ pathology.
- Ulnar abutment (impaction) syndrome.
- Fracture of the hook of the hamate.
- Ulnar neuritis.
- Dorsal ulnar nerve branch neuritis.

Central transverse wrist pain
- Kienbock's avascular necrosis of lunate (lunatomalacia).
- Scapholunate pathology.
- Ganglion.
- Mid-carpal instability.
- Arthritis.

Chapter 13

Lower limb

Lower limb trauma 430
Lower limb ulceration 433
Pretibial laceration 435
Diabetic feet 437
Lower limb reconstruction 442
Below-knee amputation 445
Above-knee amputation 448

Lower limb trauma

Plastic surgeons are frequently involved in the management of lower limb trauma assisting the orthopaedic surgeons. Do not forget EMST/ATLS/MULTI-TRAUMA resuscitation.

Assessment
It is important to consider mechanics of injury (energy imparted):
- Bone injury (fracture site, size, shape, comminution, contamination, loss).
- Soft tissue injury (periosteum, muscle, nerves and vessels).
- X-ray:
  - Fracture pattern.
  - Fracture separation.
  - Displacement.
  - Gas.
  - Soft tissue swelling.

The assessment indicates the zone of trauma, degree of injury, and devascularization of the bone and soft tissues, which are predictive of prognosis, healing, re-operation, delayed amputation, and outcome, and therefore guides treatment.

Classification
Should be determined after first debridement when full extent of defect known:
- Gustilo: does not consider bony injury.
- AO/ASIF—multi-component complex classification but covers:
  - Bone.
  - Soft tissue skin.
  - Muscle/tendon.
  - Neurovascular.

Open tibial fractures (Gustilo and Anderson 1976)
I   Wound <1 cm.
II Wound >1 cm without extensive soft tissue damage, flaps, and avulsions.
III Open segmental fracture or with extensive soft tissue damage or traumatic amputation:
  IIIA Adequate soft tissue cover.
  IIIB Soft tissue injury with periosteal stripping and bony exposure.
  IIIC Associated arterial injury.

Open tibial fractures (Byrd et. al 1985)
I   Low energy: spiral/oblique fracture with a clean <2 cm wound.
II Moderate energy: comminuted or displaced fracture with >2 cm skin laceration, with moderate muscle contusion but no non-viable muscle.
III High energy: severely displaced and comminuted fracture/segmental fracture or bony defect with extensive skin loss and devitalized muscle.
IV Extreme energy: type III with degloving or crush injuries, or vascular damage.

Management

Combined orthopaedic and plastic surgery on admission. In the UK, there are combined BOA and BAPS guidelines for the management of open fractures. The aim of management is to achieve rapid wound closure without infection and with good vascularization to ensure rapid uncomplicated union.

Principles of management
- Debridement as early as possible.
- Assessment and treatment plan formulation.
- Fracture fixation as early as possible.
- Coverage by well-vascularized soft tissues, obliterating dead spaces as early as possible.

Debridement
- Radical but preserving nerves and vessels.
- Under tourniquet.

Bone fixation
It is a good idea to be present at the initial assessment with the orthopaedic surgeon as the method of fixation and exposure incisions can be discussed. This is particularly pertinent for frame fixation, when ring, bar, and pin placement can compromise exposure for soft tissue repair.

Recipient vessel of choice
- Remote from zone of injury.
- Proximal or distal have equal outcomes, but distal is usually more accessible.
- PTA better then ATA as ATA more often injured.

Access to vessels
- Posterior midline muscle split and pass pedicle around medially (Godina et al. 1991).
- Our preferred approach is medial mid-lateral and detach soleus from tibial origin to expose PTA proximally or to go distal to PTA at ankle.

Timing of soft tissue cover
- Emergency: first 24 hours (Lister and Scheker 1988).
- Early: <3 days, less infection and less failure (Godina 1986).
- Delayed: <3 months.
- Late: >3 months (Arnez 1991).

Despite early evidence that flap success was better if performed in <3 weeks or >3 months post-injury, current techniques show no difference in flap success rates with timing of flap coverage. However, overall complications such as infection and non-union rates do increase proportionately with delay.

Current practice is for debridement and fixation on day 1 with flap coverage on day 1–5, depending on availability of plastic surgeon, theatre, and health of patient.

Soft tissue cover selection
Options are local fascio-cutaneous flaps, local muscle flaps, or free flaps.

Fascio-cutaneous flaps (local)
- Have a higher rate of complications including flap loss (partial but usually the bit you need), infection, and non-union, but may be indicated for older patients with no devascularization of the bone and little soft tissue injury.
- They are quicker to perform (but not much quicker).
- May be compromised by external fixators.
- Are restricted by the pedicle in placement, reach, and size.
- Leave ugly donor sites.

Local muscle flaps
Preferable to fascio-cutaneous flaps as provides muscle, but still;
- Restricted size, reach and volume.
- May be in zone of trauma and injured.
- Probably most applicable for low energy upper third tibial fractures when use gastrocnemius.

Free flaps
- 98–99% success rate.
- Rare partial loss so no temptation to leave it and see.
- Remote donor site.
- Adaptable for all situations.
- No restriction on placement, movement, or size.

Free flap selection
- Size, volume, contour requirements of defect.
- Level of contamination and devascularization, if increased use muscle.
- Cosmesis: reconstruction and donor sites.
- Functional deficit: reconstruction site and donor site.
- Pedicle length required.
- Donors available.
- Position of patient on table, and other simultaneous procedures planned.

Our personal preference is for muscle free flaps given the advantages:
- Better vascularity (greatest capillary density for volume tissue).
- Better ability to combat infection (Chang and Mathes 1982).
- Better compliance (greatest flexibility of tissue and pedicle).
- Better versatility in size, shape, volume (less exact planning required; with fascio-cutaneous flaps any discrepancy in size leads to tenting and creation of dead space).
- Better space-filling qualities (swells to fill available space).
- Least donor site morbidity.
- Greatest variety in donor site, size, and volume.
- Potential for functional reconstruction.

References
Arnez ZM (1991). *Clin Plast Surg* **18**, 449–57.
Byrd HS, Spicer TE, Cierney G 3rd (1985). *Plast Reconstr Surg* **76**, 719–30.
Chang N, Mathes SJ (1982). *Plast Reconstr Surg* **70**, 1–10.
Godina M (1986). *Plast Reconstr Surg* **78**, 285–92.
Godina M, Arnez ZM, Lister GD (1991). *Plast Reconstr Surg* **88**, 287–91.
Gustilo RB, Anderson JT (1976). *J Bone Joint Surg Am* **58**, 453–8.
Lister G, Scheker L (1998). *J Hand Surg (Am)* **13**, 22–8.

Lower limb ulceration

Aetiology
Venous ulcers make up 80–85% of all leg ulcers in developed countries. Other causes include arterial disease, diabetes, peripheral neuropathy, vasculitis (e.g. SLE, rheumatoid arthritis), haematological (e.g. polycythaemia, sickle cell anaemia), trauma, neoplastic, and others (e.g. sarcoidosis, pyoderma gangrenosum).

Pathogenesis and clinical features
Venous ulcers
Sustained venous hypertension, or chronic venous insufficiency caused by factors such as venous disease (e.g. varicose veins, previous DVT), impaired calf muscle pump function (e.g. immobility, joint disease, paralysis, obesity), and congestive heart failure, initiates microcirculatory changes of capillary proliferation, pericapillary fibrin deposition, leucocyte activation and trapping, and increased production of free radicals and inflammation from repetitive ischaemic reperfusion injury.

Venous ulcers usually lie just proximal to the medial or lateral malleolus in the gaiter area around the ankle, although extension to ankle and dorsum of foot can occur. They invariably occur within an area of lipodermato sclerosis and haemosiderosis.

Arterial ulcers
These are secondary to large and medium vessel disease, and may be present with other stigmata of chronic ischaemia, e.g. history of claudication or rest pain, loss of hair, atrophic skin, pale cold foot, absent or reduced peripheral pulses, gangrene.

Arterial ulcers occur distally over and between the toes or in pressure areas e.g. heels, malleoli. There are no distinguishing signs, although the ulcer base may appear pale.

Neuropathic ulcers
The majority of neuropathic ulcers are secondary to diabetes. This is covered in detail in the section on diabetic feet.

Investigations
Examination should include palpation of peripheral pulses, Trendelenburg and Bürger's tests, and measurement of ABPI to exclude arterial disease, signs of neuropathy in diabetes, and Doppler assessment of competence of the superficial and communicating veins. Duplex ultrasonography is valuable in determining location of incompetent veins, extent of post-thrombotic vein damage, and extent of arterial disease. More details can be obtained with angiography. If the vascular system proves to be normal, blood tests for systemic inflammatory disorders could be done. A biopsy is recommended for an ulcer that fails to heal to exclude malignancy.

Management

Venous ulcers
Ulceration due to pure superficial venous incompetence responds well to varicose vein surgery. Surgery need not be delayed until the ulcer has healed. Managed this way, these ulcers heal within 4 weeks of surgery.

For deep venous insufficiency or patients unfit/unwilling to undergo surgery, conservative treatment with occlusive dressings covered by compression bandages worn from the foot to the knee. Once weekly dressing change with ulcer debridement; more frequent if excessive exudate. 80–90% of ulcers heal by 12 months. Topical applications (e.g. antibiotics, antiseptics, or creams) do not affect healing time, but can cause sensitization. Patients with healed ulcers should be encouraged to wear support stockings. Recurrence rates are 25% for conservatively managed ulcers and 3% for surgically treated ulcers.

Arterial ulcers
Adequate analgesia, regular dressings to minimize exudate and hence infection, lifestyle modifications (e.g. stop smoking), search for other risk factors (e.g. diabetes), and debridement of necrotic tissue are advocated. Arterial revascularization should be considered before the end-stages of arterial disease. Amputation is performed as a final option.

Infected ulcers
Ulcers, especially venous ulcers, are frequently colonized with bacteria. *Staphylococcus aureus* is most often isolated, but coliforms, *Pseudomonas aeruginosa*, and anaerobes are also found. Streptococci of Lancefield's groups A, C, or G causes cellulitis. Group A (*Streptococcus pyogenes*) causes the most severe or life-threatening form. The use of antibiotics is indicated in frank cellulitis, but otherwise should be discouraged as they result in colonization of the ulcer with more resistant organisms.

Future
- Increasing use of growth factors as these develop (see section on factors affecting wound healing in Chapter 1).

Pretibial laceration

Definition
Injury to the pretibial region, which encompasses a wide spectrum of soft tissue damage, from superficial skin lacerations to degloving injuries.

Incidence
Very common; occurs most commonly in women over 60 years. Associated comorbid factors include peripheral vascular disease, diabetes, and peripheral oedema.

Aetiology
Skin overlying the tibia is under a higher natural tension than elsewhere in the body. The pretibial area has little subcutaneous protection and is poorly vascularized. Healing is compromised further by corticosteroid therapy.

Classification
Despite its prevalence, there are few classifications of pretibial injuries in literature. Dunkin and colleagues presented the classification shown in Table 13.1 and an algorithm for management (box opposite) based on clinical practice and best evidence.

Management
No single regimen is appropriate for all pretibial lacerations. Management should follow the basic surgical principles of asepsis, debridement, haemostasis, and wound closure. Careful handling and tension-free closure are vital to avoid compromising viable tissue. Although haematoma formation can be largely overcome by meshing the graft, patients on anticoagulant therapy should be optimized prior to grafting. Salvage of viable-looking skin from flap by defatting and laying it over the defect significantly reduces healing time compared with primary excision and grafting.

Post-operative care
Immediate mobilization is generally recommended. It does not appear to compromise graft healing, may reduce the risk of complications (e.g. DVT, pressure ulcers, pneumonia), and avoids prolonged hospital stay. Social support services should be involved early.

Table 13.1 Classification of pretibial lacerations

Type	Description
I	Laceration
II	Laceration or flap with minimal haematoma and/or skin edge necrosis
III	Laceration of flap with moderate to severe haematoma and/or necrosis
IV	Major degloving injury

Management algorithm for pretibial lacerations

Type 1	Clean, tape without tension, supportive dressing, mobilize immediately.
Type 2	Clean, debride under LA, excise non-viable skin, evacuate haematoma, dress, mobilize immediately. Review after 7–14 days and assess healing. If poor consider debridement under LA or GA, excise damaged skin and SSG, mobilize immediately.
Type 3	Debride under LA or GA, excise damaged skin and SSG, mobilize immediately.
Type 4	Debride and SSG or other reconstruction.

Diabetic feet

The diabetic foot is prone to ulceration, gangrene, and Charcot foot collapse. Treatment in the past has consisted largely of lower limb amputations; diabetics account for 50% of all lower limb amputations for non-traumatic indications. A comprehensive approach to caring for diabetic feet in a multidisciplinary setting can lower health care costs with a >90% success rate in limb preservation.

Aetiology

Peripheral neuropathy

Peripheral neuropathy affects sensory, motor, and autonomic nerves. Sensory neuropathy results in the neglect of minor injuries or infections, and predisposes to fractures and joint destruction caused by unperceived trauma and weight-bearing on an injured limb. Autonomic neuropathy causes the opening of AV shunts, allowing blood to bypass the high-resistance vessels of the skin capillary bed. The resultant increased flow through bone contributes to increased osteoclast activity and subsequent osteoporosis, increased susceptibility to fractures following minor trauma, and Charcot foot collapse. Autonomic neuropathy also causes anhydrosis (lack of sweating) and hyperkeratosis. Calluses and small fissures develop over insensate pressure areas, predisposing to infection. Motor neuropathy leads to the gradual denervation of intrinsic muscles of the foot, resulting in a claw foot from loss of metatarsal–phalangeal flexion, loss of transverse and longitudinal arches, and metatarsal head prominence. The progressive loss of nerve fibres is demonstrated in myelinated and unmyelinated fibres and Schwann cells. The pathophysiology is unclear. It is accepted as a multifactorial process and a number of hypotheses have been proposed:

- **Metabolic theory** Saturation of the glycolytic pathway shunts excess glucose into the polyol pathway, converting it to sorbitol and fructose, the accumulation of which depletes nerve myoinositol, decreases membrane Na^+/K^+-ATPase activity, impairs axonal transport, and causes structural breakdown of nerve.
- **Vascular (ischaemic-hypoxic) theory** Increased endoneural vascular resistance to hyperglycaemic blood and advanced glycosylation end-products are implicated, leading to capillary damage, inhibition of axonal transport, and axonal degeneration.
- **Oxidative stress theory** Increased free-radical generation and reduced capacity to neutralize free radicals impairs nerve function by direct toxic effect and by reducing nitric oxide.
- **Protein kinase C activation theory** Hyperactivity of the vascular protein kinase C beta-Isoform causes decreased organ perfusion and altered nerve conduction velocity.

Peripheral vascular disease

This is four times more prevalent than peripheral neuropathy and progresses more rapidly. The reason is unclear although the pathophysiology is similar. Distribution of vascular disease is also unique, affecting vessels distal to the popliteal artery and sparing the pedal arteries. Therefore it is amenable to distal bypasses to the dorsalis pedis or the peroneal or posterior tibial artery.

Depressed immune response
This is the result of diminished antibody coating of bacteria and dysfunction of polymorphonuclear leucocytes, macrophages, and lymphocytes.

Local effects
Hyperglycaemia causes irreversible glycosylation of collagen in the Achilles tendon, leading to loss of elasticity and shortening. The resultant inability to dorsiflex the foot places excessive pressure on the forefoot during walking, predisposing to ulceration and midfoot collapse.

Foot ulceration

Diabetic neuropathy and peripheral vascular disease are the main factors in foot ulceration and may act alone, together, or in combination with other factors such as microvascular disease, altered foot shape, elevated foot pressures, and increased susceptibility to infection.

Incidence
Affects 3–5% of diabetic patients, and is more common among male diabetics. 45–60% of diabetic foot ulcerations are purely neuropathic, 10% are purely ischaemic, and 25–45% are of mixed neuro-ischaemic origin.

Clinical features
- **Neuropathic ulcers** Warm foot, palpable pulses. Ulcers are wet and usually located at the site of unperceived repetitive trauma, e.g. high-pressure areas under metatarsal heads, or occasionally unnoticed foreign bodies lodged inside the shoe.
- **Ischaemic/neuro-ischaemic ulcers** Cool dry hairless foot with absent/reduced pulses. Ulcers are dry, usually painful, and have a rim of erythema. They are usually located at the toes, heels, and medial aspect of the first metatarsal head.

Investigations
- Clinical examination for 'stocking' distribution of sensory loss to one or more modalities (pain, temperature, pressure, and vibration) with absent ankle reflexes. Protective sensation is lost if foot is insensate to 10 g of pressure (applied using a 5.07 Semmes–Weinstein filament).
- Assessment of circulation, with the measurement of ABPI (indicative of ischaemia when <0.9, but often falsely elevated because of vessel wall calcification (lack of compressibility) in diabetic neuropathy). Doppler can be more useful (loss of normal triphasic waveform indicates vascular disease).
- X-ray/MRI to exclude osteomyelitis if ulcer is deep or resistant to therapy.

Management
- **Neuropathic ulcers** X-ray to assess underlying skeleton and to rule out foreign bodies, gas, osteomyelitis, fractures, or bone collapse. For superficial ulcers without cellulitis, treat conservatively with pressure-relieving footwear such as a total-contact cast which dissipates walking pressure over the whole foot. The cast is changed at 48 hr to ensure proper fit, and then weekly for 8–10 weeks until the ulcer is healed. Regular chiropody/debridement of callus and pressure sites can aid early detection of problems.

- **Infected ulcers or gangrene** Prompt treatment with surgical debridement if necessary and decompression of any involved compartment so that all potential pockets of undrained pus are opened. Broad-spectrum antibiotic therapy should be commenced after deep microbiological specimens are obtained. Close monitoring for spreading cellulitis. Reconstruction should not be undertaken until all signs of inflammation have resolved.
- **Ischaemic/neuro-ischaemic ulcers** Ulcers are unlikely to heal without revascularization if the toe pressures are <30 mmHg and $TcPO_2$ is <40 mmHg. If there is no infection, revascularize the leg before treating the ulcer. If there is gangrene or cellulitis, debridement should precede revascularization.
- **Prophylactic advice** (e.g. regular inspection of feet, appropriate footwear, regular chiropody) should be given at an early stage, especially to at-risk patients (see below).

Risk factors for ulceration
Previous ulceration, neuropathy, peripheral vascular disease, altered foot shape, high foot pressures, increasing age, visual impairment, living alone.

Debate/contentious issues
- The use of growth factors, such as becaplermin (a topical formulation of platelet-derived growth factor), or living dermal replacements (neonatal fibroblasts cultured on a bioabsorbable mesh, which are metabolically active when applied as a dressing to the wound, producing a full array of growth factors) to improve ulcer healing time.
- Hyperbaric oxygen therapy has been used to improve wound healing by improving tissue oxygenation, enhancing the killing capacity of neutrophils, and directly inhibiting the growth of anaerobic organisms.

Charcot foot collapse

Charcot neuro-arthropathy is a progressive condition characterized by joint dislocation, pathological fractures, and destruction of pedal architecture, all caused by loss of protective sensibility to the joint.

Incidence
Up to 10% of patients with neuropathy, and over 16% of those with a history of neuropathic ulceration.

Clinical features and pathogenesis
Patients present with a warm swollen foot, which may be painless. Periarticular erosions are noted to precede fractures and fragmentation. Fractures may not develop until several weeks after foot swelling. After some months, during which bone resorption continues, the swelling and warmth begin to resolve. Treatment is aimed at shortening this time in order to minimize bone and joint destruction. The midfoot is a common site of Charcot neuro-arthropathy, which can result in midfoot collapse with a plantar bony prominence and 'rocker' foot. Charcot changes have a direct effect on skin breakdown and ulceration.

Management

Rest and immobilization in a total-contact cast until disease activity has subsided. Treatment with intravenous bisphosphonate or palmidronate, directed at excessive osteoclastic activity, has been effective in some studies. Appropriate footwear is required, taking great care of the other foot because of the high risk of contralateral Charcot changes. Surgery is contraindicated in the early stages, as it may exacerbate bone resorption. At a later stage, surgery can be undertaken to remove bony prominences.

Reconstruction of the diabetic foot

Forefoot

- **Toe ulcers or gangrene** Limited amputation, preserving viable volar tissue to aid wound closure. Attempt to stay away from the MTPJ and to preserve at least the proximal portion of the proximal phalanx. The first toe is critical to ambulation, and so a conservative policy is desirable and a toe island flap from the second toe is indicated.
- **Ulcers over MTPJ without bone involvement** Osteotomy with internal fixation to maintain an anatomical metatarsal parabaloid, which avoids the development of transfer lesions inherent in the floating metatarsal osteotomy technique.
- **Deep forefoot ulcers without bony prominence** Small ulcers can be closed with a local flap, filleted toe flap, toe island flap, bilobed flap, larger rotation flap, or V–Y flap. In larger ulcers where the metatarsal head has been resected, consider a ray amputation.
- **Ulcers with exposed metatarsals** Conservative policy to preserve as much of the metatarsal bones is desirable. Consider a microsurgical free flap: fascio-cutaneous flap for dorsal defects, muscle flap, and skin graft for plantar defects. Also consider a panmetatarsal head resection if ulcers are present under several metatarsal heads, or if transfer lesions have occurred from one resected metatarsal head to a neighbouring metatarsal. Leaving the flexors and extensors to the toe intact will prevent equinovarus deformity.

Midfoot

Skin grafts are recommended for defects of the non-weight-bearing arch. Any underlying bony prominence (e.g. Charcot foot collapse) can be shaved via a medial or lateral approach, and the ulcer can be left to heal by secondary intention or closed with a V–Y flap, bilobed flap, rhomboid flap, or transposition flap if the defect is small, or with a medially based random flap or pedicled flap if it is large. Once healed, a mid/hindfoot fusion for Charcot foot collapse is recommended to reduce the recurrence of ulceration.

Hindfoot

Partial calcanectomy can permit the linear closure of small defects. Any bony spurs should be shaved. Closure with double V–Y flaps, medially based rotation flap, instep island flap, pedicled flaps, extended lateral calcaneal fascio-cutaneous flap, medial plantar fascio-cutaneous flap, abductor digiti minimi muscle flap, abductor hallucis brevis muscle flap, or muscle free flap with skin graft have been used.

Dorsum of foot

Defects are usually covered with skin grafts or local flaps if small. Pedicled flaps include extensor digitorum brevis muscle flap, retrograde dorsalis pedis flap, retrograde peroneal flap, and retrograde sural artery flap. Free flaps should be thin to minimize bulk, with restoration of sensibility and extensor function. Therefore fascio-cutaneous or skin-grafted fascial flaps are more suitable (e.g. temporoparietal fascia, dorsal thoracic fascia). Perforator flaps must be used with caution as their viability depends on the integrity of the underlying tibial or peroneal vessel.

Ankle defects

Tissue around the ankle is sparse and has minimal flexibility. Reconstruction should closely follow debridement to avoid dessication of the poorly perfused subcutaneous fat in this area, thus expanding the zone of non-viable tissue. Skin grafting is adequate if there is sufficient granulation tissue, even over the Achilles tendon. Local flaps include the lateral calcaneal fascio-cutaneous flap, dorsalis pedis fascio-cutaneous flap, retrograde sural artery fascio-cutaneous flap, peroneal retrograde fascio-cutaneous flap, and extensor digitorum brevis muscle flap. Free flaps can be either fascio-cutaneous or muscle with a skin graft.

Peri-operative care

- General:
  - Pre-operative starvation: insulin-dependent diabetics require GKI infusion (15 units of insulin, 10 mmol potassium in 500 mL 10% dextrose infused at 100 mL/hr) or sliding scale.
  - Renal disease: close monitoring of blood pressure and urine output; stop metformin for 48 hr prior to angiography to avoid lactic acidosis.
  - Care of pressure areas: use foam leg troughs and sheepskin to protect heels; prompt attention to skin breaks; regular turning.
  - Special attention should be given to the treatment of oedema, which can impair wound healing, through leg elevation and distal-to-proximal bandaging.
- Specific to reconstruction:
  - Incisions on plantar surface: no weight bearing for 6 weeks; foot can be protected in a cast if compliance is an issue.
  - Incisions on non-weight bearing surface: some dressing for protection for 6 weeks.
  - Skin graft: posterior splint or Unna boot is applied until the graft is fully vascularized.

Lower limb reconstruction

Anatomical considerations
Unique aspects of the lower limb:
- Weight-bearing:
  - Prime function of lower limb is weight-bearing. Ambulation requires a mobile ankle and forefoot/toes allowing push off. However, a fused ankle and foot can still result in a useful limb.
  - Leg muscles primarily provide ankle motion. Therefore if the ankle is fused, considerable muscle loss can be tolerated.
- Hidden contact surface reliant on sensation for protection:
  - The full force of the body is transmitted through the plantar surface of the foot during ambulation. Therefore a sensate sole is vital for normal ambulation. Loss of the posterior tibial nerve is a serious injury and is a relative contraindication to limb salvage in the trauma setting. Conversely, loss of the sciatic nerve or posterior tibial nerve, but with preservation of otherwise normal anatomy, results in a stable functional useful limb—better then a BKA or an AKA.
- Dependent position:
  - Increases oedema, reducing rate of healing and increasing stiffness.
- Increased involvement of atherosclerosis and other vascular disease,
  - Ischaemia and venous fibrosis all compromise healing and complicate reconstruction.
- Greater length:
  - Greater length-to-circumference ratios complicate resconstruction.
- Subcutaneous bone:
  - The anteromedial portion of the tibia is subcutaneous, and therefore vulnerable to exposure in trauma. Once exposed, it is difficult to cover simply.

Function of the lower limb
- Ambulation.
- Weight support on transfer.

Aetiology of lower limb defects
- Infection (e.g. osteomyelitis, necrotizing fascitis).
- Neoplasia (e.g. sarcoma, carcinoma).
- Ulcers (e.g. diabetic, radiation therapy, vascular).
- Unstable scars (e.g. after injury, burns, prosthetic joint replacement, or fracture fixation).
- Trauma (e.g. open fractures).
- Iatrogenic (e.g. post-operative wounds).
- Ischaemia.

Principles of lower limb reconstruction
- Start with a clean wound as after a 'tumour' excision. Easy after tumour excision but the same principles apply in all other circumstances including trauma and infection. Debride by excision, with a clearance margin into virginal tissue, preserving 'vital' structures as required.
- Assessment of zone of injury, and residual anatomy, function, and vascularity.

- Set aim for reconstruction and eventual functional and aesthetic outcome:
  - Aim should include filling of dead space and primary closure of wound.
  - Is it achievable? Will it be better than an amputation?
- Bone fixation/reconstruction for stability.
- Close wound and dead space.

Principles of wound closure and dead-space filling

- Assessment of site, size, anatomy, and complexity of defect.
- Assessment of available reconstructive options:
  - Are they suitable?
  - Are they viable and available?
  - Will they leave a donor site with acceptable function and aesthetics?
- Assessment of rest of leg and patient:
  - Age and requirements of the patient.
  - Vascularity.
  - Status of the foot, ankle, and other joints.
  - Other comorbidity such as IHD, metastases.
- Assessment of other requirements of the reconstruction:
  - Will radiotherapy be needed? If so, need cutaneous flap.
  - Will more orthopaedic operations be done? If so, consider future exposure, stability of reconstruction for manipulation, re-elevation.
  - Is it needed for functional reconstruction or re-vascularization?
  - Is it needed to combat infection? Muscle flaps are better for this.
  - Will it be weight-bearing? This includes amputation stumps and their weight-bearing surfaces—not necessarily their ends.
  - Does it need to be sensate?
  - Does it need to fit shoes, or a prosthesis?
- Choice of reconstruction.
- Review aim for reconstruction and eventual functional and aesthetic outcome:
  - Is it still achievable? Will it be better than an amputation?
- Reconstructive procedure.
- Assessment of achievement of aim of reconstruction:
  - Re-operation, re-reconstruction as required.
  - Change of aim.

Why is dead-space filling so important?

Dead space fills with haematoma, which readily becomes infected in open fractures and/or around prostheses (including plates and screws). Infection compromises or prevents union of bone and soft tissue, and leads down the slippery slope of complications and worsening outcome. Even if infection does not occur, haematoma is replaced by fibrosis, compromising function. Haematoma and fibrosis significantly reduce the effectiveness of post-operative therapies such as radiotherapy and antibiotics. Haematoma can be replaced by heterotopic ossification.

Thigh

- Options:
  - Rotation/advancement flaps of thigh muscles (e.g. gracilis, vastus lateralis, tensor fascia lata).
  - Fascio-cutaneous flaps (e.g. anterolateral thigh, medial thigh).

- Regional flaps (e.g. rectus abdominus).
- Free tissue transfer.
- Personal preferences:
  - THR acetabular defect—rectus femoris.
  - Groin wound—sartorius, rectus femoris myocutaneous, rectus abdominus myocutaneous.

Knee
- Options:
  - Muscle flaps (e.g. medial and lateral gastrocnemius).
  - Fascio-cutaneous flaps (e.g. saphenous, sural).
  - Free tissue transfer.
- Personal preferences
  - TKR infection or exposure use medial gastrocnemius.

Tibia
- Options:
  - Muscle flaps (e.g. medial and lateral gastrocnemius, soleus).
  - Fascio-cutaneous flaps (e.g. saphenous, proximally or distally based fascio-cutaneous flaps).
  - Free tissue transfer.
- Proximal third:
  - Medial or lateral gastrocnemius muscle flap, fascio-cutaneous flaps, free flaps.
- Middle third:
  - Free flaps, soleus muscle flap, fascio-cutaneous flaps.
- Distal third/ankle:
  - Free flaps, extensor brevis muscle flap, lateral supramalleolar flap, dorsalis pedis flap, sural neuro-cutaneous flap, fascio-cutaneous flaps.
- Personal preferences:
  - Tibial fracture wounds—free muscle flap usually gracilis.
  - Leg sarcoma defects—usually free cutaneous or myocutaneous flap.

Foot
- Options:
  - Abductor digiti minimi and abductor hallucis muscle flaps, medial plantar flap, dorsalis pedis flap, lateral calcaneal flap, free tissue transfer.
- Personal preferences:
  - Heel defect—sensate medial plantar flap. If not available, free flap medial plantar from opposite foot.
  - Sole defect—local flap if small. If not, free flap.

Bone
In general, if the skeletal defect is <6 cm distraction lengthening bone transport is suitable. For those defects >6 cm, use vascularized bone transfer using an ipsilateral pedicled fibula or preferably a free contralateral fibula or iliac crest bone flap, therefore maintaining the fibula's weight-bearing capacity and stability, and assisting in maintaining limb length and orientation.

Below-knee amputation

Indications
- Unreconstructable peripheral vascular disease (often due to diabetes) with uncontrollable infection, soft tissue or osteomyelitis, or severe rest pain due to ischaemia.
- Severe trauma: transection or IIIC tibial fracture combined with nerve injury, frostbite injury, severe foot and ankle trauma.
- Tumour: when risk of recurrence or functional result would be unacceptable with limb salvage surgery.
- Infection: due to either subsequent distal ischaemia (e.g. meningococcal) or life-threatening infection (e.g. *Clostridium difficile*).
- Congenital anomalies: amputation to allow ambulation with a prosthesis. The more proximal the amputation, the greater the energy requirement for walking. Therefore below-knee amputation is preferred.

Aims
Healed wound (primarily with no delay):
- Pain-free sensate stump.
- Tapered stump to allow easy prosthetic fitting and wearing.
- Non-adherent muscle and skin covering bone to allow prosthesis to be worn without shearing.

Planning
- Use a tourniquet.
- Give antibiotic treatment for infection, prophylaxis for clean surgery.
- Ideally, use an epidural infusion as good pain relief immediately post-operatively to reduce phantom limb pain.
- Aim to leave 12–17 cm of tibia below the knee joint (or 1 inch per foot of body height), sometimes estimated as a palm breadth (including thumb) below the tibial tubercle.
- Too short a stump reduces the leverage for the prosthesis. Too long a stump may make it difficult to fit the prosthesis and leave enough space to manufacture the ankle and foot. If in doubt, the longer the better. You can always shorten it but you cannot put it back!

Incision
- Usually a long posterior musculocutaneous flap is used.
- Skew or equal anterior and posterior flaps are also possible, especially if previous incisions/trauma compromise a long posterior flap.
- For the long posterior flap, the anterior incision is transverse at the level of the bony amputation.
- Try to avoid the incision line coming to lie at the apex of the stump.

Procedure
- Dissection proceeds to the muscle, keeping the gastrocnemius muscle attached to the skin flaps to improve vascularity and provide padding over the bone end. The deep muscles of the posterior compartment (including soleus) are excised.

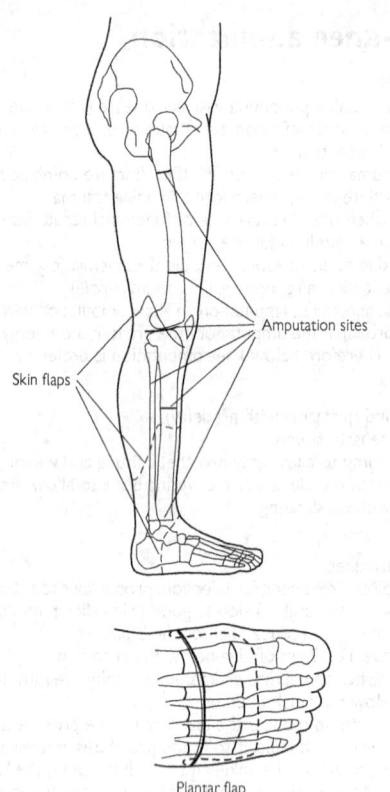

Fig. 13.1 Lower limb amputation levels.

- Neurovascular bundles are identified. The vessels are ligated. The nerves are dissected separately from the vessels and transected as far proximal as possible to the planned bone cut to avoid pain. Inject bupivacaine around the nerve stump.
- The periosteum of the tibia and fibula is incised transversely.
- Osteoperiosteal flaps can be raised and sutured to hold tibia and fibula together.
- In short amputations, a transverse screw can be placed between tibia and fibula to control abduction of the fibula.
- The bone is divided with a power saw or Gigli saw at the appropriate level and the margins smoothed with bone nibblers and a file. The anterior margin of the tibia should shelve to avoid a sharp edge. The fibula should be 4–5 cm shorter than the tibia.

Closure
- A suction drain is placed deep in the wound.
- Absorbable sutures are used to close the muscles flaps, usually to each other (stitch gastrocnemius to tibialis anterior) but in the case of soft tissue shortage to the periosteum or bone. Ensure loose muscle coverage of the bone. But not too loose!
- The skin margins are closed without tension, usually with deep sutures and an interrupted cutaneous layer. Dog ears are excised if necessary, aiming for a smooth contour.
- The wound is dressed and bandaged with light pressure.

Post-operative care
- Elevate the limb.
- Give physiotherapy to adjacent joints to prevent contractures.
- Stump bandaging can help mould the stump.
- Wound desensitization and massage follows removal of sutures at 2 weeks.
- A prosthesis can be fitted 6 weeks post-operatively, or when the wound is stable.

Complications
- Bleeding.
- Infection.
- Delayed wound healing.
- Muscle or skin necrosis.
- Stump oedema.
- Pain due to scar, palpable sharp bone ends, neuroma or pressure on nerves, and phantom limb pain.
- Joint contractures.
- Failure to mobilize with prosthesis—multifactorial.
- Stump bursa.
- Folliculitis/epidermal cyst formation at prosthesis contact with weight-bearing areas.

Above-knee amputation

Indications
- As for BKA, or when BKA not possible.
- Walking is 43% slower and expends 89% more energy than for a normal person. Easier to fit an AKA prosthesis than a through-knee amputation. However, if patient is unlikely to ambulate with a prosthesis (e.g. because they are old), a through-knee prosthesis gives them greater leverage to turn in bed.

Aims
As for BKA.

Planning
- Aim to leave 25–30 cm femur below the greater trochanter, but remove at least 12 cm above the knee to allow space for a knee mechanism in the prosthesis.
- Use a tourniquet if possible (may need to be sterile).
- Antibiotics as indicated for infection or prophylaxis.

Incision
- Use equal anterior and posterior flaps or a long anterior flap.
- Flaps are longer than the level of the bone to allow closure.
- Use a fish-mouth incision.

Procedure
- Anterior muscles are divided level with the bone transection.
- A flap of adductor muscle 5 cm longer than the bone is created.
- The femur is divided and lifted anteriorly with a bone hook.
- Neurovascular bundles are identified, vessels are ligated and divided, and nerves are divided under tension so that they retract into the muscle. Inject bupivicaine around the nerve stump.
- The remaining muscle is divided posteriorly level with the bone transection.

Closure
- A suction drain is placed deep to the muscles.
- The adductor muscles may be sutured to the femur via drill holes to prevent abduction, and the quadriceps sutured to the adductor muscles.
- Skin flaps are closed without tension.
- The wound is bandaged with light pressure.

Post-operative care and complications
As for BKA. Ambulation is less likely than after BKA.

Chapter 14

Vascular

Raynaud's phenomenon *450*
Lymphoedema *453*
Vascular anomalies *457*
Haemangiomas *459*
Vascular malformations *461*

Raynaud's phenomenon

Definition
Raynaud's phenomenon (RP) is a vasospastic condition affecting terminal arteries, classically characterized by colour change of the end-organ from pallor to cyanosis and rubor (white, then blue, then red). Blanching is followed by cyanosis due to the stasis of deoxygenated blood, and lastly rubor as a result of hyperaemic blood flow returning to the fingers.

Incidence
Female-to-male ratio 9:1. Affects 20–30% of young women, with a possible familial predisposition. It most commonly affects the digital arteries of the fingers, but can also affect the toes, ears, nose, tongue, and nipples.

Aetiology
Vasospasm of the terminal arteries is induced by exposure to cold and other sympathetic stimuli, e.g. pain and emotional stress. Other stimulants include tobacco, drugs, and trauma. The precise cause is unknown, but numerous factors are implicated including neutrophil and platelet activation, inflammatory responses, and endothelial dysfunction. Current opinion is that deficiency of a potent vasodilator in the digital nerves (a calcitonin-gene-related peptide) allows action of unopposed cold-stress-induced release of the vasoconstrictor endothelin-I.

Classification
- Primary RP (previously Raynaud's disease) occurs in the absence of any identifiable organic cause.
- Secondary RP (previously Raynaud's syndrome) is associated with an underlying disorder (Table 14.1). This diagnosis is more likely in those with late-onset disease (>30 years), or in presence of trophic changes (e.g. ulcers).

This distinction is important, as prognosis and severity can vary accordingly.

Clinical features
- Full triphasic colour change is not essential for the diagnosis of RP.
- History of cold-induced pallor and subsequent red flush is enough to support a diagnosis. Bluish discoloration in isolation is due to acrocyanosis.
- Cardinal feature: well-demarcated colour change (vs. non-pathological diffuse pallor commonly observed in cold weather). It may be asymmetrical, affecting only one or two digits on each hand. Digital pain and paraesthesia may be present.

Investigations
Objective measurements are not required unless clinical findings are vague.
- Enlarged nailfold capillaries: useful and simple diagnostic test using an ophthalmoscope at high power.
- Digital systolic BP: fall >30 mmHg (Doppler) after local cooling at 15°C is significant.
- Other investigations should be directed at differentiating between primary and secondary RP to facilitate management of the underlying condition (Table 14.2).

Table 14.1 Conditions associated with Raynaud's phenomenon

Connective tissue diseases (CTDs)	Systemic sclerosis (scleroderma)
	Systemic lupus erythematosus
	Rheumatoid arthritis
	Dermatomyositis, polymyositis
	Sjögren's syndrome
	Thromboangiitis obliterans (Bürger's disease)
Obstructive	Atherosclerosis (brachiocephalic)
	Microemboli
	Thoracic outlet syndrome (e.g. cervical rib)
Drugs	Beta-blockers
	Cytotoxics (e.g. bleomycin, vinblastine)
	Cyclosporin
	Ergotamine
	Sulfasalazine
	Interferon
Mechanical injury	Vibration (vibration white finger)
	Frost bite
Endocrine	Carcinoid syndrome
	Phaeochromocytoma
	Hypothyroidism
Miscellaneous	Haematological (e.g. cryoglobulin, paraproteinaemia, polycythaemia)
	Vasospastic disorders (e.g. migraine, Prinzmetal angina)
	Malignancy (e.g. ovarian, lymphoma)
	Infections (e.g. parvovirus, *Helicobacter pylori*)
	Reflex sympathetic dystrophy

From Block and Sequeira (2001).

Management

Medical

- Establish diagnosis and provide information about disorder.
- Consider general measures before introducing drug therapy:
  - Stop smoking.

- Consider withdrawing drugs associated with RP (e.g. beta-blockers, ergot preparations).
- Use hand-warmers, gloves, and socks.
- Consider change of occupation.
- Withdraw oral contraceptive only if there is a clear link with development of RP.
- HRT is not contraindicated in Raynaud's phenomenon and may protect against development of vascular disease.
• If symptoms are sufficiently severe to merit drug treatment, consider the following order of treatment:
  - Nifedipine (retard/slow release) 10 mg once daily up to maximum of 20 mg tds (calcium-channel blockers with antiplatelet and anti-white blood cell effects). Side-effects may limit usage (e.g. ankle swelling, headaches).
  - Naftidrofuryl 100 mg tds up to maximum of 200 mg tds.
  - Inositol nicotinate 500 mg tds up to maximum of 1 g qds.
  - Angiotensin-II type 1 receptor antagonist (losartan) has been shown to decrease the frequency and severity of attacks.
  - Iloprost® infusion (weight-related dosage given IV over 48–72 hr) is used as a last resort.
• There is insufficient evidence to recommend the use of oxpentifylline, thymoxamine, prazosin or cinnarizine in the treatment of RP.

Surgical
- Surgery may be appropriate in cases of obstructive causes or cervical rib.
- Effectiveness of cervicothoracic sympathectomy is usually short lived.
- Digital sympathectomy has been helpful in severe cases.

Table 14.2 Screening tests for detecting associated conditions

Test	Underlying pathology
Blood tests	
Full blood count	Anaemia of chronic disease
Electrolytes	Renal disease
Thyroid function	Hypothyroidism
ESR, autoantibodies	Connective tissue disease
Urinalysis	
Red blood cells, protein, casts	Vasculitis (Connective tissue disease)
Radiology	
Chest X-ray	Basal fibrosis (connective tissue disease), cervical rib

Reference
Block JA, Sequeira W (2001). *Lancet* **357**, 2042–8.

Lymphoedema

Definition
An abnormal collection of interstitial fluid because of either maldevelopment of the lymphatics or an acquired obstruction.

Anatomy
The embryological development of the lymphatics is such that they arise from endothelial sproutings of the primordial venous system in four areas: the jugulars, the iliac, the retroperitoneal, and the cisterna chyli. From here, the lymphatics develop and invade the peripheries everywhere except the brain and bone marrow.

Lymphatics are arranged from superficial to deep. There are intra-dermal lymphatics that drain into a dermal lymphatic plexus (valved). These drain into collecting channels and then into superficial fascial lymphatic trunks. Between five and eight lymphatic trunks travel with the long saphenous vein, and about four that travel with the short saphenous vein. There is a separate deep muscular lymphatic system with several channels which travel adjacent to the bone. Superficial and deep systems are independent, except for channels at the cubital fossae, the popliteal fossae, the inguinal and cysterna chylae at L1–2, and the thoracic duct and subclavian vein.

Physiology
The function of lymphatics is:
- To drain macromolecular protein loss from capillaries (50% of albumin processed every 24 hr).
- To remove bacteria and foreign material.
- Gastrointestinal transport of vitamin K and long_chain fatty acids.

Lymph is an ultrafiltrate of plasma; capillary lymphatics have no basement membrane and thus are very permeable. Flow within lymphatics occurs because the low pressure within the lymphatic vessels and valves allows unidirectional flow in response to pressure changes from intra-abdominal and thoracic respiration, arterial pulsation, and muscle activity. There may also be intrinsic lymphatic contractility.

Aetiology and classification
The aetiology of lymphoedema can be classified as follows.

Primary
Primary lymphoedema is congenital and due to abnormal anatomical or functional development of the lymphatics. Primary lymphoedema is further subdivided as follows.

- Lymphoedema congenita (Milroy's disease):
  - 10–15% of cases.
  - Present at birth.
  - Familial; females more affected then males.
  - In two-thirds affects both extremities.
  - Lower limb to upper limb ratio, 3:1.
  - Hypoplasia or aplasia of subcutaneous lymphatics.

- Lymphoedema praecox:
  - 65–80% of cases.
  - 70% due to segmental hypoplasia (obstructive), 15% due to aplasia (non-obstructive), and 15% due to hyperplastic varicose lymphatics.
  - Usually caused by incompetent valves.
  - Presents during puberty.
  - Female-to-male ratio 4:1.
  - Usually foot and ankle; 70% unilateral.
- **Lymphoedema tarda (Meige's disease)**.
  - Presents after 35 years of age.
  - Possibly a spectrum of lymphoedema praecox.
  - Inadequate drainage to meet demands.

Secondary

Secondary or acquired lymphoedema is usually due to regional lymph node pathology.

- Most common cause worldwide is elephantiasis caused by parasitic invasion by *Filaria bancrofti*.
- The other common cause is iatrogenic, following block dissection of the lymph nodes or radiotherapy.
- Other causes may be vascular (iliac artery compression of iliac vein), other infections (TB, cat scratch fever, lymphogranuloma venerium, chronic lymphangitis), neoplasm, or trauma.

In secondary lymphedema there is an increase in lymphatic pressure leading to disruption of the valve. A dermal backflow leading to fibroplasia results in a further increase in pressure, and a vicious cycle ensues.

Clinical presentation

Clinically lymphoedema presents with swelling and pitting oedema, cellulitis, or lymphangitis. Ulceration is rare (in lymphatic ulceration there is no brown discoloration as is seen with venous ulceration). There is fatigue of the limb, fibrosis, and thick hyperkeratotic skin. Differentiate from venous disease (pitting edema, stigmata of venous disease). Malignant transformation to lymphangiosarcoma is rare.

Investigation

- Doppler studies.
- Venography.
- Lymphangiogram.
- Lymphoscintigraphy (Tc^{99}-labelled antimony).
- MRI or CT scan.
- Lymph clearance using I^{132}-labelled albumin (RISA).
- Volume displacement can be used for assessment of progress or for diagnosis in mild cases where a difference of greater than 5% is significant.

Management

Conservative
Management of lymphoedema may be conservative aiming to control oedema, to prevent infection, and to watch for malignant transformation. This involves patient education, elevation of the affected limb, and external compression using stockings, pneumatic devices, or massage (four-quadrant, decongestant).

Medical
Medical intervention using diuretics and benzopyrones which promote proteolysis by increasing macrophagic activity, thus reducing interstitial proteins, may be useful. Rapid treatment of infections with antibiotics and limb hyperthermia. Diethylcarbamazepine is used for filiariasis.

Surgical
Indication
The indication for surgical intervention is functional impairment due to inability to control the size of the limb, recurrent lymphangitis, or, to a lesser extent, cosmesis.

Classification
Operations can be classified as physiological or excisional. Physiological operations aim to reconstruct or provide lymphatic drainage by a flap technique or by lymphatic reconstruction.
- Physiological.
  - Needle holes/stab wounds (LisFranc).
  - Silk thread wicks (Handley).
  - Excised strip of deep fascia (Kondoleon).
  - Cutaneous flap (Gillies).
  - Buried dermal flap (Thompson).
  - Lymph node venous shunt (Nielubowicz).
  - Omental flap (Goldsmith).
  - Lympho-venous anastomosis (O'Brien).
  - Lymph node transfer (O'Brien).
  - Lympho-lymphatic grafting (Baumeister).

The flap technique involves local rotation of lymphatic dermis deep into a deep compartment, aiming to allow lymphatic drainage from the lymphatic dermis to drain into the deep muscular compartment. The alternative is to use an omental flap brought into the lymphoedematous tissue to allow lymphatic drainage, or an ilieo-enteromesenteric flap. Lymphatic reconstruction has been attempted using silk threads, anastomosing lymphoedematous lymph nodes to veins, and performing lymphatico-venous anastomoses and micro-lymphatic grafts, none of which have proved very successful.

- Excisional:
  - Circumferential excision and SSG (Charles).
  - Partial excisional—flaps raised sub-cutaneous tissue removed (Homans or Sistrunk).
  - Subcutaneous excision and dermal flap burial (Thompson).
  - Liposuction.

Excisional operations involve excising all the subcutaneous tissue from under the skin and dermal flaps (Sistrunk) or total excision of the skin and subcutaneous tissue down to the superficial fascia layer and skin grafting that layer (Charles). A more recent alternative is to use assisted liposuction. However, the long-term benefit for this is as yet unproven.

Operation selection is important, as is patient selection. Patients must have a good understanding that this operation is not curative and the outcome may not be cosmetically acceptable. Preoperatively, attempts should be made to reduce the size of the limb by bed rest, elevation, massage, and pumping. Operatively, the procedures are best performed using a tourniquet and under cover of prophylactic antibiotics. Postoperatively, bed rest maybe required for up to a week, allowing healing prior to mobilization.

Operations performed to debulk extremely heavy limbs are the most successful.

Vascular anomalies

Vascular anomalies are given descriptive terms such as strawberry naevus, port wine stain, and cavernous haemangioma. They are very common lesions frequently found in skin and subcutaneous tissue, but can be found in all tissues.

Classification
Mulliken and Glowacki (1982) suggested a system of classification for vascular anomalies which was based on the cellular and clinical characteristics as well as the natural history of these swellings. They classified vascular anomalies as follows.

Haemangiomas
Vascular tumours characterized by a hyperplasia or proliferation of endothelial cells and increased mast cell activity.

Vascular malformations
Errors of development comprising dysplastic vessels lined by quiescent epithelium. Vascular malformations are further categorized based on their channel morphology and their dynamic blood flow characteristics:
- Slow flow.
  - Capillary malformation (port wine stain).
  - Venous malformation (venous lake).
  - Lymphatic malformation (lymphangioma, cystic hygroma).
  - Complex malformations (e.g. Klippel–Trenaunay syndrome, a capillary–venous–lymphatic malformation).
- High flow:
  - Arterial malformation (aneurysm, spider naevus).
  - Arteriovenous fistulae (AVF).
  - Arteriovenous malformation (AVM).
  - Complex malformation (Parkes Weber syndrome, a capillary–arteriovenous malformation).

Table 14.3 Comparison of haemangiomas and vascular malformations

Haemangiomas	Vascular malformations
Appear in neonatal period, 1–2 weeks after birth	Usually present at birth
Rapid, early increase in size	Growth in keeping with growth of child
Proliferate and later involute	Keep on progressing
Spontaneous regression (70% by 7 years)	No spontaneous regression
Endothelial proliferation and increased mast cell activity	No cellular hyperplasia
Firm; cannot be completely emptied	Spongy; usually possible to empty the vascular lesion completely
Non-syndromic	Associated with a large number of syndromes
Occasionally complicated by obstruction, distortion, destruction, bleeding, or aberrant physiology	Complications rare, but often ugly
Associated physiological effects in form of congestive cardiac failure or Kasabach–Merritt phenomenon	Extremely rare
Cutaneous or visceral in location	May be present in any part of the body
Management mainly conservative	Management mainly conservative
Intervention in form of steroids, laser, surgical excision	Intervention in the form of radiological embolization, excision, and debulking

Reference

Mulliken JB, Glowacki J (1982). *Plast Reconstr Surg* **70**, 120–1.

Haemangiomas

Definition
A form of a vascular anomaly characterized by the neonatal appearance of a vascular swelling, which grows rapidly during infancy (proliferative phase), reaches a plateau around 2–3 years of age, and regresses in childhood (involutionary phase).

Incidence
- Common.

Pathology
Characterized by endothelial proliferation, basal laminar becomes multi-laminated, increased mast cell activity and progressive deposition of perivascular fibrous tissue.

Clinical presentation and natural history
Classical clinical picture of a red spot at birth which rapidly develops into a growing firm vascular swelling that cannot be emptied.
- Proliferative phase: the haemangioma grows rapidly compared with ongoing body growth. The swelling appears to be dull or bright red and is firm to palpation. Often called a strawberry naevus at this stage.
- Plateau phase between the ages of 2 and 4 years, proliferative activity slows down and keeps pace with regression.
- Regression or involution phase: characterized by the skin becoming less vascular in appearance; the dermis thickens accompanied by a decrease in the size of the swelling and softening of its consistency.
- 50% of all haemangiomas resolve by 5 years, 70% by 7 years, and 90% by 9 years.
- In 50–75% of cases an aesthetic defect may be left.
- A fair proportion of resolved haemangiomas are left with residual skin stigmata in the form of crepe paper like laxity, telangiectasia, or even scarring.

Classification
- Congenital haemangioma: already proliferated and present at birth. Can be confused with vascular malformation.
- Non-involuting congenital haemangioma (NICH).
- Rapidly involuting congenital haemangioma (RICH).

Complications
Most are uncomplicated, but some may cause problems because of:
- Obstruction.
- Distortion.
- Destruction.
- Altered physiology.

Obstruction
- Visual axis (eyelid haemangioma) with subsequent amblyopia.
- Airway obstruction as with endotracheal lesions.
- Other orifice.

Distortion
When present on nasal tip, lip, or eyelid, can cause distortion of surrounding structures because of bulk and weight.

Destruction
By erosion of cartilage or skin.

Altered physiology
When present in large numbers or in the form of visceral lesions, haemangiomas can be associated with a triad of congestive cardiac failure, hepatomegaly, and anaemia.

Primary platelet trapping (Kasabach–Merritt phenomenon) is a potentially life-threatening condition characterized by multiple cutaneous haemangiomas (trunk, shoulder, thigh, and retroperitoneum), associated petechiae, thrombocytopenia (<10 000/mm^3) with an elevated PT and APTT; elevated levels of fibrin degradation products may also be detectable.

Management

The natural history of resolution of the majority of haemangiomas makes observation and reassurance of the patient and parents the mainstay of management. Intervention may be desirable if complications occur and takes the form of pharmacological manipulation, laser therapy, or surgical debulking or excision.

Laser therapy
- The flashlamp dyed pulse laser is advocated for early eyelid, nasal, or auricular lesions (premonitory spot) to prevent an increase in size and subsequent complications. Doubt exists regarding its efficacy.
- The pulse dye laser can be useful for ulcerated bleeding haemangiomas and also for residual telangectasia.

Medical
Haemangiomas causing obstructive or destructive problems can be treated with either intralesional (triamcinolone 25 mg/ml, 3–5 mg/kg) or systemic corticosteroids. Oral prednisolone (2 mg/kg/day) is given over 4–6 week cycles and then slowly tapered.

Beware the effects of steroids: growth retardation, adrenal suppression so that the patient will not respond to live vaccines, and increased infection risk. The mechanism of action is unknown. A third will respond well, a third will have a partial response, and third will not respond. Where corticosteroids have failed, caused complications, or are contraindicated, and in patients with life-threatening haemangiomas, recombinant alpha 2a interferon (2–3 million units/m^2 subcutaneous) is the drug of choice. Complications such as elevated liver transaminases, neutropenia, and anaemia are reversible, and parameters usually return to normal. Vincristine has also been used.

Surgery
Indications:
- Bleeding.
- Obstruction (debulking).
- In the reconstruction of altered or destroyed normal anatomy.
- Residual cutaneous problems (scarring).

Vascular malformations

Definition
A form of a vascular anomaly usually characterized by the appearance of some vascular swelling at the time of birth. This usually progresses proportionate with the growth of the child and shows no spontaneous clinical regression.

Incidence
- Common.
- Most common are capillary–venous low-flow lesions.

Classification
They are classified on the basis of their constituent vessels:
- Venous.
- Capillary.
- Lymphatic.
- Arteriovenous.
- Combinations.

And on their blood flow characteristics:
- Low flow.
- High flow.

Pathology
These malformations represent an abnormality of morphogenesis comprising vascular channel abnormalities. Their clinical behaviour is a reflection of their vascular anatomy and blood flow characteristics.

Clinical behaviour
These lesions are present at birth and grow commensurate with the child. Certain types, which may be deeper, may not become clinically apparent or symptomatic until late in childhood, or even in early adolescence. The natural history of these lesions is to gradually increase in size. They may cause clinical effects in the form of embarrassment or awareness, local overgrowth of tissues, problems with the constituent vessels (thrombosis), formation of phleboliths, mass effect, bleeding, and ulceration.

Complications
- Vascular malformations can cause problems by:
  - Local overgrowth.
  - Obstruction.
  - Destruction.
  - Bleeding.
  - Associated syndromic manifestations.
- Hypertrophy or localized gigantism is very common in vascular malformations (usually of the arteriovenous type), especially in the limbs. This is secondary to overgrowth of the soft tissue as well as the underlying bone.
- Macrochelia, macrotia, macrognathia, and macroglossia often complicate port wine stains.

- Obstruction can result from the presence of a swelling in any hollow structure or at the entrance to any orifice, such as a lymphangioma of the tongue, or by interfering with the function of adjacent structures like fingers.
- Lymphatic malformations, especially involving the tongue and the head and neck region, are prone to sudden episodes of enlargement following influenza-like illnesses or upper respiratory tract infections and can cause life-threatening obstruction of the airway.
- Destruction by invasion of normal structures is usually just due to expansion and pressure effect, but can lead to loss of function or pathological fracture.
- Bleeding from superficial vascular malformations that ulcerate can be dramatic, especially if arterial, and can be life-threatening if internal.
- Spontaneous thrombosis in venous malformations and even embolic phenomena causing distant gangrene are not uncommon.

Investigation
- Angiography helps to delineate the extent and the flow characteristics of the lesion.
- MRI can also help delineate the lesion.
- Plain X-ray can show phleboliths, calcification, bone destruction, mass.
- Vascular laboratory studies: Doppler, plethysmography, etc.
- Metalloproteinases are raised in the urine of patients with vascular malformation of any type. Amount is relative to size and growth of malformation.

Management
- The principles of management remain 'watchful expectancy with masterful inactivity and intervention as and when necessary'. The vast majority of these lesions will remain quiescent and only occasionally may cause problems. Regular reassurance and support of these patients is necessary.
- Intervention is greatly aided by the presence of a vascular laboratory, a radiologist who is skilled in intervention and embolization, and a team of surgeons with experience in this field. Also essential is a reconstructive surgeon when destruction or distortion of tissues has already taken place, or may occur as a result of the surgery.
- Embolization of the malformation nidus (the centre), if present, may be a definitive procedure in itself or a preoperative adjunct to surgery.
- Non-surgical intervention may take the form of injection of sclerosants or cryotherapy.

Surgery
- The proximal ligation of feeding vessels is to be discouraged, as collateral circulation re-establishes the pathology and flow characteristics of the original lesion.
- Excision.
- Debulking procedures.
- Compartmentalization (Popescu suturing) to control or minimize the malformation.

These surgical options have a role in certain circumstances. However, complete excision is often difficult to achieve and recurrence is likely. The time to recurrence may be years. On the whole these lesions are best left alone unless symptomatic or complicated.

Naevus flammeus
Present at birth or soon after; salmon patch; fading vascular patch; very common; self-resolving.

Venous malformation
Lack of smooth muscle in wall of vessel and so the vein balloons with time. Size and extent of involvement is very variable. Symptoms vary on site.

Treatment
- Direct puncture sclerotherapy with sodium tetradecyl sulphate, ethanol, or bleomycin. Not indicated if thin overlying tissue or high-flow lesion.
- Excision.

Complications
- 10% minor: pain, swelling, blistering, infection, loss of sensation and function.
- 1% major: DVT, PE, cardiac arrest, death, blindness, airway obstruction, amputation, loss of tissue.

Lymphatic vascular malformation

Classification
- Microcystic (used to be called lymphangoma circumscripta).
- Macrocystic if >1 cm.

No longer called cystic hygroma.

Treatment
- Aspiration and sclerosant.
- Surgery.

Recurrence rate is high.

Klippel–Trenaunay syndrome
- Capillary–lymphovenous malformation with limb hypertrophy.
- Limb hypertrophy is due to soft tissue.
- May present with recurrent ulceration or gigantism.
- Note that if a large area involved, the deep veins are absent. Therefore do not remove the dilated superficial veins; otherwise risk loss of limb.

High-flow arteriovenous malformations
High-flow arterial input but secondary increased outflow and venous dilatation.

Schobinger classification
1. Quiescent.
2. Progressive.
3. Symptomatic.
4. Cardiac failure.

Investigation
MRI, angiogram.

Treatment
- Embolize the nidus and then excise it.
- Excise if can control by tourniquet.
- Proximal ligation is contraindicated as it will make things worse by recruitment of collateral vessels.

Sturge–Weber syndrome
Capillary venous malformations (PWSs) in a trigeminal nerve distribution, with leptomeningeal vascular anomalies and skeletal and fibrovascular hypertrophy.

Parkes Weber syndrome
Multiple arteriovenous fistulas associated with facial hypertrophy, microcephaly, mental impairment, and seizures.

Osler–Rendu–Weber disease (hereditary haemorrhagic telangiectasia)
Arteriovenous malformations and fistulae in skin, mucous membranes, lungs, and abdominal viscera. It is AD inherited. Most other vascular anomalies are not inherited.

Maffucci's syndrome
Multiple vascular anomalies—mainly venous malformations associated with enchondromas. There is a high risk of various malignancies. The venous malformations may develop painful benign spindle cell haemangioendotheliomas.

Chapter 15

Infection

Microbiology *466*
Clostridia *468*
Osteomyelitis *471*
Prosthesis exposure or infection *475*
Necrotizing soft tissue infection *476*

Microbiology

Leprosy

Organism
Mycobacterium leprae (Hansen's bacillus-Norwegian, 1873).

Pathology
M.leprae is infectious particularly in children; adults have poor infection transmission. *M.leprae* has a predilection for neural tissue, particularly the peripheral nervous system. The bacilli enter by the endoneural blood vessels and attach to cells. The subsequent histological changes in the nerves depends on the immune status.

Classification
- Tuberculoid leprosy occurs in those with good immunity; phagocytes become epithelioid cells, leading to nerve destruction and intraneural granulomas.
- Lepromatous leprosy occurs in those with poor immunity; the phagocytes do not destroy the bacilli but carry them away giving widely disseminated lesions, but not as much nerve damage (onion skin perineurium).
- Border-line leprosy causes epithelioid cell granulomas in a more diffuse pattern than tuberculoid leprosy.
- Indeterminate leprosy.

Diagnosis
Clinical evidence of nerve or dermal involvement (plaques).

Investigation
Microscopy for acid-fast bacilli (Ziehl–Neelsen stain), lepromin.

Treatment
- ?Isolate patient.
- Medical treatment: dapsone/rifampicin.
- Surgical management of paralysed muscles and complications arising from paralysed muscles and anaesthetic skin.

Pasteurella multocida

Organism
Small genus in the group Bacillus; common in cat and dog bites.

Treatment
- Debridement.
- Penicillin.

Pseudomonas aeruginosa (pyocyanea)

Organism
A Gram-negative anaerobic bacterium producing two pigments: greenish-yellow fluorescein and blue-green pyocyanin. *Ps.aeruginosa* likes moist conditions. Other *Pseudomonas* species include *Ps.pseudomallei* which gives melioidosis and *Ps.putrefaciens* which infects ulcers and produces the hydrogen sulphide smell.

Pathology

Causes the blue-green pigmentation of bandages, dressings, and wounds. Infects necrotic ulcers and eschars; likes wounds with reduced vascularity. Occasionally prevents skin graft take.

Treatment

Topical application of acetic acid or Milton's solution was popular. This has been replaced by the use of silver sulfadiazine (SSD). Systemically *Pseudomonas* species are sensitive to ciprofloxacin.

Staphylococcus

Organism

Staphylococcus species: Gram-positive bacteria.

Pathology

Pathological conditions cause by *Staphylococcus aureus* include impetigo (superficial skin), furunculosis (acute necrotizing infection of hair follicle), caruncles (many communicating furuncles), folliculitis (infection of the hair follicle ostium), and scalded skin syndrome. It is the most common organism causing wound infections and bone and joint infection.

Classification

- Coagulase-negative: usually *Staph.epidermidis*.
- Coagulase positive: most commonly *Staph.aureus*.

Treatment

- Medical: flucloxacillin, first- and second-generation cephalosporins. IV vancomycin or teicoplanin may be needed for resistant strains.
- Surgical: remember that debridement of necrotic tissue and drainage of abscesses must be performed.

Streptococcus

Organism

Streptococcus species: Gram-positive cocci.

Pathology

Responsible for many skin infections and can be blamed for failure of skin graft take!
- Classification 1:
  - α-Haemolytic, i.e. *Strep.viridens*—partial green haemolysis.
  - β-Haemolytic, i.e. *Strep.pyogenes*—complete haemolysis.
  - γ-Haemolytic, i.e. *Strep.faecalis* (group D)—no haemolysis.
- Classification 2 goes from group A to group O, where group A = *Strep.pyogenes* and group D = *Strep.faecalis*.

Clinical conditions secondary to streptococcus include skin infections such as erysipelas (superficial skin), cellulitis (subcutaneous), impetigo, injury to skin vessels secondary to circulating erythrotoxin (scarlet fever), allergic hypersensitivity to streptococcus antigens producing vasculitis, and conditions such as erythema nodosum. Other conditions include SBE and glomerulonephritis. *Streptococcus* species are implicated as organisms involved in necrotizing fascitis.

Treatment

- Medical: penicillin.
- Surgical: debridement of necrotic tissue is essential for control.

Clostridia

Family of Gram-positive bacilli which cause numerous common infective diseases.

Clostridium welchii (C.perfringens)
- **Cellulitis** Serious septic process of subcutaneous tissue characterized by:
    - Crepitant cellulitis which spreads rapidly along fascial planes.
    - Pain.
    - Grey to reddish-brown discharge.
    - Results in thrombosis.
    - Skin necrosis and fat necrosis.
- **Myositis or gas gangrene** Similar to cellulitis but more severe:
    - Spreading gangrene and profound toxaemia.
    - Gas plus crepitus in muscles.
    - Soft swollen dark red muscle.
    - Foul-smelling brown watery exudates with gas bubbles.
    - Illness and prostration out of proportion to fever.

Peptostreptococcus and bacteroides coliforms may also cause gas gangrene.

Management
- Resuscitation.
- IV penicillin.
- Surgical debridement.
- ± Fasciotomies ± amputation.
- ± Hyperbaric oxygen therapy.

Clostridium tetani

Organism
Anaerobic Gram-positive rod; spore bearing.

Pathology
Causes tetanus, produced by powerful exotoxin. Fatal in 40–60%. Incubation 4–21days.

Tetanus-prone wounds have devitalized tissue with the reduced oxygen environment necessary for the organism. These are usually complex or crush deep wounds with contamination and denervation.

- Prodrome:
    - Restless.
    - Headache.
    - Jaw stiffness.
    - Intermittent tetanic contractions in region of wound within 24 hr.
- Tetanus:
    - Tonic spasm of skeletal muscles.
    - Trismus, risus sardonicus (classical facial distortion).
    - Episthotonos and rigidity; tonic contraction may occur from even very minor stimuli.
    - Respiratory arrest may occur during convulsions.
    - Painful contractions associated with tachycardia.
    - Increased salivation and sweating.

Management

Prevention
- ADT vaccine ± tetanus immunoglobulin.

Surgical and medical
- Surgical debridement of wound, source of infection.
- Local + IV tetanus antitoxin if established.
- IV ABs.
- Reduce external stimuli (quiet dark room, no visitors).
- Control seizures with benzodiazepines.
- ICU: circulatory and respiratory support.
- Usually die from aspiration pneumonia and respiratory arrest.

Tetanus prophylaxis
- Check patient's current immunization record. If patient has had entire immunization course, no further tetanus prophylaxis required. There used to be a 10 year recommendation, in that if no booster had been received in the last 10 years administer tetanus prophylaxis. However, this has been extended beyond 10 years to indefinitely. In a very tetanus prone wound or if in doubt, give prophylaxis.
- Prophylaxis includes surgical debridement of the wound to remove dead and dying (anaerobic) tissue!
- Tetanus toxoid in the form of ADT or tetanus toxoid adsorbed is always given if immunization status is unknown or course was incomplete.
- Additionally, consider tetanus immunoglobulin in the non-immunized with a tetanus prone wound.
- Contraindication is previous hypersensitivity to tetanus toxoid. Consider immunoglobulin (passive immunization).

Clostridium botulinum

- Botulism is acute poisoning from ingestion of toxin produced by C.botulinum.
- Characterized by progressive descending muscle paralysis.
- Block neuromuscular transmission in cholinergic fibres either by release of ACh or binding ACh at its site of release in the presynaptic clefts.
- (Home-canned foods.)
- Several strains: A–G.
- Symptoms:
    - ocular: diplopia, blurry vision, photophobia.
    - bulbar: dysphonia, dysarthria, dysphagia muscular extremities, symmetric salivation.

Investigation
- Inject stool or serum in mice: see if they die.

Management
- Symptoms IDC.
- Antitoxin.

Clostridium difficile
Produces a toxin which destroy intestinal mucosa, leading to pseudomembranous colitis.

Clostridial species
C.welchii
C.tetani
C.botulinum
C.difficile
C.bifermentans
C.histolyticum
C.fallax
C.septicum
C.sordelli
C.novyi

Osteomyelitis

Definition
Osteomyelitis is infection of the bone and bone marrow. It is classified based on the route of infection, haematogenous or contiguous focus, and into acute and chronic forms.

Plastic surgeons have a major role in the management of the dead space, in bone reconstruction, and in dealing with the affected soft tissues in osteomyelitis.

Prevalence
The prevalence of both acute and chronic osteomyelitis is 2/10 000 in developed countries. The prevalence in the developing world is likely to be higher because of a higher incidence of puncture wounds and open fractures, and less access to wound care facilities.

Aetiology
- Age:
  - Neonatal and paediatric: usually haematogenous spread.
  - Adult: usually contiguous spread.
- Routes of infection:
  - Haematogenous osteomyelitis: predominantly encountered in children; 85% of patients with haematogenous osteomyelitis aged <17 years. Affects long bones in children and vertebrae in adults. In adults there is association with intravenous drug use.
  - Contiguous focus osteomyelitis: accounts for over half of all cases. Direct inoculation occurs at the time of trauma or operation, or infection extends from an adjacent infection (e.g. from prosthesis).
  - Contiguous focus osteomyelitis in diabetic patients: the small bones of the foot and ankle are commonly involved. Predisposing factors include vascular insufficiency; motor, sensory, and autonomic neuropathy, and diminished host immune response.

Classification
Cierny classification of osteomyelitis (Fig. 15.1)
- Type 1: superficial medullary osteomyelitis with an endosteal nidus.
- Type 2: superficial cortical osteomyelitis; soft tissue compromise is common.
- Type 3: deep cortical osteomyelitis through whole thickness of cortex, often with well-defined sequestration of cortical bone. At least one side of cortex uninvolved.
- Type 4: segmental cortical osteomyelitis. Destructive lesion causing instability.

Each type is subclassified based on the host immune status:
- A: normal.
- B: minor immunocompromised state.
- C: significant immunocompromised state (diabetic, PVD, IHD).

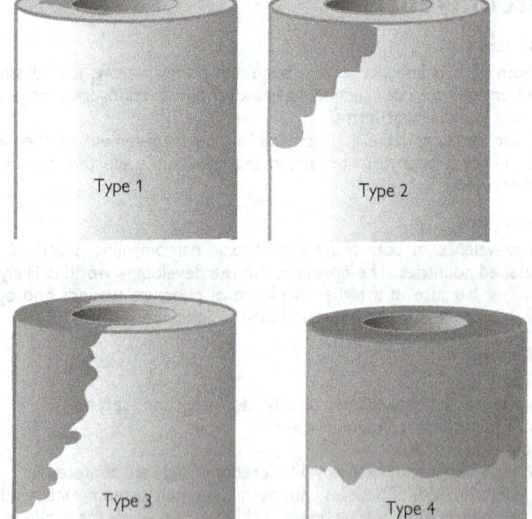

Fig. 15.1 Cierny classification of osteomyelitis.

Weiland classification
Defines chronic osteomyelitis as exposed bone, positive bone culture results, and drainage for more than 6 months:
- Type I: open exposed bone with soft tissue infection only.
- Type II: bony infection without a segmental defect.
- Type III: bony infection with a segmental defect.

Bacteriology
- Haematogenous osteomyelitis—usually monomicrobial:
  - Infants: group B *Streptococcus*, *Staph.aureus*, *Escherichia coli*.
  - Children: *Staph. aureus*, *Strep.pyogenes*, *Haemophilus influenzae*.
  - Adults: *Staph. aureus*, coagulase-negative *Staphylococcus* species, Gram-negative bacilli.
- Contiguous focus osteomyelitis—usually polymicrobial.
  - *Staph.aureus*, coagulase-negative *Staphylococcus* species, *Strep.pyogenes*, *Enterococcus* species, Gram-negative bacilli, anaerobes.
- Diabetic foot osteomyelitis—usually polymicrobial:
  - *Staph.aureus*, *Streptococcus* species, *Enterococcus* species, *Proteus mirabilis*, *Ps.aeruginosa*, Anaerobes.

Immunocompromised individuals may develop osteomyelitis with unusual organisms, as may patients who have had prolonged antibiotic therapy.

Clinical features

Acute osteomyelitis
- Infants and children:
  - Fever.
  - Lethargy.
  - Refusal to use affected limb.
  - Erythema over the affected bone.
- Adults:
  - Fever.
  - Chills.
  - Swelling.
  - Erythema over the affected bone.

Chronic osteomyelitis
- Characterized by chronic pain and sinus formation with discharge but no fever.
- If sinus closes, abscess can form and pressure can, build causing acute exacerbation with the clinical features of an acute osteomyelitis.

Investigations
- Radiographic:
  - Plain radiographs neither sensitive nor specific in acute osteomyelitis. Findings include soft tissue swelling, bony destruction, and periosteal reaction. Changes take 2–3 weeks to become apparent. Chronic osteomyelitic changes include sclerosis, new bone formation and sequestra. Difficult to distinguish active and inactive infection.
  - MRI: most sensitive and specific investigation. Anatomical detail allows planning of subsequent surgical procedure. False-positive results may be obtained in healed osteomyelitis, cancer, pressure necrosis and fracture.
  - Isotope bone scan: three-phase bone scan becomes positive after 2–3 days, and is helpful in evaluating suspected acute osteomyelitis in a patient with normal plain radiographs.
  - CT scan can give better bone detail.
- Microbiological:
  - Bone biopsy with Gram stain and culture is the diagnostic gold standard. Blood cultures may also grow the infecting organism. Biopsy should be performed before antibiotic therapy is started!
- Histopathology:
  - Findings include necrotic bone with excessive resorption flanked by an inflammatory exudate, and chronic wound changes.

Management

Medical
Acute haematogenous osteomyelitis in children is usually treated by antibiotic therapy alone. Appropriate antibiotic therapy is an important adjunct to the surgical management of chronic osteomyelitis. The duration of therapy depends on the site, severity, and degree of involvement of the bone and soft tissue, the vascularity of the bone and soft tissue, the adequacy of the excision, the method of reconstruction, the health of the patient, and the type and sensitivity of the organism(s) amongst other factors.

Surgical
Surgical treatment is indicated if there are progressive systemic or local symptoms despite antibiotic therapy, for neurological deterioration in vertebral osteomyelitis, or for the treatment of chronic osteomyelitis.

Principles of surgical treatment
- Excision debridement (tumour style) of all dead, infected, or devitalized tissue into well-vascularized unaffected tissue.
- Multiple biopsies at different sites of affected bone and tissue.
- Stabilization of the skeleton.
- Consideration of bone reconstruction: immediate or delayed. If immediate, has to be vascularized bone flap.
- Vascularized soft tissue obliteration of any dead space. and coverage of the wound.
- Antibiotic therapy as determined by infectious diseases team/microbiologists. In the interim the common empirical therapy whilst waiting for the cultures is to use vancomycin and meropenem.

Commonly, local or free muscle flaps are used to provide soft tissue cover and obliteration of dead space. The blood supply they bring with them improves oxygen, nutrient, antibiotic, and inflammatory cell delivery, and therefore aids osseous and soft tissue healing. Muscle, especially as a free transfer, is easier to conform to the dead-space complex configuration and provides better vascularity from its dense capillary network and blood flow than skin or fasciocutaneous flaps.

Complicationss
- Acute:
  - Major bone loss.
  - Vertebral collapse and neurological impairments.
  - Chronic osteomyelitis (3–40%).
- Chronic:
  - Marjolin's ulcer (malignant transformation to SCC).
  - Amyloidosis.
  - Bone loss.
  - Deformity.
  - Arthritis.
  - Amputation.
  - Ill health.
  - Development of bacterial resistance.

Prosthesis exposure or infection

Wound breakdown following arthroplasty is a serious complication. Exposure of the prosthesis results in bacterial colonization and may lead to loss of the prosthesis. Alternatively, wound breakdown may be a sign of deep prosthesis infection following implantation or haematogenous contamination. Because of its relatively superficial location, exposure of total knee replacement arthroplasty is the most common.

Aims
- To provide well-vascularized soft tissue cover and dead-space filling to aid antibiotic and host defence penetration and therefore maximize the chances of implant retention.
- In cases of implant loosening, to provide soft tissue cover and dead-space filling to clear the infection and allow later re-implantation.

Principles
- Debridement of all devitalized or infected poorly vascularized tissue.
- Stabilization of the skeleton by cement spacer, ex-fix, or plaster.
- Vascularized soft tissue coverage of the wound and any dead space.

Selection
Knee
- Medial and lateral gastrocnemius muscle flaps, or a combination of the two, can be used to cover most knee defects successfully.
- Fasciocutaneous flaps have also been reported to salvage exposed total knee replacement prostheses successfully.
- If the deficit is extensive or local flaps are inadequate or unavailable, free muscle transfer is the treatment of choice.

Elbow
- Brachioradialis or extensor carpi ulnaris can be pedicled and flipped through 180°, even using the tendon to reconstruct the triceps tendon if necessary.
- A proximally based posterior interosseous flap can be useful for exposure.
- Lateral arm flap if the previous surgical incision allows.

Shoulder
- Latissimus dorsi (muscle only or myocutaneous) or pectoralis major (muscle) are utilized.

Hip
Flaps are infrequently required because of the depth of the joint and surrounding tissues. However, if there is a very scarred bed maintaining the dead space following removal of the implant and creation of a Girdlestone hip, transposition of rectus femoris, vastus lateralis, or rectus abdominus can successfully close the dead space and wound.

Necrotizing soft tissue infection

Definition
Infection of soft tissues characterized by rapidly progressive inflammation and necrosis. Specific examples include necrotizing fasciitis, a term popularized by Wilson in 1952, gas gangrene, and Fournier's gangrene (necrotizing fasciitis of the perineum and scrotum).

Incidence
No reliable figures, but more common than believed.

Aetiology
- Predisposing factors:
  - Local: trauma, recent surgery, IV drug abuse, chronic venous ulceration, superficial skin infections.
  - Systemic: immunodeficiency (HIV/AIDS, steroid use, diabetes mellitus).

Microbiology
- Usually polymicrobial: average of 2.8 organisms per patient.
- Commonly anaerobes, skin flora, and gram-negative bacilli.
- Monomicrobial infections are usually caused by haemolytic group A streptococcus, *Staph. aureus*, or clostridial species.
- Gas gangrene is often caused by *Clostridium perfringens* which produces a lecithinase leading to myonecrosis and gas formation.

Clinical features
- Local: erythema, pain out of proportion to the inflammation, oedema, cyanosis or bronzing of the skin, induration, dermal thrombosis, epidermolysis, anaesthesia of the affected area as the cutaneous nerves become ischaemic, dermal gangrene, crepitus, vesicle formation.
- Systemic: fever, shock, acute renal failure.

Investigations
- The diagnosis of a necrotizing wound infection is clinical, and should lead to the immediate institution of a definitive management plan. No investigation should delay appropriate resuscitation and surgical debridement.
- Plain X-rays may demonstrate subcutaneous gas or a foreign body.
- MRI or frozen-section biopsy may aid diagnosis in difficult cases.

Management
Medical
Aggressive resuscitation with invasive monitoring to achieve fluid, electrolyte, and haemodynamic stability. Antibiotic therapy should be viewed as an adjunct to surgical debridement. Initial empirical antibiotic therapy should be broad spectrum and adjusted under the direction of a microbiologist in the light of the results of cultures of operative specimens.

Surgical
- **Acute phase** Surgical debridement is the mainstay of treatment, and must be performed early and aggressively—all necrotic tissue must be excised. The deep muscle should be inspected and resected if required. Debridement is adequate when finger dissection no longer easily separates the subcutaneous tissue from the fascia. The wound should be left open and packed. Patients should undergo re-exploration every 24–48 hr, earlier if indicated, until there is no further progression of the necrosis.
- **Reconstructive phase** Coverage of the wound should be delayed until the infection has clinically resolved. Methods employed include delayed primary closure, split-thickness skin grafting, local flaps, or free tissue transfer. Selection of the most appropriate method depends on the site and extent of disease.

Post-operative care
Patients should be managed in the ICU.

Prognosis
- Comorbid conditions which increase the risk of life-threatening infection are diabetes mellitus, peripheral vascular disease, malnutrition, malignancy, immunocompromised states (AIDS, steroid therapy), obesity, chronic alcohol or IV drug abuse.
- Other risk factors for death secondary to necrotizing soft tissue infection are extent of infection, delay in first debridement, and degree of organ system dysfunction at admission.

Elliott *et al.* (1996) reported a 25% mortality, comparable to the 20% reported by Meleney (1924).

References
Elliott DC, Kufera JA, Myers RA (1996). *Ann Surg* **224**, 672–83.
Meleney FL (1924). *J Exp Med* **40**, 233–52.

Chapter 16

Tumours

Fibromatoses *480*
Soft tissue sarcoma *481*
Neurilemoma (benign schwannoma) *488*
Neurofibroma *490*
Neurofibromatosis *492*
Lipoma *495*
Axillary dissection *497*
Groin dissection *500*
Sentinel lymph node biopsy *503*

Fibromatoses

Definition
- Connective tissue hyperplasia which infiltrates locally and is not malignant. They usually arise from fascia.
- Types include desmoids (rectus musculo-aponeurotic fibromatoses), nodular pseudosarcomatous fasciitis, plantar fibromatosis, aggressive fibromatosis, and juvenile digital fibromatosis.

Desmoid tumours (rectus musculo-aponeurotic fibromatoses)
- More common in females.
- Usually age 20–40 years.
- May be multifocal but are usually in association with musculo-aponeurotic fascia.
- Locally invasive and may cross fascial planes.
- Histologically see lots of collagen and fibrous spindle cells, but few mitoses. May see some mucoid degeneration.
- Aetiology unknown: trauma, hormonal (oestrogen) influence, related to Gardner's syndrome.
- Treatment is wide local excision.
- Local recurrence rates very high if incompletely excised.

Nodular pseudosarcomatous fasciitis
- Benign but worrying tumour of fibroblasts.
- Usually subcutaneous; fascial tumour rapidly growing; can be tender; can cross fascial planes and look invasive on MRI and histopathology.
- Aetiology unknown but possibly related to trauma.
- Treatment is wide excision and reconstruction. If recurrent consider re-excision and radiotherapy.

Plantar fibromatosis

Aggressive fibromatosis

Juvenile digital fibromatosis

Soft tissue sarcoma

Definition
The word 'sarcoma' is derived from a Greek word meaning 'fleshy growth'. Sarcomas are malignant tumours of mesenchymal origin, e.g. striated muscles, fat, fibrous tissue, and the vessels serving these tissues. By convention malignant tumours of the peripheral nervous system are also included.

Incidence
Relatively rare, accounting for less than 1% of malignant neoplasms; 1300 cases are seen each year in England and Wales. Can occur anywhere in the body, but most arise from the extremities, chest wall, mediastinum, and retroperitoneum. Incidence increases gradually in each decade of life, peaking in the sixties. Slightly more common in males.

Aetiology
Unknown in most cases. Many patients have a history of recent trauma, although this is thought merely to draw attention to underlying neoplasm. Can arise in lesions of inherited disorders, e.g. neurofibromatosis, multiple enchondromas. Exposure to ionizing radiation or previous radiotherapy and environmental carcinogens (e.g. phenoxyacetic acid pesticides, dioxins, and chlorophenol wood preservatives) have been implicated. Can arise in scars from thermal and acid burns and in the vicinity of prosthetic implants after a latent period. EBV has been implicated in the development of smooth muscle tumours in immunodeficient patients. Immunodeficiency has also been linked to the development of leiomyosarcomas and angiosarcomas.

Clinical features
There are no reliable physical signs to distinguish a benign mass from a malignant mass; both commonly present as a painless mass. Be suspicious when a mass is present with the following characteristics:
- Diameter >5 cm.
- Deep to deep fascia.
- Painful (especially night pain).
- Increasing size.

Classification
Earlier classifications were descriptive and based on nuclear configuration rather than type of tumour cell, e.g. 'round cell tumour', 'spindle cell sarcoma'. Recent classifications are based on the line of cell differentiation of the tumour.

Macroscopic
They enlarge in a centrifugal fashion, compressing normal tissue and giving the appearance of encapsulation. The pseudo-capsule contains an inner compressed rim of normal tissue, an outer rim of oedema, and newly formed vessels. Fingers of tumour can extend into and through the pseudo-capsule to form satellite lesions. Fascia, nerve sheath, and vessel adventitia are relatively resistant to invasion. Lymph node metastases are uncommon; lungs are the most common site for blood-borne systemic metastases.

Microscopic
Based on type of tissue formed by the tumour. The current WHO classification has 15 subtypes (Table 16.1). Further classification into high or low grade is based on cellularity, anaplasia, or pleomorphism, mitotic activity, expansive or infiltrative growth, and necrosis. Grading offers the best guide to the future risk of local recurrence, metastases and survival.

Staging
The two major staging systems used at present were developed by the American Joint Committee on Cancer (AJCC) and the Musculoskeletal Tumour Society as described by Enneking *et al.* (1980).

AJCC staging system (Table 16.2)
Based on the TNM staging system with the addition of tumour grade and depth relative to investing muscular fascia. Applicable to soft tissue sarcomas at any site. Uses 5 cm as an important dimension for determining prognosis, although this designation is arbitrary.

Musculoskeletal Tumor Society (Enneking) staging system (Table 16.3)
For sarcomas of both soft tissue and bone. With its emphasis on compartmentalization, it is best suited for extremity sarcomas. It does not include the type, size, or depth of tumour, and its grading system is probably too narrow for the wide biological range of soft tissue sarcomas.

Table 16.1 Histological classification of soft tissue sarcomas

Subtype	Classification	Example
I	Fibrous tumours	Fibrosarcoma
II	Fibrohistiocytic tumours	Malignant fibrous histiocytoma
III	Lipomatous tumours	Liposarcoma
IV	Smooth and skeletal muscle tumours	Rhabdomyosarcoma
V	Tumours of blood vessels	Kaposi's sarcoma
VI	Tumours of lymph vessels	Lymphangiosarcoma
VII	Synovial tumours	Synovial sarcoma
VIII	Mesothelial tumours	Mesothelioma
IX	Peripheral nerve sheath tumours	Malignant schwannoma
X	Primitive neuroectodermal	Neuroblastoma
XI	Paraganglionic tumours	Malignant paraganglioma
XII	Extraskeletal osseous and cartilaginous tumours	Extraskeletal osteosarcoma
XIII	Tumours of pluripotential mesenchyme	Malignant mesenchymoma
XIV	Tumours of uncertain histiogenesis	Epithelioid sarcoma
XV	Unclassified	

Adapted from Enzinger and Weiss (1988).

Investigations
Further evaluation or biopsy (or both) is indicated when a soft tissue mass arises without a history of trauma, or persists for more than 6 weeks after local trauma.

X-ray
Differentiates soft tissue and bone. Tumours adjacent to bone can cause a periosteal reaction. In most cases soft tissue sarcomas rarely invade bone, so neither X-rays nor bone scans prove helpful. Some soft tissue sarcomas show speckled calcification.

MRI scanning
Investigation of choice for delineating the anatomical boundaries of the tumour. Superior to CT scanning. Scintigraphy with tumour-seeking agents has been used, with a reported sensitivity of 56–93% using gallium or 89% using ^{99m}Tc(V)-dimercaptosuccinic acid (DMSA).

PET scanning
[^{18}F]fluorodeoxyglucose positron emission tomography (FDG-PET) allows visualization and quantification of glucose metabolism in cells (should be increased in malignant tumours). Used for identification and staging.

Biopsy
All soft tissue masses >5 cm in diameter and any new, enlarging, or symptomatic lesions should be biopsied. The choice of technique is dictated by the size, location of the mass, and experience of the pathologist: Neural and lipomatous tumours are difficult for the pathologist to diagnose accurately on small samples (needle biopsies) because of sampling error, low numbers of cells, and cellular activity. Biopsy sites should be excised with the tumour, and so should be planned and localized in conjuction with the surgeon, pathologist, and radiologist.

Fine-needle aspiration (FNA)
For sampling deep-seated tumours (e.g. retroperitoneal) under US or CT guidance. Minimizes the potential for tumour spillage in the peritoneal cavity. Acceptable for documenting local/distant recurrence in patients with a previously diagnosed sarcoma. Use is limited by difficulty in making an accurate diagnosis from a small cellular sample of aspirate.

Core-needle biopsy (trucuts or 14 gauge)
Predictive accuracy of >90% for the presence and type of soft tissue malignancy (less in lipomatous and neural tumours), and is cost effective. Limited by the small sample size (1 × 10 mm), or the tissue obtained may not be representative with consequent under-estimation of grade. Previous fears that it could cause haematoma formation and subsequent dissemination of tumour cells beyond the confines of the primary lesion are unproven.

Table 16.2 AJCC staging system of soft tissue sarcomas

Stage	Grade	Tumour size	Regional nodes	Distant metastases
IA	G1 or G2	T1a or T1b	N0	M0
IB	G1 or G2	T2a	N0	M0
IIA	G1 or G2	T2b	N0	M0
IIB	G3 or G4	T1b	N0	M0
IIC	G3 or G4	T2a	N0	M0
III	G3	T2b	N0	M0
IV	Any G	Any T	Nodal or distant metastases	

Histological grade of malignancy: G1 = well differentiated; G2 = moderately differentiated; G3 = poorly differentiated; G4 = undifferentiated.
Size of primary tumour: T1 = tumour ≤5 cm in greatest diameter; T1a = superficial tumour (entirely above fascia); T1b = Deep tumour (invasion of or entirely below fascia); T2 = tumour >5 cm in greatest diameter; T2a = superficial tumour (entirely above fascia); T2b = deep tumour (invasion of or entirely below fascia).
Regional lymph nodes: N0 = no histologically verified lymph node metastases; N1 = histologically verified lymph node metastases.
Distant metastases: M0 = no distant metastases; M1 = distant metastases present.

Table 16.3 Musculoskeletal Tumor Society (Enneking) staging system

Stage	Grade	Site	Metastases
IA	G1	T1	M0
IB	G1	T2	M0
IIA	G2	T1	M0
IIB	G2	T2	M0
III	G1 or G2	T1 or T2	M1

Grade of malignancy: G1 = any low-grade tumour; G2 = any high-grade tumour.
Size of primary tumour: T1 = Intracompartmental tumours confined within boundaries of well-defined anatomical structures (e.g. intra-articular, superficial to deep fascia); T2 = extracompartmental tumours arising from or involving extra-fascial spaces or planes that have no natural anatomical barriers (e.g. soft tissue extension, deep fascial extension).
Metastases: M0 = no regional or distant metastases; M1 = regional or distant metastases present.

Excisional biopsy
Refers to the removal of the lesion with or without a significant margin of normal tissue. Should be reserved for extremely superficial lesions, or lesions <3–5 cm in diameter. Excisional biopsies of large or deep sarcomas are undesirable as they can contaminate surrounding tissue planes and compromise subsequent definitive surgical procedure. Although sarcomas appear to be encapsulated, in reality many have a pseudo-capsule, and enucleating the tumour through its pseudo-capsule leaves gross or microscopic cancer behind.

Incisional (open) biopsy
Involves removal of a generous wedge of tissue performed through incisions which can easily be incorporated within the incision planned for future resection (e.g. orientate incision along the long axis of the extremity involved, keep buttock incisions low so as not to prejudice the posterior flap of subsequent hindquarter amputation). Attention to haemostasis minimizes haematoma formation. Drains should exit either through or near the biopsy incision, and the drain tract must be excised in continuity with the tumour if it is subsequently proven to be malignant.

Treatment

Current regimes aim to achieve effective local control with minimal functional disturbance using surgery and radiotherapy. Adjuvant chemotherapy remains controversial in most extremity sarcomas but has a role in specific intra-abdominal sarcomas (GIST).

Physical examination
Determine the size of the tumour, any fixation to adjacent structures, relation to biopsy site, functional status of the involved part and the patient, lymph node involvement, staging, and any confounding conditions that could compromise optimal surgical or radiation treatment.

Radiological imaging
CXR and chest CT scan to search for pulmonary metastases. CT scan including the liver should be added for intra-abdominal or retro-peritoneal tumours.

Surgery
The high recurrence rate following enucleation and knowledge that sarcomas initially spread along rather than across fascial planes led to excisions which included the whole musculofascial compartment (compartmentectomy). In practice, a radical wide excision is preferable, consisting of a wide excision of tumour with one intact tissue plane on all sides of the tumour. The extent of surgical resection is dependent upon the exact anatomical site defined by MRI and CT. Muscles to be sacrificed are resected from their origin to insertion whenever possible. Unless encased by tumour, large arteries are dissected free in the subadventitial plane as they are rarely invaded. Reconstruction with autologous vein graft is advocated if the artery is sacrificied. Major veins are more commonly invaded and can be sacrificed without reconstruction, with the exception of the common femoral, common iliac, and subclavian veins. Subsequent limb function will be better if these veins are reconstructed. Tumour is dissected off major

nerves, taking the epineurium. Amputation is reserved for recurrent unresectable tumours. To reduce the risk of stump recurrence, amputation is not carried out through the compartment of origin (e.g. hindquarter amputation for proximal thigh tumours, through-knee amputation for foot or ankle sarcomas).

Lymph node resection
There is no benefit in removing clinically normal lymph nodes, and lymph node dissection should only be performed in the absence of other metastatic disease.

Metastases
Curative resection of pulmonary metastases can be considered in the absence of extrapulmonary metastases. Single metastases can be considered for resection. Multiple metastases need to be treated in conjunction with the oncologist but palliative resection may be indicated.

Radiotherapy
Post-operative radiotherapy after wide local excision provides excellent local control for primary extremity sarcomas, reducing local recurrence rates significantly. Pre-operative radiotherapy is controversial; it may improve local control rates for large tumours, and in some cases shrinks unresectable tumours sufficiently to permit limb-sparing resection. Radiotherapy is more effective on untraumatized tissue because of the better blood supply and absence of scarred or fibrotic avascular dead spaces. A total of ≥ 60 Gy is required and, to avoid lymphoedema, the entire circumference of the limb must not be irradiated, i.e. a strip of skin and subcutaneous tissue away from the tumour is excluded from the treatment field. Brachytherapy offers similar benefits to external beam radiation for high-grade tumours.

Chemotherapy
No conclusive evidence that chemotherapy improves survival compared with surgery alone. Some trials have shown significant disease-free and overall survival benefit for extremity sarcomas, but the magnitude of this benefit against the significant cardiotoxic side effects must be determined on an individual basis. Nonetheless, for patients without a curative surgical option, chemotherapy represents the best currently available palliative treatment.

Isolated limb perfusion
Limb perfusion using melphalan, tumour necrosis factor-α and interferon-γ has been most effective. Although the response is usually transient, some tumours have shrunk sufficiently to permit limb-sparing surgery.

Prognosis
Grade, size, and depth are significant predictive factors with respect to survival (Table 16.4). However, the relation between these factors and prognosis is not yet defined, i.e. whether a small superficial high-grade sarcoma has a prognosis similar to a large deep low-grade sarcoma. Nodal involvement conveys the same prognosis as distant metastatic disease i.e. stage IV, and 5-year survival is 20%.

Table 16.4 Five-year disease-free survival rates by tumour size for patients with intermediate and high-grade sarcomas treated with surgery and irradiation

Tumour size (cm)	No. of patients*	% disease-free at 5 years
< 2.5	17	94
2.6–4.9	48	77
5.0–10.0	55	62
10.1–15.0	24	51
15.1–20.0	9	42
>20.0	6	17

*Only patients in whom local control was achieved were included.

From Suit et al. (1988).

References

Enneking WF, Spanier SS, Goodman MA (1980). *Orthop Relat Res* **153**, 106–20.
Enzinger FM, Weiss SW (1988). *Soft Tissue Tumors* (2nd edn). Mosby, St. Louis, MO.
Suit HD, Mankin HJ, Wood WC, et al. (1988). *J Clin Oncol* **6**, 854–62.

Neurilemoma (benign schwannoma)

Definition
This is a benign nerve sheath tumour arising eccentrically from the nerve.

Incidence
- Most common nerve tumour.
- All age groups, but most common in the age range 20–50 years.
- Equal involvement of both sexes.

Classification
- Benign schwannoma.
- Ancient (degenerated) schwannoma: large tumours of long duration with marked degenerative change.
- Cellular schwannoma: misdiagnosed as malignant in 25% of cases because of high cellularity and mitotic activity.
- Plexiform neurilemoma (5%): these grow in a plexiform or multinodular pattern which may not be clinically obvious. Less than 5% have neurofibromatosis.

Clinical presentation
- Usually present as solitary lesions; occasionally may be multiple or within the context of NF1.
- Common sites are the head, neck, and flexor surfaces of the upper and lower extremities.
- Deep-seated tumours are present in the retroperitoneum and mediastinum.
- Slow-growing tumour; usually painless and mobile perpendicular to the axis of the involved nerve.
- Occasionally causes symptoms of tenderness, paraesthesia, numbness, or weakness because of pressure/compression on nerve.

Pathology
Gross appearance
Well-encapsulated eccentric tumours which may resemble neurofibromas. The cut section may show a yellow, greyish, or a pink appearance. Secondary degenerative changes are not uncommon and help distinguish them from neurofibromas. These degenerative changes may be in the form of cystification or calcification.

Microscopic appearance
Well-marked fibrous capsule. No evidence of neurites within the substance of the tumour. Characterized by the presence of Antoni A and Antoni B areas. Antoni A areas are S-100 protein staining areas which are composed of orderly compacted spindle cells. Antoni B areas are less orderly and far less cellular. There are large irregular spaced vessels which are conspicuous in the relatively acellular Antoni B areas.

Management
- Investigation is by MRI or US.
- Malignant change is very rare and cannot be reliably detected by imaging. Suspect malignancy if >5 cm in diameter, causing pain at night, or neurological symptoms.
- Indication for excision:
  - Growing mass causing concern.
  - Symptomatic—pain, tenderness, pressure effect.
  - Neurological symptoms of paraesthesia, numbness, or weakness.
  - Mass itself causing disfigurement.
- These tumours are well encapsulated and, being eccentric, can usually be removed without sacrificing the nerve.
- The rate of incomplete excision and hence of recurrence is very small.

Neurofibroma

Definition
A benign lesion arising from within the peripheral nerve.

Incidence
- Most commont nerve tumour.
- All age groups but are most common in the range 20–50 years.
- Equal involvement of both sexes.

Classification
- Solitary cutaneous neurofibroma: single superficial neurofibroma arising outside the clinical picture of neurofibromatosis. Equal in both sexes. Common in the age group 20–30 years. Evenly distributed over body surface. Slow-growing, usually painless nodules. Rare malignant change possible.
- Peripheral neurofibroma: not associated with NF, but occurring as solitary lesion arising from peripheral nerve.
- Visceral neurofibroma: neurofibroma involving various organ systems (GIT, appendix, larynx, heart, etc.)
- Plexiform neurofibroma (elephantiasis neuromatosa): diffuse neurofibroma arising from a superficial mainly cutaneous nerve and associated with gross disfigurement. This neurofibroma is characterized by myxoid degeneration. Also termed a paraneuroma it commonly arises in children and young adults.
- Neurofibromatosis: further subclassified into Types I (peripheral) and II(central).
- Pseudo-arthrosis: neurofibroma involving the bone. Common in the tibia in growing children.
- Osseous involvement: thinning of long-bone cortex or sphenoid dysplasia.
- Acoustic neuroma: central form of neurofibroma or schwannoma involvement in NF2.
- Central involvement: optic nerve glioma, astrocytoma, and a variety of heterotopias (non-NF2).

Clinical presentation
- Usually present as solitary lesions; occasionally may be multiple especially within the context of NF1.
- Common sites are the head, neck, and flexor surfaces of the upper and lower extremities.
- Deeply seated tumours are present in the retroperitoneum and mediastinum.
- Slow-growing tumour, usually painless and mobile perpendicular to the axis of the involved nerve.
- Occasionally cause symptoms of tenderness, paraesthesia, numbness, or weakness because of pressure/compression on nerve or invasion following malignant change.

Pathology
Gross appearance
White-grey tumours lacking the secondary degenerative changes associated with neurilemmomas (schwannomas). They arise from within the structure of the nerve and tend to expand it in a fusiform manner. The normal nerve can usually be seen entering and leaving the swelling.

Microscopic appearance
Histological appearance varies depending upon the content of cells, mucin, and collagen. There are interlacing bundles of elongated cells with wavy dark-staining nuclei. A small amount of mucoid material separates these cells from adjacent strands of collagen. Neurites are visible within the substance of the tumour.

Management
- Investigation is by MRI or US.
- The incidence of malignant change is rare except in NF. Malignancy cannot be reliably detected by imaging.
- Suspect malignancy if:
  - Tumour is >5 cm in diameter.
  - Tumour is growing.
  - Tumour is causing pain at night.
  - There are neurological symptoms.
- Indication for excision or incision biopsy (needle biopsy is unreliable for nerve tumours because of the sparseness of mitoses).
  - Growing mass causing concern.
  - Symptomatic—pain, tenderness, pressure effect.
  - Neurological symptoms of paraesthesia, numbness, or weakness.
  - Mass itself causing disfigurement.
- These tumours are not encapsulated, but despite this they can usually be removed without sacrificing the majority of the nerve. They do not 'shell out' like schwannomas.
- The rate of incomplete excision and hence of recurrence is moderate.

Neurofibromatosis

Also known as von Recklinghausen's disease.

Definition
Hereditary form of multiple neurofibroma, which was considered to be a single disease for a long time, but is now recognized to be two clinically and genetically distinct entities.

Incidence
Neurofibromatosis 1 (NF1)
- 1 in 2500–3000 live births.

Neurofibromatosis 2 (NF2)
- 1 in 50 000 live births.
- Rare compared with NF1.

Classification
- Neurofibromatosis 1: previous peripheral form of the disease.
- Neurofibromatosis 2 or bilateral acoustic neurofibromatosis: previous central form of the disease.

Neurofibromatosis 1
Genetics
- Autosomal dominant with a high rate of penetrance.
- Half these patients have affected family members; the remainder represent new mutations.
- Associated with insertions, deletions, or mutations in the *NF1* gene which is a tumour suppressor gene located on chromosome 17.

Diagnostic criteria

Two or more of the following signs or factors in a single individual:
- Six or more café-au-lait macules with greatest diameter >5 mm in pre-pubertal individuals, and >15 mm in post-pubertal individuals.
- Two or more neurofibromas of any type or one plexiform neurofibroma.
- Freckling in the axillary or inguinal region.
- Optic glioma.
- Two or more Lisch nodules (iris hamartomas).
- A distinct osseous lesion, such as sphenoid dysplasia or thinning of long-bone cortex, with or without pseudo-arthrosis.
- A first-degree relative with NF1 by the above criteria.

Clinical features
- Axillary or inguinal freckling.
- Multiple cutaneous or visceral neurofibromas:
  - Present as small soft cutaneous nodules.
  - Some may be tender.
  - Neurofibromas make their appearance during childhood or adolescence and may involve any organ system (visceral or cutaneous). CNS or bony involvement is not uncommon.

NEUROFIBROMATOSIS

- Multiple café-au-lait spots:
  - >90% of patients with NF1 have café-au-lait spots and their number and size serves as a useful guide in determining the diagnosis and prognosis of this disease.
  - Patients with fewer café-au-lait spots tend to have either a late onset of palpable neurofibromas, segmental involvement with neurofibromatosis, or NF2.
  - Large café au lait spots may herald the later development of subcutaneous or deeper tissue plexiform neurofibromas.
- Tissue plexiform neurofibromas are small to massive areas of tissue neurofibromatosis:
  - Soft homogenous masses.
  - Involve all tissue planes deep to a café au lait spot which may be very pale.
  - Highly vascular.
  - Usually warm and sweaty.
  - Heal poorly.
- Peripheral nerve tumours (either neurofibromas or schwannomas) develop and may cause symptoms:
  - These tumours may be multiple and large and are confusingly described as plexiform neurofibromas by geneticists.
  - These tumours are the ones which undergo malignant transformation; however, malignancy can arise in small subcutaneous masses.
- Pseudo-arthrosis or complications therefrom may be an initial presenting feature.
- Young men with this condition may develop gynaecomastia. It is a histologically different entity from true gynaecomastia and hence has been termed *pseudo-gynaecomastia*.
- Optic gliomas and Lisch nodules are rarely detected by plastic surgeons.

Treatment

Indications for surgery include:
- Large lesions which cause mechanical problems or adverse cosmesis.
- Multiple cutaneous lesions causing problems with hygiene, cosmesis.
- Painful lesions.
- Lesions which compromise organ function.
- Lesions causing neuropathy.
- Lesions suspicious of malignancy (rapidly growing, >5 cm in diameter, situated on a deep nerve, causing pain (especially at night) or other neuropathy.

Even after so-called complete excision of these lesions, there is often clinical recurrence because the majority are ill defined.

Surgical options

- Multiple cutaneous excisions by scalpel, loop diathermy, laser.
- Debulking of tissue plexiform neurofibromas.
- Incision or excision biopsy of suspicious nerve tumours.
- Excision of pseudo-arthroses and reconstruction by free bone flap transfer.
- Wide excision of MPNST and reconstruction by nerve grafting or tendon transfers.

Malignant change
- Occurs in 2–29% of all cases.
- Malignant tumours tend to develop in patients who have manifested the disease for at least 10 years.
- Rapid enlargement or pain in a pre-existing neurofibroma usually signals the development of a neurosarcoma, and an incision or excision biopsy is mandatory.
- The prognosis after treatment of MPNST by wide local excision and/or amputation is very poor, with a 5-year survival of 20%.

Neurofibromatosis 2

Genetics
Autosomal dominant with a high rate of penetrance (95%).
Localized to changes in a gene on chromosome 22.

Diagnostic criteria
- Bilateral CN VIII masses confirmed by CT scan or MRI.
- First degree relative with NF2 and either unilateral CN VIII mass or two of the following:
  - Neurofibroma.
  - Meningioma.
  - Glioma.
  - Schwannoma.
  - Juvenile posterior subcapsular lenticular opacity.

Clinical features
Onset usually in adolescence or early adult life, with hearing loss or tinnitus. Café-au-lait spots and neurofibromas may be present, but in far fewer numbers than in NF1.

Management
- Acoustic neuromas are excised by neurosurgeons and the frequent resulting facial nerve palsy is treated by plastic surgeons.
- Neurofibromas and schwannomas are excised as indicated.

Lipoma

Definition
- A lipoma is a benign neoplasm (hamartoma) containing adipose (fat) cells of the adult type.
- A hibernoma contains fetal fat cells (brown fat). It is usually found in the first 6 months of life, mainly in the retroperitoneum.

Incidence
Very common.

Aetiology
Unknown.

Classification
Lipomas can be classified according to:
- Capsule.
    - Encapsulated.
    - Non-encapsulated.
- Anatomical location:
    - Subcutaneous.
    - Submuscular.
    - Intramuscular.
    - Subperiosteal.
    - Retroperitoneal.
    - Spinal.
    - Mediastinal.
    - Nape of neck ('buffalo hump' appearance): Madelung's disease.
- Presence of associated tissue:
    - Angiolipoma.
    - Fibrolipoma.
- Number:
    - Single—lipoma.
    - Multiple—lipomatosis.
- Associated tenderness
    - Multiple lipomas—Dercum's disease (painless).
    - Multiple lipomas—adiposa dolorosum (painful angiolipomas).

Clinical presentation
Usually well circumscribed, soft to cystic (fat is fluid at body temperature), mobile in all planes, not tethered to overlying skin.

Investigations
- Clinical examination usually suffices.
- US/MRI scan when lipoma very large, associated with vital structure, deep to deep fascia or in specific anatomical locations (head and neck, midline of back, etc.).

Management
Formal surgical excision. With soft subcutaneous lipomas an incision directly over the swelling and a squeeze usually delivers the lipoma. Larger and deeper lipomas require formal excision. Meticulous haemostasis with drains wherever required, as haematomas are a common post-operative complication.

Complications
- Pain.
- Fat necrosis.
- Calcification.
- Pressure symptoms on surrounding structures.
- Malignant change (to liposarcoma, usually with very large long-standing lipomas, deep to deep fascia, in the retroperitoneum, back, or thigh). Suspect if >5 cm diameter, deep to deep fascia, causing symptoms (especially pain).

Axillary dissection

Also known as axillary block dissection, axillary lymphadenectomy, axillary clearance.

Aim
To remove *en bloc* the axillary lymph nodes (levels I, II, and III).

Indications
- Metastatic nodal involvement with no or limited distant disease.
- Diagnosis usually confirmed by FNA.
- Not indicated in lymphoma.

Pathology
- Skin (MM, SCC).
- Breast carcinoma.

Clinical anatomy
- Apex: bounded by the outer border of the first rib medially, the posterior surface of the clavicle anteriorly, and the superior border of the scapula posteriorly.
- Base: formed by axillary fascia extending between the lower borders of the pectoralis major anteriorly and the latissimus dorsi posteriorly.
- Anterior wall: pectoralis major and minor, subclavius and clavipectoral fascia.
- Posterior wall: subscapularis above, with teres major and latissimus dorsi tendon below.
- Medial wall: first four ribs and serratus anterior.
- Lateral wall: quite narrow; forms at the convergence of the anterior and posterior walls and is bounded by the humerus, coracobrachialis, and biceps brachii.
- Contents: axillary artery and vein, brachial plexus, intercostobrachial nerves (lateral cutaneous branches of second and often the third intercostal nerves), fat, loose areolar tissue, and the axillary lymph nodes.

Axillary lymph node groups
Up to 50 (normally 15–30) arranged in three surgical groups:
- Level I: lateral to pectoralis minor.
- Level II: deep to pectoralis minor.
- Level III: medial to pectoralis minor.

Also arranged in anatomical groups:
- Anterior (pectoral) group (four or five nodes, equivalent to Level I): within the medial axillary wall along the lower border of pectoralis minor and along the lateral thoracic artery. Drains the skin and muscles of the anterior and lateral thoracic walls and the majority of the breast.

- Posterior (subscapular) group (six or seven nodes, equivalent to Level I): within the posterior element of the medial axillary wall along the subscapular artery. Drains the posterior thoracic wall and the axillary tail of the breast.
- Lateral group (four to six nodes, equivalent to Level II): lies to the medial and posterior aspects of the axillary vein. Drains the entire upper limb.
- Central (intermediate) group (three or four nodes, equivalent to Level II): lie within adipose tissue within the base of the axilla. Receives lymph from all the preceding nodes.
- Apical (subclavicular) group (six to twelve nodes, equivalent to Level III): within the apex of the axilla lying partly posterior to the upper portion of pectoralis minor and partly above this muscle. Receives lymph from all the preceding nodes.

Pre-operative planning

As for groin dissection.

Patient preparation in theatre

Supine or beach-chair with arm free draped to allow repositioning during surgery. An adjustable forearm support bar or arm board facilitates immobilization of the upper limb in the desired position. Standard skin preparation and shaving. DVT prophylaxis. Prophylactic antibiotics.

Incision

Inverted U-shaped incision (with arm abducted) with the apex of the U pointing to the deltopectoral groove. Thick skin flaps minimize risk of skin flap necrosis. There is frequently an intra-subcutaneous fat fascial plane to follow similar to Camper's fascia. Alternatively, an oblique anterior axillary incision or a zigzag incision can be made along the posterior border of pectoralis major. The U is preferred because the flap falls posteriorly, aiding exposure, and flap necrosis is rare.

Procedure

With the arm in abduction, elevate the skin flap and allow it to fall posteriorly. Delineate the boundaries of the axilla by incising the fat along the posterior border of pectoralis major anteriorly and the anterior border of latissimus dorsi posteriorly. The inferior margin is at the level of the inferior edge of the pectoralis and LD in the axilla. This inferior margin is indistinct. The lateral margin is where the fat thins as it enters the arm and where the pectoralis and latissimus converge. When the margins are defined, the fat is swept off pectoralis major taking care to preserve the lateral pectoral nerve on its deep surface. Continue elevating the fat from the medial axillary wall, preserving the long thoracic (to serratus anterior) and thoracodorsal (to latissimus dorsi) nerves. Elevate the fat from the posterior wall. Then work on the superior margin, elevating the fat from the axillary vein. The intercostobrachial nerve(s) can be difficult to identify (and thus frequently damaged) as they lie deep and roughly parallel to the axillary vein, which is a key landmark during the procedure. The surgeon should ensure that their dissection plane remains inferior to the vein. Flexing the arm to 90° allows pectoralis major to relax, thus improving access around pectoralis minor, which can be divided at its insertion to the coracoid to improve exposure. The axillary vein is skeletonized and the tributaries ligated as the fat is dissected off in a lateral to medial direction. Orientate and mark the specimen for the pathologist.

In the absence of palpable lymphadenopathy of the Level III nodes, some surgeons may elect to leave them *in situ* in order to minimize post-operative lymphoedema.

Note that if axillary dissection is performed concomitantly with a modified radical mastectomy, the breast tissue and axillary contents are usually removed *en bloc*.

If axillary dissection follows breast-conserving surgery, mastectomy, or any cancer clearance procedure, a new set of instruments, gloves, etc. must be used for the axillary dissection to avoid metastatic seeding.

Closure

Haemostasis; wound irrigation; suction drainage; tension-free skin closure. Some surgeons excise a skin strip from both wound edges prior to primary closure.

Post-operative care

Keep the drain on suction. Mobilize the shoulder as soon as tolerated to avoid 'frozen shoulder' and stiffness. Shoulder exercises and physiotherapy may be needed for some time post-operation. Mobilize the hand and arm as soon as possible to reduce lymphoedema and stiffness. A Tubigrip stocking may also help.

Complications

- Seroma/lymphocoele.
- Haematoma.
- Wound dehiscence.
- Wound edge necrosis.
- Wound infection.
- Lymphoedema.
- Paraesthesia on the medial aspect of the upper arm caused by inter-costobrachial nerve trauma. This causes much morbidity and every effort should be made to preserve the nerve.
- Chronic shoulder weakness and stiffness may be experienced; thus early post-operative mobilization is encouraged.
- Winging of the scapula may result from injury to the long thoracic nerve.
- Axillary vein thrombosis.

Groin dissection

Groin dissection, inguinal lymphadenectomy, block dissection, groin clearance.

Aim
To remove *en bloc* the deep and superficial lymph nodes of the inguinal region. First described by Basset in 1912. An ilioinguinal, or radical, groin dissection may be performed, where the inguinal, iliac, and obturator nodes are removed in continuity.

Indications
- Prophylactic (aim to remove clinically undetectable micrometastases in order to prevent further dissemination of disease). The benefits of prophylactic surgery must be weighed against the morbidity of the procedure. Current UK guidelines for the management of cutaneous melanoma do not support routine prophylactic lymphadenectomy as it has not been shown to improve survival.
- Therapeutic (when lymph node metastatic involvement is confirmed pathologically by FNA or on very strong suspicion).

Pathology
Cutaneous malignancy (MM, SCC), female genital tract (vulval SCC), male genital tract (penile SCC), gastrointestinal tract (anal SCC).

Clinical anatomy
The femoral triangle is bounded by the medial border of sartorius laterally, the medial border of adductor longus medially, and the inguinal ligament superiorly. The gutter-shaped floor is formed (from lateral to medial) by iliacus, psoas major, pectineus, part of the adductor brevis, and adductor longus. The femoral sheath (containing the artery, vein, and femoral canal) lies at the deepest part of the gutter, with the femoral nerve lying outside and lateral to the sheath. The roof is formed by fascia lata, cribriform fascia, subcutaneous tissue, and skin.

Superficial inguinal nodes
These are found superficial to fascia lata and the cribriform fascia within the boundaries of the femoral triangle. They receive afferent superficial lymphatics from the lower extremity, scrotum, penis, vulva, clitoris, anus, and the infra-umbilical region of the anterior abdominal wall. The superficial inguinal nodes can be subdivided into:
- Vertical: nodes near the long saphenous vein (leg).
- Lateral: nodes near the lateral inguinal ligament (buttocks).
- Medial: nodes near the medial half of the inguinal ligament (genitals, perineum, lower abdomen from ASIS to umbilicus).

Deep inguinal nodes
Deep to the cribriform fascia, and medial to the femoral vein, are six to eight deep inguinal nodes, the most consistent of which is Cloquet's node, located at the apex of femoral canal. The deep nodes receive afferents from the superficial inguinal nodes and the deep lymphatic trunks associated with the femoral vessels, which in turn drain the

popliteal nodes. The deep inguinal nodes drain into the external iliac nodes, which also receive direct afferents from the superficial inguinal group.

Pre-operative planning
Full clinical assessment; exclude generalized lymphadenopathy or advanced metastatic disease. In the context of clinical lymphadenopathy (as opposed to a positive SLNB) confirm pathological diagnosis by FNAC (almost 100% sensitivity and specificity with melanoma). Accurately stage disease radiologically (CT or MRI).

Patient preparation in theatre
Supine position with hip extended, abducted, and externally rotated. Standard skin preparation and shaving. Urethral catheterization optional. DVT prophylaxis. Prophylactic antibiotics.

Incision
Oblique longitudinal, or longitudinal over femoral canal and then dogleg laterally at inguinal ligament. Thick skin flaps are raised.

Procedure
Delineate the borders of the femoral triangle, superiorly the inguinal ligament, laterally the sartorius, and medially the adductor longus. Working from above infero-laterally, the femoral vessels are skeletonized. Traditionally, the long saphenous vein is divided, although preservation may reduce the risk of post-operative lymphoedema. Many surgeons perform a sartorius transposition (or 'switch') in order to protect the underlying femoral vessels in the event of a post-operative wound breakdown. The sartorius muscle is divided at its proximal insertion and the muscle belly is reflected medially (turned over like page in a book) and secured to the inguinal ligament. Orientate and mark the specimen for the pathologist.

Closure
Haemostasis; wound irrigation; suction drainage. Tension-free skin closure. Some surgeons excise a skin strip from both wound edges prior to primary closure.

Post-operative care
Controversy regarding duration of post-operative suction drainage. Some advocate early drain removal 24 hr post-operatively; others wait for drainage to fall below a specific threshold (e.g. 20 ml/24 hr), which may take some weeks. Mean inpatient stay in England is 12.8 days. Patient could go home with drain *in situ*. Early ambulation minimizes DVT risk, although may augment lymph drainage. Fit to drive approximately 4–6 weeks post surgery. Consider TED stockings or Tubigrip for DVT and lymphoedema prophylaxis.

Complications
Common and often debilitating, but rarely fatal:
- Seroma/lymphocoele formation (6–40%) is minimized by meticulous suture or clip ligation of divided lymphatics (diathermy is ineffective). Treated by percutaneous aspiration; recurrences may be managed by instillation of sclerosants such as povidone iodine, talcum powder, or doxycycline.
- Haematoma (2–4%).
- Wound dehiscence (17–65%) and wound infection (6–20%) are more frequent in elderly and the obese.
- Lymphoedema (22–80%).
- Paraesthesia due to division of lateral cutaneous nerve of thigh or femoral branch of genitofemoral nerve.
- DVT and PE.

Ilio-inguinal or radical groin clearance
- No survival benefit.
- Increased morbidity.
- Indicated in certain patients after discussion at the MDT.

Sentinel lymph node biopsy

Definition
The sentinel node is the first node in a lymphatic basin to which cells from a specific primary tumour site will drain.

Principles
Human and animal studies show well-defined lymph pathways leading from each cutaneous territory (cutaneous lymphosomes) to specific regional lymph node(s). Importantly, in melanoma, absence of melanoma in the sentinel node is very specific of the basin being melanoma free.

Uses
This technique has now been used for most solid tumours.

Indications
Melanoma >1 mm in depth. There are indications for sentinel lymph node biopsy (SLNB) in tumours <1 mm deep (e.g. high mitotic count, regression, and ulceration in a young patient). At depths <1 mm <1% of sentinel nodes are positive, at 1–2 mm 5% are positive, and at 2–3 mm 18% are positive. The overall positive rate across all depths is 18–20%. The patient should be fit and prepared to undertake potential completion regional lymphadenectomy or adjunctive trials.

Sensitivity
In experienced hands sensitivity is 95–98%. However, a figure as low as 50% has been suggested for early in the learning curve.

Technique
SLNB should be done after the excision biopsy but before the wider excision. It can be done after the wider excision, but the sensitivity drops to 85%. Mapping of the lymph channels is by a triple test. First, injection of radioactive colloid around the biopsy scar to produce a lymphoscintogram. Secondly, intra-operative injection of patent blue dye around the biopsy scar. Both injection sites will be removed by the wider excision. The gamma probe is placed over the relevant lymph node basin demonstrated by the lymphoscintogram.

Incision
Over the hot node, the incision should be orientated to permit extension for later node dissection if required.

Procedure
Deepen the incision looking for blue lymph channels. Use the gamma probe to direct dissection. Ensure that the probe is not pointing towards the primary injection site and hence picking up a transmitted signal from there. Grab the soft tissue around the hot blue node. Carefully ligaclip around the node. Bipolar can be used, but away from the node as bipolar burn can interfere with the pathology of the node. Do a target count. Check the residual count. A residual count >10% of the target should encourage the operator to search for a second node. The average number of nodes removed is 1.7. Wash out; closure with absorbable suture 4/0.

Post-operative care
Nothing specific.

Complications
Wound problems, lymphoedema (2–6%), lymhocoele.

Tips
Remember that the lymphoscintogram is two-dimensional; hence a second node can lie beneath the first.

Advantages
- SLNB gives prognostic information and currently the sentinel node status is essential for accurate staging. It can identify patients who may benefit from early lymphadenectomy and hence local control.
- Sentinel node positive status permits entry into trials of adjunctive chemo- or immunotherapy.
- Psychological benefit of a node-negative result. Low morbidity procedure.
- Very sensitive (skip lesions in melanoma 0–2%).
- Defines site of drainage in the head and neck and trunk.

Disadvantages
- General anaesthetic and complications of the procedure (see above).
- Cost implications.
- There may be harm from disrupting the draining lymph nodes and hence the body's resistance to melanoma.

Survival
There is currently no evidence that survival is increased in patients who undergo a SLNB and completion dissection as opposed to those who have wide excision, and observation, and dissection when the disease becomes palpable. It is proposed that there may be some survival benefit for certain depths of melanoma.

Chapter 17

Trauma

Extravasation 506
Frostbite 508
Traumatic tattooing 510
Degloving injuries 511
Crush injuries 513
Compartment syndrome 515
Fasciotomy 518
Gunshot and blast injuries 522

Facial trauma
Facial lacerations 524
Middle-third facial injuries 527

Hand trauma
Hand assessment in trauma 533
Nailbed and perionychial injuries 537
Flexor tendon injuries 540
Flexor tendon repair 542
Flexor tendon avulsion 544
Flexor tendon rehabilitation 546
Ring avulsion injury 548
Boutonnière deformity 549
Swan-neck deformity 551
Ulnar collateral ligament injury of the thumb MCPJ 553
Hand fractures 555
Complications in metacarpal and phalangeal fractures 570
Scaphoid fracture 573
Carpal instability 576
Distal radius fractures 579

DRUJ disorders 582
DRUJ instability 583
Ulna head procedures 584
Triangular fibro-cartilaginous complex (TFCC) disorders 585
Ulnocarpal abutment syndrome 587
Brachial plexus injuries 589
Obstetrical brachial plexus palsy 593
Sequelae of obstetrical brachial palsy 595
Volkmann's ischaemic contracture 596

Peripheral nerve
Peripheral nerve injury 598
Tendon transfers 600

Burns
Burns emergency care 602
Burns fluid resuscitation 604
Assessment of burns 606
Escharotomy 610
Pathophysiology of the burn wound 613
Burn infection 616
Burn treatment 618
Burn reconstruction 620
Burns to trunk, genitalia, and head and neck 621
Hand burns 623
Foot burns 625
Chemical burns 626
Electrical burns 628
Non-accidental injury in burns 630

Extravasation

Definition
Escape of a drug from a vessel into the subcutaneous tissues.

Incidence
In 2003 there were 365 reported incidents in the UK (via the green card system). This includes all extravasations, regardless of drug.

Aetiology
- Extremes of age.
- Lymphoedematous skin.
- Altered mental state: cannot report pain in cannula.
- Multiple venepunctures and thrombosed vessels; re-using a vein.
- Peripheral neuropathies.
- Peripheral vascular disease.
- Superior vena cava obstruction: increased pressure in arm veins.

Classification
- Pre-extravasation syndrome: severe phlebitis or hypersensitivity but little or no leakage; may progress to extravasation.
- Type I: blister, swelling around site. Usually due to injection under pressure.
- Type II: soft diffuse swelling indicating dispersal of drug.
- Drug reactions are classified as:
  - Vesicant—causes blistering or tissue necrosis.
  - Irritant—causes pain and inflammation, but no necrosis.
  - None—no reaction if administered via subcutaneous, intradermal or intramuscular route.

Pathogenesis
- Vesicants bind to DNA and may recycle locally. Therefore necrosis may progress over several weeks.
- Acids, alkalis, or fluids with osmolarity greater than plasma cause tissue necrosis.
- Irritation due to histamine release.

Clinical features
- Pain around cannula site.
- Swelling.
- Erythema or blistering.
- Increased resistance when injecting IV drug.
- Lack of return of blood from cannula, although absence of this sign does not rule out extravasation.

Differential diagnoses
Exclude the following differential diagnoses before treatment:
- Flare reaction.
- Coloured infusions.
- Vessel irritation, may cause aching or tightness. Warming the vein may help.
- Venous shock due to rapid injection of cold drugs. Again, try warming the vein.

Management

Medical
Prevention is ideal. Use a suitable site and monitor the injection. If extravasation is suspected, treat promptly:
- Stop infusion and disconnect it.
- Aspirate drug from cannula.
- Elevate limb.
- Advice on further management varies, and depends on the drug:
  - For non-vesicant drugs, elevate and apply cold compresses for 24–48 hr.
  - Specific antidotes include DMSO and sodium thiosulphate for chemotherapeutic vesicants, and phentolamine for vasoconstrictors.
  - Vesicant drugs which cannot be neutralized are dispersed. Apply warm compresses. Hyaluronidase 1500 IU in 1 mL sterile water is injected around the extravasation site to break down hyaluronic acid.
  - Saline may also be administered via the cannula and withdrawn to flush the wound; this may be combined with hyaluronidase. Ideally within 1–2 hr of injury.
  - Steroids (hydrocortisone or dexamethasone) may be given subcutaneously or systemically to reduce inflammation.
  - Antihistamines and analgesics provide symptom relief.

Surgical
- The vast majority probably heal with conservative management.
- Surgical debridement may be needed to excise vesicant drugs.
- Liposuction to the extravasation site: the area is infiltrated with hyaluronidase and then normal saline. Several stab wounds around the injury allow saline to escape and flush out the wound. Liposuction removes the subcutaneous fat and the remaining drug.

Complications
Extensive tissue necrosis; nerve, tendon, or joint damage even requiring amputation results from inadequate early treatment.

Debate
Cases referred to plastic surgery represent the tip of the iceberg. It appears that most injuries heal well with conservative treatment. Conservative management has probably improved with increased recognition of the problem, and better early management (e.g. extravasation packs on wards where chemotherapy is given). However, some injuries will progress if the drug is not adequately removed at an early stage. It is difficult to judge which cases need surgery

Frostbite

Definition
Tissue injury due to freezing.

Incidence
Unknown in general population, and hospital admissions may underestimate incidence. It is slightly more common in races from warmer climates.

Aetiology
- Age: infancy (high surface area:mass ratio), old age (reduced ability to produce and retain heat).
- Drugs, especially alcohol: loss of awareness of cold, peripheral vasodilation, loss of shivering mechanism.
- Psychiatric illness.
- Cardiovascular insufficiency: peripheral vascular disease and smoking reduce peripheral blood flow.
- Trauma: due to immobility or reduced conscious state.
- Environmental factors: wet, wind, and altitude increase the risk.

Classification
- First-degree: white waxy plaques; erythema; oedema; altered sensation.
- Second-degree: erythema; oedema; blisters with clear fluid.
- Third-degree: blood-filled blisters; full-thickness skin necrosis.
- Fourth-degree: affects muscles, tendons and bone.

First- and second-degree injuries usually recover without tissue loss.

Pathogenesis
Three aspects:
- Cold injury.
- Ischaemia.
- Inflammatory response.

Cold damages tissues by formation of intracellular ice crystals and also disrupts membranes, denatures proteins, inhibits DNA synthesis and alters pH. Slow cooling results in intracellular dehydration as extracellular water freezes, drawing water out of cells. Rewarming produces profuse oedema. Vasoconstriction, endothelial damage, and subsequent thrombosis cause ischaemia. Oxygen free radicals, prostaglandins, thromboxane A2, and proteolytic enzymes are generated, and continue the tissue damage.

Clinical features
- Site: head, hands and feet are most commonly affected.
- Cold, firm skin.
- Altered sensation: stinging, burning, or numbness.
- Severe burning and stinging on rewarming.

Investigations
Bone scans and MRI have been used to decide whether an extremity should be amputated.

Management

Medical
- Ensure rescuers and patient are safe.
- Do not rewarm until warming can be maintained—refreezing worsens the injury.
- Remove damp clothing and replace with dry clothes.
- Rewarm extremities in bath at 40–42°C.
- Do not rub extremities; it increases tissue damage.
- Elevate affected areas.
- Analgesia.
- Anti-tetanus prophylaxis.
- Alpha blockers and nifedipne have been used to increase perfusion.
- NSAIDS may reduce inflammation—induced injury.
- Management of blisters is controversial—debridement may make underlying tissue dry out, but they contain a high concentration of thromboxane A2 which may damage the underlying tissue.
- High-protein diet to enable healing.
- No smoking.
- Dressings for open wounds.
- Mobilize.

Surgical
- Escharotomy or fasciotomy as indicated.
- Amputation of ischaemic tissue should be deferred until it has clearly demarcated—usually 6–8 weeks post injury, unless there is infection.

Complications
- Tetanus (a high-risk injury).
- Burning, hypersensitivity, and cold intolerance after healing.
- Arthritis.
- Epiphyseal injury and growth disturbance in children.
- Pigment changes.
- Hyperhidrosis of the injured skin.

Traumatic tattooing

Small embedded particles implanted in the dermis or subcutaneous tissue from an abrasion will become fixed in tissue within 12 hr, resulting in permanent discoloration of the skin.

Management
- Scrubbing with a sponge or soft sterile scrub brush and surgical soap and saline rinse is adequate to remove most tattooing foreign bodies. Larger embedded particles may be surgically resected or teased out with a needle, small-jaw tissue forceps, or a pointed blade. Scrubbing is facilitated by anesthesia.
- Small amounts of ether, acetone, or xylol can be added to the cleansing solution to help dissolve any grease or oil. Polyoxyethylene sorbitan, a non-ionic emulsifying agent that is non-toxic to tissue, is useful for removing road tar.
- Cleansing has to be gentle yet thorough, and care must be taken when scrubbing not to cause more injury to the deep dermal layers, which can result in unsightly scarring.
- If particulate debris is embedded below the depth of the dermis, full-thickness excision using a scalpel or dermal punch may be necessary.
- Once foreign bodies are fixed in the tissues, formal surgical abrasion or excision is required.

Degloving injuries

Degloving injuries result from the application of a tangential force to the skin surface, with the resultant separation of skin and subcutaneous tissue from the relatively rigid underlying muscle and fascia, in the supra-fascial plane.

Incidence
Relatively common. The lower limbs are more commonly involved. These injuries usually result from entrapment between a moving vehicle and the road in road traffic accidents.

Classification
- Closed.
- Open.
- Uniplanar (simple).
- Multiplanar (complex).

Clinical features
Skin with variable amounts of subcutaneous tissue is stripped from the underlying fascia, disrupting the perforator blood supply to the skin and producing undermined flaps. These may be closed to the environment or open. When open, the laceration is often a tearing injury with untidy edges which are liable to necrosis because of the compromised circulation. The spectrum of injury can range from a simple skin flap to circumferential avulsion of integument from a limb. If the degloving extends deep to fascia, and even intra-muscular, it becomes a multiplanar complex injury. Concomitant injuries (e.g. fractures, intra-abdominal injury, head injury) are common.

Management
- Standard resuscitation protocol and management of associated injuries in order of priority.
- Assess viability of avulsed tissue by capillary return, bleeding dermal edges, and degree of trauma to skin and subcutaneous fat. Surface dermal capillary bleeding as an indicator of flap viability is advocated by some surgeons. Whole-body fluorescence (described in the 1980s) may be misleading because perfusion of the dermal plexus in acute injury can be altered by arteriovenous shunting.
- Debride necrotic or mangled tissue. Debride areas with injured subcutaneous fat even if the skin seems viable, as invariably the skin will necrose if it and the fat are left undebrided.
- Use non-viable areas of flap as full- or partial-thickness skin grafts.
- Skin graft wound.
- Place a flap on the wound where necessary.
- Provide immobilization for graft and underlying fracture, if present.
- Other techniques such as revascularization of the degloved tissue and free flap reconstruction may be neccessary.

Closed internal degloving injuries (Morel–Lavallée syndrome)

This is an uncommon but significant soft tissue injury associated with pelvic trauma in which the subcutaneous tissue is separated from underlying fascia, creating a cavity filled with haematoma and necrotic fat. It commonly occurs over the greater trochanter, flank, and lumbodorsal area and can be associated with pelvic and acetabular fractures. The presence of necrotic tissue and haematoma in the subcutaneous layers is a source of infection and the swelling could compromise the overlying skin if left untreated. Debridement should be planned with fracture fixation in mind so as to provide soft tissue coverage over internal fixation. Incisions closed primarily run a significant risk of complications (e.g. reaccumulation of haematoma, wound breakdown, infection); they should be closed over several drains after a good debridement of the necrotic and injured fat in the degloved area. This frequently converts the closed degloving into an open one with some skin loss. The defect can be left to heal by secondary intention, if small, or grafted; in some cases delayed primary closure may be appropriate.

Tips and debate

The use of a vacuum dressing device to secure the skin graft over difficult areas (e.g. degloved foot or hand) and minimize oedema under the graft has been used with some success. Debridement with the tourniquet inflated reduces blood loss and allows accurate assessment of degree of the injury. Tourniquet release after debridement confirms bleeding edges and capillary return.

Crush injuries

The sequelae of muscle crush is not confined to the direct injury resulting from the crush; but includes the more life-threatening systemic manifestations of crush injuries collectively described as the 'crush syndrome'.

Mechanism
Usually encountered in natural disasters, industrial accidents, or war. Also seen in obtunded patients who crush a part of the body with their own weight, e.g. after drug overdose or stroke. Can occur following brief severe pressure, e.g. when a limb is run over by a heavy vehicle.

Pathogenesis
- Sustained compression of muscle, damages the sarcolemmal membrane, liberating myoglobin, urate, phosphate, and potassium into the systemic circulation.
- Increased cell membrane permeability allows the influx of water, calcium, and sodium, causing muscle swelling and intravascular volume depletion.
- Precipitation of myoglobin in the renal tubules causes tubular obstruction.
- The likely mechanism of injury to the kidney is through lipid peroxidation induced by the cycling of myoglobin between its ferric and ferryl forms.

Clinical features
- Muscle: swelling, compartment syndrome.
- Circulation: hypovolaemic shock, arrhythmia, coagulopathy.
- Electrolyte disturbance: metabolic acidosis, hyperkalaemia, hypocalcaemia, hyperuricaemia, hyperphosphataemia.
- Renal: acute tubular necrosis, luminal obstruction, acute renal failure.

Indicators of severity of crush syndrome
- Peak creatine kinase > 75 000 U/L is associated with increased mortality and risk of renal failure.
- A simpler and immediate way to estimate the severity of crush syndrome is to correlate it with the number of extremities crushed, e.g. crush to one, two, or three extremities heralds a 50%, 75%, or 100% risk of developing renal failure.

Management
- Standard resuscitation protocol, with attention to possibility of concomitant injury, e.g. fractures, solid organ damage, spinal injury.
- Investigations: serum electrolytes, creatine kinase, and ABGs.
- Adequate fluid resuscitation: insert central venous catheter and urinary catheter; monitor urine volume and pH hourly; monitor serum electrolytes, osmolality, and ABGs at every 6 hr; aim for sustained increase in CVP with fluid bolus (e.g. >3 mmHg after 15 min following a 200 mL challenge).

- Alkalinization: if urine pH <6.5, give bolus of 50 mL 8.4% sodium bicarbonate.
- Enforced mannitol diuresis: Opinions differ about its efficacy. Give iv mannitol (1–2 g/kg) over the first 4 hr as a 20% solution, up to a maximum daily dose of 200g. Avoid in patients with established anuria.

Management of compartment syndrome

Remains controversial. Threshold for debridement and fasciotomy is lower in open injuries. In closed injuries, monitoring compartment pressures in the absence of neurovascular compromise is an option, especially if mannitol is administered. If the compartment pressure is <30 mm Hg beneath the diastolic pressure, proceed immediately to fasciotomy. If any symptoms arise or if in doubt, do fasciotomies. Debride all necrotic muscle or muscle which does not respond to mechanical stimuli. Delay closure of fasciotomy wounds with split skin grafts.

There are few long-term studies to confirm that early fasciotomy prevents Volkmann's contractures, or diminishes the severity of crush syndrome.

Compartment syndrome

Compartment syndrome (von Volkmann 1872) may occur in any closed anatomical space when the interstitial pressure exceeds the perfusion pressure. If untreated, compartment syndrome will lead to tissue (muscle) necrosis with subsequent severe functional impairment, renal failure, and possibly death. Compartment syndrome is most frequently observed in the extremities (which have comparatively fixed osseofascial compartment volumes), although abdominal compartment syndrome is an important clinical entity. Gluteal compartment syndrome has also been reported.

Definitions
Persistent rise in pressure within a confined compartment leading to partial or complete infarction of the contents of the compartment.

Aetiology
- Primarily trauma: long-bone fracture (open or closed), penetrating injuries (e.g. gunshot wounds with or without a concomitant arterial injury), or blunt soft-tissue trauma.
- External pressure induced by stroke, coma, or drugs can cause compartment syndrome.
- Vascular causes may be arterial (e.g. reperfusion following revascularization of an acutely ischaemic limb) or venous (e.g. deep vein thrombosis).
- Sepsis, especially meningococcal, is a rare cause.
- Uncommon aetiologies include snakebite envenomation, idiopathic muscle infarction as a complication of diabetes mellitus, or exercise-induced compartment syndrome.
- Iatrogenic compartment syndrome in the lower limb has been reported following the application of military antishock trousers (MAST), or as a result of patient positioning during prolonged surgery. Beware of tight plaster casts and circumferential limb dressing!

Pathophysiology
- At a capillary perfusion pressure (CPP) of ~25 mmHg and an interstitial pressure of ~5 mmHg, a normal cellular oxygen tension of ~7 mmHg can be achieved.
- A rise in compartment pressure occludes venous outflow, leading to venous engorgement which further raises the compartment pressure to a level that occludes capillaries and eventually arteries.
- An intra-compartmental pressure (and thus interstitial pressure) in excess of the CPP arrests capillary perfusion, resulting in local hypoxia, lowered pH, and eventually muscle necrosis (with myoglobin release). The metabolic milieu results in increased capillary permeability, thus further exacerbating the situation.

Of all the components of the compartment, muscle and nerve are the most sensitive to ischaemia. Muscle changes are seen within 2 hr but are initially reversible; irreversible changes occur by 4 hr but are recoverable as a whole. After 6 hr an increasing amount of irreversible injury occurs, and by 8 hr this becomes so extensive that the part is not recoverable as a whole. Nerve function becomes abnormal after 30 min and irreversible after 12–24 hr.

Signs and symptoms
- Pain: classically the patient presents with crescendo pain which is disproportionate to the severity of the primary injury and is unrelieved by analgesia.
- Pain on passive movement: pain is usually exacerbated by passive flexion and extension of the digits of the affected limb.
- Palpable tension in compartment.
- Paraesthesia: there may be parasthesia, diminished two-point discrimination, and vibration sense, but these are unreliable signs.
- Pallor.
- Pulselessness.
- Paralysis.

The presence of a pedal or wrist pulses does not exclude the diagnosis of compartment syndrome. Pallor and pulselessness are late signs! The limb is typically tense, firm, and tender, often with associated swelling, bruising, or fracture blistering depending on the aetiology of the primary pathology. Comparison with the unaffected limb is invaluable.

Beware of missing occult compartment syndrome in the unconscious patient (e.g. the polytrauma patient on ITU) or in the post-operative patient with a regional block *in situ*. Meticulous nursing observation of the affected extremities is essential.

Although some units electively monitor intra-compartmental pressures in high-risk cases, invasive pressure monitoring is normally reserved for cases where a degree of clinical suspicion exists. However, in view of the serious implications of missing a diagnosis of compartment syndrome, many surgeons still advocate 'diagnostic' fasciotomy if there is any clinical suspicion. If in any doubt call your senior immediately or do a fasciotomy.

Although commercially available portable pressure monitors exist, the use of a CVP line such as an 18G (green) needle attached via a saline-filled extension tube connected to a standard digital pressure transducer (readily available in all theatres and ITUs) is equally effective. The pressures of all compartments (four in leg, three in thigh, and four in forearm) must be measured and recorded in the notes. An absolute pressure ≥30 mmHg (or <30 mmHg below the diastolic blood pressure) indicates the need for immediate decompression. Beware—a normal or borderline result does not preclude the development of compartment syndrome at a later stage; if sufficient doubt exists, few would criticize a low threshold for fasciotomy. Repeat the measurements at short intervals if levels are normal but you remain suspicious although you have not yet been convinced to do fasciotomies!

Loosen tight dressings or bivalve plaster casts. Avoid limb elevation as this further diminishes arterial perfusion pressure.

Frequency
Up to 10% of lower limb trauma cases and up to 30% of limbs following vascular injury. Approximately 0.5–2% of forearm fractures result in compartment syndrome.

Pre-operative management

Depends on aetiology and anatomical site. Check serum creatinine kinase levels and renal function. Beware of myoglobinuria and subsequent acute renal failure. Keep well hydrated; some advocate the administration of IV sodium bicarbonate to induce a forced alkaline diuresis. If in doubt seek a medical opinion. The use of hyperbaric oxygen therapy has been proposed, but this must never deter from early surgical decompression.

Surgical management

The management of acute compartment syndrome is surgical: immediate fasciotomy with the aim of salvaging a functional extremity. Rorabeck and Macnab (JBJS Am 1976) demonstrated that complete functional recovery is likely provided that an adequate fasciotomy is performed within 6 hr of the development of symptoms.

In theatre the limb is free-draped and prepared with povidone iodine. Prophylactic antibiotics are administered and a proximal tourniquet applied. Unless previously undertaken, simultaneous correction of the primary pathology (e.g. ORIF of fracture) is normally performed after the fasciotomy undertaken.

Reference

Rorabeck CH, Macnab L (1976). *J Bone Joint Surg Am* **58**, 549–50.

Fasciotomy

Definition
A surgical incision in a fascial compartment normally for the purpose of relieving intra-compartmental pressure; may be performed prophylactically or therapeutically.

Indications
- Raised pressure within a fascial compartment.
- Without decompression, the resulting microvascular stasis initially alters nerve function and then progresses to soft tissue necrosis.
- Absolute values of >30 mmHg, or a difference between diastolic blood pressure and compartment pressure of <30 mmHg have been suggested as guidelines for decompression.
- Do not rely overly on measurements. Rather, if you suspect compartment syndrome have a very very low threshold to do fasciotomies.
- Clinical suspicion of compartment syndrome: history of crush or prolonged ischaemia, swollen limb, pain out of proportion to the injury, pain on passive muscle stretching, open tibial fracture grade II or higher, closed fractures, tight-feeling compartments.
- Paralysis, pallor and loss of sensation or pulselessness are signs which are too late.

Aims
- To fully release pressure within involved compartments to allow blood flow and perfusion.
- To debride non-viable tissue.

Principles
- To decompress all compartments.
- Must include the full length of the skin.
- May need to include epimysium.
- Avoid exposure of nerves and tendons.
- Arrange a second look within 24–48 hr or earlier if pain remains unrelieved.
- Avoid prolonged peripheral nerve block/epidural.

Planning
- Use a tourniquet.
- Bear in mind reperfusion injury—inform the anaesthetist when the tourniquet is to be released.

Incisions/procedure
Forearm
There are four interconnected forearm compartments:
- Superficial flexor compartment.
- Deep flexor compartment.
- Dorsal (extensor) compartment.
- Compartment containing the mobile wad of Henry (brachioradialis, ECRB, ECRL).

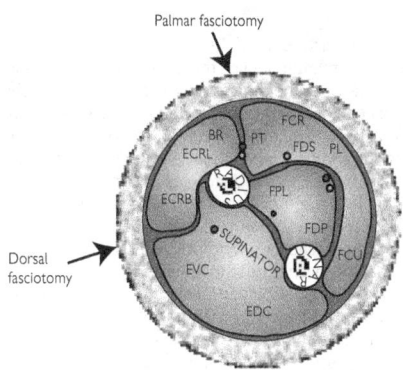

Fig. 17.1 Cross-section of forearm and proximal third showing four compartments, all of which need decompressing.

Palmar

Straight palmar incision from wrist to antecubital fossa following ulnar border brachioradialis. Decompress the lacertus fibrosus, the deep fascial compartments including FDP, pronator, FPL (by retracting FDS and median nerve laterally) and the superficial compartments of FCR, FDS, PL, FCU.

Explore the median nerve if altered function, and decompress the carpal tunnel using a zig-zag incision with the transverse limb incision at the level of the distal wrist crease such that, if swelling prevents direct closure, the apices of the zig-zag flaps can still be approximated covering the nerve and leaving secondary defects laterally where they will cause little harm. You may be able to reach the dorsal compartments via this palmar incision. However, if you cannot, do a dorsal incision.

Dorsal

Do a straight mid-dorsal incision following the ulnar border of the mobile extensor wad. Decompress the mobile wad and the deep extensor compartment.

Hand

Compartment pressures of only 15–20 mmHg are an indication for fasciotomy. Decompress the carpal tunnel as described above. Two or three dorsal incisions over the second and fourth metacarpals or over the inter-metacarpal spaces are used to decompress all 10 compartments: the dorsal interossei (four compartments), the palmar interossei (three compartments), and the adductor pollicis, thenar, and hypothenar compartments. A separate incision placed away from the main contact areas may be needed over the thenar and hypothenar eminences to decompress these properly.

Lower leg

There are four compartments of the leg:
- Anterior compartment: contains the dorsiflexors of the ankle and foot and the deep peroneal nerve (sensation to first dorsal webspace).
- Lateral (peroneal) compartment: contains the everters of the foot and the superficial peroneal nerve (sensation to dorsum of foot).
- Deep posterior compartment: contains the deep flexors and the posterior tibial nerve (sensation to sole of foot).
- Superficial posterior compartment: contains the plantar flexors of foot and the sural nerve (sensation to lateral aspect of the foot).

Approaches using one and two longitudinal incisions have been described. The two-incision approach is described here.

The anterior and lateral compartments are approached via a 15–20 cm incision 2 cm anterior to the fibula. This will lie over the septum between the anterior and lateral compartments. The superficial peroneal nerve is identified and preserved, while the fascia of both compartments is released longitudinally. The posterior compartments (deep and superficial) are approached via an incision 2 cm posterior to the medial border of the tibia. Dissect on the deep fascia to the posterior border of the tibia; retract the saphenous vein and nerve anteriorly; and release the superficial compartment. Release the soleus from the medial border of the tibia to allow a longitudinal incision in the fascia over the FDL, which releases the posterior compartment.

An alternative is an incision over the fibula, incising the fascia almost circumferentially around the fibula. The two-incision approach is prefered.

Foot

All nine compartments can be decompressed via a medial incision running from below the medial malleolus (3 cm from the sole) to the base of the first metatarsal:

Retract the neurovascular bundle. Release the fascia over abductor hallucis (the medial compartment) and FDB. Incise the fascia over the medial intermuscular septum longitudinally. Preserve the lateral plantar neurovascular bundle which runs over quadratus plantae (central compartment). The remaining compartments (central, lateral, intrinsic) can be released by blunt dissection or preferably via dorsal incisions over the second and fourth metatarsals.

Necrotic muscle is usually dark, fails to bleed when incised, and does not twitch or fasciculate on stimulation. It must be adequately debrided.

Closure

Do not close any of the wounds primarily. However, after the swelling has reduced, delayed primary closure of one of the two incisions on the limb may be possible. Split-skin grafts may be applied immediately or as a delayed procedure. Usually SSG the remaining wound when doing the delayed primary closure. Check internally for muscle necrosis first.

Wounds are dressed with a non-adherent moist dressing (paraffin gauze, then Betadine-soaked gauze). Leave the extremities exposed to allow monitoring for perfusion, sensation, and movement. Splintage of the upper limb in the position of function or the lower limb with the ankle at 90° is recommended unless otherwise indicated.

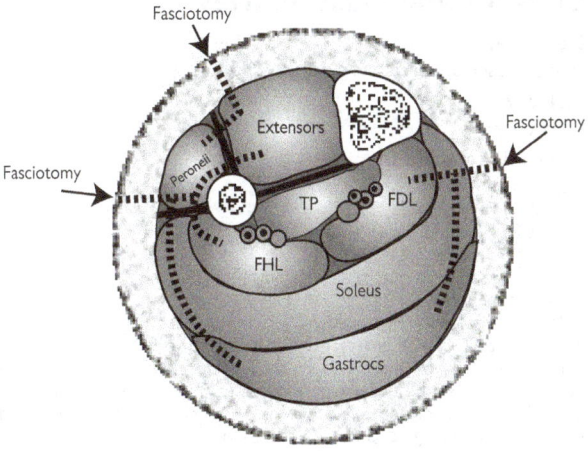

Fig. 17.2 Lower limb cross-section showing compartments and fasciotomies.

Post-operative care
- The patient should be monitored for symptoms and signs of compartment syndrome, in particular pain and altered sensation.
- If symptoms and signs of compartment syndrome persist, take the patient back to theatre and repeat the fasciotomy!
- Nerve blocks are rarely used to avoid masking symptoms of continued compression.
- Elevate the limb.
- Second look and closure usually in 48–72 hr when swelling has reduced. If not, delay further.
- Delayed closure of wounds by skin grafting is preferable to slow tension suturing.

Complications
- Inadequate decompression.
- Bleeding.
- Infection.
- Aesthetic—poor scar, SSG.
- Nerve injury.
- The complications of not doing a fasciotomy, i.e. ischaemic contracture, neuropathy, pain syndromes, growth inhibition (in children), and amputation, are much greater than those of doing one.

Results
Good in 68% when fasciotomy done within 12 hr, but falls to 8% if fasciotomy done after 12 hr.

Gunshot and blast injuries

Definition
Injuries caused by bullets and explosions.

Incidence
- Uncommon.

Mechanics of gunshot injury
Depends on:
- Velocity of projectile.
- Mass of projectile.
- Projectile movement.
- Resistance to projectile passage through body.
- Contamination.

Velocity of projectile: high vs. low velocity projectiles. Hand guns are low velocity (<2000 ft/sec). Energy transfer is related to velocity squared on entry minus that on exit: $E = mv^2/2$. Therefore energy transfer then depends on what the bullet hits; if it passes through the lung and out again there is no resistance, so there is poor energy transfer compared with the bullet hitting bone and not coming out.

A bullet has a pointed end and a blunt end, with the centre of mass at the back and air resistance at the front which encourages the bullet to tip over so that it yaws (the tip moves up and down and it also performs complex movements as it progresses forward—precession spiral movement and mutation complex spiral movement). The bullet is unstable in flight. The bullet enters tissue pointed end first, then it starts to yaw, and then travels almost vertically before exiting backwards.

This sideways movement causes large tissue injury, temporary cavitation, and ingression of contaminants. Then the cavitation expansion collapses, leaving little to be seen. Therefore if you only concentrate on what you can see, you will miss the extent of the injury. If you explore the cavitation area, you will see bruising, necrosis, and contamination.

A bullet causes injury by laceration, cavitation, and shock wave. Cavitation is caused by energy transfer to soft tissues. Generally there is a small entry wound and the size of the exit wound depends on the way the bullet is travelling on exit. Bullets are not sterile and often carry contaminants into the body.

Management
Check ABCD, neurovascular supply, compartment syndrome, and X-rays.

Low-velocity bullets
- Excise margins of wound, clean, do not close wound.
- Role of antibiotics is controversial.

Operative indications
- Vascular injury.
- Bony injury requiring reduction and fixation.
- High energy.
- ≥8 hr since injury.
- Nerve injury, but 70–80% of nerve injuries recover.

Blast injuries

Shock wave injures by three mechanisms:
- Spawling.
- Shearing.
- Blast wave.

A shock wave arises because of massive rapid expansion of solid material into gaseous material, producing a very rapid high pressure wave which, like a sound wave, has constructive and destructive interference zones. These cause injury by energy transfer bouncing off tissue, which is called spawling. Spawling causes damage at the tissue–air interface.

Shearing occurs when tissues of different density accelerate at different rates. Also, when the shock wave passes over a small air bubble the bubble expands and heats up.

The shock wave is followed by a blast wave/wind which is the fire wind: if far away, this may knock one over; if close, it may impart sufficient energy to cause amputation, etc. One may also be hit by secondary objects carried by the blastwave.

Facial lacerations

Facial injuries deserve special attention because of their enormous functional and aesthetic significance. Most soft tissue injuries of the face can await primary repair for up to 24 hr without serious risk of infection and without jeopardizing the final aesthetic result, if properly cleaned and dressed.

Preparation of wound

Basic surgical principles of cleaning, irrigation, and debridement apply. Devitalized tissue must be excised regardless of its location or former importance. Debridement should be conservative but adequate. Ragged, tangential, and severely contused wound edges are conservatively excised to leave perpendicular skin edges that will heal with minimum scarring. Parallel lacerations can occasionally be converted to a single wound by excising the skin bridge if it is thin enough. Excise any bevelled edges where possible.

Wound closure

Displaced tissue is returned to its original position. Usually the contracted displaced tissue makes the injury seem worse than it is. Reconstructive procedures should not be carried out on contused ischaemic tissue because additional planes for devascularization and potential infection may be opened. Occasionally there is an indication for immediately changing the direction of the wound by Z-plasty or for making allowance for scar contracture at the time of primary repair.

Suturing and suture removal

Close muscular and subcutaneous tissue with absorbable sutures to minimize dead space and haematoma formation with later contour irregularities. Use interrupted 5'0 or 6'0 nylon for skin closure. Sutures in the eyelid can be removed in 3–4 days, in 4–6 days elsewhere on the face, and in 10 days in the ears.

Principles

- Suture anatomical borders or junctional sites first to ensure perfect alignment of these lines, such as the vermilion border, eyelid, eyebrow edges, etc.
- Avoid distorting facial features by directly closing areas of skin loss, such as the nasal base, tip, eyelid, lip, etc. It may be preferable to apply an FTSG or a local flap, or allow healing by secondary intention.
- Scars are least conspicuous when they are in the same line as anatomical junctional areas (rather than traversing the anatomical junctions) and parallel to skin creases or skin tension lines.
- Superficial lacerations not through muscle, and consequently not gaping or under tension, can be glued using cyanoacrylate glue. Oppose the wound edges as perfectly as possible and apply glue as a continuous weld of glue material over the top of the skin including the opposed skin laceration. Do not apply glue to the dermis or subcutaneous tissue. Reinforce with tape or steristrips. An alternative is to use tape or Steri-Strips or butterfly tape alone. The principle is the same.

'Windshield' injury

This is one of the most daunting facial wounds, characterized by multiple lacerations, abrasions, gouges, and avulsion flaps. The forehead block is the preferred method of local anaesthesia. Flaps <5 mm in width and length are tacked down with single 6'0 percutaneous non-absorbable sutures. Larger flaps can be closed by using the corner technique. These flaps are prone to the 'trap-door' phenomenon where congestion, lymphoedema, and scar contracture results in a heaped-up appearance of the flap. Partial-thickness abrasions and shallow gouges (<5–10 mm wide and 1–2 mm deep) can be left to heal by secondary intention. Other lacerations are closed with percutaneous sutures.

Special anatomical considerations

Eyebrow

The eyebrow is an important anatomical feature that is always preserved as a reference point. Never shave or trim it and pay special attention to its shape and borders during repair. If macerated or devitalized tissue must be removed, excise this tissue parallel to the hair shaft.

Forehead

Repair any muscle division underneath the brow to prevent spreading and depression of the scar. A conservative excision policy should be adopted when ragged wounds are concerned; it is best to preserve as much tissue as possible by 'tacking down' ragged tissue tags so that later scar revisions can be made when conditions are more favourable. Use minimal dermal absorbable sutures because excessive tissue reaction can increase the scar size.

Eyelid

Exclude globe injury and penetrating foreign body first. Check for damage to important structures, e.g. levator palpebrae superioris muscle (traumatic ptosis, extrusion of periorbital fat from laceration of upper lid), lateral palpebral raphe, medial palpebral ligament ('cross-eyed' appearance), and lacrimal canaliculus (copious tears). Irrigate lacerations with saline. Replace avulsed tissue as an autograft. Superficial extramarginal horizontal lacerations require simple closure; lacerations perpendicular to the lid margin tend to gape and should be closed with absorbable sutures to the muscle and subcutaneous tissue prior to skin closure. Repair deep lacerations involving division of the levator palpebrae, aponeurosis, or superior rectus muscle. Intramarginal lacerations should be repaired promptly; fibrosis of the orbicularis muscle fibres and retraction of the tarsal plate makes late closure difficult. In this region, anatomically accurate approximation gives the best result and will prevent ectropion or entropion; once the tarsus and ciliary margin are accurately approximated, the remainder of the eyelid falls into place. Preserve the integrity of the lacrimal apparatus by cannulating a divided lacrimal system with a fine polyethylene catheter or suture and repairing it with fine sutures if possible.

Ears

Exclude perichondral haematoma, tympanic perforations, and basal skull fractures. Debridement should be conservative. The abundant blood supply means that narrow pedicled avulsion flaps or amputated composite tissue often survive if relocated correctly. Cartilage sutures, if necessary, should be 5'0 clear prolene or nylon.

Nose

Exclude septal haematoma, which can cause chondromalacia and subsequent loss or thickening of cartilage. Evacuation is done through a small mucosal incision.

For superficial injuries, accurate approximation of soft tissues aligning the nostril borders is adequate. For deep penetrating injuries, repair the mucous membrane first with absorbable 4'0 suture. Torn cartilage is reapproximated and secured in position by repair of underlying mucous membrane and overlying skin. Subcutaneous sutures are unnecessary if deep bites are taken through the skin with 5'0 nylon to achieve a slight eversion of skin edges.

Full-thickness post-auricular skin grafts give the best match to the nose.

Cheeks and chin

The parotid gland and facial nerve are vulnerable. Leakage of salivary fluid from the wound or bloody fluid from the parotid duct are indications of parotid injury. Test the integrity of all five branches of the facial nerve. Close superficial lacerations with percutaneous non-absorbable 6'0 sutures. In a through-and-through laceration, most commonly a bite injury through the lower lip–chin junction, the oral mucosal laceration can be left open unless it is >3 cm; close larger mucosal lacerations with 5'0 absorbable sutures.

Lips

The vermilion border, mucosal border, and orbicularis oris muscle require careful and exact apposition to achieve the best structural and cosmetic result. Repair the mucosa and orbicularis oris with 5'0 absorbable sutures, and the exposed lip and skin with 6'0 non-absorbable sutures.

Middle-third facial injuries

This term refers to injuries to the middle third of the face, including the orbits, maxilla, and nose, but tends to exclude isolated injuries to these structures. The initial management of facial trauma must include management of the whole patient according to ATLS principles, the maintenance of airway, prevention of haemorrhage, prevention of aspiration, and identification of occult injuries (e.g. eye, brain, cervical spine).

Classification
Middle-third fractures are classified by anatomical region.

Diagnosis and assessment
Evaluation for facial trauma includes examination of the skin and soft tissue, ocular function, nasal passageway, dental occlusion, oral cavity and naso-oral pharynx, integrity of the neurological system, and bony structure.

Skin and soft tissue
- Lacerations: manage isolated injuries to the skin and soft tissue according to basic surgical principles of asepsis, debridement, haemostasis, and closure.
- Ecchymosis: site, any peculiar pattern (e.g. spectacle-shaped).
- Deformity: site of any swelling, loss of malar prominence, elongation of mid-face.

Eye
- Subconjunctival haemorrhage.
- Malposition of eye/palpebral fissure: enophthalmos, inferior cant to palpebral fissure.
- Measurement of visual acuity, intra-orbital pressure.
- Extra-ocular muscle movement: diplopia, forced duction test.
- Medial canthal ligament: disruption, bone crepitation, and intercanthal distance. Any evidence of telecanthus?
- Lacrimal apparatus: copious tears.
- Infra-orbital rim: pain, localized tenderness, and palpable step.
- Zygomatico-frontal suture: step, tenderness.
- Exclude concomitant ocular injury (10–25% of orbital floor fractures have associated ocular injuries), e.g. globe rupture, hyphaema, retinal detachment.

Nose
- Deformity: deviation of septum or pyramid, depression of the dorsum, shortening.
- Obstruction in either nostril.
- Discharge: epistaxis (unilateral/bilateral), nasopharyngeal bleed, CSF rhinorrhoea.
- Exclude septal haematoma. Palpate for crepitus.

Oral cavity
- Malocclusion.
- Limited or painful mandibular excursion.
- Mobility of maxillary dental arch, or dental alveolar segments.
- Loose or fractured teeth.
- Examine the buccal cavity for intra-oral haematoma and split palate.
- Bruised or bleeding gingiva, especially extending around a tooth.
- Step, tenderness palpable along mandible.

Neurology
Examination of all cranial nerves especially the infra-orbital nerve and facial nerve.

Bony structure
Pain, localized tenderness, deformity or step/level discrepancies especially in malar, zygoma.

Investigations
- Plain films: not often employed because they do not permit sufficient detail for decision-making in general. May show opaque antrum, infra-orbital steps, mandibular fractures, displaced zygomatico-frontal stures.
- CT scan: has become the standard for diagnosing facial fractures and planning treatment. Bone and soft tissue windows, axial and coronal scans of the orbit should be done. 3D reconstructions may aid planning.

Fracture pattern
Nasal
Fractures can involve the nasal bones and/or cartilaginous septum, and are either depressed or laterally displaced. Signs include swelling, pain, nasal obstruction, epistaxis, deformity/deviation of septum, and crepitation.

Naso-orbital ethmoid
One or both frontal processes of the maxilla and the nose may be involved. Movement of the frontal process of the maxilla on direct finger pressure over the medial canthal ligament is a reliable sign; other signs include telecanthus (widening and/or asymmetry of intercanthal distance), eyelid ecchymosis, epistaxis, nasal depression/shortening, and medial canthal ligament bone crepitation. Frequently accompany Le Fort or frontocranial fractures.

Zygomatic and orbital floor
All zygomatic fractures include components in the lateral orbit and the orbital floor (except isolated zygomatic arch fractures). Signs include loss of malar prominence, inferior cant to palpebral fissure (inferior displacement of zygoma), enophthalmos (enlargement of orbital cavity). Fractures displaced at the zygomatico-frontal suture require open reduction to restore symmetry and decompress the infraorbital foramen. The most frequent orbital fracture is the 'blow-out' fracture, confined to the orbital floor medial to the infra-orbital nerve and the lower half of the medial orbit (the weakest portion of the orbit). Signs of orbital floor fracture include spectacle-shaped ecchymosis, diplopia looking superiorly or inferiorly (incarceration of fat tethered to extra-ocular muscles).

Maxillary

Fractures of the maxilla inevitably involve other bones in the mid-face:
- Le Fort I: transverse fracture which separates maxillary alveolus from the upper midface and extends through maxillary sinus.
- Le Fort II: pyramidal fracture which separates a pyramidal-shaped central segment from the upper craniofacial structure with fracture line extending through inferior orbital rims and across bridge of nose.
- Le Fort III: craniofacial disjunction with separation of the upper craniofacial skeleton from the zygoma, orbital floor, naso-ethmoid region.

Mobility of the maxilla is an important sign. Be aware of the non-mobile maxilla in the rare single-fragment Le Fort III fracture, impacted or incomplete mid-face fractures. Other signs include bilateral periorbital haematoma, malocclusion (impingement of the coronoid process of mandible), profuse nasopharyngeal bleed, periorbital and mid-facial swelling, CSF rhinorrhoea, and facial elongation. 10% of maxillary fractures are accompanied by palatal split.

Management

Midface surgical approaches

Subciliary incision
- Access: inferior orbital rim, orbital floor, zygomatico-frontal suture.
- Place incision 2 mm inferior to lash line from punctum to lateral canthus, skin muscle flap in a stairstep fashion, down to inferior orbital rim. Incise and elevate periosteum. Dissect in the subperiosteal plane to reach the orbital floor. Resuspension of periosteum is crucial in closure.

Eyelid cheek margin
- Access: Inferior orbital rim, orbital floor, zygomatico-frontal suture
- Place incision in cheek lower eyelid margin; incise directly down to inferior orbital rim. Incise and elevate periosteum. Dissect in the subperiosteal plane to reach the orbital floor. Resuspension of periosteum is crucial in closure.

Bicoronal incision
- Access: zygomatic arch, zygomatico-frontal suture, naso-orbital ethmoid region, frontal sinus.
- Make incision (straight, anteriorly curved, or zig-zag) down to galea. Elevate in the areolar subgaleal plane; in the plane between superficial and deep temporal fascia (avoiding facial nerve) over temporalis muscle. The arch is exposed by incising the fascia 1.5 cm cephalad to the arch. Resuspend the deep temporal fascia on closure.

Buccal sulcus incision
- Access: zygomatico-maxillary buttress.

Incise the mucosa of upper buccal sulcus avoiding the apex of the sulcus and frenulum. Leave a cuff of mucosa and muscle to facilitate closure. Incise through the muscle down to bone and dissect in the subperiosteal plane.

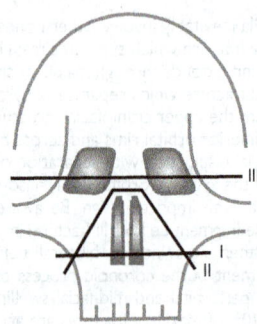

Fig. 17.3 Le Fort fracture patterns.

Management of fracture

Nasal
- Indication for surgery: displacement/deformity of nose or septum, septal haematoma
- Septal haematoma: evacuate promptly via a small mucosal incision.
- Closed reduction: reduce the septum by manipulation with an Asch forceps, completing the septal fracture and repositioning the septum in the mid-line. The nasal pyramid is reduced by 'out-fracturing' to complete the fracture, and then manipulating the nasal pyramid back into position. Reduction is assessed by palpation and visual inspection. A nasal splint is applied in the absence of skin injury and maintained for 7 days. Intranasal packing at the surgeon's discretion.
- Timing: closed reduction can be performed within 2 weeks of injury. Healed nasal fractures are treated by open reduction 6 months or more after injury, together with rhinoplasty, septoplasty for airways obstruction, and bone graft reconstruction of nasal profile as required.

Naso-orbital ethmoid
- Indication for surgery: displacement, widened intercanthal distance.
- Non-comminuted fractures: rigid fixation with plate and screws.
- Comminuted fractures: anterior and posterior transnasal wires twisted together to compress segment. If comminution extends underneath canthal ligament, it should be stripped and re-attached following bone reduction.
- Maintain or restore continuity of nasolacrimal drainage. Formal dacryocystorhinostomy can be performed if a torn lacrimal duct is anticipated. Imperfect reduction must occasionally be accepted.

Zygomatic and orbital floor

- Indication for surgery: positive forced duction test, orbital content herniation, enophthalmos, displacement of zygomatico-frontal suture, depressed malar or zygomatic arch, trismus, other significant displacement.
- Open reduction: rigid fixation with plate and screws. Some advocate that to avoid ankylosis of the coronoid process of the mandible to the zygoma, resect the coronoid process.
- Closed reduction (incomplete fractures): easier and quicker with no skin incisions, but results are less exacting and dependable. Buccal sulcus incision. Enter the maxillary antrum above first premolar tooth. Pass curved Mayo scissors into the antrum to elevate the zygoma from below. Pack the antrum with iodoform gauze to maintain reduction. As the pack is inserted, the inferior orbital rim is palpated to control fracture fragment and prevent overcorrection. Incision is left open to provide drainage, and the pack is removed after 10 days.
- Medially displaced zygomatic arch: reduce with a Kilner elevator passed through a Gillies temporal approach. Incise the scalp within the temporal hair and dissect until the temporalis muscle is visualized. Pass an elevator beneath the deep temporal fascia underneath the arch, and elevate the arch into position. Inherent stability of arch form obviates need for support. However, if unstable it can support the arch by introducing a chest tube or other similar diameter device under the arch for 1–2 weeks. Alternatively, the arch can be sutured through the skin and over an external arched splint.
- The Gillies approach and lift can also be used for medially displaced malar fractures provided that the zygomatico-frontal suture remains undisplaced. The approach is the same as above and the malar is lifted laterally and anteriorly. Once reduced, it is usually stable. However, if it is unstable it can be transfixed to the nasal bony septum with a K-wire.
- Orbital floor fractures: remove incarcerated tissue from the fracture site and cover the defect with an alloplastic sheet of silicone or thin bone graft, which may need to be rigidly fixed to the inferior rim. The periosteum is closed and the lid repaired in layers. Light perception must be checked every 6 hr for several days. Antibiotics are given at the discretion of the surgeon.

Maxillary

- Indication for surgery: all Le Fort fractures. Aim to stabilize occlusion and reconstruct mid-face width, height, and projection.
- Le Fort I: intermaxillary fixation with plate and screws ± bone graft.
- Le Fort II: rigid fixation with plate and screws ± bone graft. Intermaxillary fixation in occlusion for 4–8 weeks. Early mobilization if rigid fixation techniques are utilized. Arch bars should be left in place. Intermaxillary fixation is re-instituted or traction elastics are utilized if there is any displacement of occlusion.
- Le Fort III: reduce as in Le Fort II fractures with the addition of a bicoronal incision or anterior approach for zygomatic fractures. Teeth should be placed in best possible occlusion. Dentures or fabricated bite blocks can be wired together to achieve best possible reduction and intermaxillary relationships.

- Palate stabilization: palatal splint or open reduction and fixation with plate/mesh.
- Delayed presentation: fibrous union occurs at 3 weeks. Either surgical refracture or application of external disimpacting forces, with monoblock repositioning of bony mass and filling defect with bone grafts.

Complications
- Nasal fractures: haematoma, synaechiae, osteitis. Some degree of deformity can exist despite early reduction, e.g. dorsal hump, slight saddling of septum, septal and nasal pyramid deviation, airway obstruction, palpable step.
- Zygomatic and orbital floor fractures: blindness (up to 3%), diplopia, ectropion, convergence insufficiency (up to 21%), cavernous sinus carotid fistula (rare), trismus, ankylosis of TMJ, depression of malar eminence (untreated, inadequate reduction, or following bone resorption). Can sometimes be restored with late refracturing and reduction using open technique; adequate restoration seldom occurs with soft tissue alteration alone. 10–20% of patients with orbital fractures require a second operation for minor adjustments in globe or lid position.
- Le Fort fractures: flattened, elongated, depressed mid-face with malocclusion, usually an anterior open bite (untreated, inadequate re-duction), persistent paraesthesia of infra-orbital nerve.

Hand assessment in trauma

Principles
- The history of the injury and the patient's description should give you a prediction of the injured structures before you start examining.
- Avoid causing pain until essential, so do all the tests that will not provoke pain first, especially in children.
- Assess sensation before active movement, before palpation, before stressing the fracture and passive movement.
- Check findings with the opposite hand. Congenital anomalies do exist.

History
- Age.
- Handedness.
- Occupation.
- Exact timing of injury: time of injury is relevant for replants and open fractures.
- Mechanism of injury: this will give you a good idea of what has been injured—e.g. did the glass cut the hand as it went through the window, or the arm as it was pulled out. Were the fingers flexed gripping the knife, or were the fingers extended?
- Amputated parts: have they been transported adequately?
- Past medical and drug history, for information on anaesthetic risks and likely healing problems.
- Psychiatric history for deliberate self-harm.
- Social history: smoking will affect blood supply to fingertip flaps; patients with one arm in a bandage may need help at home. Will patient continue their therapy or wear their splint. If not, there may be no point in complicated repair.

Examination
Look, feel, move, and feel again

Remember to assess hand function in patients with arm or upper arm lacerations. The hand can be examined without removing proximal dressings.

Dressings can be left on for comfort until the majority of the assessment is done. If a dressing has been used to stop haemorrhage, leave it in place until the patient is in theatre with a tourniquet on. If it is not effective, put a tourniquet (e.g. manual blood pressure cuff) around the arm, uninflated, for use in emergency; prepare dressings; expose the wound; apply pressure with your hand proximal to the wound, and reapply a pressure dressing. Elevate the arm. Putting additional dressings over an ineffective pressure dressing is not likely to stop bleeding as the pressure will be dispersed by the first dressing. It is better to remove it and apply point pressure at the bleeding point. Do not clip anything! Do not leave a tourniquet inflated.

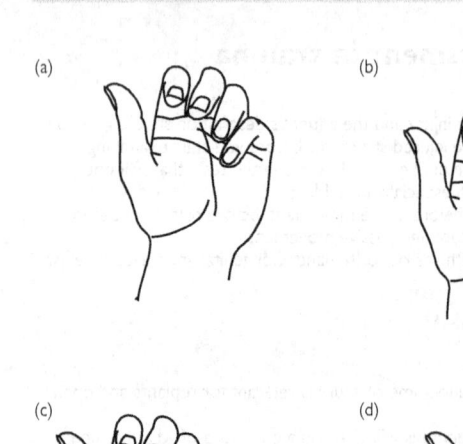

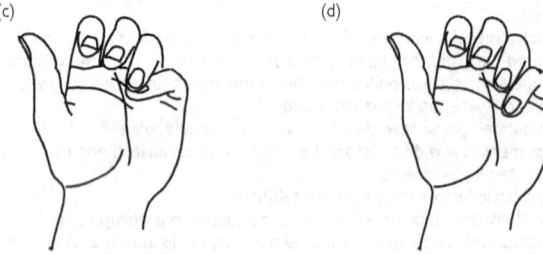

Fig. 17.4 Digital cascade demonstrating (a) normal, (b) flexor tendon injury to middle finger, (c) rotated fracture in little finger, and (d) digital nerve injury.

Look
- Assess deformity including posture of the hand and cascade of the fingers. Is there the expected amount of flexion at each joint? Compare with the normal hand.
- Assess vascularity by looking at the colour and tissue turgor (fullness of the pulp).
- Look at the fingertip wrinkling; in denervated digits they will not wrinkle (O'Riordan's test).
- Note the site and size of swelling, bruising, and wounds. What is the extent and direction of the wounds? What anatomical structures lie beneath?
- Draw a picture or photograph the wounds to save the patient repeated dressing changes.

Feel

- Sensation: check median, ulnar, and radial nerve distributions and digital nerve territories as appropriate. Compare two-point discrimination with the normal side if sensation altered but present.
- Feel the skin or draw the shaft of a pen along the skin of an area of suspected denervation. Normal sweating makes the pen drag slightly; this is lost in denervated areas (tactile adherence test).
- Check vascularity by testing capillary refill and pulses.

Move

- Can the patient make a full fist and extend their fingers? Fractures impede full movement due to pain, or occasionally tendon entrapment. Dislocated or subluxed joints will not go through a full range of motion even after pain is relieved, e.g. with a ring block. Range of movement (active and passive) should be reassessed after joint reduction.
- On finger flexion, is there a rotational deformity? Compare with the normal hand. Do all the fingers point to the scaphoid tubercle? Do all the joints flex and extend or do any lag? Is the pattern and coordination of flexion and extension normal?
- Are joints stable to lateral flexion? The thumb MCPJ should be examined in flexion, holding the metacarpal still; it has some lateral instability when extended.
- Test power of all long flexors and extensors of hand and wrist. To check FDS function, hold all fingers except the one being tested in full extension: the PIPJ should flex, leaving the DIPJ floppy. Pain on attempted use of a tendon may indicate partial division. If the patient has trouble performing the task, ask them to do it on the normal side simultaneously. The index finger may cheat in this test because of the independence of the index FDP, so ensure that the DIPJ remains loose. To check FDS function ask the patient to bend each finger in turn at the PIPJ, leaving the others straight. They can be held straight to assist. Many people have linked little and ring finger FDS tendons so that they do not move independently. Fewer have an absent FDS to little finger.
- To test the median nerve, check APB function (opposition); for the ulnar nerve, test finger abduction and adduction and Froment's test (first dorsal interosseous). Note that little finger abduction can be performed by EDM in the absence of ADM, so ensure that you palpate ADM as you test it.

Feel again

- Examine bones for tenderness, deformity, crepitus, and stability. Ensure that you are testing the bone and not mistaking joint movement for fracture instability.
- Check joints for tenderness and stability. Note which border of the joint is most tender or gives way. Remember that MCPJs are supposed to be stable in flexion and should be tested in this position, whereas the IPJs are stable in extension and should be tested in that position.

Investigations

- X-ray any tender bone or joint (including the joints proximal and distal) in two planes.
- X-ray suspected foreign bodies. If there is nothing to be seen on the X-ray, but the patient is sure that something is in there, the wound should be explored. Organic matter may not show on X-rays.
- Ultrasound, if available, can be helpful.
- Check Hb if you suspect significant blood loss.
- FBC, U&E, ECG, and CXR may be needed prior to general anaesthetic.

'Generalizations are dangerous including this one'. However, they can be useful:

- 'Bruising means broken.'
- 'Pain on tendon movement means tendon injury.'
- 'Altered sensation with an open wound means surgical exploration.'
- 'You never get sued for exploring, only for missing an injury.'

Nailbed and perionychial injuries

Incidence
- The most common hand injury.
- The middle finger, being the longest, is most often injured.
- Extremely common in children.

Aetiology
Crushing between doors (usually at hinge side against the door jamb) or between heavy objects, and saw injuries are most common.

Classification
Zook et al. (1984) classify nailbed injuries as follows:
- Simple lacerations.
- Stellate lacerations.
- Severe crush injury.
- Avulsion.

Pathogenesis
- The nailbed is crushed between a heavy object and the bone.
- Therefore most injuries also involve the paronychium or pulp.
- Half the injuries are associated with a distal phalanx fracture.
- A distal phalanx fracture can lever and cause dislocation of the nailplate, always with a nailbed laceration underneath.
- Dislocation of the proximal nailplate over the nailfold indicates an underlying basal fracture of the distal phalanx or epiphyseal injury in children (Salter-Harris type 1 usually). This is called a **Seymour fracture** and is essentially an open fracture involving the physis. It needs to be washed out, reduced, and the nailbed repaired.
- Injuries sharp enough to cut the nail usually amputate the fingertip.
- Subungual haematoma results from laceration or other injury to the nailbed, which is well vascularized, with an intact overlying nail. Painful and can lead to ischaemic injury to nailbed.

Clinical features
Subungual haematoma of >25% of the nail or avulsion of the nail from its paronychium with an adjacent perionychial injury suggests significant nailbed injury.

Investigations
Always X-ray the distal phalanx. Examine the physis; it may appear slightly wider then usual in a Seymour fracture, or the displacement may be apparent.

Management
- Small (<25% of nailbed) subungual haematomas can be decompressed with a heated paperclip or needle.
- Use local anaesthetic (ring block) with a tourniquet and loupe magnification.

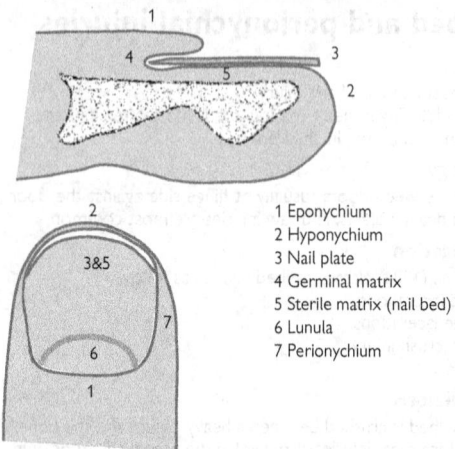

1. Eponychium
2. Hyponychium
3. Nail plate
4. Germinal matrix
5. Sterile matrix (nail bed)
6. Lunula
7. Perionychium

Fig. 17.5 Anatomy of fingernail.

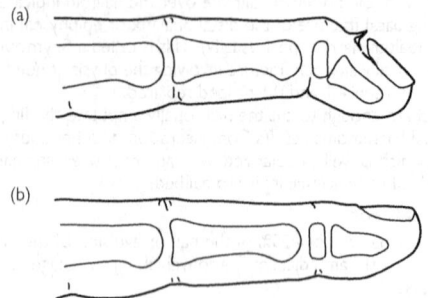

Fig. 17.6 Dislocation of the nail base can only occur if there is a bone or joint injury underneath, in this case a Salter–Harris type 1 epiphyseal fracture (Seymour fracture). This needs operative wash-out of the compound fracture, reduction, and relocation of the nail to act as a splint.

- Remove as much of the nail as required to access the injury; it is usually easier to remove the entire nail than to remove a portion of it.
- Debridement of the nailbed should be absolutely minimal.
- Explore distal phalanx fractures; debride loose or poorly vascularized bone; irrigate the open cavity with copious normal saline.
- Repair the nailbed (7/0 vicryl is ideal).

- Stable distal phalanx fractures or tuft fractures do not need fixation. A single K-wire can be used for unstable shaft fractures (i.e. those involving the FDP/EDC insertions).
- Clean and fenestrate the nail, and replace it to splint the nailfold, mould the nail to the finger, and splint the DP fracture.
- Suture the nail to the pulp tip if it is unstable and liable to fall off.
- If the nail is absent or very damaged, a foil (suture packet) splint can be fabricated.
- Straight incisions perpendicular to the nailfold can be used to allow repair of very proximal avulsions of the nailbed. However, repair these on both the deep nailfold and skin surface to avoid notching.
- Close skin with 5/0 or 6/0 non-absorbable or absorbable sutures.
- Use a non-adherent dressing.
- If the nailbed is avulsed completely, attempt to replace it as a graft (ideally still attached to the nail for easier handling and splintage).
- Nailbed loss can be replaced with a split nailbed graft from an adjacent nailbed or the great toe. Alternatively, a dermal or FTSG can be used.

Post-operative care
- Elevate the hand.
- Change dressings 12 weeks post repair; then as required.
- Start physiotherapy to mobilize the DIPJ and desensitize the tip after the first dressing change.
- Remove sutures after 2 weeks. The nail splint will fall out.

Complications
- Nail deformity/dystrophy: ridges, splits, or non-adherence due to scars or ridges in the sterile matrix/nailbed.
- Pterygium of the nailfold to the nailbed with a split in the nail.
- Tender pulp.
- Non-union of DP fracture.
- Osteomyelitis of DP.
- If untreated, a significant subungual haematoma can cause necrosis of the sterile matrix due to pressure. Substantial nailbed lacerations will lead to a deformed nail. Unrecognized open DP fractures may progress to osteomyelitis.

Nail deformity
- Beau's lines: transverse grooves due to temporary cessation of nail growth.
- Muehrcke's lines: transverse whitish lines in the nailplate (leuconychia striata) because of incomplete keratinization, so that nuclear debris or nuclei are retained. Occurs in chronic hypo-albuminaemia, chemotherapy.

Reference
Zook EG, Guy RJ, Russell RC (1984). *J Hand Surg (Am)* **9**, 247–52.

Flexor tendon injuries

Definition
An injury to the flexor tendons of the hand, usually sustained by a sharp laceration; occasionally by avulsion of origin.

Incidence
- A common hand injury.
- Index and little finger more commonly involved then ring, middle, and thumb.
- More common in males than females, and in ages 15–40 years.

Aetiology
- A sharp injury (usually knife or glass) but also follows sports or RTA injuries causing tendon avulsion.
- Occasionally an abrading mid-tendinous rupture secondary to arthritis, bone spur, or metal implant.

Classification
According to zone/level of injury:
- Zone 1: distal to FDS insertion.
- Zone 2: from the proximal edge A1 pulley to the end of FDS insertion.
- Zone 3: in the palm.
- Zone 4: under the carpal tunnel.
- Zone 5: forearm.

Zone 2 is absent in the thumb.

Clinical presentation
Presents with history of the injury and an inability to flex the affected digit or pain on attempted flexion. Determine the mechanism of the injury and hence predict the level of the distal tendon end and the degree of retraction of the proximal end. A laceration in the extended position will mark the distal tendon end at the level of the laceration. If lacerated in extreme flexion, the distal end will retract distally as the digit is extended. FDP proximal retraction is limited by the lumbrical. FPL; often retracts into the forearm.

Examination
- Examine the wound.
- Look for loss of the natural flexion cascade of digits, loss of movement.
- Check independent FDS and FDP motion.
- Be suspicious of pain on movement or triggering indicating partial injury.
- Be aware that a divided flexor tendon can still be present even if some flexion is possible because of pulling on an intact vinculum (this usually fails with time).

Management

- Extend the wound: wound extension should be sufficiently large to allow exposure of the divided ends and adequate space for their repair.
- Exploration of the wound: search for divided ends and intact structures. Explore areas of haematoma, always heading from normal anatomy towards the injury. Tendons can be differentiated from nerves by traction causing passive flexion of the appropriate digit, yellowish-white colour, no branching, muscle attached, no adherent artery, no fascicular structure, and on flexing the digit or wrist will often glide into view (beware that traction on nerves can cause some flexion).
- Identify the various divided structures: identification is assisted by knowing that the middle and ring flexor superficialis tendons lie superficial to those of the small and index finger, just ulnar and deep to the palmaris longus tendon. Tendons have different sizes and cross-sectional shapes and this can also be used to help match the ends. Traction on the distal end can help identify the distal stump. Traction on a profundus tendon will produce flexion in multiple digits in addition to the involved digit. This can be differentiated by feeling the correct tension in the digits. Once identified, the tendons should be marked with different needles or other techniques. When repaired the tendon should recreate the normal cascade of the digits and produce the normal tenodesis effect on flexion and extension of the wrist.
- Repair the tendons.

Flexor tendon repair

Repair options
- Primary repair.
- Delayed primary repair.
- Secondary repair.
- Repair by a tendon graft (either one stage or two stages).

Techniques of flexor tendon repair

Incisions
Wound extensions by Brunner style zig-zags or along mid-lateral lines. Try to avoid contact areas. Avoid scars that cause contractures.

Exposure
Use a minimal-contact atraumatic technique with fine instrumentation and magnification. Preserve the pulleys. Create an L-shaped incision in the flexor sheath over the cruciate or retinacular portions which can be more easily repaired. Create these incisions where the distal stump can be delivered for at least a centimetre through this opening (usually by flexing the DIPJ). Once the distal stump has been delivered, fix it there with a hypodermic needle.

Tendon retrieval
Deliver the proximal end by flexing the wrist and palm, assisting by externally milking the tendon from forearm to digit. If this fails to reveal the tendon it may be retrieved by passing a tendon retriever or small mosquito forceps down the flexor sheath. Care must be taken not to injure the tendon or the sheath. If this fails, create a separate incision more proximally to identify it. Retrieve the proximal tendon end. Pass an infant feeding tube from the distal wound down the flexor tendon sheath until it can be retrieved at the proximal incision. Suture it to the proximal tendon and by gentle retraction deliver the proximal tendon end through the distal wound. Fix it with a hypodermic needle in a position suitable for repair. Accurate preparation of the tendon ends for repair is vital for good result.

Relationships
Restore the FDP to FDS relationship. The FDS is divided over the proximal phalanx where the two slips wrapping around the FDP to reach their insertion will unwrap once divided. It is important to restore their orientation, otherwise the chiasma will ensnare the FDP tendon.

Tendon repair
Suture the tendon. There are many techniques for tendon repair, and many suture strengths and types are also described. The principle is for the creation of a strong repair which is sufficiently robust to withstand the tension created in mobilization, will last long enough for tendon healing to occur, and is of small enough bulk so as not to interfere with tendon healing or gliding. For early active mobilization techniques a minimum of a four-strand core suture repair of 3/0–4/0 is required, supported and neatened by a continuous 6/0 epitendinous suture (Fig. 17.8).

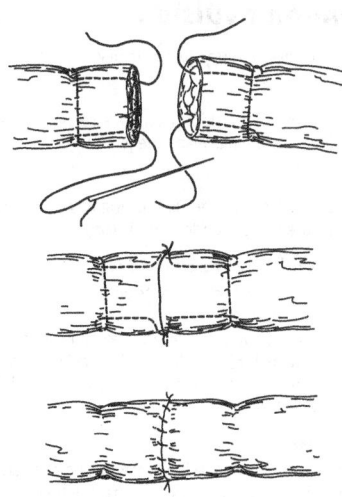

Fig. 17.7 Kessler suture and epitendinous stitch.

The most common repair technique is a modified Kessler type repair repeated (double Kessler) to give a four-strand repair with a Halstead inverting continuous epitendinous suture. Strickland described a Kessler repair combined with a mattress suture to create the four-strand core.

Sheath repair

The sheath windows should be repaired with a 6/0 nylon. Once repaired, the ability for the repair to glide through the tendon sheath, particularly the annular pulleys, must be assessed by the tenodesis test or by traction on the tendon proximally and extension passively. The advantages of sheath repair are improved tendon nutrition, reduction in adhesions, better gliding, and better remodelling. The disadvantages are constriction of the tendon repair, more adhesions, and worse gliding.

Documentation

It is important, particularly for the therapist, to document the site and type of repair, to confirm that the tendon glides through the pulleys and the repairs are strong enough for immediate mobilization.

Flexor tendon avulsion

Also known as rugby jersey injury, jersey injury.

Definition
A closed avulsion of the FDP tendon from its insertion, classically sustained whilst trying to grab a passing player by the jersey.

Incidence
The most commonly affected finger is the ring finger as it has the smallest area of insertion of the flexor tendon and is long.

Classification (Leddy and Packer 1977)
- Type 1. Tendon avulsion which retracts all the way into the palm hence has no blood supply.
- Type 2. Tendon avulsion with or without small bone fragment caught at PIPJ; hence maintains PIPJ vinculum and blood supply.
- Type 3. Bone fragment caught at A4 pulley; maintains all blood supply and no tendon retraction.

Clinical presentation
- Clinically the failure to flex at the DIPJ may not be noticed for some time.
- Tenderness or a palpable mass may indicate the level of retraction of the tendon.

Management
- Surgical re-attachment is required. In type 3 injuries there is no issue about the duration from injury to repair as the tendon does not significantly retract. However, in the other injuries repair should be performed before significant tendon shortening occurs (10–14 days).
- In type 3 injuries the fragment may be sufficiently large that the repair is essentially an ORIF of fracture.
- In the other injuries a zone 1 flexor tendon repair is needed. Similarly, in non-avulsion zone 1 injuries there may be insufficient distal stump in which to form the standard repair. In these cases the following options are suggested.

Zone 1 flexor tendon repair
Suture the proximal stump using your standard core suture technique. This can then be secured to the distal phalanx by:
- Drilling two parallel holes through the distal phalanx, exiting over the mid-nail, passing the suture ends through the drill holes (assisted by a 14 or 16 gauge hypodermic needle), and tying the ends over a button.
- Incising at the apex of the digit just below the hyponychium and passing the suture ends along the sides of the distal phalanx to be tied, through the separate apical incision, over the distal end of the distal phalanx.

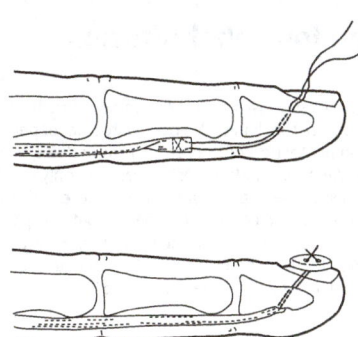

Fig. 17.8 Pull-out suture for profundus avulsion.

- A variation is to create a transverse drill hole through the tuft of the distal phalanx through which the suture is passed to make fixation more secure.
- Alternative techniques involve the use of a barbed wire suture which engages the proximal tendon stump and traverses the distal tendon stump and distal phalanx to be tied over a button on the nail. The proximal wire is left percutaneously so that when the button is removed the wire can be retracted (Jennings 1954).

References

Jennings ER (1954). *Md State Med J* **3**, 17–18.
Leddy JP, Packer JW (1977). *J Hand Surg (Am)* **2**, 66–9.

Flexor tendon rehabilitation

Introduction
Repair of the flexor tendons is only the commencement of the process in restoring function to the hand. A good outcome depends upon good rehabilitation and protection of the repair from undue strain.

Tendon is weakest 14–21 days post repair and only regains 50% of its strength at 6 weeks. The repair needs to be protected during this time period. It can be unprotected after this period but the patient should be warned not to undertake full activity for a further 6 weeks as this is the period before the tendon regains 75% of its strength. Some tension and movement are required to maximize and promote collagenous proliferation and alignment.

Classification
- Delayed mobilization: splint or cast.
- Static splint passive mobilization.
- Static splint early active mobilization.
- Dynamic.

Delayed mobilization (splint and leave)
The hand is splinted or cast in the position of function for 6 weeks. Following splint removal, mobilization commences without protection.

Delayed mobilization has advantages of simplicity and less risk of tendon rupture—can leave and forget it. It is chosen for uncooperative patients who frequently end up doing quite well, probably because they are mobilizing within their splints. Not as effective for cooperative patients.

Passive mobilization (Duran)
The hand is splinted with the wrist flexed at 20°, the MCPJs flexed at 80°–90°, and the IPJs extended. The therapy consists of passive flexion and extension only for the first 6 weeks, followed by progressive active movement and withdrawal of the splint.

Advantages are reduced adhesions, improved excursion, and improved tensile strength of repair, with less risk of tendon rupture and fewer flexion contractures compared with active techniques.

Early active mobilization (Belfast)
The hand is splinted with the wrist flexed at 20°, the MCPJs flexed at 80°–90°, and the IPJs extended. The therapy commences with passive flexion and hold with active extension for the first 2–3 weeks, followed by active flexion and extension and, after 6 weeks with progressively more independent active movement, withdrawal of the splint.

Early active mobilization has advantages in simple splint construction, a simpler therapy regime, and advantages of early mobilization in increased gliding, excursion, remodelling, and strength. Disadvantages are increased risk of tendon rupture.

Kleinert (dynamic splintage)

A protected mobilization system for flexor tendon repairs. This technique reversed the thoughts at that time about the futility of zone 2 flexor tendon repairs. It consists of a dorsal blocking splint with the wrist in neutral and the metacarpophalangeal joints between 60° and 90° of flexion with the interphalangeal joints straight. Dress hooks are glued to the fingernails, and rubber bands are attached to these to pull the fingers into a flexed position. The proximal ends of the rubber bands are attached at the level of the wrist. Variations on this theme have been described in which the rubber bands pass under a palmar bar such that the traction of the bands allows DIPJ flexion as well as MCPJ and PIPJ flexion. Another variation involves the bands passing to the dorsum of the hand through the web spaces to improve DIPJ flexion.

The therapy regime commences with active extension against the force of the rubber bands, ensuring that the IP joints achieve full extension with the MCPJs kept flexed. The finger is allowed to relax into flexion passively under the force of the rubber band. Intensive therapy supervision is required, particularly initially when the rubber band tension needs to be adjusted and the patient taught the required exercises.

Dynamic splintage has advantages in a more rapid return to tendon gliding and remodelling, and a more rapid return to tendon strength by modification of tendon healing by application of longitudinal tension. Elastic band traction reduces the risk of tendon rupture and occludes the fingers and palm, preventing inadvertent hand use. Disadvantages are complexity in construction and in the therapy regime. Risk of PIPJ contracture.

Ring avulsion injury

Definition
A digital injury caused by traction on a ring worn on that digit.

Incidence
- Sporting injury associated with goal nets in football.
- Common in industry.
- People jumping down from platforms and catching their ring on a nail.

Aetiology
Traction on a ring pulled towards the fingertip or the hand pulled away from the ring results in varying degrees of injury to the digit.

Classification (Urbaniak et al. 1981)
- Type 1. Skin laceration, circulation intact.
- Type 2. Circulation compromised, needs revascularization, no fracture/dislocation.
- Type 3. Total degloving/with or without fracture/amputation.

Clinical presentation
History and injury are characteristic.

Examination
- Examine the wound.
- Look for loss of the natural flexion cascade of digits, loss of movement, check independent FDS and FDP motion.
- Check sensation and perfusion.
- X-ray the digit.

Management
- Type 1 is treated by a debridement and closure or dressings.
- Type 2 requires revascularization, generally with interposition vessel grafts.
- Type 3 is a severe injury with poor outcome and amputation is suggested.

Surgery
Because of the avulsion nature of the injury to the vessels, the extent of vessel injury is greater than appears. Look for a red streak in the vessel wall, indicating injury, and check for in-flow after debridement. Grafts are sometimes needed to bridge the vessel from the MCPJ level to the distal DIPJ level. A separate longitudinal incision can be made over the artery just proximal to the DIPJ. Vein grafts can be harvested from the dorsum of the middle finger or palmar surface of the forearm.

Outcome
- Type 1: excellent outcome is to be expected.
- Type 2: 80% success at revascularization; 60% receive good to excellent range of movement. Most return to work in 8–9 weeks. Much better prognosis if no fracture or PIPJ injury.

Reference
Urbaniak JR, Evans JP, Bright DS (1981). *J Hand Surg* **6**, 25–30.

Boutonnière deformity

Definition
An alteration in flexor and extensor muscle and tendon balance which results in deformity with three components:
- Flexion of the PIPJ.
- Hyperextension of the DIPJ.
- Hyperextension of the MCPJ.

Incidence
- A common hand deformity.
- Occurs frequently in patients with rheumatoid arthritis/trauma.
- More common in males than females, and at ages 15–40 years.

Aetiology
The deformity results from a primary abnormality of the PIPJ (unlike swan-neck deformities which can arise at any joint). Trauma or synovial proliferation cause incompetence of the central slip.

Unable to achieve full extension at the PIPJ, a flexion posture at the PIPJ develops, the lateral bands sublux palmarly and shorten to become fixed, and the oblique retinacular ligaments shorten and cause hyperextension, limiting flexion of the DIPJ. As the flexion deformity at the PIPJ increases, the patient compensates by hyperextending the MCPJ.

Functional loss can be minimal until the late stages and so treatment in the early stages should be simple and have minimal risk.

Classification
Classified by Nalebuff and Millender (1975) as mild, moderate, or severe according to the degree of flexion, whether or not the flexion can be corrected passively, and the status of the PIPJ articular surface.
- Stage 1: boutonnière deformity (passively correctable)—only 10°–15° lag in PIPJ extension; full extension may restrict flexion of the DIPJ. DIPJ may be slightly hyperextended. MCPJ usually normal. Flexion of the DIPJ improves as the PIPJ is flexed and the functional loss is related as much to lack of full DIPJ flexion as to lack of PIPJ extension.
- Stage 2: moderate boutonnière deformity (passively correctable)—functional loss becomes significant as the flexion deformity of the PIPJ reaches 30°–40°. Patients compensate by hyper-extending MCPJ. DIPJ becomes hyper-extended with decreased flexion.
- Stage 3: severe boutonnière deformity—PIPJ cannot be extended passively.

Management
Type 1
- Operative treatment may worsen existing function.
- Steroid injection or synovectomy if synovitis present.
- Extensor tenotomy over the MCPJ to increase DIPJ flexion.
- Static or dynamic splinting to extend the PIPJ but allowing DIPJ flexion; restores balance without risking loss PIPJ flexion.

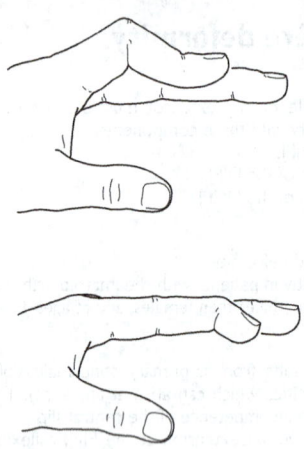

Fig. 17.9 Boutonnière and mallet deformities.

Type 2
- Extensor mechanism reconstruction if the following apply: good dorsal skin, smooth joint surfaces, functioning flexor tendons, PIPJ flexion deformity can be corrected passively.
- if present, flexion deformity of the wrist should be corrected before attempting to restore PIPJ extension.

Type 3
- Try to convert to type 2 by dynamic splinting or serial casting to restore passive extension.
- Soft tissue release (dividing transverse retinacular ligaments and accessory collateral ligaments) might be required. Surgery such as this is not often indicated.
- Fusion or arthroplasty for severe deformities with poor joint surfaces (note that loss of PIPJ flexion is compensated by the gain in MCPJ flexion).

Five types of soft tissue repair of extensor mechanism
- Anatomical (Mason).
- Tendon grafting using either a graft or a retrograde flap (Snow).
- Distal extensor tenotomy (Fowler): release lateral bands from distal phalanx so that the central slip takes up the slack and can extend the PIPJ. The DIPJ can still extend because of the functioning oblique retinacular ligaments.
- Reconstruction using lateral bands (Littler, Matev).
- Tenolysis (Curtis).

Bony repairs
Arthrodesis or arthroplasty.

Reference
Nalebuff EA, Millender LH (1975). *Orthop Clin North Am*, **6**, 753–63.

Swan-neck deformity

Definition
A digital deformity caused by musculo-tendinous imbalance characterized by hyperextension of the PIPJ and flexion of the DIPJ, and may be associated with flexion of the MCPJ. Deformity can originate from any of these joints. Functional loss is related to loss of motion at the PIPJ.

Incidence
- Common, especially in rheumatoids.
- May follow FDS division or harvest (recurvatum).
- May be congenital due to generalized laxity.

Aetiology
Depends on originating joints.

DIPJ

At the DIPJ level stretching or rupture of terminal extensor tendon produces a mallet deformity; detachment of distal insertion of extensor mechanism concentrates its action on the PIPJ and causes hyperextension.

PIPJ

At the PIPJ, laxity of the palmar plate or rupture of the FDS secondary to trauma or synovitis, results in hyper-extension at the PIPJ, in turn slackening the lateral bands and causing an extensor lag at the distal phalanx.

MCPJ

In RA ulnar palmar flexion subluxation of the MCPJ causes tight intrinsics creating hyperextension of the PIPJ. Initially positional dependent on the MCPJ (as the MCPJ position alters tension of the intrinsics), later it becomes fixed.

Classification
According to loss of motion at the PIPJ and radiographic appearances of the joint (Nalebuff and Millender 1975).
- Type 1. Deformity but no loss of motion.
- Type 2. Deformity with loss of motion according to the position of the MPJs.
- Type 3. Deformity with loss of motion regardless of the position of the MCPJ, but no radiographic changes.
- Type 4. As type 3 but with X-ray changes.

Management

Type 1
Aimed at correction of PIPJ hyperextension, and restoring DIPJ extension:
- Non-operative: ring splint, Murphy's ring, figure-of-eight ring.
- Operative:
  - DIPJ fusion.
  - Dermotenodesis of DIPJ.
  - Flexor tenodesis (FDS) of PIPJ.
  - Oblique retinacular ligament reconstruction.

Type 2
Release intrinsic tightness and correct any MCP joint disorder, usually by arthroplasty.

Type 3
- Try to convert to type 2, and restore passive motion by:
  - PIPJ manipulation under anaesthesia.
  - Skin release.
  - Lateral band mobilization.
  - Extensor tenotomy.
  - Arthrolysis.
- Then treat as type 2.

Note that if active flexion is significantly less than passive flexion, the flexor tendons should be explored for adhesion, nodules, or synovitis.

Type 4
Fusion or arthroplasty of PIPJ.

Reference
Nalebuff EA, Millender LH (1975). *Orthop Clin North Am* **6** 733–52.

Ulnar collateral ligament injury of the thumb MCPJ

Also known as skier's thumb, gamekeeper's thumb.

Incidence
- Ten times more common than the radial collateral ligament injury (RCL).
- Common as acute injury skiing, or attritional injury in gamekeepers.

Classification
- Simple incomplete.
- Complete.
- Avulsion.
- Subluxation.

Pathology
- Intra-ligamentous tear.
- Avulsion from proximal phalanx.
- May be avulsion fragment.
- Tear of capsule dorsally and volarly.

Stener lesion
In two-thirds of cases the adductor aponeurosis interposes between the torn end of the ligament and the site from which it was avulsed (Stener 1963). Thus conservative management will not allow healing, leading to weak UCL which gives weak pinch and grip and later development of arthritis.

Diagnosis
- History and examination:
    - Examine for laxity of the UCL, assess in MCPJ flexion as this should tighten the collateral ligaments, making the joint more stable.
    - Feel for end-point.
    - Assess degree of pain.
    - If too painful, protect and re-assess when swelling has reduced or try LA.
    - A Stener lesion can also be diagnosed by palpating for the end of the UCL as a mass dorsal lateral to the MCPJ.
- X-ray:
    - Comparative stress views.
    - Look for avulsion fragment.
    - Beware on examination and stress X-rays not to complete an incomplete injury.
- Ultrasound and MRI may help in detection of the stener lesion.

Treatment
- Partial tear: splint.
- Complete tear:
    - If no Stener lesion, splint.
    - If Stener lesion, explore and repair.
- Bone avulsion fragment:

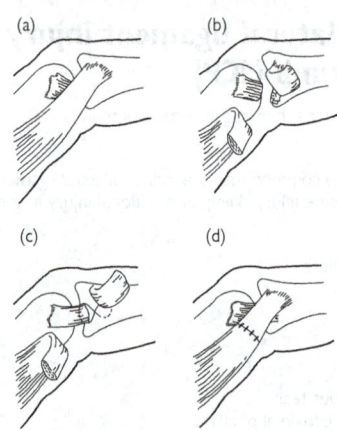

Fig. 17.10 Ruptured UCL of MCPJ thumb: (a) adductor hiding the UCL; (b) division of adductor reveals ruptured UCL; (c) UCL repaired by suture, wire, or bone anchor; (d) repair adductor.

- If undisplaced, splint.
- If displaced, open reduction and repair.
- If small fragment, suture UCL through the fragment into the bone.

Operation
- V-shaped incision on ulnar aspect of MCPJ.
- If a Stener lesion is present you will see end of UCL poking up proximal to the adductor aponeurosis.
- Divide adductor aponeurosis to expose UCL attachment site.
- Restore ligament and repair (bone anchor).
- Stabilize joint with K-wire and/or splint.

Chronic instability
- Gamekeeper's thumb (Campbell 1955): chronic attenuation of UCL.
- Other causes of chronic instability are untreated acute injury or failure to recognize Stener lesion, congenital, rheumatoid arthritis.

Treatment
Depends on status of the joint:
- If arthritic, fuse joint.
- If not, reconstruct the ligament: may need graft or use a distally based strip of adductor aponeurosis.

References
Campbell CS (1955). *J Bone Joint Surg Br* **37B**, 148–9.
Stener B (1963). *Acta Chir Scand* **125**, 583–6.

Hand fractures

- Hand fractures are one of the most common emergency problems treated by plastic surgeons.
- Most isolated hand fractures are well vascularized and heal rapidly; non-union is rare.
- Loss of function is due to loss of motion (swelling/stiffness/adhesions), malunion, or associated injuries.

Incidence
- 242/100 000 per year.
- 8% need surgery (20% in USA).
- Mainly young patients.
- Most fractures little finger and thumb. Ring, middle, and index fingers approximately equal.
- Little finger metacarpal greatest incidence at 31%.
- 17% intra-articular.
- 21% comminuted.

Fracture pathomechanics
- Elastic deformation: first part of stress–strain curve; bones normally operate in this part and when force decreases return to normal.
- Plastic deformation: second part of curve; when force is removed here, there is some residual deformity (e.g. greenstick fracture in children).
- Breaks occur in third part of the curve where force exceeds the limitation of the structure (bone).
- Fractures occur in response to compression, torsion, or tension forces. Tears on the tension side and comminutes on the compression side.
- Bone works well in axial compression, muscle and tendon take some tension.
- Fracture risk associated with state of bone (osteoporosis, age, tumour, previous deformity), proprioception (which can be trained), degree of force, direction of force, and muscle and tendon strength.

Classification
Adult or child; age and handedness of patient; open or closed; which bone involved; level of involvement; fracture pattern; intra- or extra-articular; displaced or undisplaced; stable or unstable; degree of soft tissue injury; comparison of clinical and radiological assessments. Children's fractures have their own classification.

Salter–Harris classification of epiphyseal injuries (Salter and Harris 1963)
- Type 1. Shearing separation along the physeal plate.
- Type 2. Separation of the physis with a small corner of metaphysis.
- Type 3. Fracture through the epiphysis sparing the plate.
- Type 4. Longitudinal fracture through the metaphysis and the plate and epiphysis.
- Type 5. Compression fracture of the plate.

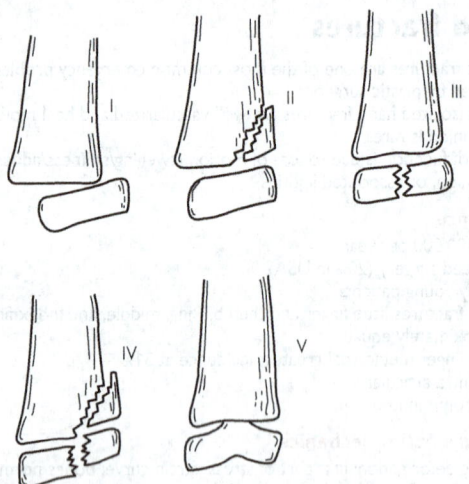

Fig. 17.11 Salter–Harris classification of epiphyseal injuries.

Consider

Fracture personality
- Direct or indirect force transfer.
- Low or high energy.
- Displacement: shift, rotation, angulation.
- Displacement: anatomical vs. clinical; i.e. is it in a position which will impair function?
- Stability: is there potential to displace during healing to a position which will impair function? Stability depends on line of fracture, comminution, impaction, soft tissue injury, bone quality.

Patient personality
- Age.
- Occupation.
- Cooperation.
- Function.
- Choice.

Surgeon personality
- Age and experience.
- Activity.
- Access.
- Choice.

In general
- Stable undisplaced—do nothing.
- Unstable undisplaced—conservative. watchful treatment, or fix.
- Stable displaced—accept displacement or reduce and splint.
- Unstable displaced—reduce and fix.

Stable fractures
Include:
- Closed impacted shaft fractures.
- Fractures with little or no displacement.
- Most distal phalangeal fractures.
- Many isolated metacarpal shaft fractures.
- Well-aligned fractures that maintain their position through a full arc of motion.

Radiographic criteria of acceptable alignment (Pun et al. 1989)
- 10° and angulation in both sagittal and coronal planes.
- 45°–50° sagittal angulation in the fifth metacarpal neck.
- 50% overlap (fracture translation) at the fracture site.
- No rotational deformity.

Direction of instability determines fixation method
- Axial = traction = lag screw, external fixator (ex-fix).
- Angular = tension or buttress.
- Rotational = torsion = pins, screws, neutralization plate.
- Translational = compression.

Management aim
United fracture with pain-free function and with sensation, mobility, strength, and stability. To accomplish this goal the surgeon must choose a treatment method that will offer the least soft tissue damage and allow mobilization as soon as fracture stability permits.

Conservative management
Most digital fractures can be treated conservatively.

Principles of conservative management
Conservative management means:
- Do nothing surgical (rather than do nothing at all).
- Splint.
- Mobilize.
- Identify displacement/slippage.
- Detect and avoid complications.
- Regularly review decision.

Indications for conservative management
- Undisplaced stable fractures.
- Acceptably displaced stable fractures.
- Some undisplaced unstable fractures.
- Shaft fractures:
  - Dorsal angulation best because of flexion forces.

- Joint fractures.
  - Undisplaced or minimally displaced, or grossly comminuted.
  - Unicondylar fractures if type 1 (see p. 564): the other types usually rotate as the fracture fragment subsides.
- Fracture dislocation.
  - Reduce and splint to keep in stable zone and mobilize within stable zone.
  - Splint, e.g. dorsal blocking, kissing splint. If persistent subluxation, then fix.

Contraindications
Multiple fractures and complex tissue involvement tend to indicate fracture fixation rather than conservative management.

Conservative management techniques
- No restraint.
- Neighbour strapping (encourages angulation and rotation).
- Flexion and extension exercises (encourages correction of angulation particularly if apex palmar/dorsally angulated).
- Splint (static or dynamic).

Complications
Stiffness, malunion, CRPS, infection, instability, non-union, arthritis, pain.

Surgical management
Remember that if you are going to fix the fracture, it must be stable enough to allow immediate functional rehabilitation to overcome the extra trauma of the fixation!

Indications for fixation of hand fractures
- Irreducible fractures.
- Open fractures (to skin or nailbed).
- Fractures with soft tissue injury (vessel, nerve, tendon, ligament, skin).
- Segmental bone loss.
- Polytrauma with hand fractures.
- Multiple hand or wrist fractures.
- Reconstruction (osteotomy, non-union).
- Intra-articular fractures.
- Subcapital fractures (phalangeal).
- Malrotation (spiral and short oblique).
- Unstable fractures.

Choice of fixation
Depends on experience, fracture pattern, and direction of instability:
- Axial instability needs traction by ex-fix, lag screw.
- Angular instability needs tension or buttress.
- Rotational instability needs torsional constraint by pins, screws, neutralization plate.
- Translational instability needs compression plate.

Principles of surgical approach
- Provide adequate exposure, extensile, avoid gliding structures, reduce scar, based on anatomy.
- Metacarpal: dorsal longitudinal, over shaft of metacarpal, deep exposure stepped slightly so that not a straight line to the bone and plate. If there are two metacarpals, go between them. If fifth metacarpal try lateral approach. Avoid a single plane from skin to tendon to plate to bone.
- Digit: mid-line or lateral. Mid-line has excellent view and is easy, but crosses gliding plane. Mid-axial or lateral is performed by dotting the tops of flexion creases and then joining the dots; less exposure but avoids gliding plane.

Internal fixation techniques

Absolute stability; gives direct bone healing with no callus formation; this is better for intra-articular fractures, short oblique diaphyseal fractures, and arthrodesis. Achieved by compression, producing friction between fragments which produces stability.

Lag screw technique
- A technique not a type of screw. Gives excellent interfragmentary compression.
- Lag screw is a technique of introducing a screw which produces compression between two surfaces.
- Lag screw gives seven times compression; using a compression plate gives three times. Produces two to three times more compression then a dynamic compression plate.
- Needs a gliding hole in the near fragment and a holding hole in the far fragment so that the screw only holds the far side and pulls it into the near side held by the screw head, creating compression.
- Compare with a *positioning* screw with both cortices drilled with threaded holes; the compression gained is only that obtained by squeezing the two bones together as the screw is inserted. No leverage advantage from the screw itself.
- Create the gliding hole by drilling at the screw thread diameter and the holding hole or thread hole at the screw core diameter.

Indications
- Ideal as sole fixation for long oblique fracture where length of fracture is greater than twice (preferably thrice!) the diameter (width) of the bone. Use two or three screws.
- To provide compression for a short oblique fracture using single screw where additional stability is given by a neutralization plate.

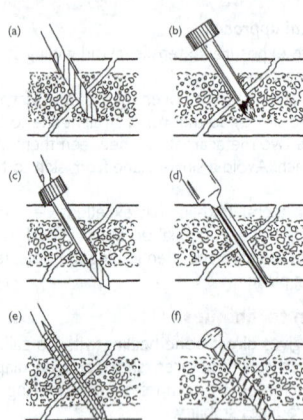

Fig. 17.12 Lag screw technique: (a) gliding hole drill; (b) insert gliding hole drill guide (AO set only); (c) drill thread hole; (d) measure depth using gauge; (e) tap if necessary, countersink if necessary; (f) insert screw, which lags and compresses the two surfaces together.

Technique

Generally do the smaller core hole first and then over-drill the near fragment. With the AO kit, which has special gliding hole drill guides, the gliding hole can be done first. There are six steps:
- Reduce and temporarily hold the fracture.
- Drill glide hole; larger drill across near cortex only.
- Drill thread hole (smaller fixation screw core diameter) across both cortices.
- Use counter-sink.
- Measure.
- Tap (tap may not be needed for the self-tapping screws).
- Insert screw.

Technical tips for lag screws
- Entry hole has to be at least two to three screw diameters from the edge to avoid microfractures of the bone fragment tip.
- Angle of screw:
  - If perpendicular to axial line of the phalanx will give best resistance to axial load, but perpendicular to fracture line will give best compression and resistance to shear.
  - If using two lag screws have one in each position.
  - An optimal screw is one angled/postioned halfway between the two.
- Drill small hole all the way first, then over-drill the near cortex/surface. Can do it the other way but unless you have a drill guide that will fit into the proximal large hole you risk eccentrically drilling the distal small hole. Also, if you fail to notice the medullary cavity you may drill all the way with your large drill, giving the screw no purchase at all.
- Measure depth using depth gauge: ensure that the tip points away from the angle.

Dynamic compression techniques
These include tension band wiring or tension band plate. Produce compression forces on flexor side and tension forces on dorsal surface, so that the flexion force is neutralized by the tension plate/wire.

K-wire and tension band
- Indications: unstable phalangeal and metacarpal fractures requiring ORIF, failed plates and screws, diaphyseal fractures with three or four fragments.
- Advantages: very stable, biomechanically sound (functional loading forces are converted into compressive loads across the fracture).
- Disadvantages: Operative exposure may be significant.

Compression plate
- Indications for metacarpal fractures:
  - Fractures with soft tissue loss.
  - Comminuted or peri-articular fractures.
  - Comminuted fractures with shortening or malrotation.
  - Fractures with segmental bone loss.
- Indications for phalangeal fractures (complex fractures):
  - Fractures with substance loss.
  - Intra-articular T-condylar fractures.
  - Some fractures with peri-articular comminution.
- Advantages:
  - Stable skeletal fixation.
  - Maintains or restores length.
  - Condylar plate lateral position permits extra-articular placement.
- Disadvantages:
  - Extreme technical difficulty.
  - Small margin of error.
  - Implant bulk is a problem with overlying tendons.
- Tips:
  - Pre-bend (over-bend the plate for the contour slightly) if you want to use as compression plate to prevent gapping at far cortex as near cortex compresses.
  - Contour the plate exactly if you want to use as neutralization plate.
  - Straight plate only with straight bone (?except locking plates).

Neutralization plate and lag screw
If both used together, fix plate first as compression followed by lag screw which will add even more compression. If screw is used first, use neutralization plate rather than compression plate as trying to compress a plate that is not well contoured can cause displacement of fragments.

Problems with plates
- Exposure and soft tissue injury.
- Adherence of tissues.
- Volume of plate makes it difficult to close wound.
- Infection.
- Requires rehabilitation and therapy.
- Stress shielding: plate tight on bone can cause necrosis of bone under the plate.

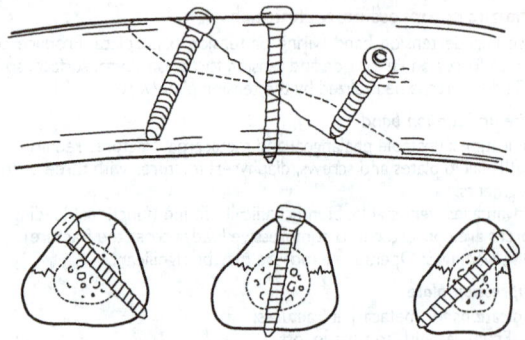

Fig. 17.13 Triple lag screw fixation of spiral fracture.

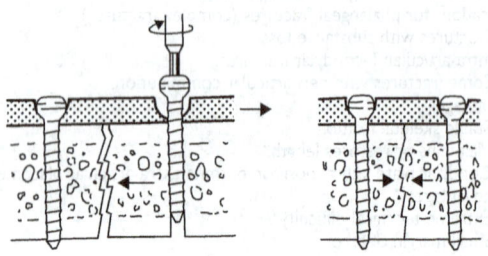

Fig. 17.14 Dynamic compression by offsetting holes in plate.

K-wires
Introduced by Kirschner in 1909.
- Advantages: percutaneous application; avoids surgical exposure and soft tissue trauma; cheap.
- Disadvantages: not easy; weak implant which is only relatively stable, and is subject to loosening and migration; wire exposure can lead to infection; if applied with wires crossing at the fracture site can distract the fracture leading to delayed union or non-union.
- Indications in phalangeal fractures: closed unstable diaphyseal, base, and neck fractures.
- Indications in metacarpal fractures: isolated shaft, neck, or base fractures (wires inserted longitudinally or transversely depending on the fracture location).
- Technical tips:
  - Diamond tipped K-wires are preferable (other tips tend to make a hole larger than diameter of the wire and so the wire hold is reduced).
  - Use low-speed driver (less heat, more control).
  - Get it right first time (tends to follow prior paths).

- Draw a line on the skin to aid direction.
- Check in three planes—visually and use intensifier.
- Know your surface anatomy.
- Irrigate the wire to dissipate heat.
- If you cannot get it right in three or four attempts, change your technique, i.e. use open approach.

Oblique K-wires and intraosseous wires
- Indications: open transverse phalangeal fractures; replantation; arthrodeses.
- Advantages: technically straightforward; minimal equipment; adequate stable fixation for early mobilization.
- Disadvantages: limited clinical application; requires surgical exposure; K-wire can limit tendon gliding.

Intraosseous wiring 90–90 technique
- Indications: open transverse phalangeal fractures; replantation; arthrodeses.
- Advantages: technically straightforward; minimal equipment; biomedically strong (second only to a plate) stable fixation for early mobilization; low-profile implant.
- Disadvantages: limited clinical application; requires huge surgical exposure; poor in osteopenic bone.

Intraosseous wiring of individual fragments
- Indications: intra-articular fractures; avulsion fractures.
- Advantages: limited exposure of the fracture fragment; maintains vascularity to the fragment; low-profile implant; technically straightforward; minimal equipment; adequate stable fixation for early mobilization sometimes.
- Disadvantages: indirect wire tightening can limit security of fixation; poor rotational control.

External fixation in hand fractures

Allows stabilization of a fracture from a distance.

Strength and stability affected by
- Distance from frame to bone: less = better.
- Distance from pins to fracture: less = better.
- Thickness of pins: thicker = better.
- Number of pins: more = better.
- Number of bars: more = better.
- Bar thickness: thicker = better.
- Inter-pin distance: more = better.
- Number of cortices held by the pins: two better than one.

Classification
- Static vs. dynamic.
- Unilateral, bilateral, ring (circular) frame.
- Clamps, pins, or tensioned wire.

Mechanism of action
- Static: bridges the injured area maintaining length and gives axial and rotational stability; allows mobilization of adjacent joints.
- Dynamic: ligamentotaxis—distraction pulls soft tissues and the bone fragments attached to them and hopefully helps reduce and unload them to aid movement. Movement further improves the position and functional recovery.

Indications
- Multiply comminuted fractures.
- Bone loss.
- Insufficient space for internal fixation.
- Contamination/infection.
- Intra-articular fractures especially if comminuted.
- Unfit patient.

Benefits
- Versatile.
- Sometimes the only solution.
- Less soft tissue dissection.

Outcome
- Static: little evidence as mainly used for complex cases—expect stiffness.
- Dynamic: mainly case series from PIPJ fracture dislocations with results reported as range of motion (ROM) 10°–90° with no pain.

Complications
- Pin-site infection.
- Loss of position.
- Tethering of soft tissues preventing movement.
- Stiffness.
- Osteomyelitis.
- Septic arthritis.
- The usual fracture-related problems: non-union, malunion, CRPS, etc.

Intra-articular phalangeal fractures

Problem is stiffness, deformity, pain, arthritis. Perfect reduction should result in less arthritis in the future.

Classification

London (1971) classification of condylar fractures
- Type 1: box.
- Type 2: short oblique.
- Type 3: long oblique.
- Type 4: bicondylar.

Weiss and Hastings (1993) classification
- Oblique palmar.
- Long sagittal.
- Dorsal coronal.
- Palmar coronal.

Note: condylar fractures are rarely uniplanar—therefore as shortens usually rotates. All complex, so use:
- Open or closed.
- Displaced or not.
- Functionally stable.
- Unstable.

Treatment of intra-articular phalangeal fractures
- Conservative.
- External fixation.
- ORIF.

Aims of ORIF
- Restore articular surface congruity.
- Joint stability.
- Tendon attachment.
- Rigid fixation.
- Mobilize as soon as possible.

Fixation technique
- Depends on size and site fracture fragment.
- Difficult.
- Completely intra-articular fragment: screw through the articular surface or use a head less screw.
- Pilon depression with extreme comminution: use ex-fix.
- If bone loss add bone graft: ex-fix provides neutralizing fixation to support minimal fixation and the bone graft.

Outcome of finger fractures

Huffaker et al. (1979) found in a series of 150 metacarpal fractures that the presence of a joint injury, tendon injury, skin loss, or more than one fracture was associated with a reduced ROM and that flexor was worse then extensor tendon injury.

Strickland reported the following features as prognostic for poor outcome.
- Patient factors:
  - Age >50 years.
  - Systemic disease (vascular, diabetic).
  - Socio-economic factors.
- Fracture factors:
  - Location (thumb less ROM than digit).
  - Intra-articular.
  - Comminuted worse than transverse.
  - Displaced worse.
  - Instability.
  - Soft tissue injury.
  - Skin and tendon injury.
  - Flexor injury worse than extensor injury.
- Management factors:
  - Recognition of injury.
  - Tissue management.
  - Fracture reduction.
  - Mobilization.

- Maintenance of reduction.
- Management of complications: 19% had complications in Strickland's series).

Some specific fractures

Metacarpal fracture (Figs 17.16 and 17.17)
Common fracture.

Classification
- Extra-articular:
  - Shaft transverse: stable if not displaced, unlikely to shorten; may rotate, but limited by intermetacarpal ligaments so treat by splint, mobilize protect; if border digit or multiple; consider ORIF (compression plate).
  - Shaft short oblique: unstable will shorten and may rotate, but limited by inter-metacarpal ligaments so treat by splint, mobilize protect; if border digit or multiple consider ORIF (lag screw and neutralization plate).
  - Shaft long oblique: fracture will shorten and may rotate, but limited by inter-metacarpal ligaments so treat by splint, mobilize protect; if border digit or multiple consider ORIF (two lag screws if length fracture is greater than twice the diameter).
  - Bone loss: treat by ORIF with bridging plate ± bone graft.
  - Neck fractures: consider the degree of angulation, shortening and rotation—usually not rotated and acceptably shortened. Metacarpal shortening of 2 mm produces 7° extensor lag, but average MCPJ can hyperextend so not noticed clinically.
- Intra-articular:
  - Metacarpal has very large surface articular area, very mobile joint.
  - Accurate and stable reduction and early movement.

Bennett's fracture (Fig. 17.18)
Intra-articular fracture of the base of the thumb metacarpal. The volar beak segment with the volar beak ligament attached is pulled off, allowing displacement of the main segment of the metacarpal. The metacarpal base moves into abduction and supination due to the pull of APL and the head moves into adduction due to pull of adductor.

Gedda and Moberg (1953) reported that 50% of 14 cases got osteoarthritis. Burton and Pellegrini (1987) reported only 2.8%, and so concluded that if <3 mm displacement reduce closed and K-wire and if >3 mm articular displacement then ORIF.

The author's preferred method is to place a wire in the thumb metacarpal angled such that advancing it would cause it to pass through the centre of the basal articular surface. Then reduce the fracture by distraction and abduction. Once reduced, ask the assistant to drive the K-wire into the trapezium whilst you hold the reduction. It is not necessary to pin the small fracture fragment, as it is relatively stable and it is sufficient to prevent the subluxation of the thumb metacarpal.

Rolando fracture
- Fracture of base of thumb in T pattern.
- Associated with dorsal subluxation.
- APL supinates proximal radially and dorsally.
- Adductors pull head of metacarpal into the palm.
- Fragment remains *in situ*; it is the distal metacarpal that displaces.
- Robert view: hyperpronated view of base of thumb metacarpal.

Treatment options
- ORIF if fragments are large.
- K-wire.

Outcome
- Grip strength 75% of other side.
- ROM 10°–15° reduced.
- X-ray narrowing of joint in 50–80%.

Fracture dislocation of PIPJ
- Look for the V sign indicating dorsal subluxation of the middle phalanx.
- Treat conservatively by extension blocking splint or K-wire (as these are stable in flexion), distraction methods (ligamentotaxis), or treat surgically by open methods.
- ORIF through the volar approach. Must reconstruct the palmar basal lip of the middle phalanx by reduction fracture, by soft tissues using advancement of the palmar plate (Eaton and Malerich 1980), or if bone loss by using autogenous composite articular bone graft from the hamate (Hastings) or navicular. Or can fuse the joint.
- Key is reduction and restoration of stability, allowing early mobilization.

Open fractures in the hand
- Wound that communicates with the fracture or the fracture haematoma.
- Common in the hand; may be 30–50%.
- Implication is that bacterial contamination has occurred, and the injury interferes with bone healing by stripping of periosteum, devascularization, creating dead space, and effects of the wound on exposure and access.
- Consider the mechanism of injury.
  - Inside out: usually low energy, less contamination.
  - Outside in: usually higher energy more contamination.

Treatment
- Prophylactic antibiotics.
- Cleaning and debridement (most important):
  - 'If a little does some good a lot may do some more'.
  - 'The solution to pollution is dilution'.
- Stabilize fracture (usually internal or external fixation, not splint or K-wires).
- Repair soft tissues.
- Closure of soft tissues.

Mobilize, rehabilitate.

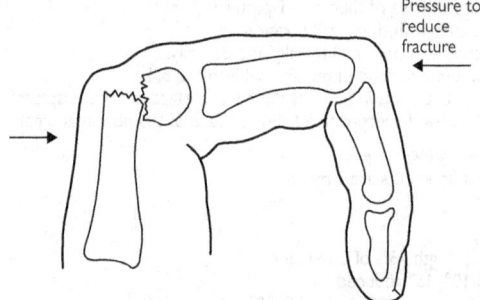

Fig. 17.15 Jahss manoeuvre to reduce fractures of the neck of the metacarpal.

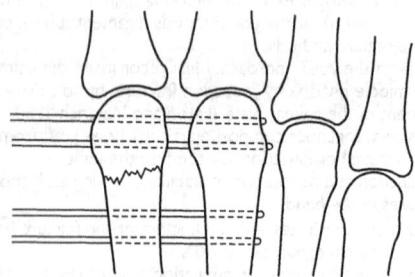

Fig. 17.16 Trans-metacarpal K-wires for fracture of the neck of the fifth metacarpal.

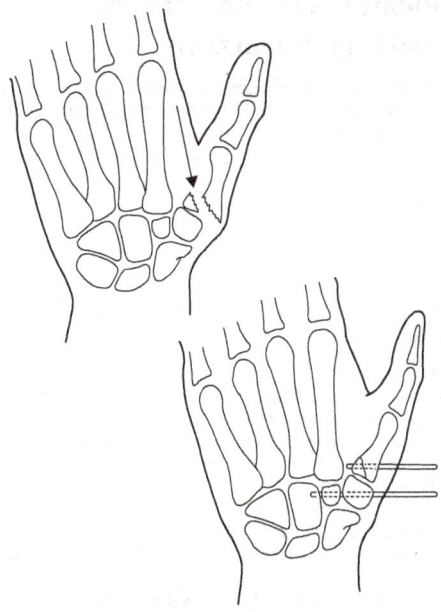

Fig. 17.17 Bennett's fracture demonstrating the displacement and the reduction and fixation with K-wires.

References

Burton RI, Pellegrini VD, Jr (1987). *J Hand Surg (Am)* **12**, 645.
Eaton RG, Malerich MM (1980). *J Hand Surg (Am)* **5**, 260–8.
Gedda KO, Moberg E (1953). *Acta Orthop Scand* **22**, 249–57.
Huffaker WH, Wray RC, Jr, Weeks PM (1979). *Plast Reconstr Surg* **63**, 82–7.
London PS (1971). *Hand* **3**, 15–18.
Pun WK, Chow SP, So YC, et al. (1989). *J Hand Surg (Am)* **14**, 474–81.
Salter RB, Harris WR (1963). *J Bone. Joint Surg* **45A**, 587–622.
Strickland JW et al. (1982). *Orthop Rev* **11**:39–50.
Williams RM, Hastings H, Kiefhaber TR (2002). *Tech Hand Up Extr Surg* **6**:185–92.
Weiss AC, Hastings H, II (1993). *J Hand Surg* 18A, 594–9.

Complications in metacarpal and phalangeal fractures

'Hand fractures can be complicated by deformity from no treatment, stiffness from over treatment, and both deformity and stiffness from poor treatment ...' (Swanson 1970).

Complications
- Non-union.
- Malunion.
- Infection.
- Stiffness.
- Pain and reflex sympathetic dystrophy.

Complications more common in intra-articular, middle-third, and open combined injuries (Ouelette and Freeland 1996).

Non-union
- Uncommon: 0.5% digital fractures.
- May be asymptomatic: usually firm fibrous union, mildly symptomatic (fibrous union), or symptomatic mobile and painful if little fibrous union (atrophic non-union). May also have large callus formation (hypertrophic non-union).
- Causes: fracture factors, surgical or patient factors.
- Most common cause is inappropriate fixation. High-energy open injuries with vascular injury complicated by infection are at greatest risk.

Treatment.
- Depends on which digit and at what level involved.
- Asymptomatic: leave alone (many of these will unite).
- Symptomatic: treat cause, debride, rigid fixation, ± bone graft, move early.
- Non-union of phalanges: may heal after 6–12 months, so best treatment is wait.

Malunion
- Healing with deformity: radiological or clinical, causing functional or cosmetic deformity.
- Causes: displaced fractures not detected and not treated, poorly reduced fractures fixed with deformity, undisplaced fractures not recognized as unstable which displace with treatment, fixation failure.
- Fractures can deform in four planes: angulate, incline, rotate, and shorten. Rarely uni-planar.
- Metacarpals go apex dorsal, proximal phalanges go apex palmar, distal phalanges go apex palmar, and middle phalanges depends on fracture relationship to insertion FDS and central slip.
- Note that in the proximal and middle phalanx the dorsal angulation (apex palmar) gives a linear reduction in the distance between joints producing a change in apparent extensor tendon length resulting in an extension lag at PIPJ or DIPJ.

Consequences of malunion (not just a bone problem!)
Loss of extension and flexion, palpable painful mass, tendon adhesion, tendon tethering, deformity, bone blocking.

Malunion tolerance
Depends on the digit, level, degree, and type (Table 17.1).

Table 17.1 The degree of malunion acceptable before intervention is indicated

Bone	Direction of malunion		
	Dorsal/palmar	Lateral inclination	Rotation
Metacarpal	Little	Lots	15°
Proximal phalanx	Less	15°	10°
Middle phalanx	Little	20°	15°

Thus the proximal phalanx is the least forgiving of malunion and the little and ring finger metacarpal is most forgiving. In border digits rotation is not so important. Note that angulation may increase joint load and increase the risk of arthritis.

Treatment
- Indicated if there is sufficient deformity and loss of function, provided that there is maximum mobility and the soft tissues are ready.
- In children deformities can self-correct. Best nearest the physis, and when young with maximum growth potential. Dorsal palmar angulation best chance, rotation least.

Timing
- If detected <8 weeks go in early and correct.
- If detected at >8 weeks leave until the fracture is firmly united, all the scar tissue is resolved, and hand mobility is maximized.

Techniques
Wedge (opening, closing or exchange)
Pivot; step cut; transverse; mixed. Planning is essential; use radiographs, clinical examination. Pre-operatively mark the skin and insert wires to help as markers and toggles/handles to judge movement before exposure and osteotomy. Technique involves osteotomy and rigid fixation. Preferably do the osteotomy at the fracture site.

Angular deformity
Do opening wedge osteotomy; then fix with bone graft (taken from Lister's tubercle) with tension band wire or plate/screws.

Rotational deformity
Do osteotomy at fracture site where possible, although some prefer doing osteotomy at metacarpal level in the case of proximal phalanx in order to avoid potential adhesions and stiffness. However, maximum rotation at metacarpal level is 19% (Gross). If metacarpal is used to correct distal deformity beware inadequate correction and double deformity. Intra-articular osteotomy is very difficult and risks necrosis; consider the possibility of extra-articular correction. If a bone spike is blocking movement, remove the spike rather than correcting malunion.

Infection
- Rare.
- Avoided by good debridement, rigid fixation, complete tension-free closure.
- Prophylactic antibiotics have no role in reducing the rate of infection.
- Treatment depends on the fixation, fracture pattern, and degree of union. If united, the fixation should be removed. If the fracture has not yet united, suppression with antibiotics until sufficient union has occurred to remove the fixation safely may be possible. If not, internal fixation should be removed and replaced by external fixation or splintage.

Stiffness
- Extremely common. Beware stiffness in uninvolved adjacent digits.
- Oedema, fibrosis, and immobilization by oedema, splinting, or pain are factors in stiffness. Stiffness can be reduced by minimizing oedema, haematoma, surgical trauma, amount of fixation, and increasing fracture stability to allow early mobilization.
- Any splintage or resting splint should minimize the effects by keeping the wrist at 20° of extension, the MCPJ at 60°, and the IPJs at 0–10°.
- Oedema control using elevation, therapy, and bandaging help to reduce stiffness.
- Treatment is time, active and passive exercises, pain control, passive and dynamic splinting.
- Occasionally operative arthrotenolysis is needed. Pre-operatively determine the cause of stiffness, including X-ray. Tendon and capsular contracture can be surgically corrected by arthrotenolysis. However, joint incongruity and bony block cannot be corrected by this approach. In these cases salvage by arthrodesis or arthroplasty may be needed.

References
Gross MS, Gelberman RH (1985). *Jnl Hand Surg* **10**:105–8.
Ouellette EA, Freeland AE (1996). *Clin Orthop Relat Res* **327**, 38–46.
Swanson AB (1970). *Orthop Clin North Am* **1**, 261–74.

Scaphoid fracture

- Most common carpal fracture 70–80%: triquetrium 17%; hook of hamate 5%.
- Usually sustained by a fall on the outstretched hand, with forced hyper-extension.

Anatomy

- Scaphoid is 80% covered by cartilage; very mobile; five joints; unstable to compression; stabilized by intrinsic and extrinsic ligaments.
- Intrinsic ligaments are scapholunate and scaphotrapezio-trapezoidal (STT).
- Extrinsic ligaments are radioscaphocapitate and long radiolunate.
- The scaphoid is the stabilizing link between proximal and distal rows. Therefore non-union means loss of kinematics, altered loads, and hence radiographic degeneration.
- Scaphoid vascularity enters distally: 13–40% risk of avascular necrosis after fracture; increased with displacement >1 mm, and with fracture position (waist 30–50%, proximal pole 50–100%).

Fracture personality

- A fractured scaphoid tends to assume a pronated posture leading to decreased wrist extension.
- Lateral intrascaphoid angle becomes greater then 45° leading to stiffness, pain, arthrosis.
- 5° of flexion of the scaphoid leads to 24° loss of wrist extension.

Diagnosis

- Have a high index of suspicion.
- Clinically tender in anatomical snuff-box and scaphoid tubercle; may have swelling, bruising. Reduced ROM, especially extension and radial deviation.
- Fracture can normally (90%) be detected on X-ray scaphoid series of four wrist views.
- If in doubt treat as if fractured and review in 14 days, with X-rays and clinical examination.
- Occult fractures leads to under-treatment, possibly resulting in non-union, malunion.
- Over-treatment leads to stiffness and pain.
- If still in doubt, MRI or CT scan.
- Beware associated injuries: 7% have radial head fracture, other carpal injuries (scapholunate ligament, carpal dislocations).

Scaphoid fracture healing
- Fracture location:
  - Distal third (10%) heal in 6–8 weeks.
  - Middle third (70%) heal in 8–12 weeks.
  - Proximal third (20%) heal in 8–12 weeks.
- At best 90% of non-displaced fractures heal in a cast if treated promptly. If delay >4 weeks non-union increases to 40%.
- No comment on re-fracture rate.
- Cast treatment is a scaphoid thumb cast. Debate about whether to include thumb, elbow, or both.

Predictors of non-union
Displacement, ischaemia, delay to diagnosis and treatment, intracapsular location, difficulty in maintaining bony coaptation, vascularity, mobility.

Surgical indications
- Non controversial: displaced, fracture dislocations.
- Controversial: proximal pole, subacute, patients with specific needs, undisplaced.
- Advantages for fixation of undisplaced fracture are less splintage, easier care. No improvement in union time or rate. In displaced fractures reduction and fixation improve union rate.

Techniques
Approaches
- Percutaneous, mini-open, open.
- Percutaneous or mini-open suitable for non-displaced or minimally displaced fractures; stable; does not need bone graft.
- Dorsal approach if proximal pole or waist fractures.
- Palmar approach done with wrist supinated and extended which tends to reduce the fracture.

Screw placement
- Centre of scaphoid, perpendicular to fracture.
- Assess thickness of cartilage.
- Anticipate compression: do not use too long a screw because as it compresses it may become too long; so use a screw 4 mm less then measured length and a drill 2 mm shorter then the measured depth.
- Use X-ray guidance.

Percutaneous
- Palmar and dorsal approaches can be done percutaneously.
- In palmar approach, the fixation is retrograde. Use a 14 gauge intravenous catheter to find STT joint and line of the scaphoid under image intensification. Then insert K-wire through the cannula. Check position of the wire in three planes under image intensification. Drill by hand. Measure depth. Insert intra-osseous cannulated compression screw (Herbert, Whipple, Accutrac, Twin Fix, AO, etc.).
- Similar for dorsal approach.

Open
- Palmar approach best for displaced humpbacked scaphoids and non-unions; sometimes may require removal of trapezial tubercle for adequate access to distal scaphoid; good access for bone grafting.
- Dorsal approach for proximal pole fractures.

Post-operative
Mobilize in removable splint immediately. Protect for 4–6 weeks.

Complications
- Screw too long.
- Screw too dorsal.
- Screw breaks through side of scaphoid.
- Non-union, malunion, infection, arthosis, pain, CRPS.
- Development of arthrosis related to non-union (SNAC) or scapholunate ligament injury (SLAC).
  - SLAC wrist type 1 with arthritis of distal scaphoid and radius is treated by styloidectomy ± scaphoidectomy.
  - SLAC type 2 with arthritis of proximal scaphoid and radius can be treated by proximal row carpectomy.
  - SLAC type 3 with arthritis also affecting capitate and lunate can be treated by four-corner fusion.

Vascularized bone graft (Roy-Camille 1965)
- The local options are pronator (Braun 1992), volar carpal (Kuhlmann et al. 1987), ulnar, 1,2 I C S R.A (1–2 inter compartmental supra retinacular artery) (Zaidemberg et al. 1991).
- May improve union rates in un-united fractures.

References
Braun C (1992). *Arch Orthop Trauma Surg* **111**, 250–4.
Kuhlmann JN, Mimoun M, Boabighi A, Baux S (1987). *J Hand Surg (Br)* **12**, 203–10.
Roy-Camille R (1965). *Actual Chirurg Orthop* **4**, 197–214 .
Zaidemberg C, Siebert JW, Angrigiani C (1991). *J Hand Surg (Am)* **16**, 474–8.

Carpal instability

Definition
Instability of the carpal bones.

Incidence
Probably more common than reported as many injuries are undiagnosed.

Aetiology
Usually caused by ligamentous soft tissue destruction or injury but occasionally due to an underlying connective tissue disorder.

Classification
- Type 1. Chronicity (acute, subacute, or chronic).
- Type 2. Constancy (static (reducible or irreducible) or dynamic).
- Type 3. Aetiology (congenital, trauma, inflammatory, arthritis).
- Type 4. Location.
- Type 5. Direction (DISI, VISI, radial).
- Type 6. Pattern:
  - CID—carpal instability dissociative (proximal row).
  - CIND—carpal instability Non-disssociative.
  - CIC—carpal instability combined.
  - CIA—carpal instability adaptive.

Scapholunate dissociation
Most common carpal instability. Common sports injury caused by a wrist dorsiflexion and ulnar deviation.

Both the scapholunate and the lunotriquetral ligaments are C-shaped, open distally. They are strong dorsally and palmarly and membranous proximally. The scapholunate ligament is associated with the radio-scaphoid ligament. The scapholunate ligament is strong compared with capsular ligaments and the dorsal segment is strongest. The palmar segment is the most important in preventing scaphoid rotation.

In instability the scaphoid tends to palmar flex and the triquetrum tends to dorsiflex; the lunate follows whichever bone it is most strongly attached to. In scapholunate injury the lunate dorsiflexes (DISI) and in lunotriquetral injuries the lunate palmarflexes (VISI).

Clinical presentation
- Presents with history of the injury and pain on wrist movement and grip. Pain is worse on extension and radial deviation.
- Differential diagnosis:
  - Dorsal impaction syndrome.
  - Dorsal ganglion.

Examination
- Watson's scaphoid shift test.
- X-ray.
- MRI and arthrograms are not very helpful.
- Arthroscopy may be helpful.
- Cine-radiography may be helpful.

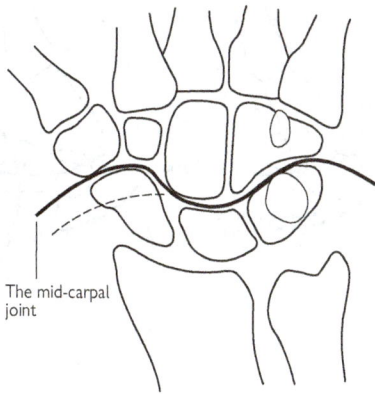

Fig. 17.18 Carpal bones and line of trans-scaphoid perilunate dislocation.

Management
- Observe.
- Cast.
- Percutaneous pin (Whipple).
- Dorsal repair.
- Dorsal capsulodesis (Blatt).
- Ligament reconstruction.
- Tenodesis (FCR).
- Arthrodesis (STT, scaphocapitate).

Scapholunate fusion is not recommended because of a high rate of non-union, probably due to high torsion force.

The paradox of Mayfield
Scapholunate dissociation produces diastasis (gapping) and malrotation. Dorsiflexion produces a better scapholunate angle but a worse scapholunate gap. Palmar flexion reduces the scapholunate gap but creates a worse scapholunate angle. Hence closed reduction is not effective.

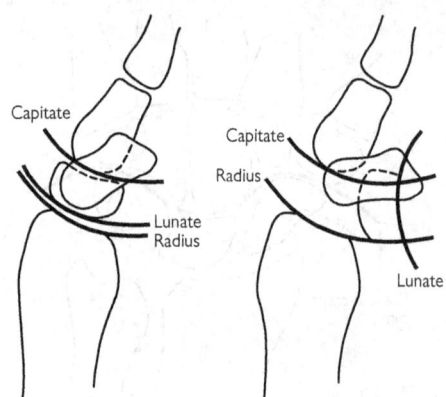

Fig. 17.19 Lateral view of carpal bones in lunate dislocation.

Distal radius fractures

Colles' fracture (first described in 1814) is just one type but is frequently used to describe all distal radius fractures.

Incidence
- 15% of all emergency room fractures.
- Two peaks of incidence:
  - 6–10 years.
  - 60–69 years (female-to-male ratio 6:1).
- Majority low energy.

Classification
Based on fracture patterns and treatment issues (Fernandez 1987).
- According to injury mechanism:
  - Bending (e.g. Colles'/Smith's).
  - Compression (e.g. die punch).
  - Shearing (e.g. Barton's/radial styloid).
  - Avulsion (rim) and radiocarpal fracture dislocation.
  - Mixed.
- Always consider distal ulna and DRUJ injury as well.
  - Type I. Stable (TFCC intact).
  - Type II. Unstable (TFCC disrupted).
  - Type III. Potentially unstable (articular disruption).

Fracture tip of ulnar styloid not significant but those at base of styloid are because of attachment of TFCC at base.

Radiology
X-Ray
Include carpal bones and the opposite wrist:
- Ulnar inclinication (normal = 22°–23°).
- Radial length (11–12 mm).
- Ulnar variance (61% ulnar neutral).
- Palmar inclination (10°–12°).

Easiest remembered as 11, 11, 22.

CT scan
- Better for complex intra-articular fractures.

Management
Considerations
- Fracture:
  - Pattern and stability.
  - Bone quality.
  - Comminution.
  - Displacement/impaction.
  - Energy of injury.

- Patient:
  - Lifestyle.
  - Medical condition.
  - Functional outlook.
  - Compliance.

Radiological features of instability
- Dorsal comminution >50%.
- Palmar metaphyseal comminution.
- Dorsal tilt >20°.

Extra-articular fractures
Impaired function if:
- >20° dorsal angulation.
- <10° radial inclination.
- >2 mm radial shift.
- Radial shortening and disruption of DRUJ.

Intra-articular fractures
- Reduce within 1–2 mm to avoid risk of reduced ROM and degenerative arthritis.

Stable fracture
- 75–80% of extra-articular fractures are stable and in an acceptable position.
- Closed reduction and cast.
- Controversy in cast position—forearm position, duration, above elbow.

Unstable fractures or stable but unacceptable position
Closed manipulation and percutaneous pinning
- Indicated in:
  - Unstable extra-articular fractures.
  - Intra-articular fractures anatomically reduced.
- Supplement with POP cast or external fixator if severe soft tissue injury.
- Bone graft if significant metaphyseal defect post reduction.

Pins and plaster
- High incidence of pin-site complications (30%).
- Not recommended.
- Kapandji through-fracture pinning versus not through fracture.

External fixator
- Complication rate 20–60%: usually pin tract infection, radial sensory neuritis, CRPS, stiff wrist.

Limited open reduction
- Indicated in two- to four-part intra-articular fractures.
- Mini-incision/reduce/K-wire or external fixator.
- Bone graft if metaphyseal defect.

ORIF/plating
- Indicated in shear fracture or complex intra-articular fracture.
- Volar approach ± carpal tunnel release.
- Dorsal approach.

Arthroscopy
- Assess/assist reduction of intra-articular fracture and carpal ligament or TFCC injury.

Distal ulna and distal radioulnar joint
- Fracture ulnar head or neck: plate/closed reduction.
- Fracture ulnar styloid: tension band wire or screw.
- TFCC disruption: repair (intra-osseous sutures), secure dorsal radioulnar ligament and ECU, and immobilize in 30°–40° supination.

Complications
- Incidence of 20–30%.
- Malunion/non-union.
- Post-traumatic arthritis in radio-carpal or radioulnar joints.
- Tendon rupture (EPL or EDC on bone spur or plate, FPL on plate).
- Peritendinous adhesions (digit stiffness).
- Stenosing tenosynovitis (De Quervain's syndrome).
- Carpal tunnel syndrome.
- Radial nerve injury associated with external fixator.
- Compartment syndrome.
- Skin necrosis, pin-site infection.
- CRPS.

Surgical approaches
- Through FCR radial to neurovascular and tendons, down to PQ which you retract off palmar surface radius.
- Via ulnar side between tendons and ulnar neurovascular bundle.
- Directly through the flexor surface between median.

DRUJ disorders

Consider two parts:
- Radioulnar joint.
- Ulnar ligamentous stability.

Definition
- Disorders affecting the distal radioulnar joint; usually post-traumatic or arthritic.
- Much overlooked and still not fully understood.

Causes
- Essex–Lopresti injury.
- Subluxation of DRUJ.
- Fracture involving DRUJ.

Examination
- Pain. Localizes to?
- Tenderness. Where?
- Range of motion.
- Manual stress test.
- Ulnocarpal stress test.
- Piano key test.
- DRUJ instability test.

Investigations
X-ray
- Ulnar variance (positive, negative, or neutral).
- Lunotriquetral cysts or OA.

Other investigations
- Bone scan.
- CT; dynamic views of both wrists, pronating and supinating.
- MRI.
- Arthroscopy.

Lesions
- Synovitis of DRUJ.
- Incongruity of DRUJ leading to OA.
- Ulnar abutment syndrome: ulna is too long and impacts on lunate especially with ulnar deviation. Cortical bruising and cyst formation can be seen in ulnar proximal corner of the lunate, especially on MRI.
- TFCC tears and detachment: lead to instability of the DRUJ with pain and reduced ROM.

DRUJ instability

Acute
- Reducible:
    - Dorsal dislocation when pronated, relocated by supination.
    - Treat by POP in supination.
- Irreducible:
    - Cannot be relocated.
    - Treat by ORIF (fix styloid fracture).

Chronic
- Intact joint:
    - Subluxed joint.
    - Treat by soft tissue reconstruction, ulna shortening, TFCC tightening.
- Deranged joint with ulna/radius malunion:
    - Treat by corrective osteotomy.
- Deranged joint with DRUJ malunion:
    - Treat by ulna head excision/prosthesis, Suave–Kapandji (ulnar head to radius fusion and ulnar neck excision).

Soft tissue procedures
- Tethering by the use of tendon transfers to stabilize the DRUJ: free tendon graft (Bunnell); ECU transfer (Hill); PL transfer (Leung).
- Strengthening using existing structures such as ECU as stabilizers.

Bone procedures
- Ulna shortening tightens the TFCC complex thus stabilizing the DRUJ.
- Ulna head excision.
- Partial ulna head excision and soft tissue interposition.
- Ulna head replacement.
- Ulna head fusion (Suave–Kapandji).

Ulna head procedures

In order of preference and least destruction
- Ulna shortening (Milch).
- Wafer procedure (Feldon 1992):
  - Indications—where ulnar variance is less than 3 mm.
- Bowers HIT (ulna head hemi-resection interposition arthroplasty).
  - Indications—as above, best for DRUJ incongruity.
  - Not indicated where cause of DRUJ instability is ulnar abutment.
  - Procedure—obliquely resect the radial half of the ulna head (and DRUJ), preserving the ulnar styloid and its ligamentous attachments.
  - Complications—ulnar styloid–carpal abutment.
- Suave–Kapandji ulna head to radius fusion and segmental ulna neck excision:
  - Indications—as above.
  - Procedure—excise DRUJ surfaces; excise a 0.5 cm segment of the neck of the ulna just below the DRUJ (try to make oblique and as distal as possible); fuse the DRUJ.
  - Complications—ulna stump instability and impingement, proximal radio-humeral OA.
- Darrach ulnar head excision:
  - Indications—chronic DRUJ instability with DRUJ derangement.
  - Not indicated in non-rheumatoids <70 years.
  - Procedure—excision of the whole ulnar head at level of neck just below DRUJ.
  - Complications—ulnar abutment, unstable ulna stump (ulna impingement).
- Ulnar head prosthesis.
  - Indications not yet confirmed, but has been used in all conditions above.
  - Procedure—excision of ulna head and replacement with prosthesis.
  - Complications—infection, dislocation, instability, exposure, pain.
- One-bone forearm reconstruction:
  - Indications—where above techniques have failed or are not possible.
  - Procedure—the distal ulna is excised, the radius is divided, and the proximal ulna stump is joined to the distal radius.
  - Complications—no forearm rotation possible, non-union, malunion.

Reference

Feldon P, Terrono AL, Belsky MR (1992). *Clin Orthop Relat Res* **275**, 124–9.

Triangular fibro-cartilaginous complex (TFCC) disorders

Consider as two components: the TFCC and the radioulnar ligaments. The radioulnar ligaments stabilize and transmit force. Two dorsal and two palmar ligaments, superficial and deep. In pronation the dorsal superficial and the palmar deep are tight and in supination the reverse occurs.

Classification (Palmer 1989)

- Type 1: Traumatic:
  - 1A. Central tear along radius.
  - 1B. Fracture ulnar styloid and tear ligamentous part (ulnar detachment).
  - 1C. Tear of dorsal radial ulnar carpal ligament from ulnar fovea.
  - 1D. 1C plus fracture (radial detachment).
- Type 2: Degenerative (usually ulnocarpal abutment):
  - 2A. Scuffing of central segment of TFCC.
  - 2B. Plus changes in lunoulna and lunotriquetral joints (chondromalacia).
  - 2C. Plus central perforation and tear on radial attachment.
  - 2D. Plus tear of lunotriquetral ligament and changes in lunotriquetral joint.
  - 2E. Plus arthritis in DRUJ.

Aetiology

Trauma
Usually fall on outstretched hand in ulnar deviation.

Degenerative
- Degenerative conditions usually relate to increased ulna length.
- Normally ulna bears 20% of load, but if ulna is 2.5 mm longer the load is 40%.
- A long ulna may result in ulnar abutment syndrome = ulnar impaction = ulnocarpal impaction. Note that this is different from ulna impingement where, following ulna head excision, the ulna stump impinges on the radius.
- Causes of a long ulna are congenital (physeal development or injury) or acquired (radius fracture and malunion, Essex–Lopresti lesion).
- Malunion of the radius, especially shortening and increased dorsal angulation, increases the ulna load. An increase of the normal dorsal angulation from 11° to 40 the ulna stump doubles the load.

Clinical presentation

Clinically TFCC problems present with:
- Ulnar wrist pain, worse on ulnar deviation or rotation.
- Ulnar swelling.
- Tenderness over the TFCC.
- Positive provocation tests (compression of TFCC and rotation DRUJ, piano key test, 'shuck test' of movement of the lunate and triquetrum).

Investigations
- Radiographs must be in the standard position of 90°–90°–0°:
  - Look at ulna length, radius alignment, ulnocarpal joint, DRUJ geometry/arthritis, lunate quality, shape, cysts.
  - Ulna length or variance measurements by articular level method or concentric circles method.
  - Note that the ulna is radiographically longer if the forearm is pronated.
- Wrist arthrography.
- MRI ± arthrography.
- Arthroscopy.

Note that 75% of perforations are asymptomatic.

Treatment
Trauma: usually immobilize in above elbow cast in neutral rotation for 6 weeks.

Non-operative
- Activity modification, splints, NSAIDs.

Operative
- Arthroscopic debridement of TFCC.
- Wafer resection of ulna.
- Ulna shortening osteotomy.
- Correction of radius malunion.

Reference
Palmer AK (1989). *J Hand Surg (Am)* **14**, 594–606.

Ulnocarpal abutment syndrome

Also known as ulnar impaction, ulnocarpal loading. Not to be confused with ulnocarpal impingement which usually refers to the ulna stump impinging on the radius shaft on rotation after ulna head excision.

Definition
A long ulna which impacts on the lunate producing pain, degeneration, and lunate cysts, and contributes to TFCC degeneration and chondromalacia.

Aetiology
Congenital and developmental
If ulna is congenitally long, why does it become symptomatic in middle age? Possibly due to a change in use or degeneration.

Traumatic
- Distal radius malunion.
- Wrist fusion.
- Galleazzi fracture.
- Essex–Lopresti lesion.

Clinical presentation
- Click.
- Loss of strength.
- Pain on rotation, especially at extremes, and in ulnar deviation.

Ulna variance is usually neutral. measured in 90°–90° view (shoulder abduction and elbow flexion) including radial and ulnar deviation, rotation, and power grip.

Differential diagnosis
- ECU subluxation.
- DRUJ pathology.
- Carpal instability.

Imaging
- X-rays in 90°–90°.
- Bone scan.
- MRI.
- Arthrography, MR arthrogram.
- Wrist arthroscopy.

Classification
Type 2 of Palmer's TFCC classification.

Treatment
Non-operative
Rest, splintage, NSAIDs.

Operative
- Arthroscopy.
- Ulnar shortening: transverse, oblique, or step cut.
- Distal ulna resection: Darrach whole head, Watson wafer, Bowers hemi-resection, or other types.

Ulnar shortening
- Pitfalls: the shape of the sigmoid notch can prevent matching of joint surfaces. Parallel joint surfaces seen on X-ray pre-operatively are obviously preferable.
- Non-union less likely with oblique or step cut osteotomies.

Brachial plexus injuries

Also known as BPI, Erb's palsy.

Definition
An injury to the brachial plexus between spinal roots and terminal branches.

Incidence
Rising because helmets preserving life in motorbike accidents; very high in Thailand which has a high prevalence of motorbike riders.

Aetiology
Traumatic: usually caused by motorbike trauma, but also falls, rugby, motor vehicle accidents, rarely sharp lacerations and gunshot injuries. Brachial plexus lesions can also occur post radiotherapy, tumour infiltration, or compression, and rarely post-vaccination, postural, 'rucksack', and compressive secondary to thoracic outlet syndrome. Can occur spontaneously from unknown cause with characteristic pain in Parsonage–Turner syndrome.

Anatomy
Brachial plexus anatomy must be learnt; it is essential to be able to diagnose the level of the injury. Sensory dermatomes and muscular myotomes must also be known to determine which muscles function and which do not and to be able to relate this to the level of injury.

Topography of brachial plexus to aid grafting
- Anterior segment roots go to lateral and medial cords.
- Posterior segments go to posterior cord.
- Cranial segment C5 goes to suprascapular nerve.
- Posterior cranial segment of C5 and C6 goes to axillary nerve.
- Anterior cranial segment of C5 and C6 goes to pectorals.

Classification
According to area, extent, and level of injury:
- Supraclavicular/infraclavicular.
- Extent of injury: complete/partial, e.g. C567 injury, C5678 injury.
- Level of injury: root avulsion, trunk rupture, cords, branches, etc.

Clinical presentation
Sensory loss, motor loss, and pain, but usually presents as multi-trauma with flail arm as one of the presenting features.

Suspect also if shoulder dislocation, fracture of transverse processes of lower cervical vertebrae, fracture of first rib, open fracture clavicle, large haematoma in supraclavicular fossa, and/or subclavian artery rupture, as all these represent significant force and distraction in this area and are often associated with BPI.

Examination
- Observe for wasting, posture (internal rotation of humerus, pronation/supination of forearm, flexion of wrist), colour change, and other sympathetic changes.
- Feel for mass in supraclavicular fossa or deltopectoral groove.
- Assess sensation in each dermatome and distinguish between each peripheral nerve.
- Assess motor function of each muscle to be able to differentiate between a peripheral nerve and a brachial plexus injury and to be able to diagnose level of injury. Try to distinguish between a supra- and infra-ganglionic lesion.

Be aware that the dural ligamentous attachments to C5 are stronger than those to C6 and 7, which are stronger than those to C8 and T1. The weaker the attachments, the more easily the root is avulsed rather than ruptured. Ruptures tend to occur between sites of origin and anchorage, e.g. the upper trunk will rupture between foramen and suprascapular nerve. 10–20% of injuries are multi-level, such as upper roots and trunks, or upper and middle roots *and* musculocutaneous or axillary nerves. Paralysis of rhomboids or serratus anterior indicates upper root avulsion, and Horner's syndrome indicates avulsion of the lower roots. Pain and phantom pain indicate root avulsion de-afferentation pain.

Imaging
- Myelograms: rather outmoded; used to visualize meningoceles and loss of rootlet shadows to diagnose root avulsions.
- CT myelograms may be better at detail.
- MRI may be helpful if positive but not if negative, i.e. specific but not sensitive.
- X-rays show fractures of neck, ribs, scapula, clavicle, or humerus.

Diagnosis
- Important to determine site (which root, trunk, division, cord, or branches) and level of injury (supraclavicular, infraclavicular, or both) and to make some assessment of its severity (avulsion, rupture, or neurotemesis, incontinuity rupture or axonotemesis, neurapraxia).
- Difficulty is in predicting the extent of the injury. This prediction is important in determining the need for surgery and the prognosis. One would not want to operate unnecessarily on someone with neurapraxia, or delay or deny a patient with a more severe injury an operative chance of repair.
- Evidence for a lesion in continuity or one more likely to spontaneously recover includes a low-velocity low-energy injury, an elderly patient (more likely to get a neurapraxia from very low energy injury), incomplete nerve lesions, signs of early recovery, nerve conduction studies.
- Evidence for a rupture with no chance of spontaneous recovery includes high-velocity or high-energy injury, wasting or involvement of posterior neck and parascapular muscles (indicating avulsion as the innervation for these muscles arises immediately after the root exits the foramen), complete nerve lesions, Horner's sign (indicates avulsion of T1 with injury to sympathetics), vascular injury.

Natural history

- Neurapraxic injuries should recover over 3 months; more extensive lesions (axontomesis and neurotemesis) will not recover.
- Sensory recovery may also give a guide to the extent of the lesion.

These are severe injuries that are significantly life-changing for the patient. Patients should be told early that their injury is significant and that they should seek alternative employment if you think that they will be unable to return to their original work. They should be encouraged to return to some form of work as soon as possible.

The neuropathic pain associated with BPI is severe and should be managed by the local acute and chronic pain service. Pain will be diminished by return to work and hobbies, and also by renervation. After 3 years, 50% will have little or no pain, 30% will have tolerable pain, and the remaining 20% will have insufferable pain.

Management

Depends on site of nerve lesion, severity of lesion, and presence of associated injuries.

Non-surgical management

- Physiotherapy to maintain joint mobility and prevent contractures.
- Psychotherapy to assist in readjustment.
- Rehabilitation advice.
- Occupational therapy to provide aids for daily life etc.
- Pain clinic.
- Splints—dynamic or static.

Operative indication

- Any severe injury in this region with BPI (Narakas).
- Failure to improve with time.

Operative principles

- Good exposure in supraclavicular, deltopectoral groove, and down medial arm. May include clavicular osteotomy. Will also include potential donor nerve grafts (back of leg for sural) or donor nerve input (intercostals for intercostal nerves).
- Determine the level and extent of injury.
- Decide on methods and plan for renervation.
- If possible, nerve graft between proximal and distal ends. If there are insufficient proximal stumps as root is avulsed, either share out remaining roots between or bring in an extra-plexural nerve source.
- Microscopic nerve repair with sutures and fibrin glue.

Donor nerve grafts

Sural, superficial radial, lateral cutaneous nerve of arm and forearm; can also use a nerve that you may have decided not to renervate (e.g. use ulnar nerve if not renervating lower trunk).

Extra-plexural nerve sources

Accessory nerve, intercostal nerves, cervical plexus, phrenic nerve, contralateral C7.

Controversies

Early versus late exploration
- Late exploration avoids unnecessary operations, the patient is stable, and it easier to tell whether a lesion in continuity found at operation is functional or not by correlating with pre-operative examination.
- Early operation: the dissection is easier, safer, and associated with better outcome (Hentz and Narakas (1988) found that the longer the delay to repair the lower the total muscle grade recovery in the upper limb). Allows patient to be given an early prognosis (so that they can commence their rehabilitation); more difficult to predict status of lesions in continuity.

Priorities for renervation
Used to concentrate on shoulder and elbow in total plexus palsies as outcome of hand renervation was poor, and so wanted to achieve a controllable arm and be able to position the hand where it could be used as a weight or assist device. Recently, moves to concentrate on hand and shoulder renervation as it is easier to perform effective transfers for elbow movement.

Reference

Hentz VR, Narakas A (1988). *Orthop Clin North Am* **19**, 107–14.

Obstetrical brachial plexus palsy

Also known as OBPP, OBP, Erb's palsy.

Definition
Brachial plexus palsy presents at birth and thought to be due to birth trauma.

Incidence
- More common in older mothers, primagravids, diabetics, large babies, past history of baby with OBP.

Aetiology
Thought to be due to failure of rotation of the shoulders once the head has passed through the pelvic brim, causing the shoulder to become trapped on top of the pubic symphysis producing shoulder dystocia. This causes distraction between the head and shoulder and traction on the brachial plexus, leading in severe cases to rupture or avulsion.

Classification
Narakas classification according to severity of presentation:
- Type 1: C5, C6.
- Type 2: C5, C6, and C7.
- Type 3: C5, C6, C7, C8, and T1.
- Type 4: Total C5, C6, C7, C8, and T1 with Horner's syndrome.

Clinical presentation
- The midwife or the mother notices the posture of the affected limb and the lack of movement.
- The classic posture is the 'waiter's tip' position with the arm internally rotated, the elbow extended, the forearm pronated, and the wrist flexed.
- With complete total plexus palsy may have the forearm supinated and the wrist extended under the action of gravity.
- Look for the presence of Horner's syndrome and a phrenic nerve palsy.
- Look for the extent of bruising, swelling and the presence of fractures of the clavicle, scapula, or humerus.
- Assess for torticollis.
- Do a neurological examination of the contralateral limb and the legs.

Management
- Regular assessment.
- Physiotherapy to maintain joint flexibility, especially shoulder external rotation, abduction and adduction, and supination.
- Indications for operation are debatable:
  - Gilbert—failure for good biceps recovery by 3 months.
  - Toronto—Toronto grading score that fails to progress.
  - Complete plexus palsy at birth associated with Horner's syndrome and phrenic nerve palsy.

- Surgery comprises exploration and assessment with repair of ruptured nerves by nerve grafts.
- Nerve grafts are usually sural, but some use superficial radial, medial cutaneous of forearm, or even the ulnar nerve if it is not going to be re-innervated.
- Where root avulsions are present the graftable roots are either spread out to the distal nerves (intra-plexural transfers) or a combination of extra-plexural and intra-plexural transfers are performed. For example, a ruptured C5 but avulsed C6 with intact C7, C8, and T1 may be repaired by using the accessory nerve to neurotize the suprascapular nerve, and the C5 root to neurotize the rest of the upper trunk, or if more distal the anterior and posterior divisions of the upper trunk.
- Post-operatively, a baby with poor head control is fitted with a cowl to stabilize the neck and head for a few weeks. Physiotherapy recommences after 4 weeks.
- Regular observation to assess recovery and watch for the sequelae of OBPP.

Sequelae of obstetrical brachial palsy

Shoulder
Incidence of secondary shoulder problems is 10%.

Aetiology
- Internal rotation contracture of the shoulder is thought to be due to muscle imbalance (Babbitt and Cassidy 1968) or cross innervation (Chuang and Wei 1998).
- Shoulder developmental dysplasia is not associated with severity of the brachial plexus lesion. Aetiology maybe muscle imbalance or epiphysiolysis (Zancolli) or neonatal dislocation (Dunkerton). Prognosis is poor if undetected.

Clinical presentation
Shoulder contracture and developmental dysplasia present with humeral shortening, axillary skin webbing, deep axilla, clicking on shoulder movement, fullness of the posterior shoulder, subluxation, coracoid hypertrophy, and hypoplasia of the humeral head. Rapid loss (within a month) of external rotation to 65°.

Classification of the shoulder deformity (Waters and Peljovich, 1999).

Investigation
Plain radiology is of little use; ultrasound and CT may be useful (Torode and Donnan 1998).

Treatment
- Anterior release by subscapularis lengthening (Carlioz and Brahimi 1971).
- Posterior release of subscapularis.
- If external rotators weak or inactive external rotation muscle tendon transfers using latissimus dorsi.
- Pearl (1998) recommended release before transfers as activity of the external rotators was impossible to determine.

References
Babbitt DP, Cassidy RH (1968). *J Bone Joint Surg Am* **50**, 1447–52.
Carlioz H, Brahimi L. (1971). *Ann Chir Infant* **12**, 159–67.
Chuang Wei (1998). *Plast Recon Surg* **101**:686–94.
Pearl (1998). *Jnl Bone Jt Surg* **80**:659–67.
Torode I, Donnan L (1998). *J Pediatr Orthop* **18**, 611–15.
Waters PM, Peljovich AE (1999). *Clin Orthop Relat Res* **364**, 144–52.

Volkmann's ischaemic contracture

An ischaemic contracture and paralysis of the upper limb first reported by Volkmann in 1881.

Definition
Chronic flexion contracture of the upper limb as a result of untreated or late treated compartment syndrome of the forearm.

Aetiology
- Usually post-traumatic or extravasation injury, but can occur after sepsis (meningococcal), burns, external pressure after coma/stroke.
- The worst affected muscles are flexor digitorum profundus and superficialis, flexor pollicis longus and pronator teres. The best preserved muscles are the wrist flexors and extensors (the more superficial muscles). The median nerve is more affected than the ulnar which is more affected than the radial.

Clinical presentation
- Mild or localized if only some of the flexor profundus muscles are affected.
- Clinical picture is usually of flexion contracture in two or three fingers.
- Moderate or classical if all the FDPs and FPL are involved with some superficial flexors also affected.
- Clinical picture is then one of flexion contractures of all the fingers, thumb, and wrist.
- Severe if in addition to the flexors being involved there is severe neurological disturbance, and some of the extensors are also affected.
- Very severe if there is no motor or nerve function.

Classification
Volkmann's contracture (Lipscomb)
- Mild: no nerve, minimal muscle deficit; treat by flexor slide.
- Moderate: no nerve, some dysfunction in muscle; treat by flexor slide.
- Severe: nerve deficit and little residual muscle function; treat by resection, neurolysis, transfers.
- Very severe: complete nerve deficit with no residual muscle function; treat by free functioning muscle transfer.

Treatment
Conservative
- Dynamic splinting.
- Physiotherapy.
- Functional training.

Surgical
Neurolysis
Neurolysis of the median and ulnar nerves may allow some recovery, especially in the median nerve.

Nerve grafts (image of sural nerve harvest to go opposite)
Excision and grafting of the nerves if they are very fibrosed may be helpful in restoring sensation. Nerve grafts may also be used to provide innervation for free functioning muscle transfers.

Muscle dissection, excision
Muscle dissection and excision if very fibrosed.

Tendon lengthening
- Flexor (Zancolli) slide: medial epicondyle release of flexor origin (flexor slide) will release mild contractures giving 2–3 cm of lengthening.
- Musculo-tendinous lengthening (Zancolli FAR: flexor aponeurotic and intermuscular fascial release): releases the muscle at the intermuscular fascia and musculo-tendinous junction. This will release mild contractures, providing 2–4 cm of lengthening.
- Tendon lengthening (FDP to FDS transfer) by dividing FDP tendons very proximally and the FDS tendons very distally and joining the ends providing length of 10 cm and using the better preserved FDS muscle to power FDP movement.

Tendon transfers
Free functioning muscle transplantation usually using gracilis or gastrocnemus from medial epicondyle to FDP and FPL.

Surgical indication
Depends on severity of the contracture, and the degree of functional loss.

Peripheral nerve injury

Nerve pathophysiology and assessment of injuries.

Diagnosis of nerve injury
- History.
- Loss of function.
- Tinel's sign.
- Tactile adherence.
- Immersion.
- Electrodiagnostic testing.
- Iodine–starch/ninhydrin/electrical skin resistance/thermography.
- Systematic examination with good knowledge of neural anatomy.

Classification

Table 17.2 Classification of nerve injury

Seddon	Sunderland
Neurapraxia	I Loss of conduction
Axonotmesis	II Loss of axon continuity
	III Including endoneurium
	IV Including perineurium
Neurotmesis	V Complete severance

Consequences of injury

Distal nerve:
- Wallerian degeneration.
- Schwann cell/macrophage debris removal.
- Schwann cell proliferation/organization.
- Schwann cell production of trophic factors.
- Endoneural collagen tube.

Nerve healing
- Initial delay.
- Site delay.
- Axon growth to endpoint.
- Functional recovery.
- Neurotropism:
  - The inherent ability of a regenerating nerve to find its correct pathway.
  - A motor nerve will preferentially move to a distal motor branch.
- Neurotrophic:
  - Nerve growth factors (NGF, laminin, aFGF, gangliosides, pyrogens, T3, steroids, cAMP).

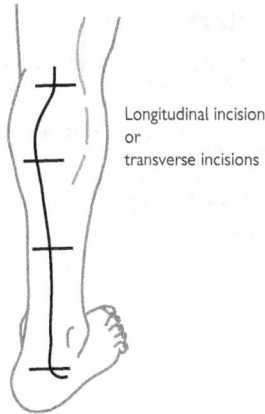

Fig. 17.20 Sural nerve harvest.

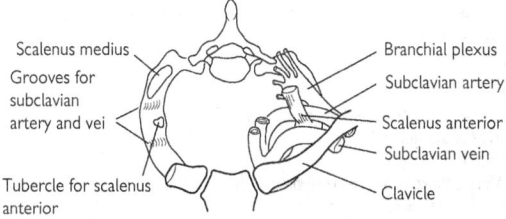

Fig. 17.21 Thoracic outlet: first rib and structure closing it.

Tendon transfers

- The tendon of a functioning muscle is detached from its insertion and then reattached to another tendon or bone to restore function of a paralysed muscle or injured tendon.
- The transferred tendon remains attached to its parent muscle with an intact neurovascular pedicle.
- Tendon transfers correct instability, imbalance, and lack of coordination not by addition but by redistribution of remaining muscular forces.

Indications for tendon transfer

- Restore function of paralysed muscles due to peripheral nerve, brachial plexus or spinal cord injuries.
- Restore function following tendon ruptures or tendon injuries.
- Restore balance to the deformed hand.

Principles

- Recipient.
- Donor.
- Technical.

Recipient

- Good joint mobility.
- Good bed (tissue equilibrium: no inflammation/infection/scars).
- Good cover.
- Good patient.

Donor

- Power (3.65 × cross-sectional area).
- Active/available/active.
- Amplitude:
  - Wrist flexors and extensors, 33 mm.
  - Finger flexors, 70 mm.
  - Finger extensors, 50 mm.
  - Thumb flexors, 50 mm.
- Two ways of augmenting effective amplitude:
  - use of tenodesis effect.
  - freeing fascial attachments to muscle.
- Expendible.
- Dynamic tenodesis.
- Synergistic.
- Independent.
- One tendon for one function.
- Wrist arthrodesis to provide additional donor tendons.

Technique

- Remote incisions.
- Strong insertion.
- Adequate tension.
- Straight line of traction.

Low ulnar nerve lesions
- Intrinsic clawing:
    - Zancolli (FDS) loops.
    - PL and grafts.
    - ECRB and grafts.
    - EDQ/EI.

High ulnar nerve lesions
- As for low ulnar nerve lesions + FDP tenodesis.

Low median nerve lesions
- Thumb opposition:
    - FDS.
    - FCR.
    - PL.

High median nerve lesions
- Thumb opposition: EI/ECRL.
- Thumb flexion: ECU/BR.
- Index/middle finger flexion: other FDPs.
- Pronator: Zancolli biceps.

Low median and ulnar nerve lesions
- Intrinsics: many tailed ECRB, FDSs, EDQ/EI.
- Thumb opposition: FDS, FCU.

High median and ulnar nerve lesions
- Thumb opposition: EI.
- Thumb flexion: BR.
- Finger flexion: ECU/ECRL.
- Intrinsics: ECRB.

Radial nerve lesions
- Wrist: PT.
- Finger: FDS(IV)/FCR/FCU.
- Thumb: PL to EPL; FDS(IV)/FCR to APL.

Burns emergency care

- Rescue the patient while ensuring safety of the rescuer.
- Give first aid.
- Stop the burning process:
  - For flame burns, roll the patient on the ground.
  - For scalds, remove wet clothing which will otherwise continue to heat the skin.
  - Remove burned clothes (unless stuck to the skin), watches, jewellery, and belts.
- Cool the burn wound:
  - Ideally cool, running water between 8 and 25°C for 20 minutes.
  - Spraying or sponging the wound also works; wet towels are less efficient and should be changed regularly.
  - Ensure the patient does not become hypothermic; if necessary, stop applying water and wrap the patient.
  - Do not use ice, which will vasoconstrict the skin and cause further damage.

Primary survey: ABCDEF

- **A**irway maintenance with C-spine control. Clear the airway of debris. Open the airway with chin lift and jaw thrust.
- **B**reathing and ventilation. Check for chest expansion. Intubate and ventilate if needed. Always give supplemental oxygen. Consider carbon monoxide poisoning, and circumferential chest burns (may need escharotomy).
- **C**irculation with haemorrhage control. Elevation and direct pressure to bleeding points. Check capillary refill <2 sec distal to burned areas. Circumferential, full-thickness burns may need escharotomy.
- **D**isability: neurological status.
- **E**xposure and environmental control: keep the patient warm; size of burn can be estimated.
- **F**luid resuscitation: Insert two large bore IV cannulae, preferably through unburned skin. Take blood for FBC, U&E, clotting, amylase, carboxyhaemoglobin. Start fluid resuscitation. Insert urinary catheter; monitor ECG, pulse, BP, respiratory rate, pulse oximetry as needed. NG tube for large burns to decompress the stomach.
- X rays: lateral C-spine, chest, and pelvis for burns associated with trauma.

Secondary survey

This proceeds according to ATLS guidelines:
- A full history of the burn is required—place, mechanism of burn, duration of exposure, and resuscitation given.
- Give tetanus prophylaxis.
- Reassess adequacy of resuscitation.
- Dress the burn simply. Plastic cling wrap is ideal as it allows inspection of the wound. If not available, a sheet will do. Keep the patient warm. Do not use topical antimicrobials, which make further assessment of the wound difficult.

Burns unit referral

All complex burns should be referred to a burns unit. These include:
- Extremes of age: <5 years or >60 years.
- Special sites: face, hands, feet, perineum, flexure surfaces, circumferential burns.
- Inhalation injury.
- Chemical, electrical, or radiation injuries.
- Large burns: >5% TBSA in children, >10% TBSA in adults.
- Coexisting medical conditions.
- Other injuries.

If in doubt, refer!

Burns fluid resuscitation

Principles
- Burn injuries cause release of inflammatory mediators resulting in vasodilatation and increased vascular permeability in tissues around the burned area. In burns over 20% TBSA (total body surface area), this can effect the entire body. Fluid moves from the vasculature into the interstitial spaces causing oedema. Lack of circulating fluid volume causes organ failure (especially renal failure) and death.
- The surface of the burned skin also loses protein-rich fluid by evaporation. The loss of protein exacerbates oedema.
- Fluid shifts due to vascular permeability are maximal in the first 24 hr, especially the first 8 hr following a burn injury. After 8–24 hr, colloid can be used as the resuscitation fluid; most units use crystalloid initially.
- Burns units vary in their fluid resuscitation guidelines. Fluid resuscitation with crystalloid (Hartmann's solution) according to the Parkland formula is described here.
- Resuscitation should be closely monitored and adjusted according to results.

Indication
Intravenous fluid resuscitation is required for:
- Children with burns >10% TBSA.
- Adults with burns >15% TBSA.

Method
- Place two large-bore IV cannulae, preferably through unburned skin.
- Calculate the percentage total body surface area (%TBSA) burned.
- Weigh the patient (or estimate their weight).
- Estimated fluid requirement.
  - **3–4 mL Hartmann's solution/kg body weight/%TBSA burn**.
  - Half the above fluid in the first 8 hr from the time of injury (not from the time assessed); second half over the next 16 hr.
- Children should have maintenance fluids of 4% glucose or 1/5 normal saline in addition to the above. Over 24 hr, give:
  - 100 mL/kg for first 10 kg body weight plus.
  - 50 mL/kg for 10–20 kg plus.
  - 20 mL/kg for each kg over 20 kg.
- Adult maintenance fluids as required.

Monitoring results
A urinary catheter should be passed. Aim for:
Adults: 0.5 mL/kg/hr or 30–50 mL/hr.
Children: 1.0 mL/kg/hr (0.5–2 mL/kg/hr).
- If urine output is inadequate, give boluses of 5–10 mL/kg, or increase the next hour's fluid by 50%.
- Monitor Hb, U&E, and arterial blood pH.
- Acidosis usually reflects inadequate fluid resuscitation. Consider tissue injury, e.g. electrical burns and crush injuries (look for myoglobinuria), and need for escharotomy.

- Hyperkalaemia occurs as a result of tissue injury in electric burns. Bicarbonate or glucose and insulin may be needed.
- Extensive tissue damage releases myoglobin and haemoglobin into the blood, to be filtered by the kidneys. The urine looks a dirty red colour. Deposition of haemochromogens in the proximal tubules of the kidney causes renal failure. Check the urine for myoglobin/haemoglobin. Increase urine output to 1–2 mL/kg/hr. Consider adding bicarbonate to the resuscitation fluid (to alkalinize urine and reduce deposition of haemochromogen crystals), or mannitol.
- For larger burns or patients with significant injuries consider central monitoring of CVP and an arterial line for blood pressure.
- Extra fluid resuscitation is often needed in:
  - Children.
  - Inhalation injury.
  - Electrical injury.
  - Delayed resuscitation.
  - Dehydration.

Assessment of burns

Burns need to be assessed with respect to their thickness (which reflects the duration, temperature, and mechanism of heat transfer) and the area of body skin involved as well as the involvement of the respiratory system. Commonly described as first-, second-, or third-degree burns, which is a laypersons assessment of the depth of the burn. Medically these are described as superficial, superficial–partial, partial or dermal, deep dermal, and full thickness. Burn surface area is reported as a percentage of total body surface area.

Estimation of depth of burn
- All burns contain areas of different depths.
- The history will give you a clue as to the depth.
- Look for colour, blisters, capillary return, and sensation within the burn area.
- Blisters indicate separation of dead skin from intact dermis by inflammatory exudate.
- Fixed staining (i.e. non-blanching erythema) indicates damage to dermal capillaries.
- Lack of sensation implies damage to pain receptors; therefore a deep burn.
- Superficial burns heal spontaneously by re-epithelialization from intact adnexal structures. They may be epidermal or dermal.
- Deep burns may heal spontaneously, but will leave significant scarring. They are deep dermal or full thickness

Table 17.3 Signs and symptoms of differing depth of burn

Depth	Colour	Blisters	Capillary refill	Sensation	Common causes
Epidermal	Red, may be shiny and wet	No	Brisk	Painful	Sunburn, flash burns
Superficial dermal	Pink, may be dry	Yes, small	Yes, may be slow	Painful	Flame, scald, chemical burns, brief contact burns
Mid-dermal	Dark pink	Yes, larger	Slow	May be absent	
Deep dermal	Blotchy red	May be present	Absent	Absent	
Full thickness	Thick, white, leathery	No	Absent	Absent	Flame, electrical burn entry/exit points, prolonged contact burns

Assessment of percentage total body surface area (%TBSA)

- Important as it guides further treatment, but is often done poorly, with a lack of consensus even among experts.
- Large burns tend to be underestimated, small burns overestimated.
- Try subtracting percentage non-burned tissue from 100% to obtain a more accurate assessment.
- Erythema is not included in %TBSA burned.
- Remember to turn the patient and assess the back.

Methods

- Palm of patient's hand represents 0.8% TBSA. Useful in very large or very small burns. For children or patchy burns, cut a template of the hand out of paper and see how many times it fits in the burn area
- Wallace rule of nines: this is quick but less accurate for children. Use it to check your calculation, e.g. a burn of one arm cannot be >9%.
- Lund–Browder chart: the most accurate method, allowing for change on shape with growth. Shade in burned areas on the picture and use the chart to compute TBSA.

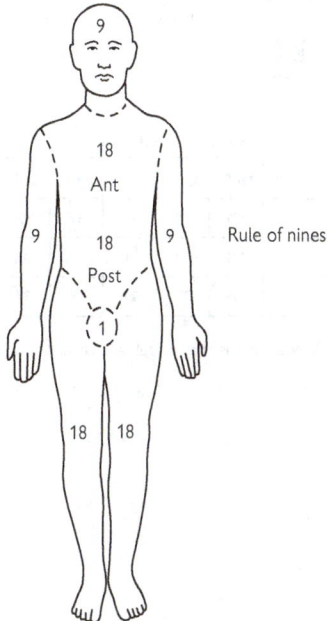

Fig. 17.22 Wallace rule of nines.

DATE: Weight:
          Age: 7½ years to Adult

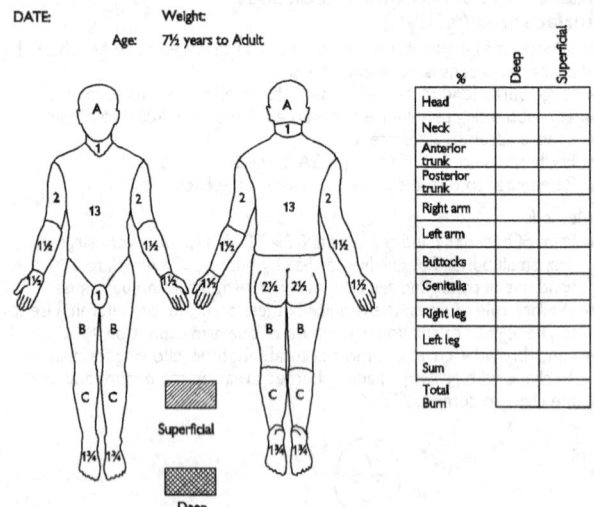

Fig. 17.23 Lund–Browder burns charts: adult and child.

Date: Weight:
Age: Birth to 7½ years

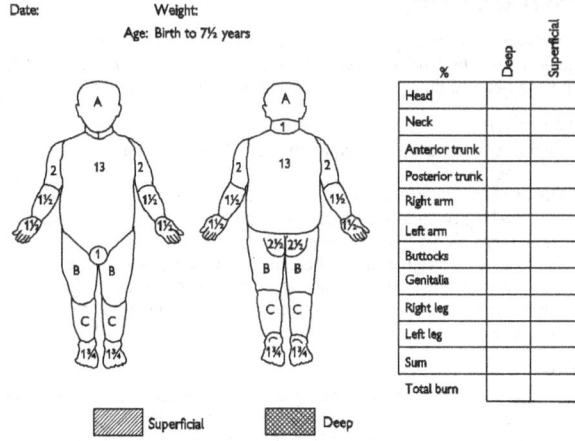

Relative percentages of areas affected by growth

Area	Age 0	Age 1	Age5	Age10	Age 15	Adult
A = ½ Of head	9½	8½	6½	5½	4½	3½
B = ½ Of one thigh	2¾	3¼	4	4¼	4½	4¾
C = ½ Of one leg	2½	2½	2¾	3	3¼	3½

Fig. 17.23 (*Contd.*) Lund–Browder burns charts: adult and child.

Escharotomy

A limb- and life-saving procedure to prevent compartment syndrome caused by the inelasticity and constricting effect of burnt skin in association with the oedema due to the capillary permeability and burn response.

Indications
- Circumferential or near-circumferential full-thickness burn to digit, limb, chest, or neck.
- The combination of the non-expansile full-thickness burn and oedematous swelling of underlying tissue may cause ischaemia of muscle and other tissue within 6 hr of injury.
- Full-thickness circumferential chest burns stop excursion of the chest wall, increase the work of breathing, and decrease the lung capacity.
- Full-thickness abdominal burns increase the risk of intra-abdominal hypertension, reducing renal perfusion.

Aims
To divide the burned tissue, allowing the skin to expand to accommodate underlying oedema, thereby preventing compartment syndrome and ischaemia of underlying and distal structures and allowing movement.

Planning
- Resuscitation is the priority, and should be under way before doing escharotomies.
- Perform within 6 hr of injury, ideally under GA in an operating theatre in a burns unit.
- Have blood available.
- Patient supine with arms on arm boards.
- If the ideal is not available, do not allow that to delay escharotomy.

Incision
Best with a scalpel, but bleeding can be profuse and is easier to control with monopolar diathermy.

Procedure
- Limbs: incise along mid-lateral line, and if necessary central axial line as well. Pass anterior to medial epicondyle at elbow and anterior to head of fibula to avoid ulnar and common peroneal nerves.
- Fingers: incise one lateral border—radial of little, ring, and thumb; ulnar of index and middle to avoid the leading edges.
- Hands: incise dorsum of first, second, and fourth compartments, and perform fasciotomies of the small muscles if required.
- Chest: a shield shape running down both anterior axillary lines with a connecting chevron across the lower border of the ribs.
- Abdomen: continue down medial and lateral sides.
- Neck: lateral longitudinal incisions. Be careful of underlying structures.

All incisions should be deep enough to allow the skin to split open and joints should move freely. Include deep fascia if muscle compartments swollen and tight. If in doubt do fasciotomies. Always extend incisions into non-burned skin; otherwise the burned margin may produce a tourniquet effect.

Closure
Paraffin gauze such as Jelonet (or alginate dressing such as Kaltostat) are suitable to cover the wounds, then gauze covered by the same dressing as the rest of the burn.

Post-operative care
- Elevate involved arms and legs.
- Check Hb within 24 hr.
- Physiotherapy for burned limbs, especially hands; resting splints for hands.
- Dressing changes will depend on the management of the rest of the burn.
- The wounds will need to be skin grafted, again in conjunction with the other burned skin.

Complications
- Bleeding.
- Damage to underlying structures, in particular nerves.
- Inadequate escharotomies will leave the patient at risk of ischaemic damage and ultimately ischaemic contractures.
- Escharotomies performed late subject the patient to reperfusion injury from necrotic metabolites.

Tips
- Use finger switch diathermy with cutting and coagulation modes and a pair of forceps in the other hand to control bleeding vessels.
- In extensive burns, do the chest escharotomies first—it will make ventilation easier.
- Oedema due to a burn generally increases over 48 hr, and so the effects of an inadequate escharotomy may not be apparent immediately.

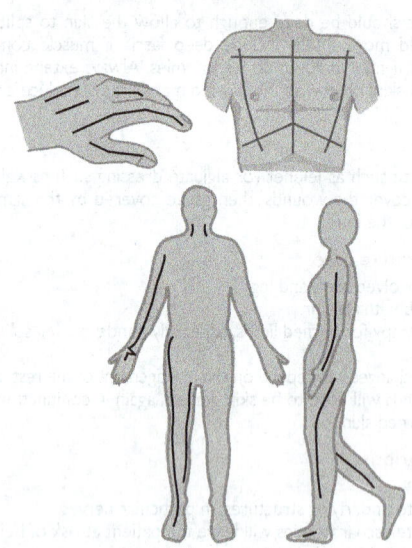

Fig. 17.24 Design of escharotomies in various regions.

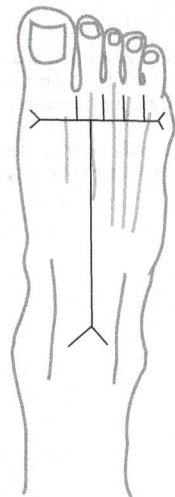

Fig. 17.25 Design of suggested foot escharotomies.

Pathophysiology of the burn wound

Initial insults
- Heat-induced injury: immediate; proteins denatured; cells damaged. Depth of burn depends on temperature and duration of contact. Wet burn (scald) travels through skin more quickly than dry burn (flame).
- Inflammatory injury: days 1–3 post burn. Inflammatory mediators cause further tissue damage and increase tissue permeability.
- Ischaemic injury: injured capillaries in viable skin adjacent to the burn thrombose due to mediator injury, causing more tissue to necrose.
- Delayed insults: inflammation continues due to mediators released from breakdown of eschar, bacterial colonization, wound exudate, and trauma to the open wound. The effects of inflammation are only understood in part. Specific to the wound.
- Neutrophils damage adjacent tissue by producing proteases and oxidants; and by using oxygen contribute to ischaemia.
- Proteases, particularly metalloproteases, are increased in open burn wounds. They injure newly forming tissue and deactivate local growth factors.
- The delay to healing stimulates excess collagen synthesis, resulting in increased scarring.

Jacksonian model of the burn wound
Described by Jackson in 1947:
- Zones correspond to current understanding of histopathology of burn wounds.
- Zone of coagulation: necrotic tissue, irreversible injury.
- Zone of stasis: surrounds zone of coagulation in three dimensions. Contains injured but viable cells.
- Zone of hyperaemia: peripheral to zone of stasis; inflammatory mediators cause vasodilation. Usually recovers fully. In a 25% burn, this zone may involve the entire body.

Local factors
Conversion (of zone of stasis to necrosis) is increased by local factors:
- Reduced blood flow.
- Increased inflammation.
- Dessication.
- Exudate.
- Mechanical or chemical trauma, e.g. from dressings.
- Systemic factors:
  - Septicaemia.
  - Hypovolaemia.
  - Excess catabolism.
  - Chronic illness.

Burn shock
Initially hypovolaemic shock due to fluid loss from the wound. Reduction in plasma volume, cardiac output, and urine output follows. Haemoglobin concentration and haematocrit are raised. Cardiac output is also reduced independent of fluid loss; this may be due to inflammatory mediators released at the burn wound.

If shock is untreated, sympathetic stimulation and hypovolaemia result in release of catecholamines, ADH, angiotensin II, and neuropeptide-Y, causing arteriolar vasoconstriction and eventually end-organ ischaemia.

Hypovolaemic shock is maintained by development of burn oedema.

Burn oedema
- Within an hour of injury, the water content of the burned tissue increases rapidly.
- In the first 12–24 hr after a burn, fluid extravasation continues more slowly in both burned and non-burned tissue.
- It is thought that capillary permeability in the burn wound increases, allowing proteins to leak from plasma. The hydrostatic pressure in the burn tissue interstitium drops, possibly due to altered integrin function. Fluid rushes out of the vasculature and into the burned tissue down hydrostatic and osmotic pressure gradients. Hypoproteinaemia and increased capillary permeability account for the oedema in non-burned skin.
- Tumour necrosis factors, interleukins, histamine, kinins, serotonin, thromboxanes, and prostaglandins have all been implicated as mediators of burn shock and oedema.

Effect of burn on immune system
All injuries, including burns, are immunosuppressive. The mechanism is not known, but the extent of immunosuppression is related to the size of the burn. The inflammatory response to a burn follows the usual pattern in response to injury, i.e. activation of inflammatory cascades locally; migration of neutrophils and then macrophages into the wound; and an attempt to clear the injured tissue by phagocytosis. Specific deleterious effects include:
- Ratio of T_4 (helper) to T_8 (suppressor) lymphocytes is reversed.
- T_4 lymphocytes alter receptor profile and become less effective.
- Cytokine production by macrophages appears to become overactive.
- Neutrophils release toxic contents of phagolysosomes into surrounding tissues, causing necrosis, rather than killing bacteria intracellularly.
- Products of arachidonic acid cascade are skewed to increase levels of prostaglandin E_2 and thromboxane B_2. The result is increased capillary permeability and immunosuppression.

Hypermetabolic response to a burn
- Metabolism is slowed for 2–3 days post burn, and then increases to up to three times normal rate.
- Levels of catecholamines, cortisol, insulin, glucagon, and prolactin rise.
- Consequences include increased body temperature (to ~38.5°C), increased oxygen and glucose consumption, increased CO_2 production; and breakdown of glycogen, protein, and fat stores.

- This stress response appears to be maladaptive in the context of a burn, and results in recycling of energy stores which are very rapidly depleted.
- The hypermetabolic state may last for 9 months.
- Erosion of lean body mass, muscle weakness, immunosuppression, and poor wound healing are long-term consequences.

Treatment of burns

Unfortunately, despite improved understanding of aspects of burn pathophysiology, few treatments have been demonstrated to improve outcome. However, the following do save lives:
- Early aggressive fluid resuscitation.
- Early enteral feeding.
- Early excision of the burn.
- Warming the environment to 33°C reduces the hypermetabolic response.

Burn infection

Prior to the 1970s, the majority of patients with burns over 50% TBSA died from sepsis, usually originating from the burn wound.

Aetiology
Barriers to infection are violated as a result of the injury or its treatment. The innate and adaptive arms of the immune response are depressed.

Portals of infection
The burn wound is an excellent culture medium, surrounded by a zone of ischaemia which compromises immune surveillance of the wound. Transfer of organisms or endotoxin into the circulation causes sepsis:
- Respiratory tract: inhalation injury, reduced chest wall compliance, intubation, and ARDS contribute to risk of infection.
- Gastrointestinal tract: bacterial translocation is increased by ischaemic damage, and lack of early enteral feeding.
- Urinary tract: indwelling catheters.
- Intravascular cannulae.

Clinical features
- Signs of an infected burn wound include:
  - Increased erythema.
  - Slough, exudate, or frank pus.
  - Progression of the burn to involve the zone of stasis.
  - Pain.
- Signs of systemic infection include:
  - Hyper- or hypothermia.
  - Hypotension.
  - Tachycardia.

Investigations
- CRP is usually raised in a burn so may not be helpful in diagnosing infection.
- White cell count may not increase because of immune suppression.
- Chest X-ray.
- Tissue microbiology: $>10^5$ organisms per gram of burn tissue (burn wounds are usually colonized).
- Tissue biopsy to show histological evidence of invasion of infecting organisms into viable tissue adjacent to the burn.
- Microbiological culture of sputum or bronchial washings, urine, faeces, and catheter tips (urinary or intravascular).
- Common infecting organisms in burns sepsis include *Pseudomonas aeruginosa*, *Staphylococcus aureus*, *Klebsiella pneumoniae*, *Escherichia coli*, *Enterobacter* spp. and *Candida* spp.

Management
- Preventative measures include fluid resuscitation, early excision of the wound, early enteral feeding, continued nutritional support, chest physiotherapy.
- Antimicrobial dressings reduce colonization of the wound.
- Antibiotics for sepsis.
- Supportive management for systemic effects of sepsis.
- Toxic shock syndrome:
  - Rare consequence of burn; more common in young people.
  - Symptoms include nausea, vomiting, diarrhoea, muscle pains, headache.
  - Signs include fever, hypotension, rash, cutaneous desquamation. The burn may look normal.
  - It may progress rapidly to multiple organ failure and death.
- Pathogenesis:
  - The burn is colonized with an exotoxin-producing staphylococcus.
  - The exotoxin is absorbed into the blood, and causes a massive inflammatory response.
  - Treatment is supportive with antibiotics to attempt to reduce the bacterial colonization.

Burn treatment

Conservative

Indications
- Superficial burns: mixed superficial and deep dermal burns that will heal in <2 weeks.
- Patient request.
- Burns with uncertainty of depth. Review after 48 hr of dressings.

Management
- Once decision to treat conservatively, change the dressings infrequently to allow healing.
- Review to ensure aim of healing within 2 weeks. If breaches, consider change of plan.

Dressings
Aim is to:
- Reduce pain.
- Prevent infection.
- Absorb fluid and allow healing.
- Allow mobility.

First layer is simple non-adherent dressings either tulle gras (paraffin gauze) or mepitel. Second layer is gauze to absorb exudate. Third layer is bandage, tape, or Tubigrip to secure. SSD cream can be applied to smaller burns. It has a topical microbial action but alters the colour of the burn, so should only be used when the depth of the burn is known or deemed unimportant. Hands can be dressed in bags filled with SSD cream or glycerine to permit movement and physiotherapy.

Surgical

Indications and aims
- Immediate life- or limb saving procedure.
- Prevention and control of infection.
- Preserve viable tissue.
- Maintain function.
- Reduction of scar.

Timing of surgery
- Immediate: escharotomy, fasciotomy, amputation, tracheostomy, cut down.
- Early (<5 days): early burn excision and graft.
- Delayed (>5 days): delayed excision and graft and scar revision.

Types of excision
- Direct excision of full-thickness burns to viable tissue.
- Tangential excision using a skin graft knife or scalpel to shave off the burnt tissue until it is excised.
- Avulsion excision is the late excision of slough in the plane of natural separation.

Types of closure
- Direct closure is not usually recommended because of the high infection risk. Split-skin graft can be autograft (either harvested or via cell culture), allograft (cadaver or family member), xenograft, or artificial.(e.g. Integra^{TM}). The skin graft is usually meshed 1:1.5 where there is no donor shortage; the mesh ratio can be increased where there is a shortage of skin.
- Full-thickness graft is usually used in specialized areas (e.g. hand, face or neck.
- Flaps can be used for exposed bone, vessels, nerves, and viscera.

Burn reconstruction

The quantity and quality of burn reconstruction is determined to a large extent by the initial treatment of the burn injury and patient. Burn reconstruction is mainly concerned with the effect of burn scarring and contracture, and to a lesser degree with reconstruction of parts and function lost in the burn injury.

26–63% of burns scars are hypertrophic. If the wound heals in less than 21 days it is less than half as likely that a hypertrophic scar will occur. If healing takes longer then 14 days, a hypertrophic scar is likely (Deitch et al. 1983).

Principles
- Prevention:
  - Early burn wound management and closure.
  - Pre operative splinting and compression.
  - Post-operative splinting, compression and scar management.
  - Mobilization and return to activity.
- Team approach: surgeon, nurse, psychologist, occupational therapist, physiotherapist.
- Timing: when scars have matured unless severe functional deficit, pain or deformity.
- Aims: prevention of deformity, restoration of function, aesthetic considerations.
- Plan: review burn as a whole, assess each problem area and options for reconstruction and then prioritise.
- Psychology: pre-operative discussion and involvement of patient in decisions. Be realistic about outcomes.

Conservative management
Pressure garments for 24 months or until it is clinically apparent that scars have matured. If deformity is increasing consider early surgical intervention.

Surgical management
Release
- Ensure that this is complete in width and depth. If necessary extend into normal skin or deeper tissue. Significant contractures may have shortening of underlying vital structures, such as tendon, nerve, and artery.
- Incision is usually adequate. However, excision may be necessary to restore movement or function. Excision of deep scar causing tendon or joint adherence may be necessary.
- The resulting defect, even in incision alone, can be surprisingly large.

Repair
If there is no deficiency of tissue and some lateral laxity consider direct closure or lengthening procedures such as Z-plasty and Y–V advancement. If there is a deficiency of tissue, skin grafting (split, full, or composite) or flaps should be considered. In the cases where deeper structures are involved flaps (local, distant, and free) and tissue expansion can be used.

Reference
Deitch EA, Wheelahan TM, Rose MP, Clothier J, Cotter J (1983). *J Trauma* **23**, 895–8.

Burns to trunk, genitalia, and head and neck

Breast
- Conservative management: the nipple–areola complex should be allowed to demarcate. This does not effect breast development but secondary surgery may be needed.
- Surgical management: treat burnt breast skin as non-specialized area.
- Secondary surgery: multiple breast releases may be required to assist development. Despite this there may well be contour deformities. Release incisions are infra-mammary, superior, and lateral as necessary. In deep burns formal breast reconstruction will be required.
- Deep burns or burns to the breast can result in galactorrhoea.

Perineum
- Conservative management: treatment of choice for patchy full-thickness and superficial burns. If there is no urethral involvement the patient can be catheterized. If there are urethral burns a suprapubic catheter should be used.
- Surgical management: reserved for larger full-thickness burns.
- Secondary surgery: perineal webbing can occur and is treated with Z-plasties. Penile contractures are treated with incision and FTSG. Perianal stenosis requires colorectal surgical involvement, with release and eversion of unburned tissue from the anal lining. Total penile reconstruction may sometimes be required.

Burns to head and neck
- Conservative management: observe all but the most blatant FT burns for 2–3 weeks. Sit up to reduce swelling and apply topical antimicrobials, e.g. Polyfax, Betadine. Compression masks may be needed during or after healing.
- Surgical management: reconstruct in aesthetic units, a larger reconstruction can cover more than one aesthetic unit. Early reconstruction should be considered to preserve function and prevent contracture.

Eyelids
If there is corneal exposure, this is a priority. For extrinsic lower eyelid ectropion (ectropion caused by contracture of the facial tissues), the contracture is released 1–2 mm inferior to the lower eyelid margin. If necessary, it can be extended medially and laterally above the canthal line. The orbicularis is released and a crescent-shaped FTSG that acts as a sling is placed on the defect. For upper eyelid release the incision is 7–10 mm superior to the lash margin, extending laterally above the lateral canthal line.

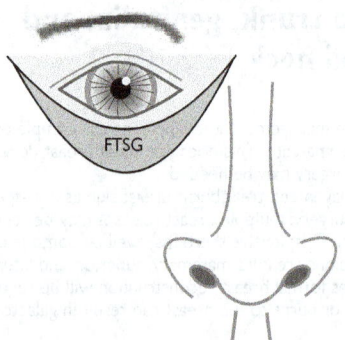

Fig. 17.26 Burn ectropion release; release extends beyond the borders of the eyelid.

Mouth and lips
- Classification: intrinsic (contraction of component parts) and extrinsic (contraction of face and neck tissue).
- Principles: correction of microstomia first; therefore address commissures before lips and vermilion. For vermilion loss and commissure webbing, use mucosal advancement procedure. The lower lip is best excised as an aesthetic unit, leaving the prominence to highlight the chin. On the upper lip the columella can be lengthened with fork flaps. Scar excision should be of aesthetic units, with the seam of the skin graft along the philtral column.

Neck
- Consider the influence of the chest contracture on the neck.
- Deformities: single vertical band is treated with Z-plasty or incision and graft. Partial or complete involvement of neck skin requires formal release including platysma scar. Reconstruction with FTSG, tissue expansion or flaps, and post-operative splinting.

Nose
- Deformities: eversion of nares, thin skin on dorsum, and loss of cartilaginous support.
- Principles: consider aesthetic units and assess as for nose reconstruction.

Ear
Lowest priority area on the face. See ear reconstruction.

Scalp alopecia
Best managed by serial excision, rotation or transposition flap, or tissue expansion.

Hand burns

Approximately 30% of burns are on the hand.

Conservative management
In partial-thickness or mixed picture burns give hand burns the benefit of the doubt and allow to heal conservatively. Elevate and dress in a Flamazine or glycerine bag to allow movement and physiotherapy, with night splinting as required. Prevention of deformity and joint contractures is essential and requires proactive management using splinting, therapy, and in some instances surgical joint fixation or release to maintain optimal joint positions.

Primary surgical management
Escharotomies will be needed in circumferential full-thickness burns. Tangential excision and skin graft under tourniquet control (remember to mark burn area before application of the tourniquet). Flap cover is required if vital structures are exposed or for improved function of specialized areas such as fingertip or web-space burns.

Post-operative care
For the first 7 days splint in position of function, allowing any graft to heal. Thereafter physiotherapy during the day and night splinting in position of function. K-wires can be used for joint or first web-space contractures to maintain correction or position. Compression garments to control scarring. These may need inserts, moulds, or special modifications to enable pressure to be applied to the complex contours of the hand.

Secondary management
Syndactyly
This can be managed conservatively in some cases with specialized pressure garments with spacers and web straps. Surgical management with division of the syndactyly and reconstruction of the web space is indicated when there is limitation of abduction, loss of independence of the syndactylized digits, persistent skin breakdown in the syndactylized webs, limitation of extension, or inability to wear rings. Syndactyly techniques are varied, but in principle consist of a web-space reconstruction using local flaps, and release and breaking up of the scar by interdigitating flaps or grafts.

Joint contractures
The MCPJ is usually contracted in an extended position. A dorsal release is indicated, extending beyond the axial lines with FTSG or flap to defect. PIPJ contractures are usually into flexion, which in addition to release of flexor skin and soft tissue may also require release of accessory collateral and check rein ligaments.

Boutonnière deformity
Can result from burn destruction of the central slip or flexion contracture of the PIPJ. Difficult to treat once established. Treatments are not different for burn aetiology.

Nailfolds

These are best left for 6 months to assess nail growth. Dorsal scarring can cause eponychial fold retraction, and this should be treated with a dorsal release, transposition flap, and/or FTSG. Severe nailbed burns may need formal nailbed reconstruction or excision of remaining nailbed. Nail prostheses can be used if the bed is flat.

Other concerns

There is an increased incidence of peripheral neuropathy in hand burns. In 2–3% of patients there is para-articular ossification. More extensive reconstructive procedures are required in extreme burns with loss of digits and thumb. These do not differ from traumatic loss of other aetiologies.

Foot burns

Conservative management
Elevation, splinting, and dressings will suffice for partial thickness burns. Early mobilization is encouraged. Sole burns usually heal with dressings alone.

Surgical management
In deeper burns tangential excision and skin graft followed by elevation and splinting until the graft is stable. Thereafter gradual mobilization with pressure garments. Orthopaedic shoes and splints should be used to prevent contracture. With exposed tendon, bone, or joint, assess the viability of the foot. Flap cover will be needed if the foot is viable and worth keeping.

Secondary surgery

Dorsal burn contracture
This gives hyperextension and subluxation of the toes, with syndactyly and a rocker bottom foot. It is treated with a horizontal release extending medial to the first toe and lateral to the fifth, with extensions for the web spaces and ascending the foot longitudinally for width depending on severity (see Fig. 17.25). The defect can be reconstructed with a graft or flap. Post-operative management as above.

Plantar burn scar
This leads to a cavus deformity which in mild cases can be released and grafted, but in severe cases will require an Ilizarov fixator and osteotomies.

Equinus deformities
In mild cases these can be treated with capsulotomy and tendon lengthening. If the skin over the Achilles tendon is very scarred, this may need to be accompanied by flap replacement of the skin over the operative site. In severe deformity a combination of Ilizarov fixator for distraction and arthrodesis to maintain position is indicated.

Unstable skin or soft tissue
This will require excision and free flap cover. Functional units may need to be replaced to locate the junctional scars in areas with less shear and movement.

Amputation
Except for toes this should be considered as a last resort (two-consultant decision).

Chemical burns

Epidemiology
Minority (1–4%) of burns admissions are chemical. Most (95%) are <10% TBSA and are treated conservatively. Alkali burns are the most common.

Pathophysiology
The chemical causes damage until it is neutralized by the tissue. Tissue damage depends on the concentration, toxicity, temperature, and quantity of the chemical, surface area and duration of contact, exothermic reaction, ease of absorption, and systemic effects.
- Acids cause coagulative necrosis (like thermal burns).
- Alkalis cause liquefaction necrosis.

Sites of chemical injury
Skin, cornea, gastrointestinal (swallowed), respiratory (inhaled), and systemic (absorbed).

Treatment
- History of incident and of chemical (data sheet).
- Examination: ABC etc., exclude concomitant injury.
- Management:
  - Extensive lavage, initially 2 hr for acid burns and 12 hr for alkali burns, but continue until pain subsides and pH (litmus paper) returns to normal.
  - Ensure removal of lavaged fluid.
  - Apply an antidote only for the commonly used chemicals, as there can be difficulty in controlling the concentration and exothermic heat generation from the reaction.
  - Fluid resuscitation for large BSA burns.
  - Involve other teams early (e.g. respiratory and gastrointestinal) and refer corneal burns early.
  - Contact poisons centre re chemical composition.

Acids

Sulphuric, nitric, and hydrochloric acids
Sulphuric acid burns are second most common chemical burns. Treat with copious irrigation, wiping away resulting soapy solution. Early excision and grafting.

Hydrofluoric acid
Irrigation and calcium gluconate gel every 4 hr for 3–4 days. Injections of calcium gluconate around the burn area. Continue until pain relieved. Local calcium injections have also been used. Early excision and repair, especially in >1%TBSA as there is high morbidity and mortality.

Chromic acid
Very toxic; produces renal failure in 1%. Lethal dose is 5–10 g. Treat with lavage and rinsing with sodium hyposulphate solution. Unless obviously superficial proceed to urgent excision and grafting (<2 hr). Involve a medical team early due to high systemic toxicity.

CHEMICAL BURNS

Phenol
Rapid systemic absorption; therefore copious irrigation and wipe off with vegetable oil. Urgent excision.

Alkalis

Sodium hydroxide and potassium hydroxide
Sodium hydroxide burns are the most common chemical burns. Irrigation alone or phosphate buffer soaks changed hourly for 24 hr.

Cement
Depending on length of contact tends to produce full-thickness burns which require excision and grafting.

Bitumen
Irrigate if within 30 minutes of contact. If it remains in the skin leave *in situ* and it separates as an eschar. Can remove with arachus or vegetable oil as necessary.

Electrical burns

Epidemiology
3% of burns.

Classification
- Low voltage <1000 V.
- High voltage >1000 V.

Pathophysiology
- Low-voltage burns mimic thermal burns.
- In high-voltage burns, heat is produced as the current passes through the body. The amount of heat is directly dependent on the current, resistance, and duration of contact (Joule's law). The amount of tissue damage is related to the above plus the surface area of contact and the pathway through the body. Tissue resistance increases in the order nerve, vessels, muscle, skin, tendon, fat, bone.
- Two theories of the progressive tissue necrosis found in electrical burns.
  - Periosseous core of necrosis is due to the bone generating the most heat as it has the highest resistance or due to the prolonged elevation of the bone temperature. Muscle damage is due to the delayed thrombosis of vessels or the irreversible microscopic damage to muscle at the time of the burn.
  - Electroporation is tissue necrosis in the absence of the heating effect. The current exceeds the critical limit which leads to cell membrane breakdown.

Types of burn
- Contact: entry and exit.
- Flash, arc: exit and re-entry.
- Thermal: ignition of clothing and nearby structures.

Immediate management
- Remove from danger; rescue and resuscitation at the site.
- History: best from an observer; ascertain site of injury, voltage of source, associated injuries.
- Examination: ABC and spine; B (pneumothorax often associated), C (including cardiac rhythm); neurology and conscious state; full secondary survey as 10–15% have associated trauma.
- Burn assessment: percentage burn, site, entry and exit (check on scalp), viability of limbs. Assess the need for escharotomy or fasciotomy. If in doubt, do it.
- Investigations: urinalysis (myoglobinuria), U&E (renal failure), LFT (visceral function), FBC, cardiac enzymes, rhythm strip and ECG, X-ray and arteriography as indicated.
- Resuscitation: as previously. Fluid requirements exceed surface wound estimates. Maintain high urine output (50–75 mL/hr in adult). Increase to 100 mL/hr if myoglobinuria. Consider osmotic diuretic, e.g. mannitol.

Surgical management
- Immediate: escharotomy, fasciotomy, nerve decompression, and debridement.
- Early: excision, skin graft, and flap cover.
- Late: as in other types of burn.

Complications
- Burn wound: muscle fibrosis, peripheral neuropathy. The neuropathy may appear late and be at sites remote from the obvious injury.
- Non-burn wound: cerebral haemorrhage, personality change, paralysis, cataract formation.

Prognosis
Mortality 8–14%.

Non-accidental injury in burns

Child abuse is thought to be the cause of up to 20% of paediatric burns. A checklist of indicators is below:
- Child brought in by unrelated adult.
- Greater than 12 hr delay in presentation with no explanation.
- Inappropriate parental affect.
- Blame apportioned to child or siblings.
- History and burn not consistent with injury.
- History incompatible with developmental age.
- Previous history of NAI of patient or siblings.
- Differing histories of the incident.
- Injury to perineum, buttocks, or genitalia.
- Pattern of injury:
  - Mirror image injury to the extremities.
  - Implying forced immersion.
  - Deliberate contact burn.
- Unrelated other injuries.
- Inappropriate affect of the child.

Any one of these should raise suspicion; two or more give a 60% risk of non-accidental injury. Any suspected cases should be managed with a team approach, including a specialist nurse, paediatrician, surgeon, and social worker.

Be suspicious of cigarette burns, burns with clear demarcation/borders, burns with consistent depth.

If you suspect NAI, document the history and examination of the burn carefully and fully, and record the affect and behaviour of the child and parents. Ask another doctor to repeat the above. Photograph the injuries. Obtain medical records from the hospital, the hospital local to the child's home, and the GP's records to determine number, frequency, and types of admission to hospital or medical contact. Discuss your concerns with the senior staff and nurses. They will repeat the history and examination, and discuss matters with social services and the paediatricians. A multidisciplinary meeting will be held. The issue will be discussed with the parents, usually individually. The concerns will be explained and the parents asked for their explanation. A surprising number of parents admit to the NAI.

Increasingly awareness has been raised of NAI to dependent adults, particularly the elderly. The above checklist can be modified and used in such cases.

Chapter 18

Metabolic, endocrine, degenerative

Rheumatoid arthritis *632*
Scleroderma, CREST syndrome, systemic sclerosis *636*
Osteoarthritis *638*
Gout *640*

Rheumatoid arthritis

Definition
Chronic systemic autoimmune disease causing inflammation and proliferation of synovium.

Incidence
- 1%, fairly consistent worldwide.
- Female-to-male ratio 3:1.

Aetiology
- Multifactorial and uncertain; possibly an environmental agent in genetically susceptible individuals, with hormonal modulation.
- Genetic: concordance of 20% in monozygotic twins (increased in severe disease); five times higher than in dizygotic twins. High prevalence in certain American Indian tribes. Increased risk in relatives of those with severe seropositive disease. Increased risk for certain HLA types: *DR1* has doubled risk; *DR4* has sixfold risk.
- Environmental: rare in rural sub-Saharan Africa, but prevalence similar to that in Europe in urban African populations. <50% concordance in monozygotic twins. Appears not to be present in antiquity; therefore may be due to a relatively new antigen, possibly infective.
- Hormonal: often settles during pregnancy, to be followed by flare after the birth (although this may be immune mediated). Evidence is building for a role for oestrogen in mediating inflammation.

Classifications
- By number of joints affected:
  - Monoarthropathy—one joint.
  - Pauciarthropathy—two to four joints.
  - Polyarthropathy—more than four joints.
- By clinical course:
  - Polycyclic—80% cases. Intermittent flares cause progressive joint destruction, with eventual quiescence.
  - Explosive onset—10%; usually men over 55 years. Rapid onset, severe polyarthropathy, but may have minimal long-term sequaelae.
  - Progressive—5% cases. Inflammation, joint destruction, muscle wasting, and systemic disease progress inexorably.
  - Monocyclic—rare, or possibly not diagnosed. One or two episodes; then subsides.
- By stage of the disease:
  - Stage 1—proliferative. Inflammation of synovial membranes, reversible.
  - Stage 2—destructive. Erosion of articular cartilage, bone, joint capsule and ligaments; tendon ruptures.
  - Stage 3—reparative. Fibrosis of tendons and joints leads to fixed deformities.

Thumb deformity
Nalebuff classification:
- Group 1: boutonnière—flexed MCPJ.
- Group 2: flexed MCPJ with metacarpal adduction.
- Group 3: Z-shaped thumb, zig-zag thumb, or swan-neck deformity—CMCJ and IPJs flexed; MCPJ hyperextended.
- Group 4: gamekeeper's thumb—CMCJ subluxed due to attrition or rupture of UCL.

Pathogenesis
Auto-immune: 70% of patients have rheumatoid factor in blood (antibody–antigen complexes to native IgG). Plasma cells in subsynovium synthesize immunoglobulins (predominantly IgM and IgG), which form complexes with native IgG. These activate complement and cause leucocyte infiltration around the involved tendon or joint. Synovium proliferates and invades tendons, periarticular soft tissues, articular cartilage, and bone.

Clinical features
A heterogeneous disease, with a variably relapsing and remitting course. May present in children (juvenile rheumatoid arthritis), or more commonly in adults between the ages of 25 and 50 years. Various systems may be effected. Extra-articular disesase is more common and more severe with high titres of rheumatoid factor.

Joints
Distal, symmetrical, polyarthritis of small joints. PIPJs, MCPJs, wrists, MTPJs, ankles, knees, and cervical spine commonly affected. Any synovial joint may be affected, including crico-arytenoid and temporo-mandibular joints. Also bursae. Symptoms are of pain and stiffness, often worse in the morning and evening. Examination reveals tenderness, swelling, warmth, and redness over joints, which may have reduced passive and active movement.

Tendons
Tenosynovitis of the palm may cause trigger finger, over the extensor and flexor surfaces of the wrist may cause tendon ruptures, and may lead to nerve compressions. Tendons are swollen, red, and tender, with pain and crepitus on movement.

Rheumatoid nodules
Subcutaneous and intra cutaneous nodules occur in 25% of patients. Rheumatoid nodulosis is the rare phenomenon of nodules without associated joint disease. Nodules are macroscopically discrete, firm, and non-tender swellings in various sites, including over the olecranon, forearm, dorsum, and palm of hand. May cause ulceration of overlying skin, or pain due to pressure (especially on the palms). Histology shows central fibrinoid necrosis with surrounding palisades of fibroblasts and chronic inflammatory cells. May also develop in eye, pleura, pericardium, heart and lung parenchyma, and vocal cords.

Vasculitis
Splinter haemorrhages, nailfold infarcts, and Raynaud's phenomenon.

Blood
Normochromic normocytic anaemia is a common finding. Platelet count is often raised in active disease, but may be low due to marrow suppression by drug treatment. Felty's syndrome (RA, splenomegaly, and leucopenia) develops in <1% and causes increased susceptibility to infection.

Lungs
Pleurisy, lung nodules, pulmonary fibrosis, and obliterative bronchiolitis may feature. Caplan's syndrome (massive pulmonary fibrosis with pulmonary nodules) develops on exposure to coal dust or inorganic dusts. Patients are rheumatoid factor positive, but may not have joint disease.

Heart
Pericardial effusions, inflamed heart valves, and patchy myocardial fibrosis may cause pericaditis, valvular incompetence, and conduction defects.

Eyes
Episcleritis and scleritis. Sjögren's syndrome, inflammation of exocrine glands (including lacrimal), affects 20%. Brown's syndrome is a rare cause of diplopia due to stenosing tenosynovtis of the superior oblique tendon.

Nerves
Peripheral entrapment neuropathies of carpal, cubital, and radial tunnels due to tenosynovitis. Polyneuropathy rarely.

Muscles
Myositis is rare; muscle wasting is usually due to disuse because of joint pain. Also consider cervical spine and nerve compressions.

Liver
Mild hepatosplenomegaly is common, but liver function is rarely significantly reduced.

Kidneys
Renal amyloidosis may result.

Diagnosis
American College of Rheumatology criteria for diagnosis of rheumatoid arthritis (four or more of these indicate RA):
- Morning stiffness >1 hr.
- Arthritis of three or more joint areas.
- Arthritis of hand joints.
- Symmetric arthritis.

The above should be present for at least 6 weeks.
- Rheumatoid nodules.
- Serum rheumatoid factor positive.
- Typical X-ray changes in hand and wrist.

Investigations
Blood tests show raised ESR, CRP, and platelets in active disease; rheumatoid factor in 70%; antinuclear antibodies in 30%. X-ray changes typically include:
- Soft tissue swelling.
- Periarticular osteoporosis.
- Reduced joint space due to loss of articular cartilage.
- Periarticular bone erosions.
- Joint deformities.

Management

Aims to stop synovitis, prevent deformity, reconstruct unstable or deformed joints, and rehabilitate the patient.

Medical

- Analgesics such as paracetamol and codeine for pain.
- NSAIDs also improve pain and stiffness, but may have significant GI side-effects. COX-2 inhibitors avoid these.
- Disease-modifying drugs include methotrexate, sulfasalazine, gold, penicillamine, antimalarials, azathioprine, cyclophosphamide, and chlorambucil. They reduce synovitis in many patients, but have significant side-effects, and so blood count, renal and liver function should be monitored. Methotrexate is currently the most popular first-line drug.
- 'Biologics' (e.g. infliximab) are TNF-alpha blockers and are currently used in severe RA which does not respond to the above. Their side-effects include susceptibility to infections which may be overwhelming, or atypical, e.g. extra-pulmonary TB.
- Steroids: injections for localized synovitis or disease limited to a few joints. Systemic steroids are used sparingly (because of side effects) for acute exacerbations.
- Splintage: reduces inflammation, relieves pain, and protects joints and tendons.
- Physiotherapy: passive exercises are used in acute exacerbations to preserve range of motion. Strengthening the muscles around a joint improves function and reduces pain.

Surgical

Aims to relieve pain, improve function, prevent deformity, and improve cosmesis. In a painless deformed hand, function is the paramount consideration and should not be sacrificed to improve cosmesis. Surgery involves a selection of:

- Synovectomy and tenosynovectomy.
- Tendon surgery—repair, transfer, grafting, or repositioning.
- Nerve decompression or transfer.
- Arthroplasty—excision or replacement.
- Arthrodesis.

In general, proximal joints are operated on before distal (as surgery to the proximal joints may affect function of the distal ones). An exception is the PIPJ in Boutonnière deformity, which should be corrected before surgery to MCPJs as the flexed PIPJ affects MCPJ function. Lower limbs are treated before upper limbs, except when procedures such as wrist fusion are needed before lower limb surgery to allow mobilization with crutches.

Before surgery, consider the C-spine and temporo-mandibular joint (may make intubation difficult), whether disease-modifying drugs should be stopped to improve wound healing and reduce risk of infection, and potential drug interactions with anaesthetic agents.

Scleroderma, CREST syndrome, systemic sclerosis

Definition
A connective tissue disease which causes damage to small blood vessels and fibrosis of skin and internal organs. Scleroderma refers to the thickened skin characteristic of the disease.

Incidence
- 2/100 000 per year.
- Female-to-male ratio 4:1; increased in women of child-bearing age.
- Slightly more common and more severe in African Americans than in Caucasians.
- Occurs worldwide.
- Peak onset 30–60 years of age.

Aetiology
- Thought to be environmental and genetic.
- Organic chemicals, epoxy resins, toxic oil, silica, foam insulation, and some drugs have been implicated.
- May be related to HLA type.
- There is no evidence that silicone breast implants cause scleroderma.

Classification
- Systemic sclerosis: thickened skin with internal organ involvement.
- Limited cutaneous scleroderma (CREST): calcinosis, Raynaud's phenomenon, oesophagitis, sclerodactyly, telangiectasia. Affects skin of hands, face, and feet only. Internal organs involved late.
- Diffuse cutaneous scleroderma: diffuse skin involvement with early internal organ involvement.
- Scleroderma sine scleroderma: internal organs affected; may have Raynaud's phenomenon; no skin changes.

Pathogenesis
Thought to be due to autoimmune activation of fibroblasts with excessive connective tissue deposition.

Clinical features
- Skin: thickened, tight, and shiny; hypo- or hyperpigmentation; telangiectasia.
- Hands: Raynaud's phenomenon; calcium deposits in finger pulps; ulceration; resorption of distal phalangeal tufts.
- Gastrointestinal: microstomia; dry mouth (sicca syndrome); reflux oesophagitis; bowel hypomotility; anal sphincter incompetence.
- Respiratory: pulmonary fibrosis; pulmonary hypertension.
- Cardiac: pericardial effusion; myocardial fibrosis and myocarditis causing heart failure and arrhythmias.

- Renal: renal failure; sudden-onset malignant arterial hypertension; microangiopathic haemolytic anaemia.
- Patients may be impotent, develop trigeminal neuralgia, or suffer hypothyroidism.

Investigations
- Antinuclear antibodies, topoisomerase I, anticentromere antibodies, fibrillarin antibodies, anti-ThRNP and anti-PM-Scl may be present and predict which type of scleroderma the patient has (and therefore likelihood of internal organ involvement).
- Doppler echocardiography, pulmonary function tests, and renal function (creatinine, urine microscopy, and creatinine clearance) are monitored with frequency depending on the type of disease.
- Nailfold microscopy in patients with Raynaud's phenomenon may reveal a row of capillary loops at the nailfold which predict subsequent systemic sclerosis.

Management
Medical
- Skin care: emollients; protect from trauma; hand and foot warmers.
- Arthralgia: aspirin; NSAIDs.
- Skin thickening: D-penicillamine, methotrexate; interferon gamma, cyclophosphamide.
- Heartburn and abdominal pain: antacids, H2 blockers, proton pump inhibitors, prokinetic agents, octreotide, laxatives.
- Raynaud's phenomenon: calcium-channel blockers; GTN patches; SSRIs; prostacyclin infusions.
- Hypertension and renal disease: ACE inhibitors.

Surgical
- Skin ulcers may need debridement or terminalization of the digit.
- Digital artery or lumbar sympathectomy for Raynaud's phenomenon.
- Calcinosis may need excising.

Osteoarthritis

Definition
Disease of synovial joints characterized by focal loss of hyaline cartilage and increase in marginal and subchondral bone.

Incidence
10% of adults over 60 have symptomatic OA. Most people over 70 have radiological evidence of OA.

Aetiology
- Age: reflects the time taken for OA to develop.
- Obesity.
- Genetic: tends to run in families; concordance of generalized OA in monozygotic twins.
- Sex: site of OA differs, being more common in knees and hands in females, developing after menopause. Equal sex incidence for hip OA.
- Inflammatory or infective arthritis.
- Trauma: fracture, soft tissue injury, or repetitive trauma.
- Developmental deformity: mainly hip disease (DDH, Perthes disease, slipped upper femoral epiphysis).
- Metabolic: Paget's disease, ochronosis, haemochromatosis, Wilson's disease.
- Endocrine: acromegaly, diabetes.

Classification
- Primary: no obvious cause.
- Secondary: following a demonstrable abnormality.

Pathogenesis
Poorly understood, but thought to be due to disparity between stress applied to cartilage and ability of cartilage to withstand stress. Initially, cartilage metabolism is altered so that the balance of proteases and protease inhibitors moves to favour breakdown of cartilage. Fibrillation (erosion of the cartilage surface) follows. Chronic inflammation develops, further destroying cartilage. Bony overgrowth appears to be an attempt to stabilize the joint. The pain probably relates to capsular fibrosis, pressure on underlying bone, and spasm of muscles around the joint, as the cartilage and synovium themselves have no nerve supply.

Clinical features
Usually presents after middle age, although may present earlier if secondary to joint disorder or injury. Pain, swelling, stiffness, and weakness are the main complaints. Pain is worse after activity; stiffness is worse after rest. Examination reveals tender joints, effusions, bony swelling due to osteophytes, reduced ROM and crepitus. Muscle wasting is a feature of long-standing OA. Affects weight-bearing joints and the hand.

Typical changes in the hand are:
- Pattern of disease, involving DIPJs and base of thumb.
- Heberden's nodes—bony swelling of DIPJs.
- Bouchard's nodes—bony swelling of PIPJs.

Investigations

X-rays typically show:
- Narrowed joint space.
- Subarticular sclerosis.
- Bone cysts.
- Periarticular osteophytes.

Management

Medical

Aims to relieve pain, reduce the load on the joint, and improve mobility.
- Splints and modification of activities rest affected joints.
- Physiotherapy can improve ROM and power.
- NSAIDs or COX-2 inhibitors.
- Intra-articular steroid injections.

Surgical

Usually for pain relief. Options include:
- Osteotomy to realign joints.
- Ligament reconstruction.
- Arthroplasty—excision, interposition or replacement.
- Arthrodesis: most useful procedure for the DIPJ, reducing pain and instability.
- Options for thumb CMCJ:
  - Osteotomy of metacarpal.
  - Ligament reconstruction.
  - Trapeziumectomy—the defect can be filled with FCR or palmaris longus tendon; a spacer device, or left free.
  - Joint replacement.

Gout

Definition
An inflammatory arthropathy due to deposition of monosodium urate monohydrate (MUM) crystals.

Incidence
1%; male-to-female ratio 10:1.

Aetiology
Hyperuricaemia due to either under-excretion or over-production of uric acid. However, most people with hyperuricaemia do not have gout, and patients with gout may not have hyperuricaemia at presentation. Under-excretors have reduced ability to clear urate from the kidneys. Rarely, over-producers have an inherited defect in purine metabolism, but in most the cause is unclear. Severity of disease depends on level of serum uric acid. Women have a lower incidence and the disease presents later because of the protective effect of oestrogens, which have a mild uricosuric effect.

Classification
- Primary: mostly men; often give family history.
- Secondary: due to diuretic drugs, cyclosporin, alcohol abuse, renal insufficiency, lead poisoning, and hypothyroidism. Equal sex prevalence.

Pathogenesis
MUM crystals are gradually deposited in and around around synovial joints. The crystal's surface, exposed because of alterations in uric acid levels, activates inflammatory pathways. Chronic inflammation produces joint damage in long-standing gout.

Clinical features
Usually presents at age 30–60 years with acute synovitis. A slowly progressive arthropathy or tophi may develop without an acute attack. Tophaceous deposits can develop in joints already affected by OA, e.g. in Heberden's nodes. The disease progresses through four phases:
- Asymptomatic hyperuricaemia, for 10–20 years.
- Acute attack: involves first MTPJ (podagra) in 50% of first attacks and 70% of all attacks. Mild irritation rapidly progresses to a hot, red, swollen, and extremely tender joint. May have fever and malaise. Resolves over 2 weeks.
- Intercritical periods: asymptomatic periods. In most cases, the next attack occurs within a year, and they gradually increase in frequency and severity.
- Chronic tophaceous gout: large crystal deposits produce firm chalky nodules around joints, tendons, bursae, and the helix of the ear (rarely, eye, eyelids, tongue, larynx, and heart). Characteristically asymmetrical. May ulcerate and discharge chalky contents with pus, despite lack of infection. If untreated, progresses to joint destruction causing pain, crepitus, reduced motion, and joint deformities, especially of MTPJs, mid-foot, small finger joints, and wrists.

Gout is commonly associated with kidney stones. It is also associated with, but does not cause, hypertension, diabetes, hyperlipidaemia, and coronary atherosclerosis.

Investigations
- Serum urate: joint aspirates yield crystals which are negatively birefringent on compensated polarized light microscopy. X-ray changes depend on the stage of the disease:
  - Acute attack: soft tissue swelling (rarely with juxta-articular osteopenia).
  - Chronic disease: narrowed joint space, sclerosis, cysts, and osteophytes. Similar to OA.
  - Gouty erosions: uncommon but specific to gout, these are asymmetric, eccentric, para-articular 'punched out' bone defects; they have well-defined sclerotic margins, and contain overhanging hooks of bone.
  - Tophi may have patchy calcification.

Management
Medical
- Drug treatment may be avoided by weight loss, reducing alcohol intake, and stopping diuretics.
- High-dose NSAIDs reduce pain and inflammation during the acute phase. If hypo-uricaemic drugs are started, they will prolong the attack.
- Oral colchicine is usually avoided because of its side effects: nausea, diarrhoea, and abdominal cramps.
- Allopurinol reduces uric acid synthesis by inhibiting xanthine oxidase.
- Uricosuric drugs (e.g. probenecid) prevent renal tubular resorption of urate, but are contraindicated in renal impairment.

Surgical
Other than debridement of discharging or painful tophi, surgery follows similar principles to treatment of OA.

Differential diagnoses
A wide variety of crystals may be deposited in or around joints. Calcium pyrophosphate causes pseudo-gout. Presents in sixties and seventies, and is more common in females. Often associated with OA. May be entirely asymptomatic, or present as acute synovitis or chronic arthritis. The crystals are positively birefringent on light microscopy. Treated with joint aspiration, steroid injections, NSAIDs, or colchicine.

Chapter 19

Miscellaneous disorders

Pressure sores *644*
Complex regional pain syndrome *647*
Hidradenitis *649*
Hyperhidrosis *651*
Gender reassignment *653*

Pressure sores

Definition
Tissue loss resulting from pressure. Note that a decubitus ulcer is one resulting from lying down (from the Latin *decumbere*). Therefore not all pressure sores are decubitus ulcers.

Incidence
Between 3% and 10% of hospitalized patients have a pressure sore and 2.7% will develop one during their stay. Prevalence in nursing home patients is between 3% and 33%. Between 25% and 85% of young patients with spinal injuries will develop a pressure sore; 7–8% die as a direct result of a pressure sore.

Aetiology
- Intrinsic factors: see Waterlow assessment.
- Age: two-thirds of pressure sores in hospital are in the over-seventies. Skin changes in the elderly increase susceptibility to shear and reduced blood flow.
- Reduced mobility: risk increases as mobility decreases; quadriplegics have higher risk than paraplegics.
- Mental state.
- Reduced sensation due to lack of protective feedback.
- Malnutrition: low serum total proteins, albumin, haemoglobin, and lymphocyte count are associated with higher rates of pressure sore formation, although the evidence for healing when these are corrected is less clear.
- Over- or underweight.
- Other predisposing illness.
- Extrinsic factors:
  - Pressure. Arterial capillary pressure is 32 mmHg; venous capillary closing pressure is 8–12 mmHg. Animal models show that constant pressure for over 2 hr produces irreversible skin changes.
  - Shear: may be more important in closing capillaries than direct pressure.
  - Friction.

Classification of pressure sore (National Pressure Ulcer Advisory Panel)
- Stage I: non-blanching erythema of intact skin.
- Stage II: partial thickness epidermal or dermal loss, presenting as abrasion, blister, or shallow crater.
- Stage III: full-thickness damage or necrosis down to, but not through, underlying fascia; may have undermined adjacent tissue to produce a crater.
- Stage IV: full-thickness damage or necrosis involving underlying muscle, bone, tendon, or joint, including osteomyelitis or septic arthritis.

Pathogenesis
The pressure ischaemia theory states that pressure sores are caused by continued pressure sufficient to prevent blood flow to soft tissues. In a supine patient, pressure is greatest over the sacrum, heel, and occiput at 40–60 mmHg; when prone, chest and knees are under greatest pressure at 50 mmHg; when sitting, the ischial tuberosities are exposed to 100 mmHg (Lindan et al. 1965). Muscle appears to be more susceptible to pressure than skin and fascia, possibly because of its higher metabolic requirements. Epidermis, which can tolerate long periods of low oxygenation, shows signs of pressure late.

Investigations
- Hb and serum albumin to check nutritional state.
- ESR and WCC if raised may indicate osteomyelitis.
- X-ray, bone scan, MRI, and bone biopsy if osteomyelitis is suspected.

Management
Medical
- Prevention is key. Prophylactic measures should allow all stage I and II ulcers to heal, and many stage III or IV ulcers:
- Regular pressure relief, every 2 hr when supine or every 15 min when seated, until tolerance is demonstrated (by lack of redness of skin after longer periods of pressure).
- Mattress or cushion to minimize pressure. Examples include air-filled alternating-pressure mattress, sponge-rubber egg-crate mattress, silicone gel or water mattress, air flotation mattress; Roho wheelchair cushion.
- Keep skin clean and dry. Consider urinary catheter or faecal diversion.
- Optimize nutrition.
- Minimize sedation.
- Physiotherapy to improve mobility and posture, and to relieve contractures.
- Treat spasticity with baclofen or diazepam.
- Treat infection with debridement. Use antibiotics for surrounding cellulitis or sepsis, but also debride the wound.
- Stage III and IV ulcers may require debridement, but this can be done without surgery either by dressings or with sharp debridement on the ward.

Surgical
- Patient selection is important to avoid failure of healing. Intrinsic risk factors must be optimal. Patients must be able and prepared to cooperate with pressure area care.
- Debride ulcer cavity using bursectomy method: the cavity is packed with methylene-blue-soaked gauze or sponge and excised as a tumour. Residual blue areas indicate inadequate excision.

- Infected joints or bony prominences should be debrided to bleeding bone. This may require joint disarticulation, e.g. Girdlestone arthroplasty for infected hip. Ischial tuberosities should not be over-excised, as this puts increased pressure on the opposite ischial tuberosity. If both are excised, perineal pressure sores result.
- Direct closure is rarely an option because of tension on the suture line. Keep suture lines away from the pressure area.
- Pad bone stumps and fill cavities with flaps containing muscle or fascia.
- Choose flaps which can be re-advanced if ulceration recurs, and which do not violate the territory of salvage flaps.
- If it is possible to bring in sensate skin, this may reduce re-ulceration.
- Commonly used reconstructive options for different sites include:
  - Ischial sore: gluteal thigh fascio-cutaneous flap (based on inferior gluteal artery), hamstring muscle flap, posterior thigh skin flap or skin plus biceps femoris, TFL flap, inferior gluteus maximus flap.
  - Sacral sore: rotation or V–Y advancement of gluteal skin, or gluteus maximus musculo-cutaneous flap. Bilateral flaps may be needed.
  - Trochanteric sore: TFL flap; vastus lateralis flap; anterior thigh flap.
- Total thigh flaps and hemicorporectomy are used as a last resort in patients with uncontrollable infection with no other reconstructive options. Both have a high morbidity.

Post-operative care
- Suction drainage of the wound.
- Pressure-relieving mattress.
- Gradual progression to sitting, with careful observation of pressure areas.

Complications
- Surgery:
  - Haematoma.
  - Seroma.
  - Infection.
  - Wound dehiscence; if this fails to heal within a week or so, suspect inadequate debridement.
  - Recurrence: up to 80% in paraplegics.
- Chronic pressure sores:
  - Urethral or bowel fistulae.
  - Malignant degeneration (Marjolin's ulcer).
  - Death.

Contentious issues

Is a fascial flap more resistant to pressure than a muscle flap? Although muscle flaps have a theoretical increased risk of ischaemic necrosis over fascial flaps, they are a useful space-filler, provide well-vascularized tissue, and pad the area.

Reference
Lindan et. al. (1965). *Arch Phys Med Rehab* **46**:378–85.

Complex regional pain syndrome

Also known as causalgia, Sudek's atrophy, reflex sympathetic dystrophy (RSD), sympathetically maintained pain, CRPS.

Definition
A term describing a variety of painful conditions following injury or operation, which exceed in both magnitude and duration the expected clinical course of the inciting event. There is a predominance of abnormal findings distal to the injury, often resulting in significant impairment of motor function and showing variable progression over time.

Has previously had multiple synonyms but the current term CRPS arose from a consensus workshop held in 1993.

Incidence
- Common, but often mild.
- More common in anxious and neurotic patients.

Classification
- CRPS type 1 (RSD).
- CRPS type 2 (causalgia).

In both types there is an initiating noxious stimulus (though this may be very mild): in type 1 the noxious stimulus is not clearly a nerve injury, whereas in type 2 a nerve injury can be clearly identified. In both types this is accompanied by spontaneous pain or allodynia/hyperalgesia which need not be limited to the territory of a single peripheral nerve, and is disproportionate to the inciting event. There is or has been evidence of oedema and skin blood flow abnormality, or abnormal sudomotor activity (increased or decreased sweating/hair growth/skin markings) in the region of the pain since the inciting event.

This diagnosis is excluded by the existence of conditions that would otherwise account for the degree of pain and dysfunction.

Management
- Early recognition is very important.
- CRPS is more responsive to treatment in the early stages.
- Remove the noxious stimulus. This may mean exploration and nerve repair or grafting or neuroma transposition.
- Analgesia.
- Reassurance and patient education.

Specific options
- Pharmacological:
  - Antidepressants (amitriptyline).
  - Gabapentin (Neurontin).
  - Sympatholytic drugs (alpha adrenergic blockers (e.g. prazosin).
  - Somatic nerve blocks.
  - Stellate ganglion blocks.
  - Corticosteroids.
  - NSAIDS.
  - Calcitonin sprays.

- Physiotherapy.
- Psychological support.
- Surgery:
  - Removal of stenosis of subclavian vein (Albrecht Wilhelm).
  - Implantation of electrodes for electrical stimulation (Cooney).

Physiotherapy
Treatment priorities are:
- Stop pain and oedema.
- Maintain or gain mobility.
- Rebuild strength.
- Restore function.

Patients need to know that some pain is to be expected in the early treatment stages but will diminish with perseverance. TENS, analgesia, and physical treatment (hot/cold packs) may help.

Allodynia or hyperalgesia can be managed with contact adhesive dressings or gloves. Oedema may respond to compression gloves, elevation and movement.

Mobility and range of motion are best treated by functional exercises such as Kirk Watson's stress-loading programme with simple activities like scrubbing, polishing, and carrying which can be adapted for even the most severe cases so that real functional activity can be started immediately.

The author's personal preference for treatment is to eradicate the stimulus, educate and reassure, and then to commence the patient on NSAID, gabapentin, and amitriptyline (at night). Refer for intensive physiotherapy to use the affected part as much as possible.

Hidradenitis

Definition
A chronic inflammatory condition of follicular epithelium within apocrine-gland-bearing skin resulting in abscess and sinus formation.

Incidence
- 4%, 1/300.
- Female-to-male ratio 3:1.
- Peak prevalence in twenties and thirties.

Aetiology
Exact aetiology unclear. Many factors have been indicated:
- Deodorants.
- Depilatory products and shaving.
- Obesity probably exacerbates the condition in those who have a propensity by increasing shearing forces.
- Androgenic affects have been suggested, but androgens have been shown to have little effect on apocrine, unlike sebaceous glands.
- Keratin hydration favours occlusion and this is more likely in areas of increased sweating such as groins and axillae.
- Smoking exacerbates the problems associated with hidradenitis by impairing healing.
- A genetic link has been proposed which would be autosomal dominant but with a variable penetrance.

Classification
According to the area of body affected and:
- Type 1: solitary or multiple, isolated abscess formation without sinus formation.
- Type 2: recurrent abscesses, single or multiple widely separated lesions, sinus tract formation, and cicatrization.
- Type 3: diffuse or broad involvement, multiple interconnected sinus tracts and abscesses.

Pathogenesis
Two types of sweat glands, eccrine (salt) and apocrine (fat, cholesterol, and salt). Apocrine found in axilla, groin, peri-areolar, perianal.
The primary event appears to be:
- Occlusion of apocrine ducts draining into hair follicles by a keratinized stratified squamous epithelium plug.

This in turn leads to:
- Apocrinitis and subsequent local inflammatory response which is worsened by dilatation.
- Rupture of apocrine glands due to the occlusion. The spilled contents, including keratin and bacteria, account for the odorous discharge associated with this condition and form a vigorous chemotactic stimulus for an inflammatory cellular infiltrate consisting of neutrophils, lymphocytes, and histiocytes.

- Abscess formation occurs which worsens local tissue destruction and leads to the formation of sinuses and progression to a chronic state. This chronic state demonstrates dermal inflammatory cells, giant cells, sinus tracts, subcutaneous abscesses, and fibrosis.

Clinical features
Pain, malodorous discharge, abscesses, and sinuses affecting one or more areas of the body including groin, axillae, perineum, perianal, sub-mammary, pubis, scrotum, labia, periumbilical, external ear canal, and eyelids.

Investigations
Clinical diagnosis, no specific investigation is warranted.

Management
Medical
- General: weight loss; stop smoking, loose-fitting clothing which limits shear.
- Antibiotics: may be helpful in treating super-added infection and prevention of secondary infection by long-term use (clindamycin 300 mg twice daily). Does not treat primary problem of occlusion; cannot treat sinuses.
- Anti-androgens (cyproterone acetate): case reports of short-term remission. However, high side-effect profile (e.g. hair growth and fetal androgenization).
- Retinoids have also been used with mixed success.
- Radiotherapy: early success with significant symptom relief but not widely investigated.

Surgical
Mainstay of treatment of established disease; only treatment likely to have effect after sinus formation has occurred.
- Incision and drainage of abscess for symptomatic relief.
- Laying open sinus tracts.
- Tumour style clear margin excision of the affected area with primary closure (primary closure is associated with increased recurrence rate), dressings and secondary intention healing, skin grafting, or local flap cover. With regard to recurrence rate there is no clear benefit of one technique over another, cf. primary closure.
- Laser treatment: CO_2 laser ablation and secondary intention healing. Early stages of assessment; proponents claim shorter healing times with a quicker return to work and less pain and scarring.

Hidradenitis suppurativa is not primarily an infective condition but rather one of apocrine gland occlusion leading to local inflammation and subsequent abscess formation. Non-surgical treatment is appropriate to limit disease progression and possibly lessen recurrence but will not address established disease.

Hyperhidrosis

Definition
Sweating in excess of the body's homeostatic requirements, causing discomfort and social embarrassment. Bromidrosis is body odour caused by the bacterial degradation of apocrine sweat gland secretion.

Aetiology
The cause of primary hyperhidrosis, which occurs in isolation, is unknown. Secondary hyperhidrosis occurs because of an underlying organic cause, e.g. endocrine disorders (hyperthyroidism, diabetes, obesity, menopausal change), malignancy, trauma, chronic infection, psychiatric disorders, iatrogenic causes, nerve injury, and medication (gonadorelin analogues, tricyclic antidepressants).

Incidence
Mild hyperhidrosis is common; severe hyperhidrosis affects 1% of the population. Primary hyperhidrosis has a familial tendency. It presents in childhood or adolescence and may last for life.

Clinical features
The symptoms of hyperhidrosis affect the palms, axillae, soles, face, neck, and torso in decreasing frequency. Sweating may be episodic, continuous, or seasonal, and can be precipitated by anxiety. In contrast, secondary hyperhidrosis induces generalized sweating, apart from localized hyperhidrosis related to local trauma or nerve injury.

Investigations
Diagnosis is based on history and visible signs of excessive sweating. Gravimetric sweat tests can provide an objective parameter of severity before treatment; the iodine starch test charts the area for treatment.

Management and complications
Most treatments are directed locally (medical/surgical); systemic treatments are reserved for patients with more generalized symptoms. Treatment for secondary hyperhidrosis is directed at the underlying cause.

Non-surgical
- Antiperspirants: aluminium-based compounds (e.g. Driclor®) which cause sweat to thicken and clump, plugging the pores. Regular reapplications are needed as the sweat plugs dissolve. Mostly used for axillary symptoms. Use limited by rash, stinging sensation, irritation.
- Iontophoresis: Involves immersion of sweating area in a solution and use of low intensity DC electrical current to drive charged ions in the skin, temporarily disrupting function of sweat glands. Devices (e.g. Idrostar®) for home use are commercially available. Multiple weekly sessions needed; therefore it is time-consuming and inefficient. Mild irritation, which responds well to hydrocortisone, is commonly reported; otherwise safe. Not to be used in pregnancy or in presence of cardiac pacemaker or metal implants.

- Anticholinergic drugs: inhibit acetylcholine receptors on sweat glands, stopping sweat production. Limited by widespread cholinergic side-effects. Glycopyrolate (Robinul®) is available by private prescription.
- Alpha-adrenergic blocker drugs: alpha-blockers such as those used in the management of hypertension (prazosin) can effectively reduce the degree of sweating.
- Botulinum A toxin–haemagglutin complex: prevents acetylcholine release at the axonal synapse for 4–14 months (dose-dependent). Administered by multiple intradermal injections. Effective first-line treatment for axillary hyperhidrosis, which can be repeated. Antibody formation to toxin can limit long-term efficacy. Use in palmar hyperhidrosis is limited by toxin-induced local muscle group paralysis. Rash, burning sensation, and compensatory sweating are rare.

Surgical
- Excision of affected skin: wide elliptical excision of the apex of axilla is limited by poor cosmesis, abscess/sinus formation, and hypertrophic/constrictive scarring. Can overcome some of these by excision and local flap reconstruction.
- Local denervation of affected skin: excision of subcutaneous tissue or undermining of adjacent tissue in subdermal plane to denervate sweat glands through cruciate or two parallel incisions (Skoog procedure).
- Open surgical sympathectomy (cervical or lumbar): interrupts the sympathetic chain. Effective for palmar, axillary, and facial hyperhidrosis, but rarely used now because of the extensive and traumatic dissection required.
- Transthoracic endoscopic sympathectomy (TES): performed via one or two 10 and 5 mm chest portals through the ipsilateral hemithorax. Achieves satisfactory control of symptoms in 95%, 85%, and 75% of patients for palmar, facial, and axillary symptoms, respectively. Compensatory hyperhidrosis (trunk and groin) affects 50–70% of patients; up to 11% of patients regret the TES procedure. Rebound sweating (an unexplained temporary recurrence of sweating) affects up to 31% of patients; patients should be warned to avoid anxiety that procedure has failed. Other complications include pneumothorax (up to 2.3% requiring chest drainage), haemothorax, surgical emphysema (up to 2.7%), pleural effusion, atelectasis, Horner's syndrome, gustatory sweating, pleuritic chest pain, intercosto-brachial neuralgia, long thoracic and thoracodorsal nerve injury, and recurrence of sweating. Deaths have followed massive intrathoracic haemorrhage from trocar insertion, and severe and unrecognized hypoxia due to anaesthesia. Contraindicated in pulmonary disease and keloid scarring.

Gender reassignment

Definition
Transsexualism is the desire to live and be accepted as a member of the opposite sex, usually with the wish to make the body as similar as possible to the preferred sex with hormone treatment and surgery. This identity has to be present for at least 2 years; the disorder is not due to an underlying mental disorder or chromosome abnormality.

Incidence
1/30 000 males and 1/100 000 adult females seek gender reassignment surgery; the prevalence of transsexualism is higher at 1/11 900 males and 1/10 400 females in one study.

Management
A combination of hormones, real-life experience, and surgery, not necessarily in that order.

Medical
- Hormone treatment is usually given after real-life experience as the opposite sex for 3 months, or psychotherapy for 3 months.
- Females are given testosterone.
- Males are given a combination of oestrogen, progesterone, and anti-androgens.
- Effects of treatment may increase over 2 years.
- Males may find that breast enlargement is not reversible.
- Females may find deepened voice, clitoral enlargement, breast atrophy, increased facial and body hair, and male pattern baldness are not reversible.
- Side effects in males include increased risk of venous thrombosis, benign pituitary prolactinomas, infertility, weight gain, emotional lability, liver disease, gallstones, somnolence, hypertension, and diabetes.
- Side effects in females include infertility, acne, emotional lability, increased sexual desire, increased risk of cardiovascular disease, and liver disease including malignancy.

Surgical
Breast surgery
- Real-life experience for 3 months and a psychiatric review are advised before breast surgery.
- For males, 18 months of hormone therapy is also advised, as breast enlargement may be adequate without surgery.
- Females may require mastectomy, skin excision, nipple and areolar reduction, and repositioning of the NAC.

Genital surgery
- Hormone therapy for 12 months, real-life experience for 12 months, and two psychiatric reviews are advised.
- Males may have orchidectomy, penectomy and vaginoplasty.

- The neovagina is usually created from inversion of the penile shaft skin, and placed posterior to the prostate; skin grafts or pedicled colon may also be used.
- Part of the glans may be preserved pedicled on its neurovascular supply to form a clitoris.
- Labia minora are formed from penile or prepucial skin; labia majora from scrotal skin.
- Females may have hysterectomy, salpingo-oophorectomy, vaginectomy, metaidoioplasty, scrotoplasty, urethroplasty, testicular prostheses, and phalloplasty.
- Vaginal mucosa may be used to lengthen the urethra; bladder and buccal mucosal grafts are alternatives.
- Metaidoioplasty involves release of the clitoris to create a neoglans with a skin flap from the labia minora to cover the shaft. This produces a sensate microphallus which is not usually large enough for sexual penetration.
- Phalloplasty involves free tissue transfer (usually radial forearm flap) designed so that a neo-urethra is formed from one side of the flap, and the neophallus is rolled around it. Erogenous sensation is achieved by nerve anastomoses. Erectile function may be achieved at a second procedure with an implanted prosthesis.
- A neo-scrotum may be fashioned from the labia majora and testicular implants.

Adjunctive procedures

In female to male transsexuals these include liposuction of hips, thighs and buttocks; rhinoplasty; chin and jaw augmentation; and calf or pectoral implants.

In male to female patients, procedures include thyroid cartilage reduction; liposuction of the waist; rhinoplasty; genioplasty; jaw reduction; face lift; blepharoplasty; scalp advancement; brow elevation; contouring of orbital rim; cheek augmentation and lip augmentation.

Post-operative care
- Long term follow-up improves outcomes.
- Patients taking hormones long term should be monitored for side effects.

Complications

Persistent regret is rare: <1% for female to male and 1–1.5% for male to female. The rate appears to be reducing, possibly because of improved psychological and surgical care.

Key reference

The Harry Benjamin International Gender Dysphoria Association produces a 'Standards of Care' document, which includes minimum eligibility criteria and readiness criteria used worldwide in advising people on gender reassignment treatment.

Chapter 20

Aesthetic

Aesthetic surgery 656
Assessment of a patient for aesthetic surgery 657
Facial ageing 660

Breast
Bra and breast sizing 661
Aesthetic breast surgery assessment 662
Breast reduction surgery 664
Breast augmentation 670
Breast ptosis 674
Inverted nipples 677
Tuberous breast 678
Gynaecomastia 679

Skin
Non-surgical aesthetic techniques 682
Skin-lightening methods 685

Facial
Blepharoplasty 686
Brow lift 692
Rhinoplasty 694
Submucous resection 698
Facelift 700
Augmentation of the facial skeleton 704
Genioplasty 706

Body contouring
Body contouring 709
Arm reduction 711
Abdominoplasty 713
Thigh and buttock contouring 717
Medial thigh lift 719
Calf augmentation 720
Liposuction 722

Aesthetic surgery

Also known as cosmetic surgery.

Definition
Plastic surgical procedures have long been classified into reconstructive and aesthetic (Greek *aesthetikos*, perceptible by the senses) procedures.

Procedures
Reconstructive procedures were considered to be those which attempted to return to normal what was abnormal as a result of birth defects, disease, trauma or following excisional surgery. Aesthetic procedures, on the other hand, were considered to be those that attempted to surpass the normal.

Pure aesthetic surgery can now be considered to be that dealing with the appearance rather than the mechanical function of a part of the body. This includes:
- Congenital abnormalities with cosmetic consequences only (correction of prominent ears, excision of accessory auricle).
- Cosmetic improvement of normal appearance (breast augmentation).
- Correction of deformity secondary to trauma or previous procedures (secondary rhinoplasty, scar revision).
- Rejuvenation after the effects of actinic damage and the ageing process (rhytidectomy).
- Removal of excess fat (liposuction).
- Removal of excess skin (abdominoplasty, mastopexy).

All plastic surgery procedures contain elements of aesthetic and functional improvement. The relative ratios of these elements determine the perception of the procedure as aesthetic. Procedures with a predominantly aesthetic benefit are considered aesthetic. They may still have considerable psychological and other functional benefits but these may be difficult to measure and quantify, and hence may be under-appreciated.

Assessment of a patient for aesthetic surgery

Introduction
The initial consultation should assess both the physical and psychological suitability of a patient for aesthetic surgery. Documentation should be meticulous.

The varied responsibilities of the aesthetic surgeon include: physician, technician, artist, psychologist, and counsellor.

Psychological benefits of aesthetic surgery
It is well recognized that appropriately selected patients can gain significant psychological benefit from aesthetic surgery. Published evidence demonstrates improved body image, reduction of self-consciousness, less avoidance of exposure during sexual activity, and improvement of patient's psychosocial function. However, poorly selected patients will not be satisfied and operating on such patients will harm both the patient and the surgeon!

History
- Listen closely to the patient; show insight and empathy for their concerns. Establish a good rapport and the trust of the patient.
- Observe mannerisms and non-verbal communication, such as eye contact.
- The patient should be able to clearly delineate their perceived aesthetic concern.
- Determine the true motives for the surgery. Be wary when the reasons are to improve personal or social relationships.
- Are the expectations reasonable? Note in particular expectations that are emotional rather than physical.
- Has the patient had any previous aesthetic procedures. How many consultations have they had for this particular concern?
- Does the patient have a history of any psychiatric conditions.
- Take a full medical history to determine fitness for surgery.

Examination
- Is the problem perceived by the patient apparent and correctable?
- Is there any other associated finding that has bearing on the index condition and also needs to be addressed as part of the treatment?
- Undertake a full examination to determine their fitness for surgery.

Discussion
Discuss the findings of the history and examination. Talk about the complications from the procedure, the limitations and any areas of uncertainty.

Psychological assessment
- Does the patient have a realistic expectation of what can be achieved?
- Does the patient have a personality disorder? Manipulative, demanding, impulsive, flighty, reactive, depressed, helpless, obsessive, talk forever, never-ending questions. These patients have inadequate personalities and may disguise the real reason for surgery. Personality disorders cannot be corrected with surgery. The risk of litigation is higher in such patients.
- Is there any history of a psychotic disorder e.g schizophrenia? Confused thoughts, emotionally flat, unable to establish rapport, no sense of humour. Even surgery which would be entirely appropriate in others should be undertaken with great caution in such individuals. Suspiciousness of others, feelings of persecution, excessive concern with self. These patients require full psychiatric assessment before surgery.
- Is the patient a surgery addict or suffering from dysmorphophobia. This is a condition characterized by an unreasonable intense dislike against one's own bodily parts or features. They have often had repeated procedures by different surgeons. Avoid these patients. Refer them for psychiatric assessment.
- Is the patient deceptive? Do the findings bear no resemblance to the extent of their concerns? Falsify and exaggerate symptoms for pecuniary gain from insurance companies or by faking post-operative symptoms to avoid payment.
- Note these patients may display a lack of cooperation with an examination and inconsistency between symptoms and examination findings.
- Is the patient neurotic? Often this is anxiety and with effective counselling surgery can be successful in these patients.

Physical assessment
Is the patient fit enough to undergo the procedure? If not can they be optimized with further medical input?

Surgeon assessment
Do you have the experience and expertise to carry out the required procedure in keeping with accepted success rates?

Options after consultation
Select for procedure. Defer pending further investigation and assessment. Refer for a second opinion or to another surgeon for treatment. Reject.

Second consultation
This takes place after an adequate gap (the cooling-off period). Ensure that the patient is well informed and all questions are answered. Take photographs and ensure that all consultations are meticulously documented.

Post-operative disappointment
- Is there just cause for disappointment? If so ensure that this is rectified at no cost to the patient.
- Complications often surprise patients even if they have been well counselled.
- Despite the surgeon's best attempts at counselling and consent, some patients will be unjustifiably dissatisfied.
- Listen long and carefully to such patients and show concern. Clearly delineate their exact concern. Do not be defensive, but empathetic. A significant proportion of such patients have become accustomed to their new body shape and will have forgotten their pre-existing complaint. Discussion with pre-operative photos will often be all that is required to reassure them.
- Secondary procedures must be given the same attention with regard to counselling and consent as the initial surgery. The trust between patient and surgeon must remain. Good colleagues who are able to offer a second opinion should be consulted in certain cases.
- By demonstrating understanding and with explanation and regular review, patients' dissatisfaction as a result of unrealistic expectations usually resolves in time.

Litigation
- Risk of litigation is reduced by careful patient selection.
- Well-selected patients are not litigious prior to their surgery but become so as result of unfulfilled expectations.
- Reject or refer to others for a second opinion those with unrealistic expectations/psychological problems/poor rapport.
- Patients must be well informed pre-operatively.
- Sometimes litigation is justified. In such cases, it exposes poor quality surgery and may result in and improvement in standards.
- Where it is unjustified:
  - Do not take criticism to heart.
  - Do not argue with the patient.
  - Try to understand the patient, however much you may disagree.
  - Try to be understood by patient as far as this is possible.
  - Rely on the judicial process.

Summary
- Prevent future problems by listening, counselling, and establishing good rapport.
- Recognize those patients who are psychologically unfit for surgery.
- Remember that the surgeon has no obligation to operate.
- In selected patients, psychological symptoms, well managed, do not necessarily imply poor psychological prognosis.
- Well-selected patients who are well informed and with a good surgical result will enjoy great psychological benefit from aesthetic surgery.

Facial ageing

Aetiology

Mechanical
Gravity acts on facial features, resulting in chin and brow ptosis, sagging of the cheek and the jawline forming jowls, and deepening of the naso-labial folds and the orbital sockets.

Physiological
The ageing process of the skin and subcutaneous tissue (intrinsic) and the results of chronic actinic damage (extrinsic) result in a generalized lack of tone, wrinkling, and irregularities in pigmentation.

Microscopic changes
These consist of changes in the epidermis, the dermo-epidermal junction, and the dermis:
- Epidermal dysplasia (sun damage—extrinsic).
- Flattening of the dermo-epidermal junction (ageing—intrinsic).
- Reduced number of Langerhans cells (ageing—intrinsic).
- Dermal elastosis (sun damage—extrinsic).
- Decrease in the amount of glycosaminoglycan: ground substance (ageing—intrinsic) decrease in the amount of collagen, especially type 3 (ageing—intrinsic).

These cellular changes result in the gross appearances described earlier which take the following form:
- Thinning of the skin.
- Decreased resistance to shearing forces.
- Decreased elasticity.
- Increased susceptibility to ultraviolet radiation damage.
- Increased susceptibility to developing skin cancers.
- Decreased ability to regenerate/repair damaged cutaneous structures.

Genetic
Certain syndromes can cause early ageing, e.g. cutis laxa, pseudoxanthoma elasticum, Ehlers–Danlos syndrome, progeria.

Management
The mechanical effects can be corrected by surgical procedures (facelift, blepharoplasty, brow lift, etc.), whereas the intrinsic effects of sun damage and physiological ageing are best dealt with by resurfacing techniques (peels, dermabrasion, laser). Some genetic conditions can be improved with surgery (cutis laxa, pseudoxanthoma), but surgery should not be contemplated in others (Ehlers–Danlos syndrome, progeria).

Bra and breast sizing

Bra sizes are nominated as a number and a cup size, e.g. 32B, 34C. The number corresponds to the chest circumference in inches measured at the level of the infra-mammary fold.

The cup size is not an absolute measure but is proportional to the chest circumference. It is based on the difference in circumference around the chest and breasts at nipple level and the chest circumference, in increments of 1 inch or 2 cm. For example, if the chest circumference is 32 inches and the chest/breast circumference is 34 inches, the bra size would be 32B, and if the chest circumference was 32 inches but the chest/breast circumference was 38 inches, the bra size would be 32F. An AA cup indicates no difference or less than 1 inch difference between chest/breast measurement and infra-mammary chest circumference.

There are enormous differences in cup size notation between manufacturers. This is especially true in sizes above D in the USA, UK, Australia, and New Zealand. In general, sizes between AA and DD are fairly standard, but once above this there is little or no coherence. Some manufacturers use size DD but then continue with E, F, G, H, I, J, etc. Others use DDD to represent an E, and some go on to use E, EE, F, FF, G, GG, H, HH, etc.

European manufacturers use chest circumference in centimetres and the cup size increments in 2 cm steps. They also tend to use a standard AA, A, B, C, D, E, F, G, H scale, thus avoiding the DD, DDD, EE confusion. Apart from the differences in cup size notation, there is another major possible difference in international bra sizes: US standard cup sizes tend to be calculated on half-inch increments, whereas UK manufacturers tend to use one inch increments. However, to confuse the issue further, some US manufacturers use one inch increments.

Breast volume

The volume of breast in each cup size varies with chest circumference, but a 32 inch chest has a cup volume of approximately 100 g/cup increment. A 34 inch chest has a volume of approximately 120–140 gm/cup increment. A 36 inch chest has an increment of 180 g/cup and a 38 inch chest has an increment of 200 g/cup.

These volume approximations may help in implant sizing, although alternative techniques can also help such as asking the patient to borrow a bra of the size they would like to be (ensure that it is a full cup bra and not a balcony bra!) and fill the cup with a plastic bag with water in it. They can adjust the volume of water until they are happy with the size, and then measure and record the volume. Alternatively, some institutions have sizers that their patients can try in their bras under tight T shirts or jumpers. Implant sizing can also be based on chest wall dimensions such as height and width of breast base.

The above chest circumference can also be a useful measurement to determine the fullness of the breast upper quadrants.

Aesthetic breast surgery assessment

History
- Establish the patient's concerns with her breasts and the motives behind her request for surgery. What is her current bra size? Has it changed? Determine what size and shape breasts she wants after surgery? Has she noticed any differences between her breasts?
- Are there any physical symptoms due to the breast? Breast reduction patients will often complain of neck ache, back ache, bra strap indents, intertrigo, and poor posture. Breast pain will not be cured by aesthetic breast surgery.
- Does her breast problem interfere with daily activities such as exercise and clothing choice?
- Does she receive any comments with regard to her breast size or shape?
- What is her partner's opinion of her breasts? Are there any psycho-sexual problems due to the breast size (inability to undress in front of the partner, difficulty in sexual relations)?
- Are there any other psychological problems brought on by the breast size, such as lack of confidence and reduction in social interaction?
- Does the breast size change with the menstrual cycle, weight change, or the oral contraceptive pill and if so by how much? If it does it will continue to do so after the surgery. Is the breast size static or changing? Best to consider surgery only on breasts of static size.
- Is her weight steady or is she planning to gain or lose weight? This may affect her post-operative breast size.
- Has she had any children? Has she completed or is she planning a family? Does she wish to breast feed in the future? Any surgery done before children has a greater chance of requiring revision after children.
- Is there any nipple discharge? Is the sensation to the nipple normal and how important is that in her sexual relations? Nipple sensation may be lost in any form of breast surgery.
- Has she had any breast lumps, cancers, or previous breast surgery?
- Is there any family history of breast disease or cancer?
- Past medical history: previous surgery and scarring. How did the scars settle? Are there any medical problems?
- Drug history: particularly important in gynaecomastia patients.
- Smoking: many surgeons will not do breast reduction or mastopexy operations on smokers.

Examination
Look for any spinal curvature or chest wall deformities and visibility of the ribs. Note shoulder guttering. Examine the skin of the breast for intertrigo, skin conditions, and stretch marks. Note the nipple height, areola size, infra-mammary fold level and volume distribution on the breast. In particular, record any asymmetry in the above. Assess the lateral extent of the breast. Note the position and symmetry of the nipple.

Feel Check for any lumps or masses. Assess skin turgor and pinch test for skin and breast thickness and breast density. Assess nipple sensibility.

Measure nipple distance from sternal notch, inter-nipple distance, nipple to infra-mammary fold, width of the breast and length of the infra-mammary fold, chest circumference at level of infra-mammary fold and at nipple height.

In breast augmentation, patient's other measurements are required to determine correct implant size. Breast width is important, as implant width is equivalent to the desired breast width minus thickness of the breast. Implant height depends on the nipple to sternal notch distance. If >21 cm a full height implant should be considered. If <21 cm a low or medium height implant is best. The projection of the implant is based on the laxity of the skin and the patient desires. Requests for larger breasts need fuller projection implants.

Breast reduction surgery

Indications
- Breast hypertrophy, either developmental (virginal) or secondary to weight gain, pregnancy, and breastfeeding.
- Breast hypertrophy causing embarrassment, inability to exercise, intertrigo, shoulder denting from bra straps, neck and back pain, postural problems, upper limb symptoms including paraesthesia and pain.
- Unilateral: either developmental breast asymmetry or symmetrizing after breast reconstruction or partial mastectomy.

Aim
Relieve symptoms by reducing breast volume leaving symmetrical, smaller breast more in proportion with the body habitus.

Anatomy
Breast tissue comprises a ductal system in a lipomatous stroma. There are supportive ligaments (of Cooper) extending from the chest wall through the stroma to the skin. The ideal breast lies over the ribs 3–7 anteriorly between the parasternal and anterior axillary lines. The nipple lies over the fourth intercostal space slightly lateral to the mid-clavicular line about 2–3 cm below the mid-humerus level.

The blood supply to the breast is via perforators from the internal mammary (internal thoracic) (60%), branches from the lateral thoracic (30%) and a small contribution from the intercostals, and branches from the axillary, thoracodorsal, subscapular, and pectoral arteries.

Lymphatic drainage is mainly to the axillary nodes, but there is some drainage to the internal mammary chain and an even smaller drainage to the subdiaphragmatic lymphatics and intra-abdominal nodes.

The nerve supply to the breast is via the anterior branches of the second to sixth intercostal nerves and the lateral branches of the third to sixth intercostal nerves. The major supply is from the fourth lateral branch.

Assessment
See section on breast assessment.

Planning
Pre-operative mammogram in patient >40 years; FBC; mark breast and key landmarks pre-operatively with patient standing.

Surgical options
Liposuction (alone or in combination with breast tissue excision technique).

Breast reduction techniques are distinguished by the resulting scar and by the design of the pedicle of breast tissue used to retain the nipples' attachments to the chest wall. Historically every scar type has been tried with every pedicle.

Skin incisions
- Periareolar.
- Keyhole/inverted T/Wise (1956) pattern.
- Vertical (Lejour et al. 1990).

- B shape (Regnault 1980).
- L shape.
- Periareolar and infra-mammary.

Pedicles
- Medial.
- Inferior (Robbins 1977).
- Superior (Weiner).
- Horizontal bipedicle (Strombeck 1960).
- Lateral (Skoog).
- Vertical bipedicle (McKissock 1972).
- Central mound (Balch 1981).
- None (free nipple graft technique). The free nipple graft technique (Thorek 1931) involves amputation of breast tissue and application of the nipple as a composite graft on de-epithelialized skin. This technique is usually reserved for massive breast reductions in the elderly.

Complications

Bleeding, haematoma, and abscess requiring re-operation. Fat necrosis. Asymmetry, dog ears. Nipple sensory change (increased/decreased) and nipple numbness. Nipple loss (partial/complete). Inability to breastfeed (all pedicles except central mound and inferior). Wound infection, wound dehiscence (especially at T junction in Wise pattern skin incision). Rarely, large areas of skin necrosis and loss. Discovery of occult carcinoma resulting in future mastectomy (1%). Suture spitting. Scar hypertrophy/keloid, problems most likely at the medial and lateral end of the inframammary scar. Change in shape over time including re-enlargement with weight gain or drugs (OCP or HRT) or shrinkage with weight loss. Warn about bottoming out of the breast (inferior pedicle techniques). Secondary procedure to remove dog ears, especially in vertical scar techniques.

Tips

- Nipples placed too high are difficult to correct.
- Ensure that the skin envelope is not over-reduced or too tight otherwise you will have to over-reduce the breast to fit it in or close it under tension with consequent skin necrosis or dehiscence.
- Complications are reduced significantly in patients with lower BMIs (<30).
- Breast tissue should be sent for histological assessment. Unsuspected malignancy occasionally diagnosed.

Vertical scar medial pedicle breast reduction (Hall-Findlay 1999)

Indications
Initially for small to medium reductions; as experience grows can use for larger breasts.

Aims
Breast reduction with reduced scarring.

Planning
Warn the patient that breast shape will be unusual for the first 3 months (prominent superiorly, flattened inferiorly). Mark the breast meridian on the breast and the infra-mammary fold. Project the infra-mammary fold onto the breast Place the nipple 1–2 cm lower than this line and in the meridian of the breast. Draw a 16–18 cm mosque-shaped opening, starting at a point 2.5 cm higher than the new nipple position. Swing the breast medially and draw a line from the end of the mosque to the infra-mammary fold. Do the same laterally. Depending on the extent of the resection leave 2 cm(<400 g), 4 cm (400–800 g), 6 cm (800 g) of skin superior to the fold and join up the medial and lateral limbs. The pedicle is medially based, with half the base in the areola opening and a length to breadth ratio of 1:1.2.

Incision
Along the markings, preserving the pedicle.

Procedure
De-epithelialize the pedicle. Deepen the incision around the pedicle directly to the chest wall, making the pedicle full thickness and attached to the chest wall as well as medial skin. Remove the breast tissue en bloc inferiorly, laterally, and to a lesser extent superiorly. Remove enough superiorly to inset the pedicle adequately. Ensure inferiorly that the skin is only 0.5–1 cm thick. Rotate the pedicle into the areola opening and place one suture to close the areola opening. Stitch the medial pillar (which is in fact the rotated inferior border of the pedicle to the lateral pillar (residual breast tissue on the lateral incision) with 3/0 PDS. Tailor laterally and inferiorly with liposuction as required.

Closure
Use interrupted 3/0 monocryl to the dermis. Then a running 3/0 monocryl, cinching (rucking) in the lower third of the incision to close the skin. Drains if necessary. Tape to the wounds.

Post-operative care
Non-underwired bra for 6 weeks; tape wounds for 3 months.

Complications
10% will require revision of dog-ear of scar.

Tips
Do not take too much skin. Do not take too much tissue superiorly. It is very hard to over-resect and the breasts can be slightly larger with this technique than the inferior pedicle techniques.

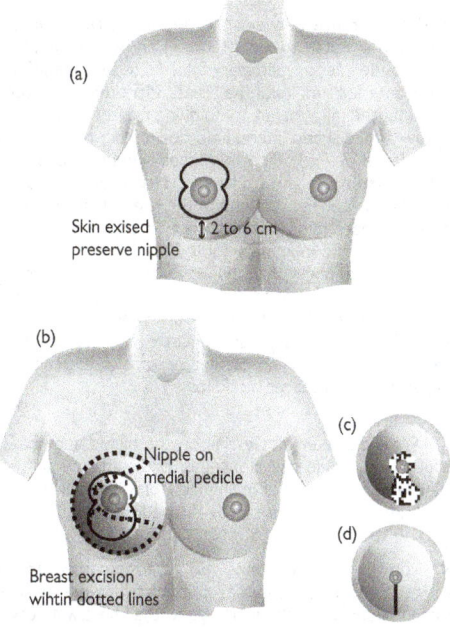

Fig. 20.1 Vertical breast reduction. (a) Pattern: excise skin within figure-eight pattern preserving the NAC. (b) Undermine the skin flaps. Excise breast within dotted line. Maintain NAC on medical pedicle. (c) Close superior hole of figure-eight pattern around the nipple. (d) The inferior hole is a vertical scar beneath the NAC.

Inferior pedicle breast reduction (Wise pattern/ invertedT)

Indications
Any size breast. Most reliable technique for nipple sensation and ability to breastfeed post-operatively (50%). Good for unilateral reduction in asymmetric breasts as can adjust both the horizontal and vertical difference.

Aims
Smaller, aesthetically pleasing breasts with minimal interruption in sensation and function.

Planning

Note any size difference between the breasts. Mark the midline of the chest (from sternal notch to xiphisternum) and vertical midline of each breast down to the inferior mammary fold. Transpose the infra-mammary fold onto the anterior surface of the breast. Mark the new nipple position at the point that the infra-mammary fold line transects the vertical breast midline. Draw a medial and lateral limb down from the new nipple position for a distance of 7 cm. The two limbs should be at an equal angle from the breast meridian and usually not create an angle of more than 90° between them. Connect the end of the lateral limb to the lateral end of the infra-mammary fold. Connect the end of the medial limb to the medial end of the infra-mammary fold. The length of these two transverse lines should be longer than the length of the infra-mammary line as they will be sutured together at the end. The pedicle is based inferiorly, is at least 10 cm in width, and is centred on the midpoint of the infra-mammary fold and ascends to and encircles the nipple. Pre-operative local anaesthetic and adrenaline use is a personal preference. There may be soft evidence that it reduces blood loss.

Incision

Centre a 4.5 cm diameter nipple ring on the nipple and draw round it. Incise through the epidermis along this circle and de-epithelialize the pedicle. Cut along the inferior mammary fold (epithelium only for the pedicle) and the markings. Incise along the pedicle margin.

Procedure

Cut down from the medial, lateral, and superior edge of the pedicle to the chest wall. Beware under-cutting and narrowing the pedicle. Deepen the inferior incisions along the markings to the chest wall leaving a layer of fat and fascia over pectoralis major. Then raise the superior skin flaps with a thickness of 1 cm to the margins of the breast. Remove the breast tissue, starting medially, moving superiorly and finally laterally. Trim and tailor the pedicle as necessary. Weigh the tissue and send for histology.

Closure

Close the breast by connecting the tip of the medial limb and the tip of the lateral limb to the midpoint of the infra-mammary fold. Then suture the new infra-mammary fold and the vertical wound (3/0 and 4/0 absorbable). Ensure that you de-tension the T-junction. Centre the nipple ring over the superior point of this vertical line. Cut around it and deliver the nipple. Close the NAC wound with 4/0 absorbable sutures. Drains depend on bloodiness of wounds and on personal preference, but there is no evidence for their use.

Post-operative care

Tape the wounds and support in a bra with gauze laid in it to catch any ooze. Dressing check at 1–2 weeks. Advise patient to wear a bra non-stop for 6 weeks. Tape the wound for 3 months.

Complications

See above.

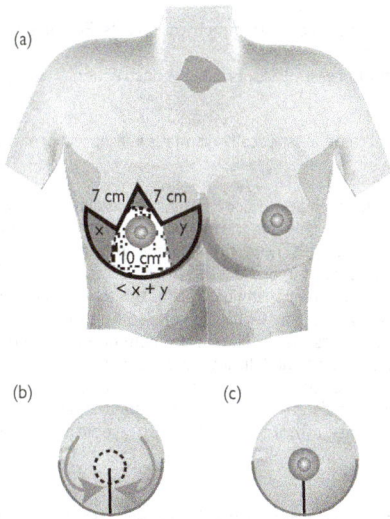

Fig. 20.2 Wise pattern breast reduction. (a) Pattern: 7 cm from new nipple point to new infra-mammary crease. Length of superior flaps should be equal to or slightly longer than the infra-mammary incision. Maintain 10 cm dermal and subcutaneous fat and breast pedicle. Excise breast medial and lateral to this pedicle. (b) Close superior flaps together to create vertical scar and to close infra-mammary fold. (c) Excise 4 cm disc to allow nipple–areolar out.

Tips

This technique tends to bottom out over time so placing the nipple 1 cm lower than the infra-mammary fold is a good idea. During the marking check the medial and lateral limb length by swinging the breast and making sure they reach the midline. Reduce the angle between the lines for a more tension-free closure.

References

Balch CR (1981). *Plast Reconstr Surg* **67**, 305–11.
Hall-Findlay EH (2002). *Aesthet Surg J* **22**, 185–94.
Lejour M, Abboud M, Declety A, Kertesz P (1990). *Ann Chir Plast Esthet* **35**, 369–79.
McKissock PK (1972). *Plast Reconstr Surg* **49**, 245–52.
Regnault P (1980). *Plast Reconstr Surg* **65**, 840–5.
Robbins TH (1977). *Plast Reconstr Surg* **59**, 64–7.
Strombeck JO (1960). *Br J Plast Surg* **13**, 79–90.
Thorek M (1931). *Med J Rec* **134**, 474.
Wise RJ (1956). *Plast Reconstr Surg* **17**, 367–75.

Breast augmentation

Indication
- Congenital: small breasts, asymmetrical breasts, Poland's syndrome, tuberous breasts.
- Acquired: mild breast ptosis, breast reconstruction.

Aim
To attempt to create aesthetically normal symmetrical breasts.

Implant choice
The implant shell is made of silicone; the surface may be smooth or more commonly textured. This integrates with the body and reduces the risk of capsular contracture. The content of the implant is either silicone or saline. Virtually 100% of implants used in UK contain silicone filler. This is usually cohesive gel rather than liquid gel as this lowers the risk of capsular contracture and gel bleeds. Cohesive gel also holds its shape and is used in anatomical implants. Saline fill is more common in the USA, Australia, and France and for trans-umbilical placed implants.

The implants are either round or anatomical (teardrop, bio dimensional). Factors that determine choice are patient and surgeon preference. If the patient wishes a more prominent upper pole then round implants are preferred.

Planning
Good information exchange with the patient, especially in determining the size and shape of the breast required, and informing her of all the risks. Preoperative marking is important. Asking the patient to place her hands on her head can reveal the elevated post-implant nipple position. Draw a line from this nipple position to the midline over the sternum. Measure the half-height of the implant down from here to give the new infra-mammary fold level. Mark the same distance superiorly for the upper limit of the pocket dissection. Mark the new breast width (implant width + skin pinch thickness); this gives the pocket dimensions. Mark the midline. Preoperative flucloxacillin or cephalosporin antibiotics.

Incision
- Infra-mammary: good exposure for the important area of pocket dissection. The most common scar, but can be visible. Depending on the size of the implant, the scar ranges from 4.5 to 6 cm long. The medial end is placed equal to the medial areola.
- Axillary: for subpectoral placement. More difficult dissection, particularly of the important inferomedial area. Scar is off the breast and very well hidden.
- Periareolar: scar disguised by areola–skin junction. Nipple sensory changes are risked and dissection through breast tissue may increase risk of infection and other complications.
- Umbilical: remote dissection risks bleeding complications. Excellent scar. Expandable saline implants only.

Exposure
The pocket is usually made under direct vision with haemostasis using diathermy, all assisted by using a lighted retractor. Submuscular pockets are an easier plane to dissect, except when releasing the pectoralis origin from the inferior ribs.

Placement
Subglandular
Continue deep to breast tissue, superficial to pectoralis major. Once above the nipple the dissection becomes easier. Proponents suggest that subglandular implants look more natural than those placed in the subpectoral plane. No risk of pectoralis major atrophy. Less risk of implant distortion or displacement by muscle activity. Better for ptotic breasts. Less risk of bleeding. Less post-operative pain.

Partial submuscular
A small subglandular pocket is made up to the level of the areola. Incise through the pectoralis muscle along the fourth rib and continue deep to pectoralis major, superficial to pectoralis minor. Advantages are quicker surgery and smoother implant and breast appearance, especially to upper pole. Reduced incidence of capsule formation. Implant rippling less apparent especially in small-breasted women. Method of choice in slim women. Mammography more accurate.

Total submuscular
Used in breast reconstruction. Deep to pectoralis major for the most part. Inferiorly, deep to the fascia of rectus abdominis. Laterally, deep to serratus anterior.

Subpectoralis fascia
Raise the pectoralis fascia off the muscle; this gives an extra layer to cover the implant.

Closure
Drains only if concerned. Closure of Scarpa's fascia to chest wall at inframammary fold with 3/0 absorbable. Deep dermal and skin suture 4/0 absorbable.

Postoperative care
Day case or overnight stay. Keep arms moving in full range but no strenuous activity for 2 weeks. Straight into non-underwired bra for 6 weeks non-stop.

Complications
- Scar.
- Wound healing problems.
- Haematoma requiring evacuation.
- Infection and abscess requiring explantation, delay, and re-insertion.
- Nipple numbness (10%) and breast and nipple hypersensitivity (may take 3–6 months to settle).

- Implant rupture or deflation. Ruptures may be intra-capsular in which case they may be asymptomatic, or extra-capsular in which case the patient will notice deflation.
- Gel diffusion (bleed) of minute quantities of silicone may occur but are usually not problematic.
- Silicone foreign body granulomas may form in the tissues or lymph nodes. These are usually asymptomatic but may raise concerns of being a malignant mass and need to be biopsied.
- Rotation of anatomical implants (1%).
- Interference with mammography.
- Asymmetry, stretch marks, and change in appearance over time.
- Rippling palpable creases.
- Implant replacement variously recommended as early as 8 years after implantation to whenever/if they become symptomatic. Prostheses that were explanted as part of the silicone scare showed gel bleed in 50–65% of cases, most of which were asymptomatic.

Capsular contracture

The body places a connective tissue wall around the implant. This becomes activated and contracts in 8% of cosmetic enlargements (20% of reconstruction patients). This contraction starts in the first 3 years in 80% of patients. Risk and degree of capsular contracture is reduced by a factor of 6–10 by using textured implants (Coleman *et al.* 1991), by washing the pocket with povidone iodine (Betadine), and by placing the implant subpectorally.

Capsular contracture may be due to subclinical infection, foreign body reaction, ordinary scarring.

Baker classification (1975)
- Class I: no capsular contracture.
- Class II: palpable capsular contracture.
- Class III: palpable/visible capsular contracture.
- Class IV: palpable/visible/painful capsular contracture.

Management

There is no clinical urgency to intervene unless the patient requests usually with aesthetic or symptomatic concerns. Breaking the capsule by manipulation (closed capsulotomy) has been used but risks implant rupture. The most reliable method is removal of capsule and implant and replacement (capsulectomy). The skin is often thin and the key is to get to the capsule and dissect the tissues off it with the implant in situ. Try and use a different implant in a different plane where possible. Capsular contracture may recur after capsulectomy.

Silicone controversy

- In 1982 Van Nunan reported three cases of connective tissue disease in women whom had silicone breast implants.
- This started a media frenzy and legal cases. Several high-profile cases in the USA were granted enormous sums of money on spurious evidence linking their connective tissue disease to their implants. Silicone breast implants were banned in the USA, Australia, and France amongst other places. They were not banned in the UK. Saline breast

implants were the most commonly used alternatives. These still have a silicone outer shell!
- Several studies subsequently show no increased risk of connective tissue disease in patients with silicone breast implants.
- In 1998 a UK Department of Health independent review group found No link between silicone implants and auto-immune or connective tissue disease.
- In 1999 a report from the Institute of Medicine of the National Academy of Science of the USA found no evidence of a link between silicone implants and systemic disease.
- No proven risk of induction of breast cancer.
- Several animal studies report a reduced incidence of cancer in the presence of an implant, perhaps because of alterations to blood supply.
- Silicone (polydimethyl siloxane) is an almost universal product with wide application in medical devices, including needle coatings, valves, joints, and testicular and penile implants.
- No evidence of silicone in breastmilk of implanted breastfeeding mothers causing problems. One study showed no increase in silicone levels.

Reference

Coleman DJ, Foo IT, Sharpe DT (1991). *Br J Plast Surg* **44**, 444–8.

Breast ptosis

Definition
Sag or droop of the breasts following ageing, breast involution, or weight loss.

Aetiology
The common causes are increasing age, post childbirth, post breastfeeding, and post weight loss.

Classification
This was first described by Regnault in 1973 and was based on the position of the nipple relative to the infra-mammary fold:
- Type A: minor—nipple at infra-mammary fold.
- Type B: moderate—nipple below infra-mammary fold (1–3cm) but above the most projected part of the breast.
- Type C: major—nipple below infra-mammary fold (>3 cm) and lying at the lowest part of the breast.
- Pseudo-ptosis—nipple above and gland below the infra-mammary fold.

Principles
It is important to determine the patient's concerns. If she is concerned that her breasts are too large, reduction techniques are employed. If she is concerned that her breasts are too small, augmentation, either alone or in combination with mastopexy, will be needed. When the patient is happy with her breast size mastopexy alone is used. Once the extent of scarring is explained, the patient may refuse the surgery or choose a lesser technique with lesser results. This must be clearly defined prior to operating.

Management
- Type A: minor ptosis/normal volume:
  - Periareolar or short vertical scar mastopexy.
- Type A: minor ptosis/hypoplasia:
  - Breast augmentation.
- Type B: moderate ptosis/normal volume:
  - vertical scar or inverted T mastopexy.
- Type B: moderate ptosis/hypoplasia:
  - Augmentation mastopexy. Usually lesser scarring is possible using a small vertical scar for mastopexy and implant access.
  - Periareolar mastopexy with the implant placed via an infra-mammary incision.
- Type C: major ptosis/normal volume:
  - Inverted T mastopexy.
- Type C: major ptosis/hypoplasia:
  - Augmentation with inverted T mastopexy.
- Pseudo-ptosis/normal volume:
  - Horizontal excision of tissue along the infra-mammary fold.
- Pseudo-ptosis/hypoplasia:
  - Breast augmentation.

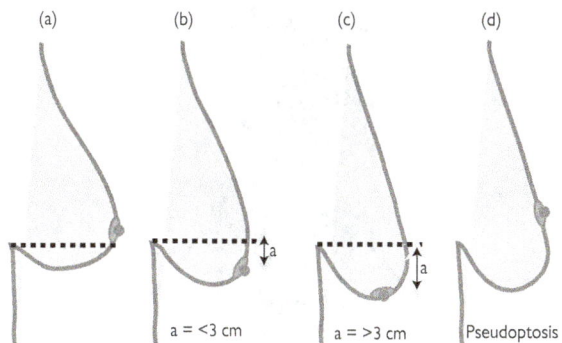

Fig. 20.3 Regnault's classification of breast ptosis.

Mastopexy techniques

All forms of mastopexy can be dermal alone or involve breast gland suture and rearrangement. The principle behind breast rearrangement is to maintain the nipple viability on a pedicle and move more breast tissue behind the nipple to give a longer lasting result, with more projection.

Periareolar (doughnut) mastopexy

This procedure removes tissue in a vertical and horizontal plane by de-epitheliazing tissue in an elliptical fashion superior to and around the areola, elevating the areola to the superior margin of the ellipse and taking up the excess in a purse string fashion leaving a circumferential areola scar.

Short vertical scar

This technique allows nipple areola transpositon with reduction in areola size if necessary. The ellipse is drawn and de-epithelialized as above but once the areola is elevated, the tension and skin excess is mainly taken in the short vertical scar.

Inverted T and vertical scar principles

Please see breast reduction. These techniques use similar incisions and leave similar scars, but rather than removing breast tissue, the lateral breast pillars are centralized to narrow and elevate the base of the breast, increasing projection.

Augmentation mastopexy

This is a difficult procedure. The best approach is to augment first, elevate the patient to the sitting position whilst anaesthetized, and make final adjustments to the nipple and areola position intra-operatively by which ever technique is appropriate.

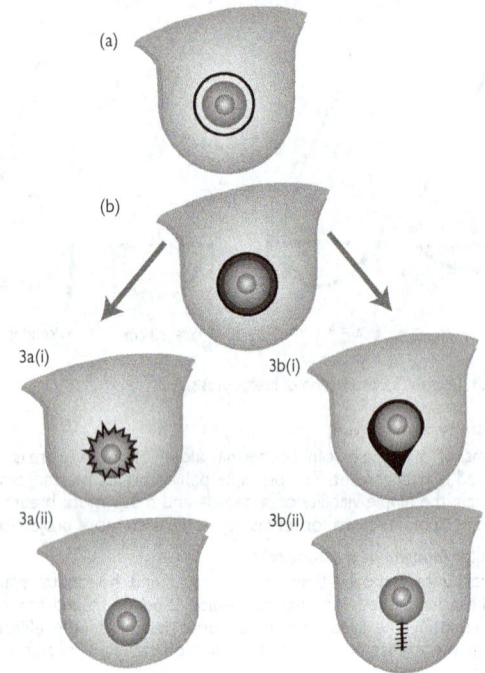

Fig. 20.4 Periareolar mastoplexy: (a) doughnut periareolar excision of skin; (b) defect; 3a(i) purse string closure; 3a(ii) periareolar scar; 3b(i) tissue retracted below nipple to lift and create short vertical scar closure; 3b(ii) Short vertical scar.

Further reading

Whidden PG (2003). *Can J Plast Surg* **11**, 73–8.

Inverted nipples

Definition
A reversal of normal nipple projection, in which it is retracted beneath the areola.

Incidence
Common: females > males.

Aetiology
- Decreased areola subcutaneous tissue.
- Short hypoplastic lactiferous ducts and fibrotic bands tethering the nipple. Post-mastitis fibrosis.

Classification (Han and Hong 1997)
- Grade 1: minimal fibrosis. Easily correctable manually. Maintains position without traction.
- Grade 2: moderate fibrosis. Correctable manually but position not maintained after release of traction.
- Grade 3: Severe fibrosis. Difficult to correct manually.

Clinical features
- Nipple retraction.
- Interference with breastfeeding.
- Psychological distress.

Treatment
Non-surgical
- Suction devices: simple devices, e.g. shortened plastic syringes (plunger removed), placed on nipple and suction applied.
- Commercial devices such as the Niplette (McGeorge 1994).

Surgical (Hamilton 1980; Teimourian and Adham 1980)
- Grade 1: Traction and a single purse string suture.
- Grade 2: Blunt dissection to release fibrotic bands without division of lactiferous ducts. Purse string suture to maintain position.
- Grade 3: Sharp division of fibrotic bands and lactiferous ducts through transverse nipple and areola incision (Pitanguy) or through star-shaped circumferential nipple base incision utilizing de-epithelialized dermal flaps from the star limbs to replace soft tissue loss, and bridge under the nipple. The star limb defects are closed directly further giving the nipple support.

References
Hamilton JM (1980). *Plast Reconstr Surg* **65**, 507–50.
Han S, Hong YG. (1999). *Plast Reconstr Surg* **104**, 389–95.
McGeorge DD (1994). *Br J Plast Surg* **47**, 46–9.
Teimourian B, Adham MN (1980). *Plast Reconstr Surg* **65**, 504–6.

Tuberous breast

Also known as tubular breast.

Definition
Breast deformity where the breast has a tubular or tuberous shape with a narrow base.

Incidence
Unknown, as many mild unreported cases exist and never present for treatment. Severe cases presenting for treatment are uncommon. Unilateral is less common than bilateral.

Aetiology
Congenital cause. Thought to be due to absence of superficial fascia over the breast allowing it to herniate anteriorly.

Clinical presentation and assessment
Patients present requesting breast enlargement, or are embarrassed about their breast shape and asymmetry. Rather than the pyramidal or wide-based conical shape of the normal breast, these breasts have a narrow constricted base and herniation of the breast towards the NAC, giving in extreme cases a 'tennis ball in a sock' appearance. The NAC tends to be larger then expected. It has a pouting appearance with a tight fibrous ring at the circumference, and herniation of breast tissue under it, pushing it forward. This can give the breast a double-bubble appearance. The breasts are generally hypoplastic and small.

Classification
- Type 1: inferior medial hypoplasia.
- Type 2: inferior medial and lateral hypoplasia.
- Type 3: as above plus sub areolar skin shortage in circumferential plane.
- Type 4: severely constricted base.

Surgical management
Augmentation in the submammary pocket with disruption of the fibrous ring at the base of the breast corrects mild deformity. This may need to be combined with a doughnut-type peri-intra-areolar excision to reduce the size of the areola. The implant can be introduced through the same incision.

In more severe cases an expandable implant may be needed to gradually overcome the skin shortage. The alternative is using a flap to introduce skin along the infra-mammary meridian from NAC to and across the infra-mammary fold. This flap may be a large Z-plasty or a transposition thoraco-epigastric flap.

Some have tried internal breast flaps to rearrange the internal breast anatomy and fill out the inferior deficiency.

Outcome
Rarely perfect but usually much improved. The pouting of the NAC tends to recur.

Gynaecomastia

Definition
Abnormal overdevelopment of the male breast.

Incidence
60% of newborns, 65% of boys at puberty, 8% by age 17, 30% in older men.

Aetiology
- Physiological: neonatal, pubertal, old age.
- Pharmacological: spironolactone, digoxin, diazepam, methyldopa, cimetidine, metoclopramide, steroids, theophylline, marijuana, oestrogens, anti-androgens (cyproterone acetate).
- Pathological: malnutrition, hypogonadism (congenital or acquired), Klinefelter's syndrome (XXY), thyroid disease, cirrhosis, malignant tumours secreting steroids/human chorionic gonadotrophin (testicular, pituitary, renal, adrenal, hepatic, bronchogenic), carcinoma of the male breast, idiopathic.

Classification (Simon et al. 1973)
- Grade 1: small enlargement, no skin excess.
- Grade 2A: moderate enlargement, no skin excess.
- Grade 2B: moderate enlargement, with extra skin.
- Grade 3: marked enlargement, with extra skin.

Histology
- Florid: increased ductal and vascular tissue.
- Fibrous: acellular fibrous stroma, few ducts.
- Intermediate.

Clinical features
Overdevelopment of breast tissue, in the male. Some have just breast disc development, but others also have associated fatty stromal hyperplasia as well. Most patients are asymptomatic. Some patients experience breast tenderness.

Investigations
Always examine genitals, secondary sex characteristics, and possible causes. LFTs, thyroid function tests, hormone screen, other investigations directed by clinical features, e.g. chromsome analysis, USS/CT/MRI liver, US testes, CXR.

Medical treatment
- Most gynaecomastia is physiological and does not need treatment. Pubertal physiological gynaecomastia resolves within 2 years.
- Danazol, tamoxifen, or clomiphene are sometimes useful in pubertal gynaecomastia.

Surgical treatment

Indications
Indicated when medical treatment has failed, persistent physiological pubertal gynaecomastia for >3 years and into patient's twenties, resistant to weight loss, and causing functional or psychological problems.

Surgical techniques
Liposuction (Rohrich et al. 2003)
Ultrasound-assisted liposuction (UAL) for dense breast tissue and standard liposuction for fatty tissue (grades 1 and 2A and grade 2B if good skin) depending on the pros and cons of UAL for breast tissue.

Excision
- Webster's procedure: semicircular incision along inferior areolar margin, excision of breast tissue (grades 1 and 2A and grade 2B if good skin).
- Doughnut-shaped skin de-epithelialization around nipple (grade 2B and moderate grade 3) The lower half of the de-epithelialized skin is removed to permit access to excise the breast tissue. The nipple stays alive on a superiorly based dermoglandular flap. The circumareolar incision is then closed over de-epithelialized skin, cinching in the excess.
- It is important not to overdo the resection, leaving a saucer-shaped deformity or recessed nipple.
- Formal reduction with scar limbs extending onto the breast from either side of the nipple to extending to Wise pattern reduction (severe grade 3).
- Drainage as required.

Post-operative care
Compression dressings are worn for a week; can go home with drains in place if there is excess drainage.

Complications
Bleeding, haematoma, and re-operation. Abscess, wound infection, wound dehiscence, nipple loss, numbness and indentation, saucer deformity, asymmetry, recurrence. Seroma formation requiring frequent aspirations and possible further surgery. Most common complaint is insufficient reduction, but it is easier to repeat excision then to try to correct a saucer deformity.

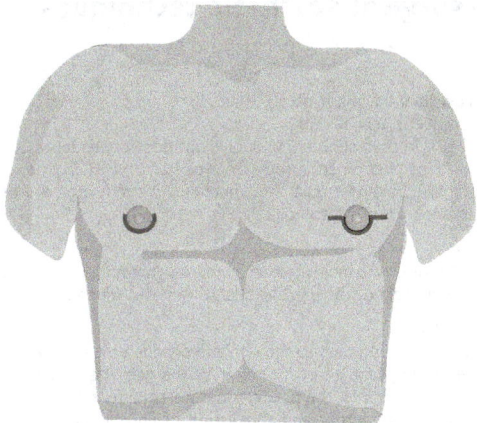

Right nipple showing areolar inferior hemicircumferential incision

Left nipple showing extensions

Fig. 20.5 Gynaecomastia incisions: (right) with inferior hemicircumferential periareolar; (left) with lateral extensions.

References

Simon BB, Hoffman S, Kahn S (1973). *Plast Reconstr Surg* **51**, 48–52.
Rohrich RJ, Ha RY, Kenkel JM, Adams WP, Jr (2003). *Plast Reconstr Surg* **111**, 909–23.

Non-surgical aesthetic techniques

Chemical peels

Agents
- Salicylic acid and alpha hydroxy acids.
- Trichloroacetic acid 10–50%.
- Phenol 50% in soap solution: phenol is not dose dependent but an all-or-nothing phenomenon (beware liver toxicity and cardiac arrhythmias). Baker formula: 3 mL phenol; 2 mL tapwater; 8 drops liquid soap; 3 drops croton oil.

Indications
Fine facial wrinkles (rhytids), blotchy skin pigmentation, pre-cancerous skin lesions, and acne scarring. Deep facial wrinkles (phenol).

Method of action
Chemical peels are applied to the skin and produce a controlled chemical injury. Depending on the concentration of the peel the necrosis extends from the epidermis into the papillary dermis to differing depths. Healing results in a new epidermis and stimulation of fibroblasts to form a new extracellular matrix. The collagen is laid down in a more compact and parallel fashion. The epidermis usually heals within a week and the overall change is visible after 2 months.

Complications
Hypo-pigmentation/de-pigmentation, hyper-pigmentation, erythema, milia, hypertrophic scarring, ectropion, sun sensitivity.

Dermabrasion

Indications
As for peels, in particular for perioral rhytids in darker-skinned patients.

Method of action
Mechanical removal of epidermis and superficial dermis. The depth is controllable and produces less bleaching.

Carbon dioxide laser

Indications
As above.

Method of action
See laser. In this context similar to chemical peel.

Retin A (tretinoin 0.05%–0.1% cream)

Indications
Early signs of ageing and sun damage. Minor skin irregularities.

Mode of action
Increases collagen formation, removes atypia and microscopic keratoses, leaving a normal epidermis.

Dose
Nightly application and daily sunscreen. Results after 4–8 months.

Hydroquinones (2%–4% cream)

Indications
Uneven pigment due to sun damage.

Method of action
Inhibits tyrosinase which converts tyrosine to melanin. Hence bleaches the skin and produces an even skin colour. Commonly used on the face and dorsum of hands.

Dose
Daily with results at 3–6 months.

Non-autologous fillers

Agent
There are over 70 fillers on the market today. The two most common are hyaluronic acid and collagen.

Indications
Facial lines such as upper lip, naso-labial fold, oral commissure.

Method of action
The filler is injected intradermally to fill fine to moderate lines and creases. This gives an immediate, but temporary, result which will need to be repeated every 6–9 months.

Complications
Minimal. Collagen can give an allergic reaction. Otherwise, redness, bruising, itchiness, and discoloration are the main problems. Over-filling can give instantly recognizable pouting lips.

Autologous fillers

Agent
Fat graft.

Indications
Forehead and glabellar creases, lip creases and augmentation, malar augmentation.

Method of action
The fat is harvested from the lower abdomen using a 3 mm cannula and is then centrifuged (Coleman fat transfer) or washed with normal saline until no blood discolours the solution. It is placed in the subdermal plane under the relevant skin crease. The bevelled end of the needle is used to break up the connections between dermis and deeper layers, so creating a clear plane 5 mm wide under the crease. The fat is injected, over-correcting to allow for absorption.

Complications
Resorption is the greatest problem and re-injection may be required.
NB Lipofilling large amounts (100–200 cm^3) to augment a flap post breast reconstruction uses the same technique.

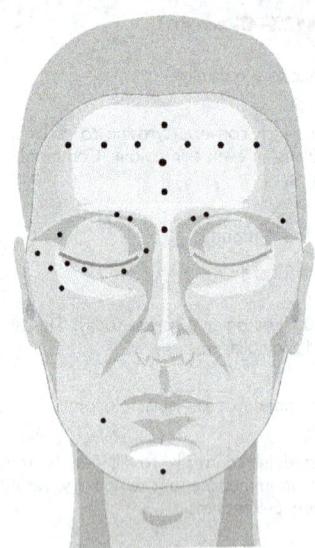

Fig. 20.6 Botulinium toxin injection points for facial wrinkles.

Botulinum toxin

Indications
Glabellar and forehead lines, crow's feet, lateral and medial brow lift.

Method of action
Clostridium botulinum produces eight exotoxins. Type A exotoxin has a commercial license. It inhibits the release of acetylcholine at the neuromuscular junction, causing a temporary flaccid paralysis. Under no or topical anaesthesia the toxin is injected into the muscle (or onto the muscle at the crow's feet) at pre-planned sites. It takes 24–48 hours to work and lasts for 1–6 months depending on site dose and patient.

Complications
Bruising, under- and over-correction, headache, diplopia. Upper lid ptosis occurs in 0.5–5%. This is usually a 1–2 mm droop and reverses with time. Upper lid ptosis (crow's feet).

Skin-lightening methods

Benign hyper-pigmented lesions such as lentigo and chloasma frequently cause embarrassment, and requests for de-pigmentation agents or methods are common. Benign hyper-pigmented lesions are treated by topical applications, lasers, or surgery. Determine the cause by investigating the history of the patient. Look for aetiologies such as:
- Drugs (hormonal).
- Photosensitizing agents.
- Post-inflammatory hyper-pigmentation.
- UV exposure.
- Systemic diseases (liver, Addison's disease), pregnancy.

Hydroquinone

A phenol catechol chemical agent that is readily available in non-prescription forms for skin lightening. It is one of most effective inhibitors of melanogenesis, and acts by inhibiting cell metabolism. The effect is non-specific but melanocytes become more sensitive. May take 4–6 weeks before effect is seen, then continues to improve for 4–6 months.

Hydroquinone 2% can be compounded with other skin lightening agents such as retinoic acid and dexamethasone (Triluma). More effective if combined with tretinoin.

Side effects: contact dermatitis, rarely ochronosis (sooty darkening of skin with degeneration of collagen and elastic fibres).

There is a monobenzyl ether form that gives irreversible depigmentation. There is also a glycosylated form called arbutin.

Other chemical agents

- Mequinol (4-hydroxyanisole): similar to hydroquinone; cytotoxic to melanocytes. Used in combination with retinoic acid.
- Azelaic acid and kojic acid: Naturally occurring acids that inhibit tyrosinase. Effective but cause local irritation.

Laser

- Q-switched ruby or Nd:Yag laser: best for treatment of hyper-pigmented lesions. The melanin in the lesion acts as a chromophore absorbing the energy destroying it. The wavelength determines the depth of penetration and the chromophores targeted. Adverse reactions are pain, irritation, post-inflammatory hyper-pigmentation.
- Intense pulse light: high-intensity pulsed light with broad wavelength (515–1200 nm) is delivered to the skin and absorbed by the chromophores. Adverse reactions are pain, irritation, post-inflammatory hyper-pigmentation.
- Fractional photothermolysis (Fraxel): creates thermal damage to the epidermis and dermis. Variant of laser; delivers 15–20% skin resurfacing in a single treatment. Adverse reactions are pain, irritation, post-inflammatory hyper-pigmentation.

Blepharoplasty

Definition
Plastic surgical procedure performed on the eyelids, usually with the aim of reversing the ageing process.

Indications
- To restore a youthful appearance to the peri-orbital region and hence to the rest of the face.
- To relieve mechanical visual field obstruction caused by excess skin, especially over the upper eyelid.
- As an adjunct to a facelift as a means of restoring a youthful appearance to the ageing face.

Aims
- To get rid of excess eyelid skin and eliminate wrinkles.
- To re-create symmetrical supratarsal folds.
- To address fat protrusions without creating a hollowed-out appearance.

Anatomy
See eyelid anatomy, Chapter 3.
- Orbital fat has two upper pockets and three lower pockets (Castannares 1951).
- Lid crease 8–10 mm centrally but 5–6 mm medial and lateral.
- Males: crease is lower (otherwise look female), so make the incision straighter.
- Asian eyes: preseptal fat goes right down because orbital septum inserts into the distal expansion.
- Asian lids may wish creation of double-eyelid fold vs occidentalism, epicanthal folds, lateral cantholpexy.

Pathophysiology
- With age the orbicularis becomes hypotonic, relaxes and descends, producing the fold overhanging palpebromalar crease. The adaptation of the lower lid to the globe diminishes, producing epiphora.
- The supporting structures relax with age, producing ectropion, elongation of the lower eyelid, descent of the lateral canthus, ptosis, and shallow lower fornix with possible entropion.
- The skin becomes thinner, and the elastic fibres less resilient. The fat atrophies. The septum relaxes, allowing the fat to herniate anteriorly and the globe to retract.
- Four factors contribute to eyelid bags:
  - Intraorbital pressure (e.g. ↑fat volume).
  - Weakness in septum orbitale.
  - Descent of globe (due to laxity of orbital musculo-fascial structures e.g. Lockwood's ligament).
  - Relaxation of orbicularis and skin.

Types of blepharoplasty
- Upper eyelid.
- Lower eyelid.
- Combined (four lid).

Patient assessment
Concerns
The patient should clearly define their concerns. In particular, are the wrinkles of concern mimetic or static? If mimetic they will not be helped by surgery. On the lower eyelid, bagginess of the lower lids must be separated from malar bags. Assess what the patient does not like. Too much skin? Puffy lids? Looking tired? Dark circles around the eyes? (May be pigmented.) Tendency to squint often means an over-active orbicularis muscle that will need to be addressed. Asians may want to look occidental or just have a lid crease.

Ocular history
Previous eye or eyelid surgery or trauma. Eye conditions such as cataracts, use of glasses and contact lenses, dry eye (do you get dry eyes on aeroplanes?), tears, and inflammatory eye conditions.

Drug history
In particular aspirin or warfarin.

Medical history
Hypothyroidism, diabetes, bleeding disorders. Take a skin history, in particular of infections such as herpes.

Examination
Eyelid frame
Take in the proportions of the whole face. Look for asymmetry and point it out. Palpate the bony anatomy. Assess the position of the brow, especially for ptosis (it should overlie the supra-orbital ridge). If ptosis exists, the upper eyelid skin should be examined with the eyebrow held in the correct position. Beware adapted ptosis where constant frontalis action hides the brow ptosis, but once the blepharoplasty is done the need for frontalis activity will reduce, making the brow ptosis apparent. Assess supra- and infra-orbital rims.

Eyelid: qualitative and quantitative
On the upper lid assess the skin excess. Does it exist with the brow in a normal position? There should be 8 mm of pretarsal skin on straightforward gaze. Does overhanging skin cover this? Is there any ptosis? Assess eyelid ptosis. The upper eyelid should lie 1 mm below the limbus (edge of the iris/cornea). Assess the fat bulges (medial and central) and the prominence of the lacrimal gland (lateral). These can be accentuated by gentle pressure on the globe with the lids closed. Do the tension test and Flower's test: eyelid downward retraction.

Assess the orbicularis. Assess obicularis tone:
- Finger feel tone test—feel tone on forceful contraction.
- Pinch test—pinch orbicularis at rest and on contraction.
- Squint test—to evaluate hypertrophic muscle, oblique lateral thickening downward; also evaluates pretarsal muscle.
- Squinch test—assesses festoons.

Assess and measure the eyelid aperture (usually 7–11 mm), the distance from lateral canthus to tail of eyebrow, and the angle of the palpebral fissure to the transverse axial line.

In the lower lid assess the skin excess, palpebral and malar bags, and nasojugal folds. Look for lid laxity using the snap test. Pull the lower lid inferiorly as far as possible; it should snap back in a fraction of a second. Look at lid position. The lid should lie at the limbus (edge of the iris/cornea) and the vertical opening of the eye should be 10–11 mm. Scleral show (sclera between limbus and lid) is undesirable. Do Schaefer's test—lower eyelid pull (normal is 3–5 mm, certainly <8 mm with involution up to 10–12 mm). Look for fat herniation (medial, central, lateral) or depression above the infra-orbital rim. If the snap test is poor avoid a blepharoplasty or do a minimal skin excision and a lateral canthal suspension or a trans-conjunctival fat removal. Do the bags diminish on tightening eye closure? Are the bags due to herniating fat or muscle festoons? Malar bags are due to oedema and cannot be corrected by blepharoplasty.

Vector
From above, assess the vector of the eye and cheek. This is the angle between a line dropped vertically from the cornea and one that joins the cornea to the prominence of the cheek. A positive vector is one where the cheek lies anterior to the eye. Beware a negative vector in which the cheek prominence lies posterior to the cornea, which is usually due to proptosis or a recessed cheek. These patients often have scleral show and the risk of ectropion is high.

Eye function
Do a general eye examination (VA, ROEM, PERLA) Look for any conjunctival reaction. Check extra-ocular muscle movement. Also test pupillary reaction and visual acuity, as 2% of amblyopia is not previously documented. Ensure that the patient has had an eye test in the last year. Watch blinking, usually 10–15 blinks per minute moving tears lateral to medial. Assess levator function. To do this immobilize the head and measure the distance between the eyelid on maximum downward gaze and maximum upward gaze. Normal is 15 mm; >8 mm is good; <4 mm is poor. Perform Schirmer's test to assess tear production. Take photographs.

Operative principles and planning
- Correct brow ptosis first! Correct periorbital ptosis first (by facelift).
- Plan procedure depending on clinical findings and patients desires.
- If redundant skin, plan skin and orbicularis excision. Raising the skin only or raising a myocutaneous element.
- If bags/fat herniation plan fat excision or redraping the retroseptal fat (Hamra 2004).
- If eyelid ptosis consider levator shortening and supra-tarsal fixation.

- If lacrimal gland ptosis do dacroadenopexy.
- To create supra-tarsal fold (in Asians) do supra-tarsal fixation.
- In the lower lid, if severe skin redundancy or orbicularis is hypotonic consider orbicularis plication or suspension.
- If eyelid redundancy consider wedge tarsectomy or lateral canthoplasty.
- Entropion or ectropion will need to be treated.

Anaesthesia

LA with sedation or GA. Minimal infiltration with a very fine needle (~1 mL 2% lidocaine with 1:200 000 adrenaline) to avoid distortion of eyelid. If under LA, then topical use of ocular prilocaine and placement of corneal shield.

Upper blepharoplasty

- *Aim of procedure* To create a nice upper eyelid crease without overhanging skin, or bulging fat. To clear vision if obscured. May reduce weighty feeling of upper eyelid.
- *Planning* Mark with patient supine. Place the lower mark on the tarsal crease and with the eye closed pinch with forceps to see how much skin can be removed. Then mark upper incision; extend laterally and medially with superior curve at each end. Ensure enough skin remains between lash and eyebrow.
- *Incision* Incise through markings down to muscle (Fig. 20.7(a)).
- *Procedure* Remove skin and subcutaneous tissue. If removing a strip of orbicularis, do so carefully with sharp scissors. Ensure meticulous haemostasis throughout. If fat is to be removed, make a small incision in the orbital septum and remove fat from central and medial fat pads. Gently dissect the fat, retract under minimal tension, and remove with cautery ensuring coagulation of all vessels. Note that lacrimal gland is grey-brown, eye fat is yellow, and nasal fat pad is white. Closure using 6/0 subcuticular monofilament suture. Steristrips for wound dressing. Suture removal at 5 days. BEWARE the lateral bulge of the lacrimal gland, which can be mistaken for a fat herniation. Lacrimal gland reduction can also be undertaken as part of the operation.
- *Variations* Septal contraction with cautery; septal incision using button-hole or open sky; suture fixation of crease to levator.

Lower eyelid

- *Aim of procedure* Restore cheekbone contour, remove dark circles, and improve shape of fissure.
- *Planning* Mark the incision extending laterally from the lower punctum along a subciliary route until the lateral canthus, merging it with one of the wrinkles or crow's feet.
- *Incision* Initial small incision laterally. Incise with scalpel or cut along the marked incision with a pair of sharp serrated scissors (Fig. 20.7(b)).
- *Procedure* Leave the pretarsal orbicularis intact. Below this, develop a myocutaneous plane with scissors down to the infra-orbital rim. Stay within the limits of the eyelid and do not extend onto the cheek. Incise the orbital septum. Remove the fat, starting with the central compartment and moving medially than laterally, as above. Gently pressing on the globe will produce bulging if there is excess fat to remove. Drape

the skin back in a lateral direction and excise the excess (usually <3 mm). Closure: 6/0 monofilament suture and Steristrips; remove at 5 days. BEWARE the excision of excess skin. Preserve resected skin for 10–14 days in case it is required for a gross post-operative ectropion)
- *Other options* Rather than fat removal, fat redraping. Drape the excess fat to avoid hollowed out or concave appearance and to fill medial nasojugal fold (Hamra 2004). Capsulo-palpebral fascial plication in a vertical direction can also be used. If bags are caused by muscle festoons, these can be plicated laterally.
- *Transconjunctival blepharoplasty* with an incision halfway between the fornix and the tarsal plate. This allows fat removal only. Laser to the lower eyelid skin produces skin tightening if required.

Complications

Most commonly slightly dry gritty eye, conjunctivitis, protracted swelling, excess bruising, conjunctival bruising for 2–3 weeks, and persistent skin excess on upper lid. Less likely, infection, bleeding, wound dehiscence, keloid or hypertrophic scarring, epiphora, hyper-pigmentation, residual bags, asymmetry, hollowed-out eye from over-excision of fat, ptosis, diplopia, dry eye syndrome, inflammation of the lid margin (blepharitis), conjunctival swelling (chemosis), scleral show, ectropion from over-excision of lower lid skin. Rarely, lower lid lag, retrobulbar haematoma, blindness (0.04%).

Management of complications

- Eyelid haematoma must be drained.
- Orbital (retrobulbar) haematoma must be treated with extreme urgency. Remove sutures on the ward and drain the haematoma. Consider a lateral canthotomy. Prescribe acetazolamide and mannitol. Decompress the orbit and seek an ophthalmology opinion.
- Dry eye should be managed by lubricants, taping, and humidification. Consider a temporary Frost suture.
- Lid malposition may resolve in 4–6 weeks by a massage and taping.
- Excessive skin removal can only be treated by skin grafts.

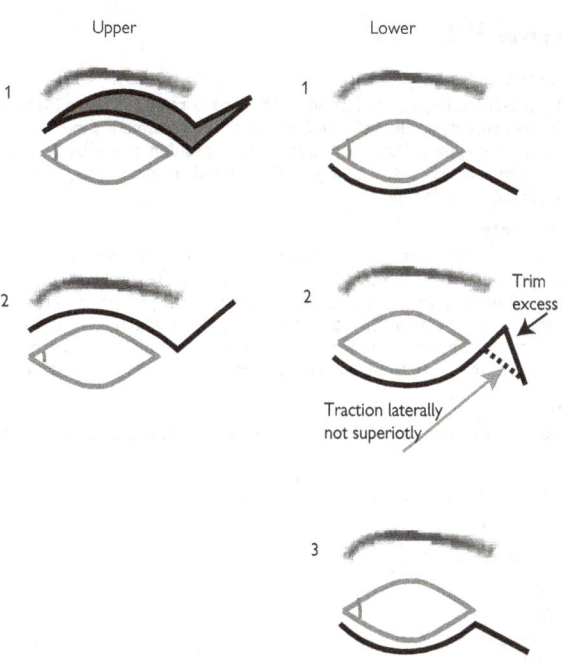

Fig. 20.7 (a) Upper eyelid blepharoplasty: (1) design and excision; (2) closure. (b) Lower eyelid blepharoplasty: (1) subciliary incision continued in high crow's feet line; (2) skin flap elevated, and tensioned laterally not superiorly; suture the sub-ciliary margin then excise excess laterally; (3) closure.

References

Castanares S (1951). *Plast Reconstr Surg* **8**, 46–58.
Hamra ST (2004). *Plast Reconstr Surg* **113**, 2124–41.

Brow lift

Assessment
May present as request for face lift and be incorporated in facial rejuvenation Usually presents as an eyelid problem, and the assessment should include that for a blepharoplasty. In addition, assess position of the brow at rest and with frontalis activity, height of forehead, hairline shape, and hair distribution and density.

Anatomy
The medial brow lies level with the medial canthus and the alar. It arches to its highest point two-thirds along its length, in a vertical line above the lateral limbus. In men the eyebrow lies along the supra-orbital rim and in women the high point of the arch lies just above the rim. The distance from the mid-pupil to the top of the brow is 2.5 cm. The distance from the top of the brow to the hairline is 6 cm in men and 5 cm in women.

Aims
Return of the brow to its natural position with good shape and symmetry.

Indications
Eyebrow ptosis due to ageing or facial nerve palsy.

Approaches
Open or endoscopic.

Open
- Bicoronal:
  - High.
  - Low.
- Mid-brow.
- Supra-brow.

The latter two approaches are for men with deep forehead wrinkles and male pattern baldness. Bicoronal approaches can be at the hairline or in the hair. Hairline approaches are good for those with a high forehead, as skin resection shortens the forehead. Approaches in the hairline (usually 5 cm behind the hairline) are useful in those with hair cover to hide the scar. The open approach leaves a long scar, numbness, and possible hair loss, but is effective. The skin excision is decreasingly effective as one moves the incision from the brow. An excision of 1 cm from the supra-brow will elevate the brow 1 cm; however, an excision of 3 cm is required to achieve the same elevation from a bicoronal approach.

Procedure
Dissect in subgaleal plane centrally and superficial to deep temporal fascia laterally. Mobilize the lateral eyebrow off the supra-orbital rim avoiding the supra-orbital and supra-trochlear nerves. Resect the corrugator. Drape the skin back and resect, being conservative in the central portion, to achieve the anatomical ideal. Drain.

Closure
Two-layer absorbable.

Endoscopic

Uses shorter scars. Less nerve trouble and less hair loss, but is less effective: '80% of the result for 20% of the scar'. It is not suitable if the brow is very ptotic or very heavy.

Incisions
Three to five vertical incisions in hair line.

Procedure
Tunnel endoscopically, subperiosteally centrally and superficial to the deep temporal fascia and laterally to the brow ridge. Resect corrugator muscles, avoiding the supra-orbital and supra-trochlear nerves. Fix the brows by lateral fascia sutures to temporalis fascia, and fix mid-laterally with glue or with sutures anchored to screws or through a bone tunnel. Do not over-lift centrally. Drain.

Closure
Two-layer absorbable.

Complications

- Supra-orbital, supra-trochlear, or frontal nerve injury.
- Alopecia.
- Numbness.
- Asymmetry.
- Hairline elevation.
- Recurrent ptosis.
- Temporary itching.
- Scarring.

Rhinoplasty

History
The patient should clearly define the area of concern. If there is more than one they should prioritize. Be wary if they just do not like their nose! Specific nasal history problems of epistaxis, allergic rhinitis, and nasal obstruction should be sought. Previous nasal trauma or surgery should be documented. The use of medications which promote bleeding are also important to note.

Examination
Relative to face
First examine the nose in relation to the other facial features. Sometimes a prominent nose is in fact a retruded chin!

Internal nasal examination
Look at the septum, turbinates, nasal valves, and mucosa. Ensure that there is no septal deviation, enlarged turbinates, or defective valves. Cottle's test is test of collapse/narrowing of the lower lateral cartilages, producing narrowing of the mid-nose on forced inspiration, which can be exaggerated by occluding the nostril. If inspiration is made easier by stretching the cheek laterally this is a positive test. This can be reconstructed with spreader grafts (Sheen 1984).

External nasal examination
Assess the nose in a systematic fashion from front, lateral, and worm's eye view.
- **Skin** Assess the skin quality and variation over the nose. If thick and sebaceous, the skin will not re-drape well over any skeletal change.
- **Deviation** Look for obvious nasal deviation.
- **Radix** The nasofrontal angle, which should be level with the upper lid eyelash line on straight forward gaze.
- **Bridge** Examine the nasal bones and the upper lateral cartilages looking for variations in width and height. The width of the nasal bones should be 75% that of the alar base. Look for a dorsal hump.
- **Supra-tip** Note the landmarks of the supra-tip break, i.e. where it starts and the projection of the supra-tip relative to the bridge and the tip.
- **Tip** Where is the tip defining point. Tip projection, shape, symmetry.
- **Columella** Examine the columella, assessing its relationship with the lip (columella–labia angle usually 90°–105°) and the alae. The columella should hang just inferior to the alar rims.
- **Alar** The alar base should be the same width as the intercanthal distance. The worm's eye view of the nose should show the nasal base as an equilateral triangle with the tip as the apex.

Document all findings meticulously. Photograph front, lateral, oblique, and worms' eye views as a minimum.

Indications

- To alter the appearance of any or a number of the constituents of the nose.
- To add definition to the nasal dorsum: augmentation rhinoplasty.
- To reduce the height and /or prominence of the nasal dorsum: reduction rhinoplasty.
- To alter the appearance of the nasal tip or alar domes, or the width of the nose: tip rhinoplasty.
- To correct any form of lateral nasal deviation.

All the above can be combined with a septoplasty (to correct a deviated nasal septum or nasal obstruction) or osteotomies to shape the osteocartilagenous vault.

Aims

To create or reshape a nose that is in proportion to the facial features according to the patient's desire. If performed in connection with nasal obstruction, the aim is to relieve obstruction.

Planning

Computer image analysis can help in pre-operative planning and consent, but can create unrealistic expectations. Drawings to illustrate the principles and expected changes can be better, and ensure that the surgeon and patient have the same idea about the requirements. Surgical planning should include a step-by-step analysis and correction of each component of the nose.

Anaesthesia

Local anaesthetic as a nasal block and then subcutaneously and submucoperichondrial to elevate the skin and the nasal mucosa. A topical vasoconstrictor such as cocaine paste or spray is put intranasally. Clean the inside of the nose and remove nasal hair with the scalpel.

Incision

There are two approaches to a rhinoplasty, internal (closed) and external (open).

Closed

The internal incisions can be:
- Inter-cartilaginous (between upper and lower lateral cartilages).
- Trans- or intra-cartilaginous, (through the lower lateral cartilages).
- Infra-cartilaginous (caudal border of lower lateral cartilage).
- Marginal or rim incisions.

If wide exposure of the nasal tip is needed inter- and infra-cartilaginous incisions with delivery of the cartilage are used. The incision continues down behind the columella in the coronal plane separating it from the septum. The closed approach is best for patients who require a minimum of adjustment to the tip. The incisions can be varied depending on the deformity, and post-operative recovery and operative time are shorter. However, exposure is limited.

Open

An external approach combines a trans-columella step or V-ncision at the narrowest part of the columella, which is usually the mid-portion, with a marginal or infra-cartilaginous mucosal incision. The advantage of open rhinoplasty is good exposure of the nasal framework without distortion, and it is particularly useful for significant tip surgery and for severe post-traumatic or congenital deformity. However, the operative time is longer, there is an external scar, and the nasal swelling is prolonged.

Exposure

The soft tissues are dissected off the cartilage in a submuscular plane, stopping at the inferior aspect of the nasal bones. Here the periosteum is incised and the plane is changed to subperiosteal. Raise the skin off the osseocartilaginous vault dorsally. Dissect and expose the lower lateral and upper lateral cartilages. Separate the mucosa from the upper laterals.

Procedure

Debate exists about whether to address the tip before the dorsum or vice versa. The author's personal preference is the principle of skeletal stability before soft tissue correction.

Small dorsal humps (<5 mm) can be reduced with the rasp alone. Larger humps require excision. An Aufricht's retractor is introduced to elevate the nasal soft tissue off the osteocartilagenous vault. The excessive dorsal prominence of the septal and upper lateral cartilages are cut transversely with cartilage cutting scissors. A guarded osteotome is introduced with its cutting edge transversely oriented in the gap created by the cartilage scissors and abutted against the nasal bones. The bony excess is now removed. The resected hump tissue should be wrapped in saline-soaked gauze in case any augmentation needs to be performed.

In some cases the nasal dorsum appears to be flattened and the normal triangular relationship amongst the nasal bones needs to be restored. This is done most commonly by performing osteotomies on the lateral aspects of the nasal bones (in-fracture). On occasions a dorsal on-lay graft will be used.

Osteotomies are performed to straighten nasal bones, restore the bony triangle, or narrow the nasal bones. This may be done externally via small stab incisions around the medial canthus (and, if necessary, in the nasal cheek border) and then introducing a periosteal elevator to carefully elevate a subperiosteal tunnel down the nasomaxillary angle. Then, with a fine osteotome 1–2 mm, the bone is perforated down the intended fracture line like a postage stamp. Digital pressure will then create the fracture. Alternatively, an internal osteotomy can be done through a small incision through the mucosa on the piriform fossa. Preserving the periosteum, the osteotome is tapped, cutting through the bone of the frontal process of the maxilla. As the sound changes the thinner cephalic bone may be fractured with digital pressure causing a greenstick fracture. Depending on the direction of fracture chosen by the surgeon, osteotomies have been classified as 'low to low', 'low to high', or 'high' relative to the nasomaxillary angle.

The techniques to improve tip projection are columella struts, crural suture techniques, and on-lay grafting. The first two are used in preference as grafting has a revision rate of approximately 30%. Bifid tips can be sutured together following excision of the connective tissue between the crura. A bulbous or prominent tip can be reduced by excising a wedge from the alar and/or excising the cephalic coronal edge or half the alar cartilage.

The columella and alar base are addressed. A nasolabial angle of 95°–105° is aimed for by trimming the caudal septum. If the tip hangs over the columella, the septum and columella are augmented by a cartilage graft from the septum. Alar resection is done for alar flare or a widened alar base.

Spreader grafts are cartilage grafts placed in a submuco-perichondrial pocket parallel to the dorsal septal margin and medial to the free edge of the upper lateral cartilage. They are designed to hold the upper lateral cartilage from the septum.

Other procedures which may need to be carried out include septoplasty, turbinectomy, and graft harvest. Where grafts are required, the nasal septum is the preferred donor. Auricular and rib cartilage may be also used.

Closure
5/0 rapid absorbable suture for mucosa and 6/0 nylon to skin. Taping (Steristrips) to nose and internal and external splints.

Post-operative
Splints remain for 1 week, suture removal at 5 days.

Complications
- Resulting from the procedure:
  - Bleeding (1–4%).
  - Infection (2–3%).
  - Distorted sense of smell.
  - Sinusitis.
  - Septal perforation.
  - Prolonged swelling.
  - Sensory disturbance to nose or anterior upper incisors.
- Undesirable aesthetic sequelae:
  - Under- or over-correction.
  - Lateral deviation.
  - Supra-tip deformity.
  - Contour irregularities.
  - Palpable osteotomy site(s).
  - Nasal vestibule webbing.
  - Nasal valving.
  - Nasal asymmetry.

The reported revision rate of rhinoplasties is up to 18%.

Reference
Sheen JH (1984). *Plast Reconstr Surg* **73**, 230–9.

Submucous resection

Also known as septoplasty or septal cartilage graft harvest.

Airway obstruction
Caused by:
- Septal deviation.
- Enlarged or persistently congested inferior tubinates.
- Polyps.
- Internal valve collapse.
- External valve collapse.
- Rhinitis.

Definition
Submucous resection (SMR) as initially described by Freer and Killian (1902–1904) included resection of the septal cartilage and bone (vomer and ethmoid), retaining the dorsal and caudal margin for nasal bridge, tip and columella support. SMR is now synonymous with septoplasty, which is a more conservative resection of limited areas of the septal cartilage alone. The zone resected is usually limited to the buckled area. The dorsum and caudal struts are retained.

Indications
- An adjunct to rhinoplasty when the septum is deviated causing nasal obstruction.
- May be performed as a sole procedure for nasal obstruction caused by a deviated septum, or to harvest septal cartilage for graft.
- Occasionally indicated in chronic epistaxis as a deviated septum can obstruct view of the bleeding point or cause air turbulence, leading to drying and cracking of mucosa.

Septal deviation
- Congenital or growth related? Related to trauma, micro trauma.
- Trauma with septal fracture in any plane.

Procedure
Local anesthetic with adrenaline injection and cocaine pledgets or spray.

Incision
Incise vertically on the convex side of the septum about 0.5–1 cm posterior to anterior margin septum (Killian incision). If the anterior septum is also buckled, then the septum can be approached via the transfixion incision that has been made posterior to the columella for exposure in the closed rhinoplasty approach. If an open rhinoplasty or no rhinoplasty is being performed, this can be a hemi-transfixion incision through one mucosa and the septum, leaving the opposite mucosa intact. In an open rhinoplasty the septum can also be approached from the dorsum. If a transfixion or dorsal incision is used, the septal resection must still leave dorsal and anterior struts for support!

Dissection/resection

Dissect the mucosa from the cartilage in the subperichondral plane. This is assisted by hydrodissection with local anaesthesia with adrenaline. Carefully incise through the septum to the other side but not through the contralateral mucosa. Place this incision 1 cm posterior to the anterior margin of the septum. Leave a 1 cm dorsal strut as well. Dissect the opposite (concave side) perichondrium and mucosa from the septal cartilage. Then resect the septal cartilage in the area of deformity using scissors or a swivel knife (Ballenger knife). This cartilage can be reversed or remodelled by scoring and replaced, but more commonly is discarded. The cartilage can be minimally resected in the caudal margin and the majority left in place but remodelled by scoring.

The mucosa is closed with absorbable sutures. Small mucosal holes can be left to heal provided that they are not directly opposed, creating a through-and-through perforation. Large holes or through perforations are closed with mucoperichondral flaps. One or two through-and-through sutures are used to quilt the mucoperichondrium to prevent septal haematoma.

The nasal cavity is packed lightly for 24 hr, or until discharge.

Complications

Early
- Septal haematoma: needs to be drained to prevent cartilage necrosis.
- Epistaxis.
- CSF leak due to damage to cribriform plate; usually self-resolves.
- Infection.

Late
- Persistent nasal obstruction.
- Synaechiae between septum and turbinates.
- Septal perforation.
- Collapse of septal bridge (dorsal saddle deformity).
- Retraction of columella.
- Drooping tip.
- Alar widening.
- Anosmia.

Facelift

Definition
Rhytidectomy is the surgical rejuvenation of the ageing face.

Classification
According to the plane of dissection and structures addressed.

Indications
Ageing face, facial palsy. Deep lines such as deep nasolabial folds are not removed by facelift.

Pathophysiology
Causes
- Photo-ageing.
- Developmental laxity.
- Atrophy of underlying structures.

Signs of an ageing face
- Descent brows.
- Deepening glabellar furrows.
- Horizontal forehead lines (attempt to elevate brow).
- Nasolabial folds.
- Descent of cheek skin and fat to overlie the mandible, forming jowls.
- Banding of the anterior neck due to laxity of skin and muscle.
- Vertical lines around the lip.
- Longer upper lip.
- Corner of mouth turns down.
- Lips thin.

Patient assessment
Clearly define the patient's concerns and ask the patient to prioritize them:
- What does the patient want to achieve?
- Have they got realistic expectations?
- Why is the patient doing this?
- Are they doing this for someone else?

History
Particularly to include smoking (12 times increased risk of skin necrosis), NSAID use, hypertension, and any haematological defect which may increase bleeding risk.

Examination
- Must take in the whole face.
- Look for any signs of asymmetry, however small, and point them out to the patient.
- Assess the skin quality and wrinkles. Is any adjunctive resurfacing procedure required?
- Assess the soft tissues, looking for laxity of the support structures of the face.
- Look at fat deposition and determine whether liposuction will be required (neck) or fat augmentation needed (malar and lips).

- Assess the underlying skeleton. Would mentoplasty, mandibular osteotomy, malar implants, or advancement assist?
- Systematically examine the face starting at the forehead and finishing with the neck. Will adjunctive brow, eyelid, or neck lift be required? How are the nasolabial folds and perioral wrinkles?
- Adjust the patient's face to see which direction of pull will create the desired effect and make a note of it.
- Discuss goals of surgery with patient, including photographs and a realistic expectation of results.

Anatomy

A detailed knowledge of facial anatomy is required. The superficial musculoaponeurotic system (SMAS), a continuous fibromuscular layer investing and interlinking the muscles of facial expression with fibrous septa that extend through fat to attach to dermis (Mitz and Peyronie 1976) (term coined by Tessier) is continuous with the platysma and superficial parotid fascia lying over the parotid gland. The facial nerve vertically approaches the skin 1 cm below and anterior to base ear and branches deep to the SMAS. Facial nerve branches lie beneath this, apart from the frontal branch which is almost periosteal at the level of the zygomatic arch, then it lies in SMAS as it crosses zygomatic arch, and then between two layers of temperoparietal fascia over the forehead. BEWARE frontal nerve 1 cm lateral to lateral eyebrow, and marginal mandibular 1 cm below mandible, crossing jaw with the facial vessels.

Anaesthetic

Can be LA (usually with sedation) or GA.

- *Incision* Extends from temporal region to post-auricular/occipital or a part thereof (Fig. 20.8).
- *Temporal* 2–3 mm within the hairline.
- *Prehelical* Curved incision parallel to the helix within the colour change area of helix–face junction.
- *Tragal* May be pre- or post-tragal. Pre-tragal leads to easy access and closure. However, if significant skin excision predicted, colour mismatch is likely as colour and texture of the skin change towards the nose. Post-tragal proves slightly more difficult for access and closure; however, the scar is more hidden. Surgery may advance hair-bearing skin onto tragus and this is overcome by excision and electrocautery to hair bulbs on the underside of the skin; tension must be avoided.
- *Ear lobe* 2–3 mm distant from the inferior edge of the earlobe to avoid a webbed deformity.
- *Post-auricular* Within the retro-auricular sulcus towards occiput. At level of tragus, a posterior direction of incision. If >1.5 cm of skin excision is predicted, the direction should follow the hairline; otherwise a straight posterior extension should be used.

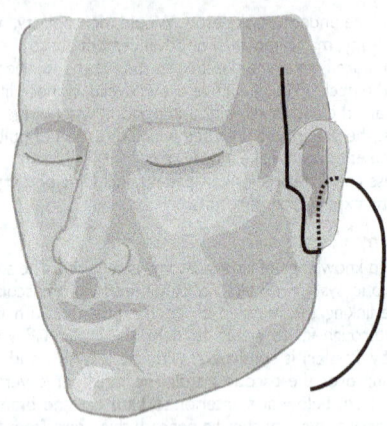

Fig. 20.8 Facelift incision.

Procedure

Dissection proceeds subcutaneously, elevating a skin flap with 2–3 mm of subcutaneous fat as far forward as the anterior edge of the parotid. Continue down into the neck, avoiding the greater auricular nerve which lies in the mid-portion of the sternocleidomastoid 6.5 cm below the external auditory meatus. The SMAS–platysma can be addressed in several ways: excision, plication, imbrication (folding back onto itself and suturing). Imbrication has the benefit of augmenting the zygomatic arch as well as providing a SMAS lift. Plication has a similar lifting effect, without the benefit of the zygomatic arch augmentation but with a lower complication rate as regards nerve injury. For SMAS excision, start 1 cm anterior to the tragus. From this point incise horizontally for ~3 cm parallel to the zygoma and extend distally up to 5 cm below the lower border of the mandible. Taking care to avoid the marginal branch of the facial nerve and the external jugular vein, pull the SMAS upwards and excise the excess. Then close the SMAS. With all techniques of addressing the SMAS, the correct vector of pull on the SMAS is important to give the desired result. This will produce a lift not only to the face but also to the neck.

Neck procedure is done once the SMAS–platysma flaps have been sutured. Liposuction subcutaneously and subplatysma may be sufficient. However, a 3 cm submental incision, splitting the platysma in the midline, allows direct fat excision. The platysma can then be resected if excess, or closed or imbricated if more fullness is required.

Tension-free **skin closure** is the goal and has been helped by the addition of the SMAS suture. Ensure that the head is in a neutral position. Place the temple suture and the occipital suture. Advance the skin flap over the ear. Mark and trim the excess. Closure with subcuticular sutures. Drains are usually used and come out in post-auricular incision.

Post-operative care

Strict care not to compress the facial flaps, which leads to necrosis. Avoidance of excessive neck flexion or head turning. Minimize increased head and neck venous pressure (e.g. by coughing, straining, and bending over). Dressings should be minimal to allow for observation and to limit pressure. Removal of sutures at 7–10 days.

Complications

- Haematoma.
- Facial nerve injury.
- Sensory nerve injury (greater or lesser auricular).
- Wound dehiscence, skin necrosis (1% chance) or slough.
- Alopecia.
- Infection.
- Asymmetry.
- Windswept appearance.
- Hypertrophic scars.
- Little lumpy bits under skin—take time to settle.
- Ear lobe deformities such as webbing.
- Prolonged oedema or ecchymosis.
- Submental depressions.

Other facelift techniques

Skoog raised the SMAS as a composite with the skin flap, which has the benefit of augmenting the skin flap blood supply. However, the disadvantage is a more limited skin re-draping than if the SMAS layer is dissected separately. SMAS lift gives excellent neck and jawline but can deepen nasolabial fold because the skin not pulled up, and this was why the deep plane facelift was developed. However, other techniques are safer.

A face lift is a two-layer procedure. It can be likened it to a sheet and blanket. Cannot just tidy sheet. Have to turn down sheet and tidy blanket. Therefore dissect subcutaneous to nasolabial fold and pull skin, and under this pull the SMAS.

- SMAS plication is the goal of the minimal access cranial suspension (MACS) lift, which also benefits from a shorter scar. In this technique the SMAS is suspended with non-absorbable sutures. Can be compared with the S' lift—little undermining, two sutures to plicate the SMAS. Benefits from being very quick to do and quick to recover, but does not last.
- Subperiosteal facelift.
- Composite and deep plane facelift (Hamra 1992).
- Circum-oral rejuvenation: take out triangular upper corner of mouth; lip lift rarely indicated; may need to inject fat or other filler for volume.
- Nasolabial fold: elevate and lift skin, inject fat or other filler.

Secrets of success

- Keep it simple.
- Pre-plan.
- Pick your patients.

References

Mitz V, Peyronie M (1976). *Plast Reconstr Surg* **58**, 80–8.
Hamra ST (1992). *Plast Reconstr Surg* **90**, 1–13.

Augmentation of the facial skeleton

Implants can be used to improve facial proportions or reconstruct defects. Implants may be autologous tissue, allogeneic or alloplastic material.

Indications
Congenital
- Cosmetic.
- Congenital facial clefts.
- Cleft lip and palate:
  - Alveolar bone grafts.
  - Alar base augmentation.
- Hemifacial microsomia.
- Craniofacial syndromes:
  - Pierre Robin sequence—chin hypoplasia.
  - Crouzon's and Apert's syndrome—mid-face hypoplasia.

Acquired
- Trauma:
  - Orbital floor.
  - Nose.
  - Malar.
- Radiotherapy in childhood causing bony hypoplasia or osteo-radionecrosis.
- Romberg's disease (progressive hemifacial atrophy).
- Treacher Collins syndrome, Crouzon's syndrome.
- First and second branchial arch syndrome.
- Cosmetic (ageing):
  - Genioplasty (described in next section).
  - Malar augmentation.
  - Nose augmentation (bridge or tip).

Complications
- Infection.
- Malplacement leading to mobility and asymmetry.
- Nerve injury.
- Ectropion: lower lid or lip.
- Seroma.
- Demineralization of bone.
- Corneal injuries.
- Contour imperfection (in the chin leading to genio-mandibular sulcus).
- Extrusion or exposure of the implant.
- Asymmetry if bilateral implants.
- Over/under-correction.

Malar and cheek augmentation

Cosmetic implants to increase the prominence and projection of the cheekbones. are the most common reason for augmentation in the face. However, not infrequently, cheek defects from hemifacial atrophy are treated with free tissue transfer of omentum or dermal fat flaps. More recently, buccal hollowing from antiretroviral medication has instigated a range of procedures to correct this deformity, the most common being injectable alloplastic augmentation.

Anatomy of the malar region
The prominence of the malar is formed by the maxilla and zygoma. The infra-orbital foramen is 1 cm below the infra-orbital rim in line with pupil, emitting the infra-orbital nerve.

Profile evaluation and planning
Reference lines such as the zero meridian. Radiographs and cephalometric studies can be used to quantify lack of projection but more commonly this is done with the use of 1:1 photographs (AP and lateral). MRI and 3D CT scans can also be useful. A trial prosthesis (moulage) can be used to size and site the implant.

Implants
Commonly silicone, but Gore-Tex, Medpor, Mersilene, and autologous bone or cartilage are also used.

Malar implant procedure
Intra-oral approach
Create a 2–3 cm incision through the buccal mucosa in the upper buccal sulcus perpendicular to the upper first premolar tooth. Go through the periosteum of the maxilla. Create a subperiosteal pocket just large enough for the implant.

Subciliary
Similar to a lower lid blepharoplasty skin–skin/muscle stepped incision. Then down to infra-orbital rim and proceed sub-periosteally.

Facelift
Through the facelift incisions as an adjunct to facelift. This is the favoured approach for free tissue transfer, allowing access to the defect and the facial or pre-auricular vessels for anastomosis.

BEWARE of the zygomatic branch which is vulnerable in the oral and rhytidectomy approach, the frontal nerve which is vulnerable in the pre-auricular and temporal approaches, and the infra-orbital nerve which is vulnerable in all approaches.

Genioplasty

Techniques to alter the shape and prominence of the chin.
- Options to increase the prominence of the chin:
  - Alloplastic implant.
  - Autograft implant—bone/cartilage.
  - Sliding advancement osteotomy.
- Options to reduce the prominence of the chin:
  - Resection or sliding recession osteotomy.

Anatomy
Mandibular region
- Mental foramen is 2.5–3.5 cm lateral to the midline, 1.2–1.8 mm above the inferior mandibular border and directly beneath the second premolar. The mental nerve is directed supra-medially.
- The central mentum is the area between the two mental foramen. Implants here increase AP projection.
- Mid-lateral mandibular: mental foramen to mid-point between angle to mental tubercle. Implants here increase the breadth of the lower third of the face.
- Postero-lateral mandibular: posterior third of mandible to the angle, and including the inferior third of the ascending ramus. Implants here modify posterior jaw contour and can be isolated or extended to include central or lateral.
- Submental: space below anatomical border of the mandible. Implants here increase the vertical dimension of the lower third of the face and the contour of the mandible.

Profile evaluation and planning
Reference lines such as the zero meridian. Radiographs and cephalometric studies can be performed to quantify lack of projection but more commonly this is done with the use of 1:1 photographs (AP and lateral).
A trial prosthesis (moulage) can be used.

Chin implants
- Commonly silicone, but Gore-Tex, Medpor, Mersilene, and autologous bone or cartilage are also used.
- Ousterhoudt (1975) extended implants, increased lateral breadth, and overcame adjacent jawline contour defect associated with isolated central mental augmentation. The projection increase ranges from 4–9 mm. These implants, known as revision D, have little or no central projection but 5–8 mm projection 2.5–4 cm lateral to the midline.
- Genio-mandibular sulcus: this is a groove lateral to the central mental projection. It can be secondary to the ageing face, due to lateral jowl, or secondary to isolated central mental augmentation.

Approaches

Mandibular

Submental

Reserved for cases when incision is otherwise planned for this area, i.e. platysmaplasty, or if excessive technical difficulty is anticipated. There is a decreased infection risk as all approaches and dissection are extra-oral. Dissection continues to a pre-mandibular subperiosteal plane. Ensure that the pocket is created over cortical bone (not dento-alveolar). The periosteum is lifted with an elevator laterally; care is taken around the mental foramen to displace the nerves in their tough sheath. Fingers placed inferior to the mandible prevent the formation of a false tunnel and also protect against the risk of marginal mandibular nerve injury. A false tunnel can lead to contour problems, asymmetry, and persistent implant mobility. Centralization of the implant is aided by careful posterior palpation and utilization of a blue line marking the midline of the implant. Care should be taken to ensure that no twist or buckling occurs.

Intra-oral approach.

Central transverse incision 1.5–2.5 cm long, 1 cm from the inferior labial sulcus with scissors. Vertical separation through the median raphe of musculature to periosteum. The subperiosteal plane is then developed laterally through this vertical incision, sweeping in an upward direction and using the contralateral fingers to protect and direct from the inferior mandibular border. The implant is carefully placed with regard to midline and twist, and is securely held in place by the overlying musculature.

Outcome of implants

Polytetrafluoroethylene carbon (Proplast) (Whitaker 1987):
- 176 implants over 6 years for malar augmentation.
- Infection 2.3%.
- Implant removal or reposition 8.5%.

Tips

- Placement of the chin implant depends on the distance between lip and chin: if short, place the implant lower and vice versa.
- Malocclusion or marked microgenia is best treated by osteotomy.
- In intra-oral insertion there is a tendency for the implant to be placed too high, especially in the short mandible.
- Be wary in those with a shallow sulcus, as there may be loss of the labiomental fold or the production of a palpable mass in labial sulcus.

Horizontal (transverse) advancement osteotomy (Hofer 1942)

Principle is to osteotomize the lower anterior mandible and slide forward: jumping or sliding advancement genioplasty.

Procedure
- GA or LA with sedation.
- Intra-oral degloving exposure.
- Limited subperiosteal dissection.
- Oscillating saw: mark bone midline osteotomy.
- Be careful of tooth roots and the mental nerve.
- Fixation: wires (three), miniplates, or screws.
- Bone grafting may be required for large movements.

References
Whitaker LA (1987). *Plast Reconstr Surg* **80**, 337–46.

Body contouring

Body contouring surgery is performed to remove excess skin and fat and improve the patients body contour.

According to Regnault and Daniel (1984), 'the fundamental principle of total body contouring is the excision of as much redundant tissue as possible with minimal undermining and moderate tension'. Tension can be reduced by repairing or suspending the superficial fascial system. The length of incision should be as great as required to remove the excess.

- **Causes** of excess skin and fat include obesity, weight loss, pregnancy, post-traumatic defect, congenital deformity.
- **Classified** as skin only or skin and fat: localized, regional, or generalized.

Pathophysiology

As people age, fat accumulates and redistributes. Fat accumulates not by an increase in the number of cells, as these stop replicating at puberty, but by an increase in individual fat cell size. Fat accumulates on the abdomen and flanks in men, and on the abdomen, hips, and thighs in women.

Most fat is supplied by vertical perforators that travel with vertical fascial septa. Lockwood (1991) described the superficial fascial system (SFS) as a horizontal layer of fascia in the fat which interconnects with the vertical septa. Its function is to support and shape the fat. Lifting and securing the SFS can help the lifting and reduce tension on the skin. Lockwood also describes zones of adherence of the SFS which, if not released, prevent the transmission of the tension of the lift and reduce the result. Zones of adherence are the upper abdomen, medial thigh, and lateral thigh.

Cellulite is the result of extrusion of subcutaneous fat into the reticular dermis, and distension by fat and tethering of the superficial fascial system of radial and longitudinal fibres. Primary cellulite occurs with obesity, and secondary cellulite from laxity after weight loss or liposuction (the stretched skin ligaments sag and hang due to gravity). The pattern of connective tissue differs between males and females. Males have more radial fibres and so fat deposits are different. Women have a diffuse pattern of regular and discontinuous connective tissue immediately below the dermis, but this is smooth and continuous in men. As the fascia cannot be removed by liposuction, the only way to remove cellulite is by direct excision of the involved area.

Patient assessment

History

Ascertain the exact areas of concern and the patient's goals; weight loss and gain, dieting, eating disorders; pregnancy history and family history in relation to skin disorders and laxity; smoking. Avoid operating on smokers.

Examination
Weigh and assess BMI. Do not operate on the obese or those with fluctuating weight. Patients who have had gastric banding/bypass surgery should have had a stable weight for 6 months. Assess the body as a whole, as reduction in one area can make a deformity elsewhere seem worse. Assess the skin for striae and tone. Record areas of fat deposition.

Investigations
Gastric bypass/band patients require a full dietetic assessment and bloods before proceeding to surgery.

Management
- Localized deposits are suitable for liposuction.
- Regional and generalized deposits, especially those with redundant skin are best suited to excision and redistribution of adjacent skin and fat into defect.
- Plan a staged approach if multiple problems. If doing an abdominoplasty do this with/without a thigh and buttock lift before a medial thigh lift.
- Regnault and Daniel (1984) based their approach on the location of the major redundancy. If it is anterior, perform an abdominoplasty. If anterolateral, a 'batwing torso lipectomy that incorporates a thoracobrachioplasty is performed'. A circular deformity requires a 'sloping ring belt lipectomy'.

Contraindications
- Obesity.
- Smoking.
- Unrealistic expectations.
- Vascular disease.
- Lymphoedema.
- Comorbidity.

Complications
Serious complications death, DVT, PE, fat embolus occur in less than 0.1%. Major wound necrosis in 3%. Minor complications are more likely (20%). Haematoma, seroma requiring frequent aspirations, minor wound healing problems, wound dehiscence, suture spit, infection, irregularity, poor scarring (wide or hypertrophic), numbness, dog ears, asymmetry, lymphoedema. Rate of complications linked to BMI.

References
Regnault P, Daniel R (1984). *Aesthetic Plastic Surgery*. Little Brown, Boston, MA.
Lockwood TE (1991). *Plast Reconstr Surg* **87**, 1009–18.

Arm reduction

A body contouring technique directed at improving arm contour, especially to correct 'batwing arms'. Described originally by Correa-Iturraspe and Fernandez (1954), from the 1970s onwards there have been numerous revisions and improvements, most recently by Lockwood (1995).

Indications
Moderate or severe skin laxity of arms extending from the olecranon to the axillary fold with or without fat excess.

Aims
Restore arm contour with a hidden scar and normal axilla.

Planning
Patient sitting with arms abducted 90° and elbows flexed 90°. Pinch the inferior dependent fold of skin, estimating the possible width of skin that could be excised. A vertical ellipse of redundant tissue is marked leaving the scar in the bicipital groove or more posteriorly. In moderate to severe cases the excision will extend to the medial epicondyle. The excess in the axilla is dealt with by a T-plasty, fish tail, L-plasty, or Z-plasty closure, the medial limb of which sits at the axillary fold. General anaesthetic, supine, free draped arms below the elbows, arms 90° abducted.

Incision
Along markings do axillary and inferior arm incision only as intraoperative modification is possible, particularly in varying the length of the arm excision.

Procedure
Remove the skin and subcutaneous fat down to the axillary fascia. Deepen the arm incision through the superficial fascia system (SFS). Raise the tissue to be resected in the sub-SFS plane using a combination of blunt and sharp dissection. Minimal undermining. Before resecting the excess skin on the arm, temporarily suspend the SFS off the axillary fascia. This may lead to an adjustment in the amount of tissue to be removed from the arm. Final tailoring of the excess to be removed from the arm. Drains.

Closure
Superficial fascial closure starts in the axilla with 1/0 non-absorbable sutures, 3/0 absorbable to dermis, and 4/0 absorbable to skin.

Postoperative care
Bulky dressings and bandages from hands to axillae initially. Once wounds are healed, light compression garments for 2–4 weeks with gradual return to normal activity, avoiding abduction initially.

Complications
- Damage to axillary structures: lymphatics, veins and nerves.
- Wound: dehiscence secondary to necrosis, or infection.
- Scars: widening, prominence or hypertrophy.
- Asymmetry.
- Over/under-correction.
- Contour deformity due to over resection in the centre and under resection proximally and distally.
- Transverse cutaneous folds.
- Lymphoedema.

References
Correa Iturraspe M, Fernandez JC (1954). *Prensa Med Argent* **41**, 2432–6.
Lockwood T (1995). *Plast Reconstr Surg* **96**, 912–20.

Abdominoplasty

Operative procedure to reduce the over-hanging fat or redundant lower abdominal wall. Commonly known as a 'tummy tuck'.

Assessment
A careful review is necessary to advise as to the correct operation and prevent post-operative disappointment

History
Delineate the exact patient concerns. Current medication, coexisting disease, previous abdominal surgery or pregnancy, and smoking history are important in determining what you offer to the patient. Ensure that weight and health are stable in a weight-loss patient.

Examination
Calculate the BMI. Assess the quality of the skin, including its elasticity, scars, striae, and stretch marks, and the amount of overhang in both the lying and standing position. Test for pre-existing patches of numbness. Determine where the excess fat lies on the abdomen. Examine for any hernias, especially umbilical, and the degree of divarication of the rectus muscles. Point out any existing asymmetry.

Avoid operating on the obese, smokers and those with significant comorbidities. Ideally, smoking should cease 6 weeks and oral contraceptive medication 4 weeks pre-operatively.

Options
- *Liposuction* alone: this is a good option if the skin quality and muscle tone are good, and the overhang is minimal.
- *Mini-abdominoplasty*: if the laxity and excess is lower abdominal, with good contour in the upper abdomen, this is a good option. It can be combined with liposuction to the upper abdomen if fat excess is the only problem in this area.
- *Formal abdominoplasty*: where laxity exists over the whole abdomen this is the operation of choice. Some authors will do limited liposuction of the abdominal pannus in conjunction with this operation. However, this is risky, increases the complication rate and should only be done in a conservative manner by experienced surgeons.
- *Combined procedures*: any of the above can be done in conjunction with liposuction to hip rolls or flanks, or extended as a belt lipectomy or thigh lift.
- *Apronectomy*: excision of the abdominal apron without undermining or redistribution of the remaining abdominal skin and fat or plication of the recti. Used in higher-risk patients as this is a less traumatic and quicker procedure, with a lower incidence of complications, particularly wound problems.

Operation
- *Aims* To improve the contour and external appearance of the abdomen with a well-placed scar and a natural umbilical appearance.

- **Indications** Excess abdominal wall skin and subcutaneous tissue with or without musculo-aponeurotic laxity.
- **Planning** Pre-operatively plan the areas requiring excision, which will determine the excision (abdominoplasty) design. Mark the incision with the patient standing and lying. Ensure that it lies under the patient's favoured underwear. Measure and check for symmetry. Take photographs. Subcutaneous heparin and TED stockings; GA, catheter. Intraoperatively prepare and drape the patient from above xiphisternum to upper thighs. IV antibiotics. Pneumatic foot or calf compressors. Position the patient on the operating table so as to be able to 'break' or bend the table at the hips to de-tension the inferior abdominal skin closure. Tattoo or mark the midline.
- **Incision** A variety of incision designs, mostly variations on a curved suprapubic extending laterally. Rarely, a superior subcostal incision is used for upper abdominal laxity. Most common incision modification is the transverse suprapubic with lateral extensions in an open W design (Regnault 1975). The lateral extensions can be continued posteriorly in the case of a belt lipectomy or truncal resection, giving a body lift. The other common design is the inverted T or fleur-de-lys pattern which can be used for excess medial tissue resection (Castañares and Goethel). A circular incision around the umbilicus is used, and a semi-circle (smile), V, or linear incision is made to reset the umbilicus in the repositioned abdominal skin.

Procedure

The incision is made vertically through to the abdominal muscle fascia. The abdominal pannus is raised off the anterior abdominal wall in the supra-fascial plane as far as the costal margin and xiphoid process, taking care to isolate and preserve the umbilical stalk. Diathermy the perforating vessels above the rectus sheath as they can retract into the rectus muscle causing bleeding. Musculo-aponeurotic laxity (divarication) is addressed by plication of the rectus sheath in the midline with non-absorbable sutures (0 nylon), taking care not to render the umbilicus ischaemic. The sutures are placed in the anterior rectus sheath anterior to the rectus muscle, so pulling the rectus together Particular attention should be paid to the depth of sutures, as this should be solely within the anterior rectus sheath, hence avoiding intra-abdominal perforation. This may be interrupted figure-of-eight sutures or a running suture. Redrape the abdominal skin with slight caudal traction and flexion of the hips and excise the excess. Refashion the umbilicus in the midline at the level of the upper part of the iliac crest.

Closure

Close the skin over suction drains starting with Scarpa's fascia (2/0 absorbable); then use a layered skin closure with absorbable sutures. Pleat the superior skin excess into the lower abdominal skin, creating most of the rucking in the suprapubic zone. Occasionally the umbilical defect is not excised, and must be closed as a vertical midline scar. This sometimes creates an inverted T-scar through which the midline excess of the superior skin can be excised.

Post-operative care

Use knee bolsters or pillows to maintain hip flexion. Commence early mobilization within realms of comfort maintaining a flexed position. Anti-embolic measures should continue until the patient is mobile. Return to light activities in 2–3 weeks; stressful activities and exercise from 4–6 weeks. Longer with muscle plication.

Complications

- Wound problems, including infection, suture spitting, granuloma, minor skin necrosis and dehiscence.
- Dog ears.
- Haematoma or seroma: requires repeat surgery or aspiration.
- Significant skin necrosis and loss: requires 3 months of healing and revisional surgery including SSG.
- Umbilical necrosis.
- Umbilicus too small or too large.
- Asymmetry.
- Numbness of the abdomen or thighs.
- Fat necrosis leading to lumpy abdomen or prolonged discharge.
- Hypertrophic scarring.
- Upward traction of the mons leading to a high pubic hairline and traction on the genitals.
- Necrotizing fasciitis.
- DVT, PE.
- Fat embolus.
- Recurrence of deformity.

References

Castañares S, Goethel JA (1967). *Plast Reconstr Surg* **40**, 378–83.
Lockwood T (1995). *Plast Reconstr Surg* **96**, 603–15.
Pitanguy I (1975). *Clin Plast Surg* **2**, 401–10.
Regnault P (1975). *Plast Reconstr Surg* **55**, 265–74.

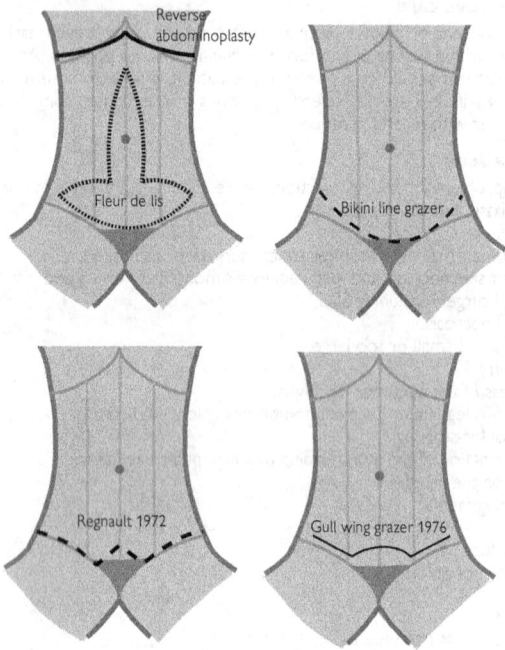

Fig. 20.9 Abdominoplasty incisions.

Thigh and buttock contouring

The original description was by Pitanguy (1964) for the excision of trochanteric fat. Thigh and buttock reduction refers to the excision of skin and fat from the thighs and buttocks with or without resuspension of the superficial fascia system (SFS) in order to improve the contour of the thighs and buttocks.

Indications

Moderate or severe laxity and lipomatosis of trunk/thighs, buttock ptosis, or a combination of the two.

Aims

Resection of excess tissue. Placement of stable aesthetically acceptable scars. This is related to clothing position (e.g. bikini lines) and the areas of excess and lax tissue.

Planning

- Note is taken of the position of intended closure, i.e. final scar placement, and the areas and direction of maximal tissue excess. Thigh-only laxity can be excised as a vertical medial ellipse similar to the brachioplasty in design and procedure.
- Thigh and buttock and flank/abdominal excess and laxity is usually excised in transversely directed ellipses, which are centred on the midlateral lines. Closure of lateral ellipses elevates the thighs and tightens the flanks. Therefore the procedure is sometimes called thigh/flankplasty. These ellipses may coalesce anteriorly or posteriorly or even extend circumferentially (belt lipectomy).
- With the patient standing, an estimate of superior skin resection and inferior skin resection is made and marked (up to 4–5 cm and 10–18 cm, respectively, above and below the bikini line laterally).
- GA with patient laterally placed; hips are flexed to 30°–45° and thighs abducted to 30–45 cm separation at the knees. If liposuction is required, this is carried out first.

Incision

Through the marked incision line and superficial fascia.

Procedure

Undermining continues inferiorly deep to the SFS to release adherence zones. Superiorly only minimal undermining. Distally undermine beyond the tissue to be resected, preserving the tissue over the buttock posteriorly and staying lateral to the femoral triangle anteriorly. Discontinuous cannula undermining is performed more distally if the deformity extends further down the thigh. The redundant tissue is then excised, being careful to leave more skin than SFS as this results in a tension-free skin closure and hence stable scars. The anterior skin incisions often meet across the midline, incorporating an abdominoplasty. Drains.

Closure
Closure of SFS with 1/0 or 2/0 nylon or absorbable suture. Dermis 3/0 and skin 4/0 absorbable suture.

Post-operative care
Hips flexed 15°–20° and thighs abducted for 12 weeks. Return to limited work at 3 weeks, regular activity at 6–10 weeks.

Complications
- Asymmetry.
- Over/under-correction.
- Scar instability or stretch.
- General surgical complications such as dehiscence, infection, haematoma etc.

Reference
Pitanguy I (1964). *Plast Reconstr Surg* **34**, 280–6.

Medial thigh lift

Indications
Medial thigh skin laxity.

Aims
Excess tissue resection and stable aesthetic scars.

Planning
With the patient standing, the extent of medial thigh redundancy is marked distal to the thigh/groin crease. The incision is marked along the perineal thigh crease, posteriorly stopping at the buttock crease. Anteriorly the marking ascends vertically at the pubic tubercle. Assess the need for adjunctive liposuction. General anaesthetic, supine patient, legs free-draped.

Incision
Deep liposuction as indicated. Incision through skin only.

Procedure
Anterior to the pubic tubercle undermine in subcutaneous fat leaving skin flaps approximately 1 cm thick, thus preserving lymphatics. Posterior to the tubercle undermine deep to SFS, superficial to the adductor longus down the thigh for 2–3 cm distal to the planned resection to allow for SFS tensioned closure and therefore de-tensioning skin closure. Skin resection is likely to be 5–7 cm. Colles fascia is identified in the lateral mons pubis. Resect the tissue and anchor the Colles fascia to the thigh SFS. Not usually drained.

Closure
1/0 non-absorbable to fascia; 3/0 dermis and 4/0 skin.

Post-operative care
Light dressings; gradual return to normal activity.

Complications
- Asymmetry.
- Over/under-correction.
- Scar instability.
- Mons pubis lymphoedema and general complications of surgery.
- 35% risk of delayed wound healing; worse if combined with other procedures or if liposuction used in thigh.

Further reading
Lockwood TE (1988). *Plast Reconstr Surg* **82**, 299–304.
Lockwood TE (1991). *Plast Reconstr Surg* **87**, 1019–27.

Calf augmentation

Definition
Subcutaneous implant-based augmentation to improve the aesthetic quality of the leg. Initial report of six cases (Carlssen 1979).

Classification
Medial, lateral, or total.

Indications
- Augmentation of a hypoplastic limb, e.g. secondary to trauma, polio, or scleroderma.
- Cosmetic augmentation.

Planning
Implant placement is usually in a subfascial plane. More recent reports have placed the implants in a submuscular plane below gastrocnemius or soleus, but these are very small series. GA, lateral or prone position. Prone is preferable for bilateral placement.

Incision
Popliteal crease transverse 4 cm.

Procedure
Dissect through fat and incise popliteal fascia. Continue with blunt dissection in a bloodless subfascial plane to form the implant pocket. Similarly, the lateral pocket can be created by dissecting from the original incision lateral to the median raphe and hence producing distinct pockets. Ensure the implants are flat against gastrocnemius and not folded or buckled. Layered closure as indicated.

In the grossly hypoplastic limb a tissue expander may be required which is larger than standard augmentation implants. Pocket dissection is as above but placement of the implant is aided by the use of a Keith needle and the suture is tied to the distal pole of the implant. This allows appropriate careful distal implant placement. The needle is then advanced through the skin and removed, and the sutures are cut under tension.

Post-operative
12–24 hr bed rest and elevation. Compression hosiery for 4–6 weeks post-operatively.

Complications
- Compromised skin vascularity secondary to inappropriate pocket dissection superficial to the deep fascia, or too large an implant.
- Compartment syndrome.
- Infection.
- Extrusion.
- Wound dehiscence.
- Incorrect implant placement, i.e. position or buckling.
- Migration due to inadequate or excessive pocket dissection.
- Sensory change, probably neurapraxia of sural or saphenous nerves, must be closely monitored for compartment syndrome risk.
- Capsular contracture—very rare.

Reference
Carlsen LN (1979). *Ann Plast Surg* **2**, 508–10.

Liposuction

Definition
Suction-aided subcutaneous fat removal.

Classification
- Deep (leaving 8–10 mm of superficial fat) or superficial (leaving 2–4 mm of superficial fat).
- Syringe suction or machine suction.
- Ultrasound assisted, mechanically assisted, or manual.
- Dry, wet, super-wet, or tumescent.

Principles
Removal of fat cells in a region by mechanical trauma and suction to restore aesthetic contour with avoidance of superficial irregularity and asymmetry.

Uses
- Minimal to moderate localized fat deposits not managed by diet or exercise under areas of minimal skin laxity and good skin elasticity.
- As an adjunct to reconstructive surgery, particularly of the breast.
- To reduce bulky fat fasciocutaneous flaps.

Indications
- Cosmetic removal of fat, alone or as an adjunct to other surgery (e.g. abdominoplasty or facelift).
- Lipomas.
- Flap contouring.
- Harvesting for fat injection/graft.
- Gynaecomastia.
- Breast reduction.
- Extravasation injuries.
- Lymphoedema.

History
- Assess patient expectations and areas of concern.
- History of dieting and weight gain/loss.
- Family history of fat deposits distribution.
- Bleeding disorders/bruising history.
- Past operations/trauma/scarring.

Examination
- Record BMI.
- Assess the skin looking for striae, accordinization, pinch test, and retraction speed.
- Look at the fat for the size, location, and extent of fat deposit, pre-existing dimples, waves, and fat fractures.
- Define asymmetry and assess the effect of contracting the underlying muscle on the fat deposits.

Planning
Fully prepared patient with a realistic expectation of results. Goals of treatment established. Pre-operative marking with the patient standing to map out contour irregularities. Show the markings to the patient in the mirror and gain their agreement. Photographs before and after marking. Larger areas require pre-operative FBC and U&E.

Requirements
LA or GA. The appropriate suction cannulae and liposuction system. Large cannulae are faster but are likely to leave more contour defects, so tendency to use smaller cannulae. Pneumatic compression for GA cases or those lasting >1 hr.

Options
Infiltration
- Dry: no wetting solution, historical only.
- Wet: 100–300 mL of wetting solution per area of treatment.
- Superwet: 1 mL of wetting solution per expected 1 mL of aspirate.
- Tumescent: infusion of wetting solution to achieve skin turgor, typically 3 mL per 1 mL of aspirate.

Cannula choice
Single or multiple ostium. Multiple ostium can be basket type or tubular.

Suction choice
- Syringe (Tulip) or wall suction (1 atm).
- US-assisted, mechanical, or manual.

Level of liposuction
Superficial (Gasparotti) or deep.

Wetting solution
Physiological crystalloid, usually normal saline, with adrenaline 1mg/500 000 to 1 mg/million and local anaesthetic such as lidocaine or bupivicaine in the appropriate dose. Lidocaine doses of up to 55 mg/kg have been reported as safe. However, an upper limit of 35 mg/kg is generally used. Peak lidocaine plasma levels occur 8–14 hr after surgery.

Method
After infusion of the wetting solution the suction cannula is introduced through small stab incisions oriented so as to allow passes of the cannula through the area to be treated. Some advocate pre-tunnelling, i.e. passing the cannula through the tissues to be treated without suction at first.

Cross-tunnelling is the concept of treating an area in more than one direction. Feathering is the treatment of the periphery of the area in order to achieve a smooth transition into untreated areas.

Liposuction
Pass the cannula backwards and forwards through the fat deposit in centrifugal rays from the incision and in different planes (fan technique). Have the cannula tip aperture pointed deep. Classically liposuction addresses the deep fat plane. However, superficial liposuction has been

advocated (Gasparotti 1992). Care must be taken not to create skin dimpling or visible tunnel depressions when superficial to the fascia. Pinching the skin during surgery assesses the amount removed. Check the fat aspirate (yellow, pink, red) and move to a new tunnel when the aspirate becomes more blood-stained.

US-assisted liposuction

Adopts US energy to disrupt the adipose tissue and emulsify it. This can be delivered externally or internally, and is usually 1 MHz. US energy is thought to work by three mechanisms: cavitation, micromechanical disruption, and thermal damage.
- External: the energy is delivered via a probe, which should be moved continuously in a circular motion over the skin to avoid over-treatment and complications due to overheating. The emulsified fat is then evacuated either by syringe or vacuum.
- Internal: the energy is delivered via dedicated probes, or more commonly via hollow cannulae, and probably works mainly by cavitation. Complications include the need for larger incisions for access to reduce local thermal injury and skin injury by 'tip hits'.

The emulsified fat is usually removed via the hollow shell of the cannula. The increased risk of seroma as well as the incidence of thermal injury has led to these techniques being less commonly practised than when they first appeared. (At the time of writing the sale of US-assisted devices is no longer licensed in the UK).

Mechanically assisted liposuction

A cannula is mechanically moved forwards and backwards, typically by 2–4 mm. This mimics the movement of the surgeon, consequently amplifying the effects. The side-effect profile appears to be the same as for standard liposuction techniques and therefore would appear to be preferable.

Coleman liposuction system

A centrifuge is used to spin down the fat after removal, it can then be used for re-injection to augment other areas. The centrifuge treatment aims to prolong the duration of this augmentation. Access incisions can often be closed with Steristrips alone.

Post-operative care
- Meticulous monitoring of volume status (urinary catheterization, non-invasive haemodynamic monitoring, communication with anaesthetist). After large volume liposuction (>2 L) patients should have their fluid balance and FBC monitored for 24 hr.
- Compression garments worn for at least 6 weeks; preferably 3 months for the best results.

Complications

- Early:
  - Shock from third-space fluid shifts and losses or less likely blood loss.
  - Bleeding requiring open drainage.
  - Haematoma or seroma.
  - Swelling.
  - Thermal injury (particularly with US-assisted techniques).
  - Entry/exit friction burns.
  - Liposuction can injure or enter any structure or cavity in the body (e.g. bowel perforation).
  - DVT/PE.
  - Fat emboli.
  - Infection.
  - Skin necrosis.
  - Bruising.
- Late:
  - Surface contour irregularities (furrows, wrinkles and dips)—visible or palpable.
  - Numbness.
  - Discoloration.
  - Asymmetry.
  - Insufficient removal of fat.
  - Over-removal of fat, exaggerating adjacent areas.
  - Lax baggy skin.

Reference

Gasparotti M (1992). *Aesthetic Plast Surg* **16**, 141–53.

Chapter 21

Reconstruction

The reconstructive ladder 728
Direct closure (primary intention) 729
Secondary intention 734

The reconstructive ladder

This is a simple aide memoire for remembering the various options for reconstructing a defect.

The initial plastic surgeons' philosophy was to do the simplest possible treatment, and where this was not possible to proceed up the ladder to the next most complex procedure. The ladder is as follows, from simplest procedure to the most complex:

- Secondary intention healing/conservative treatment:
    - Simple dressings.
    - Vacuum dressing.
- Primary closure.
- Graft:
    - Split-skin graft.
    - Full-thickness skin graft.
    - Composite graft.
- Local tissue transfer.
- Tissue expansion.
- Distant tissue transfer.
- Free tissue transfer.

In modern practice the type of reconstruction depends on an analysis of the following:

- Defect: size, site, depth, exposed structures and function.
- Donor: size, site, function and aesthetics.
- Patient: preferences, expectations, impact on quality of life and systemic health.
- Environment: hospital facilities, post-operative care, complication rate, insurance system.
- Surgeon: ability and preferences.

The reconstructive menu

Many surgeons are opposed to the concept of a 'reconstructive ladder' as it encourages the simplest rather than the optimal reconstructive option. They prefer the concept of a reconstructive menu from which any item can be chosen, allowing personal preference, but like any menu always with a view to the cost and value delivered by each item.

Direct closure (primary intention)

Definition
Opposition of the skin edges of a wound following a full-thickness breach to the skin.

Pathophysiology
See wound healing.

Methods of closure
Suture, staples, glue, tape.

Principles
- If creating the wound:
  - Place the incision in relaxed skin tension lines, muscle contraction or joint creases, or along anatomical boundaries.
- If treating a traumatic wound:
  - Adequate debridement.
  - Clean wound.
  - Possibly reorient wound to favourable lines by Z-plasty/W-plasty.
- Atraumatic technique (do not pinch the wound edges with the forceps as more trauma = more scarring).
- Minimize dead space by closure of fascial layers.
- Tension-free closure of the epidermis (by tension-relieving deep dermal sutures).
- Fat will not relieve tension. Do NOT suture fat to relieve tension. Loose sutures to reduce dead space are OK.
- Eversion of skin edges (so that the eventual scar will be flat).
- Avoid the skin edges overlapping as the waterproof epidermis and contact inhibition will prevent healing.
- To avoid dog ears at the corners ensure that sutures are placed to match the opposing skin edges without translation and to share out any length discrepancy evenly throughout the wound closure. This may be helped by the *halving technique*. Place the sutures in the middle of the wound, halving it, and repeat this until the wound is closed.
- Sutures are a foreign body, so use the least amount of the finest suture possible for the tension.

Sutures
- Absorbable sutures maintain deep wound strength, depending on type, for varying lengths of time from 2 weeks to 6 months. They may be used as individual or continuous deep sutures or as running intra-dermal (subcuticular) sutures.
- Choice of suture depends on strength of suture required, handling characteristics, period the suture is required to act, period for suture to absorb, and further choices regarding needle size and shape.

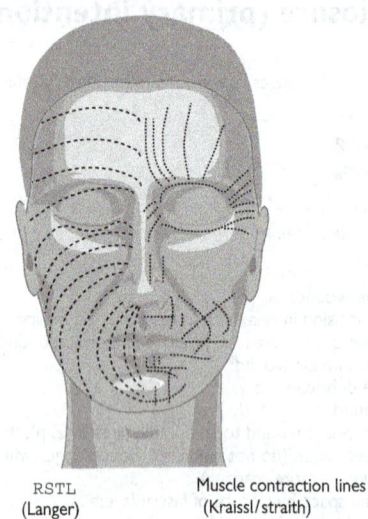

RSTL (Langer)   Muscle contraction lines (Kraissl/straith)

Fig. 21.1 Facial relaxed skin tension lines on the patient's right and muscle contraction creases on the left.

- Non-absorbable sutures are used for skin closure, and are removed once early healing has commenced. They are also used when permanent fixation is needed, such as suspension of tissue or repair of tendons.
- Choice of suture depends on strength of suture required, handling characteristics, colour, braided or monofilament structure and needle choices.

Stitch mechanics
- As they are tied, all interrupted sutures try to assume the shape of a circle as the suture tensions. Entry and exit points will match up as the skin edges are drawn together, emphasizing the need to be exact in the placement of these points.
- Continuous sutures will try to assume a straight line as the suture is tensioned; they will be prevented from this by the interposing tissue, but the resultant tension holds the wound together. Again, entry and exit points will match up as the skin edges are drawn together, emphasizing the need to be exact in the placement of these points.

Method of fascial stitch
- Fascia closure by absorbable suture, either interrupted or continuous.
- Suture strength depends on size and site of fascia.
- Do NOT stitch fat; suture tension causes fat necrosis.

Method of deep dermal stitch

Deep dermal stitch uses an absorbable suture. The knots are buried deep to minimize risk of stitch palpability, abscess and exposure. Use only enough sutures to create eversion and oppose the skin edge.

Start at the deep aspect of the dermis. Take a bite of dermis either vertically or horizontally. Whichever direction is chosen, try to have the bite include some dermis more superficial to the entry point as the needle extends outwards. Go back to the same depth as the entry point as the needle re-enters the wound. This has the effect of everting the wound as the suture is tied. A good suture will evert and draw the skin edges together so that there is no tension at the epidermal edge.

Method of skin stitch

Types of skin stitch

Simple interrupted, vertical mattress, horizontal mattress, half-buried mattress (MacGregor stitch), running, intra-dermal (subcuticular).

Simple interrupted skin closure technique

- The aim is to close the wound with eversion of the wound edges.
- Place the needle through the skin at an angle of 90°, taking a greater quantity of dermis than epidermis.
- Take an equal bite from the other side of the wound.
- The exit point of the needle should be the same distance from the wound surface as the entry portal.
- Sutures should be spread evenly along the length of the wound ~5 mm apart.
- After the suture is tied the wound edges should be just touching to permit post-operative swelling.
- Final tiny adjustments of epidermal alignment can be achieved by knot positioning. The knot side will sit slightly higher as the knot causes the suture circle to have a slight teardrop shape.

Continuous intra-dermal (subcuticular) suture

- The aim is to close the wound with eversion of the wound edges.
- Depending on the suture used a knot may be required to commence the stich.
- The stitch is inserted at the mid to deep level of the dermis.
- As the suture is inserted, the dermal bite should be angled towards the epidermal surface before turning to return to the cut dermal surface at the same level as the entry site.
- Insert the suture in the opposite side at the same level from the epidermal surface as the exit point to ensure accurate opposition of the edges.
- Do not double back, but enter the opposite side directly opposite the exit point.
- Repeat the dermal suture again, angling it towards the surface, before it turns and heads back and deeper to be retrieved at the cut surface.
- In cross-section this looks as if the suture makes a V, U, or keel shape.
- This ensures eversion as the suture tightens and flattens.

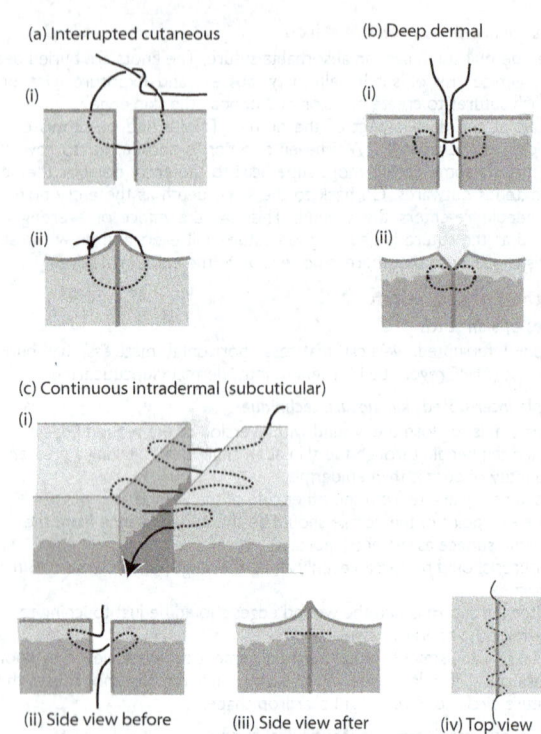

Fig. 21.2 Suture techniques. (a) interrupted cutaneous suture. Note the larger bite of dermis than epidermis, causing eversion as the suture circle closes.
(b) Deep dermal suture. Note the buried knot and the shape of the dermal bite.
(c) continuous intradermal or subcuticular suture. Note the shape of the suture similar to the keel of a boat.

Post-operative care
Secure wound with tape or Steristrip, if possible. Keep dry for 24 hr; then shower not bath. Remove sutures on face after 5–7 days, and elsewhere after 7–14 days; re-secure with tape for a further week. In areas of tension such as the shoulder, tape for 3 months. When healed apply moisturizing cream to scar. Protect from sun for 6 months.

Complications
- Incorrect suture placement can cause failure of primary wound healing.
- Infection, bleeding, and knot or suture failure can cause wound dehiscence, resulting in prolonged healing and more visible scar formation.
- Adverse scarring, producing stretched, hypertrophic, or keloid scars.
- Stitch abscess: sterile or infected.

Suggested protocol
- Face: 5/0 or 6/0 deep medium-acting absorbable suture and 6/0 or 5/0 to skin removed at 7 days. Micropore tape for 2 weeks.
- Body: 3/0 or 4/0 deep medium- to long-acting absorbable suture and 4/0 or 5/0 subcuticular absorbable or non-absorbable (removed at 2 weeks) to skin. Micropore tape for 3 weeks.

Delayed primary closure
Also known as tertiary intention. The wound is initially dressed for a period and sutured later.

Secondary intention

Also known as conservative management.

Definition
This is the process of wound healing when no form of direct closure, graft, or flap is used. Split-skin graft donor sites heal by secondary intention; however, the term has more relevance to a full-thickness area of skin loss that heals by granulation and epithelialization from the edges.

Pathophysiology
See wound healing.

Uses
Certain wounds by preference are left to heal by secondary intention:
- Burns: superficial partial thickness and small areas of deep partial thickness and full thickness burns.
- Trauma: grazes, small areas of skin especially fingertip loss (<1 cm^2).
- Elective: shave excisions, full-thickness excision of small lesions particularly on the nose and inner canthus, after partial take of skin graft, small pre-tibial lacerations.

Advantages
- No surgical intervention, particularly in the frail.
- No scars or minimal scars if a shallow defect.
- No donor defect.

Disadvantages
- Dressings and changes.
- Prolonged healing.
- Risk of infection.

Principles
- The key is the selection of the appropriate injury or lesion and the dressing regime. For some patients the healing time with dressings will be similar to that with surgery and the results will be better.
- Dressings should be chosen to provide a moist comfortable environment whilst being easy to apply and care for. Cost is an important consideration, given the minimal difference a dressing makes in healing time or quality.
- Dressings should be undisturbed as long as possible, provided that they remain intact and comfortable.
- A decision to proceed with secondary intention healing should be an active decision and be reviewed. If it is failing to achieve the desired result, the decision should be reconsidered.

Chapter 22

Flaps

- Flaps *736*
- Flap terminology *739*
- Classification of flaps *741*
- Free tissue transfer *743*
- Lessons in free flap transfers *746*
- Flap monitoring and care *748*
- Advancement flaps *750*
- Pivot flaps *756*
- Rotation flaps *758*
- Distant flaps *760*
- Fascio-cutaneous flaps *762*
- Muscle flaps *764*
- Vascularized bone 'graft' *766*
- Venous drainage in reverse flow flaps *769*
- Venous flaps *771*
- Z-plasty *773*
- W-plasty *776*
- Rhomboid flap *778*
- Dufourmental flap *780*
- Bi-lobed flap *781*
- Horn flap *783*
- Banner flap *785*
- Dorsal nasal flap *787*
- Nasalis flap *789*
- Nasolabial flap *791*
- Cervico-facial flap *793*
- Jejunal flap *795*
- Omental flap *797*
- Lateral arm flap *799*
- Medial arm flap *801*
- Radial forearm flap *803*
- Ulnar forearm flap *806*
- Dorsal ulnar flap *808*
- Posterior interosseous artery flap *810*
- Fingertip flaps *813*
- Kite flap *816*
- Flag flap *819*
- Brunelli dorsal ulnar thumb flap *821*
- Neurovascular island flap *823*
- Cross-finger flap *826*
- Moberg flap *828*
- Thenar flap *830*
- Dorsal finger flaps *832*
- Forehead flaps *835*
- Temporalis flap *839*
- Temporo-parietal flap *841*
- Auriculo-temporal flap *843*
- Delto-pectoral flap *845*
- Pectoralis major flap *847*
- Scapular flap *850*
- Parascapular flap *853*
- Trapezius flap *855*
- Gluteus maximus flap *858*
- Rectus abdominis flap *861*
- VRAM (vertical rectus abdominis myocutaneous) flap *863*
- TRAM (transverse rectus abdominis myocutaneous) flap *865*
- DIEP (deep inferior epigastric perforator) flap *868*
- Latissimus dorsi flap (and TAP flap) *870*
- Serratus anterior flap *873*
- Gracilis *876*
- Groin flap *878*
- DCIA (deep circumflex iliac artery) flap *880*
- TFL (tensor fascia lata) flap *882*
- Anterolateral thigh flap *884*
- Biceps femoris flap *886*
- Soleus *888*
- Medial and lateral gastrocnemius flaps *890*
- Medial plantar flap *892*
- Toe transfer *894*
- Great toe wrap around flap *896*
- Fibula flap *898*
- Sural flap *901*
- Leg fascio-cutaneous flaps *903*

Flaps

Definition
A flap is a unit of tissue of variable composition which, when transferred from a donor to a recipient site, *brings its own blood supply* and intrinsic circulation.

Classification
The three methods of flap classification are based on flap characteristics: vascularity, movement and composition.

Blood supply
- Random.
- Non-random:
  - Axial.
  - Fascio-cutaneous.
  - Septo-cutaneous.
  - Perforator.
  - Reverse flow flaps.
  - Venous flaps.

Movement
- Local:
  - Advancement:
    — Single pedicle.
    — Bipedicle.
    — V–Y.
    — Y–V.
  - Pivot:
    — Rotation.
    — Transposition.
    — Interpolation.
- Distant:
    — Pedicled.
    — Tubed.
- Free.

Composition
- Cutaneous.
- Fascio-cutaneous.
- Musculo-cutaneous (myocutaneous).
- Osseo-cutaneous.
- Muscle.
- Bone.
- Fascia.
- Tendon.
- Digit.
- Various combinations of the above.

Notes

A random flap is a flap with no significant bias in its vascular pattern. Vascularity is based on the subdermal plexus. There is no defined pedicle and as a consequence the length-to-breadth ratio is limited to 1:1 on the body and 4:1 on the face. Non-random flaps are based on a known vascular directional pattern. The vessel can enter and travel through the flap in different planes giving rise to the subclassification.

Local flaps make use of tissue adjacent to or in close proximity to the defect and remain attached to the donor site by a pedicle.

Distant flaps are those that use tissue at some distance from the defect. They either have no attachment to their primary donor site (e.g. free flap) or may retain their attachment via the pedicle. This pedicle may require division once the flap has inset, i.e. developed its own blood supply from the recipient bed. The pedicle can be buried (tunnelled under skin and soft tissue) inset, becoming a component of the skin and soft tissue, or exteriorized.

Movement of flaps can also be described as single stage or multiple stages (e.g. second stage to divide a pedicle).

Flap design and incisions

Incisions must aim to provide excellent exposure, whilst protecting the pedicle of the flap on closure. There must be the option for extension proximally, distally or laterally as required.

In the case of a pedicle flap, the design must accommodate sufficient flap length and width to fill the defect without tension. Design it larger, especially longer, than you will need. When covering a joint always check joint movements to ensure that these do not compromise the stability and tension on the flap.

It is very important to consider the zone of injury and scarring, as these zones may be unsuitable for re-vascularization of a free flap or for basing a pedicle flap (the stiffness of the tissues may prevent transposition, for example).

It is very important that the vascular pedicle is protected by adequate soft tissue from exposure, tension, internal compression, or external pressure.

Why do flaps die?

Flaps die due to compromise of their vascularity. This may occur for the following reasons.

Flap design and raising

- A flap may be designed or raised extending outside the area supplied by the pedicle.
- A pedicle will have a primary and secondary areas of supply, and the secondary areas may be more sensitive to a reduction in perfusion pressure from systemic causes or from local causes such as tension or compression of the pedicle.
- As the flap is raised the pedicle may be injured.

- Lack of knowledge of the area of supply or poor skills may lead to a flap being raised without a blood supply.
- Venous drainage of a flap may be different to arterial supply.

Flap inset
- Pedicle compromise by twisting, tension, kinking, or external compression such as over-tight closure or bandage will reduce or stop blood flow, perfusion, and/or venous outflow.
- Flap compromise by insetting under tension, which may only become apparent post-operatively when oedema becomes established, or when the part starts to be mobilized.
- Flap tension most commonly occurs from poor design by underestimating the size of flap or length of pedicle required for the transposition and defect.
- If a pedicled flap becomes compromised following transposition and cannot be rectified by attention to the details above, then return it to whence it arose to minimize stress upon its pedicle and maximize its perfusion. It will 'delay', and 2 weeks later may tolerate transposition.

Flap choice

Being aware of the reasons why a flap may fail leads to processes to avoid failure and find flap success. All the above features must be checked and re-checked at all stages of flap choice, design, and execution. Flap choice depends on
- Knowledge and awareness of flap options.
- Experience and skills.
- Patient.
- Local details and needs.

There are usually many suitable choices for each defect. Each of these will have benefits and drawbacks, some of which will be very individualized to the surgeon and patient.

Flap terminology

Flap prefabrication (vascular induction)
Implantation of a vascular pedicle into a new territory, followed by a period of maturation and neovascularization, and the subsequent transfer of that tissue based on its implanted pedicle (Shen 1981).

Flap prelamination
Implantation of tissues or devices into a vascular territory before it is transferred. The blood supply is not manipulated (Pribaz et al. 1999). Examples include pre-flap expansion, the implantation of cartilage under radial forearm fascia in ear reconstruction.

Free style flap
A perforator (usually free) flap in which the perforator is found by Doppler or by exploration at operation and then followed proximally until the vessel size becomes sufficient on which to perform anastomoses or to base the flap.

Flow-through flap
A free flap in which the arterial pedicle is used to re-vascularize the limb/part as well as vascularize the flap. Ideally type C flaps (e.g. radial forearm flap) with a largish artery flowing through the septum feeding the flap by perforators and the additional anastomosis performed at the distal end of the artery revascularizes the limb.

Chimeric flap
A flap with separate components linked by having the same pedicle. An example is latissimus dorsi and serratus anterior, both on the subscapular vessels. Can also be similar to the flow-through flap except that the distal end is used to revascularize another free flap.

'Crane' principle
If a defect that is unsuitable for grafting is temporarily covered with a flap (10–20 days), when the flap is removed the defect will have granulated sufficiently to permit grafting.

Pin cushioning flap
A complication in which the flap contracts to bulge above the surface of the surrounding tissue like a pin cushion. Thought to be due to excess flap size for defect, and scar contracture in the deep and circumferential plane squeezing out the flap. Avoid by careful sizing of flap, avoiding circular defects and flaps, breaking up the circumferential scar by Z-plasty, prevent haematoma in the deep plane by quilting sutures.

Super-charged flap
Flap in which the arterial or venous supply is augmented by an additional anastomosis. e.g. a large-volume/size TRAM flap that has been pedicled superiorly on the superior epigastric vessels for breast reconstruction. To augment the blood supply and drainage the inferior epigastric vessels are anastomosed in the axilla.

Super-drained flap
Flap in which an additional venous drainage anastomosis is performed draining to a different venous network.

Supra-fascial
Dissection occurs in the plane just superficial to the fascia.

Sub-fascial
Dissection occurs in the plane just deep to the fascia.

Pedicle
Vascular and/or neural connection from the body to the flap.

Neurocutaneous flap
Flaps based on the principle anatomical finding that peripheral nerves are accompanied by an artery. The pattern of which varies from having a long artery that accompanies the nerve (proximal to distal throughout its length anastomosing with another artery following the nerve from distal to proximal), or being accompanied by arcades of arteries supplying segments of nerves (e.g. like those that supply segments of bowel). The arteries that pierce the deep fascia with the nerve tend to be the long type. Those that do not accompany the nerve through the deep fascia tend to be the arcade or chain type. A nerve that crosses an artery will usually pick up branches of the artery. When a nerve crosses a fixed skin site it frequently picks up its next vascular companion. These neurovascular relationships present the basis for neurocutaneous flaps. Many existing axial flaps are in fact neurocutaneous flaps.

References
Pribaz JJ, Fine N, Orgill DP (1999). *Plast Reconstr Surg* **103**, 808–20.
Shen (1981). *Zhong Wai Ke Za Zhi* **19**:692–5.

Classification of flaps

Classification of muscle flaps (Mathes and Nahai 1981)

Based on anatomical relationship between muscle and its vascular pedicle and the intra-muscular anastomoses. Aids flap selection and usefulness.

- Type 1: one vascular pedicle (tensor fascia lata, gastrocnemius, rectus femoris).
- Type 2: one dominant and minor pedicle(s) (gracilis, trapezius, soleus, biceps femoris, abductor digiti minimi).
- Type 3: two dominant pedicles from different sources, either of which can support the whole muscle (gluteus maximus, rectus abdominis, serratus anterior, temporalis).
- Type 4: segmental supply each of which only supplies its segment and an immediately adjacent segment (sartorius, sternomastoid, tibialis anterior, flexor and extensor digitorum).
- Type 5: one dominant pedicle near the insertion which can supply the whole muscle and several minor pedicles near the origin which can also supply the muscle (latissumus dorsi).

Classification of fascio-cutaneous flaps

Based on the route to reach the skin and directness of supply of the vascular pedicle. Aids flap selection and usefulness

- Type A (broad base with perforators unseen): multiple perforators at flap base, vessels orientated longitudinally along flap axis (Ponten, Becker).
- Type B (perforator/axial): single consistent perforator feeding a fascial vascular plexus which may run along flap axis (medial arm, perforator flaps, antecubital forearm, Quaba, groin).
- Type C (ladder type): longitudinal septal vessel sending multiple perforators to fascia and skin as it travels (posterior interosseous, lateral arm, radial forearm, ulnar forearm).
- Type D (osteo-fasciocutaneous): type C with bone (radial forearm with radius, lateral arm with supracondylar ridge humerus, ulnar with ulna).

Classification of fascio-cutaneous flaps

- Type A (axial): vessel runs under then over deep fascia into skin (groin, sural, forehead, temporo-parietal fascia, dorsal metacarpal art.).
- Type B (septo-cutaneous): vessel(s) to skin branch from deep inter-muscular longitudinal vessel travelling along intermuscular septum (radial forearm, lateral arm, ulnar, anterior lateral thigh, PIA).
- Type C (musculo-cutaneous): vessel to skin travels through muscle (anterior lateral thigh, delto-pectoral, gastrocnemius, gracilis, DIEP).

References

Cormack GC, Lamberty BG (1984). *Br J Plast Surg* **37**, 80–87
Mathes SJ, Nahai F (1981). *Plast Reconstruct Surg* **67**, 177–87.

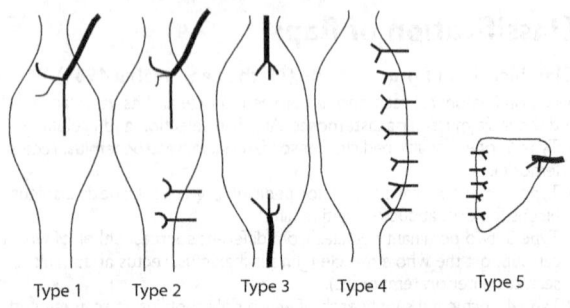

Fig. 22.1 Classification of muscle flaps (Mathes and Nahai 1981).

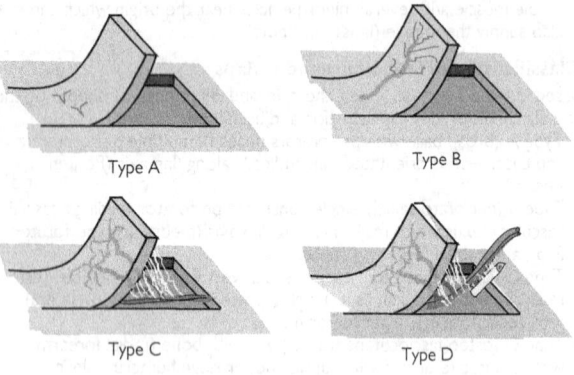

Fig. 22.2 Classification of fascio-cutaneous flaps (Cormack and Lamberty 1984).

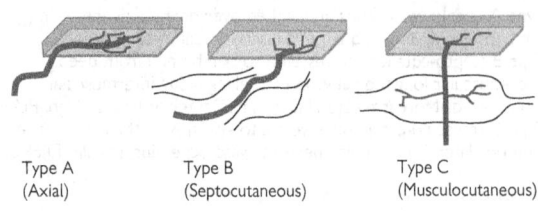

Fig. 22.3 Classification of fascio-cutaneous flaps.

Free tissue transfer

Definition
This is an autotransplant. Tissue is removed from one part of the body with its supplying artery and draining vein, and transferred to another part of the body where the artery and vein are anastomosed to recipient vessels.

Classification
By tissue composition (see flap classification).

Pathophysiology
Free tissue transfer generates a period of ischaemia and hypoxia. Different tissues can tolerate different periods. The length of time can be prolonged by cooling (skin and subcutaneous tissue, 4–6 hr warm and 12 hr cold; muscle, 2 hr warm and 8 hr cold; bone, 3 hr warm and 24 hr cold). Anaerobic metabolism in the tissue during ischaemia increases production of superoxide radicals. Following reperfusion, free-radical scavengers (e.g. superoxide dismutase) attack the radicals, injuring the cells. This causes endothelial swelling and fluid leakage into the interstitial space, further narrowing the vessel lumen. Intravascular platelet aggregation then occurs. This is known as ischaemia-induced *reperfusion injury* and gives rise to the *no-reflow* effect. Clinically, this appears as initial flap perfusion which gradually tails off as the effect takes place and results in irreversible flap ischaemia.

Indications
General indications are post-tumour resection, trauma, congenital defects, or chronic wounds where free tissue transfer would give the optimum aesthetic and functional result (any defect). Specific indications include:
- Need for a certain tissue, e.g. bone especially if defect is greater then 6 cm.
- Where there is no local option, e.g the foot and the distal third of the leg, head and neck.
- Massive defects.
- Defects requiring complex reconstruction of multiple tissue types.
- Areas where freshly vascularized tissue is required, e.g lower limb trauma.

Advantages
- Single stage procedure.
- Variety of donor tissues.
- Large amounts of tissue can be transferred.
- Donor defects can be hidden in cosmetically acceptable areas.
- Less immobilization than pedicled flaps.
- Improved vascularity of flap and to the recipient area.
- More aesthetic than local flaps.

Disadvantages
- Lengthy operation.
- Recipient vessel may be unavailable, damaged, or atherosclerotic.

- Donor site morbidity (see individual flaps); problems such as scar, loss of function, poor healing, and herniation.
- Thrombosis and flap loss can occur.

Planning

Preoperative

- Recipient site: size and tissue composition of flap needed after resection or debridement, available vessels, zone of injury/surgery/radiation. Consider need for arteriogram (previous free flap loss, extensive zone of injury) or Doppler.
- Donor site: best flap in terms of size, composition, pedicle length, vessel diameter match, donor site morbidity, special features, e.g. fascia neurosensory etc., ease of raising, ability for two surgical teams to operate. Doppler of donor vessel or perforators may be helpful.

Patient assessment.

- Age: infants and old age are not a contraindication.
- General health, concurrent illness, cardiovascular status, smoking (encourage patient to stop at least 10 days prior to surgery) do not affect flap survival but wound healing is impaired.
- Previous radiation therapy is not a contraindication but there may be wound healing problems.
- Medications are not a contraindication.

Investigations

Baseline U&E, FBC, clotting, cross-matching (≥ 2 units), and more advanced investigations and X-rays as indicated.

Operative

See individual flaps.

Post-operative

See flap care.

Complications

General

These can occur with any surgery but are particularly common in prolonged procedures. Anaesthetic, positional (neurapraxia and pressure sores), DVT and PE, respiratory problems, and cardiac overload.

Specific

Intra-operative

- **Failure of flap perfusion** This is the major complication and patient factors as well as local factors must be considered. Ensure the patient is warm, with a good blood pressure and urinary output indicating good blood flow. Ensure that this good blood pressure is not being produced by vasoconstricting agents used by the anaesthetist. Locally, check no clamps are left on, the artery is not kinked, too loose, or too taut, and the anastomosis is patent (do patency test on the vein *not* the artery). If everything else is in good order then vessel spasm is the most likely cause and 2% lidocaine placed around the vessels with no interference for 5–10 min should produce an improvement. If no sign

of perfusion the anastomosis should be redone and the inflow checked. If there are no technical or patient/anaesthetic reasons for lack of blood flow, the anastomosis seems patent, and blood flowing in the pedicle but the flap not perfusing, the no-reflow effect has to be considered. Flap salvage with thrombolytics or prostacyclin will be needed. The problem may not be anastomotic; check for an intimal injury at the site the pedicle enters the flap.
- **Failure of venous drainage** Again spasm, an errant clamp, kinking of the recipient vein, or anastomotic problems may be the cause. If there is any doubt, the anastomosis should be redone. It may be necessary to find different recipient vessels.

Post-operative
The first 72 hr are most critical but flap failure may occur up to 7 days following transfer. Early signs of decreased perfusion or venous engorgment should provoke a return to theatre. Whilst waiting to return, loosen the bandage, remove sutures, and elevate or lower the limb. Do not be deceived by a temporary improvement. Haematoma tends to indicate venous occlusion causing bleeding out of the flap which keeps the flap in good colour for a while. On return to theatre explore the anastomosis, the lie of the vessels, and the flap. Determine why thrombosis or cessation of flow occurred. There is little point in just revising the anastomosis without correcting the cause of the problem. Some surgeons formally anticoagulate their patients following an anastomotic revision. Extensively thrombosed vessels may occasionally be salvaged by embolectomy and intra-flap thrombolytic. However, most of these will necrose or, if salvaged, will have patchy necrosis compromising the aim of the original procedure.

Other complications
Partial flap loss, poor healing, blood loss, bulky or poor aesthetic result. Donor site problems. For specific complications see individual flaps.

Success rates

Flap survival rates of 95–98% for routine procedures are expected. There is an operator learning curve. Free tissue transfer is being undertaken for increasingly complex cases.

Lessons in free flap transfers

Definition
Personal lessons in free flap transfers that may help you avoid failure.
- Debride, debride, debride before you cover.
- Call the orthopaedic surgeon if in doubt about bone fixation, bone viability, or bone defect.
- Do not close under tension.
- Big option is better.
- Use a larger flap than the hole to fill the hole.
- Better vessel exposure eases the microsurgery. If you are having technical problems with the anastomosis, extend the wound.
- Use muscle flap for infection or contaminated cases, as they have better vascularity, better dead-space filling capacity, and more pliability/versatility with fewer fitting constraints than fascio-cutaneous flaps.
- Flow through rather than AV fistula or AV fistula with flap coming off it and separate venous drainage for flap.
- Wait 30 min before closure to check anastomosis/outflow etc. Use this period to close the donor site, complete inset of the flap, harvest the skin graft, etc.
- If in doubt about perfusion after closure, re-open and check the lie of the vessels/pedicle/anastomoses again. They may be getting kinked on closure.
- Always use a microscope.
- Always protect the flap from avulsing the pedicle by securing it to the body.
- Inset the flap before adjusting the pedicle length, tension, and lie.
- Do not trim or throw away excess flap until it has been re-vascularized and you are sure of the final inset and position.
- Do not traumatize the vessels by over-dissection of its length or adventitia.
- Check arterial downflow, and venous outflow before anastomosis in cases where there may be proximal obstruction, e.g. lower limb trauma, DVT, osteomyelitis, radiotherapy.
- Kinking or a twist will propagate and occur at the branch closest to the anastomosis, so move from the fixed point to the anastomosis point when checking that there is no twist.
- Veins in particular shorten once divided, so ensure that they are tensioned to length before anastomosis to avoid kinking due to excess length.
- Try to avoid having the anastomosis at the apex of any bend in the vessel's path.
- If the flap is not perfusing well do not warm it, as this will raise the metabolic demand of the tissue, causing more ischaemic injury. Warm the patient and the limb instead.

Poor downflow may be spasm, proximal injury, or a systemic problem. To treat poor downflow and spasm, optimize anaesthesia, dissect the recipient vessel more proximally with a minimal touch technique, and *in extremis* use vasodilators such as papavarine or plain lidocaine 2%. In some cases, despite poor downflow, the anastomosis should be performed, the wound closed, and the patient woken up, which somehow alleviates the spasm. Spasm is thought to be partially due to unclipped or uncoagulated bleeding branches of the vessel, so ensure that any branches encountered are diathermied or clipped.

In the case of cessation of flow across an anastomosis, which is usually due to poor technique or a platelet thrombus, it is important to clamp the vessel downstream of the anastomosis before touching it. This is to avoid any platelet showers heading downstream and embolizing within the flap, causing no reflow. Once the clamps are placed to protect the flap, place a clamp upstream to prevent inflow, take the anastomosis down, and identify the cause: a pedicle may be too long, too short, kinked, or twisted, the anastomosis may be technically poor, or there may be poor inflow due to local or systemic causes. In all these cases correct the cause and redo the anastomosis. If it was previously an end-to-side anastomosis, consider a change to an end-to-end.

Flaps can be salvaged but only if taken back to theatre promptly, so if in doubt return to theatre.

Flap monitoring and care

The approach to caring for flaps can apply to local and free flaps. The flap is most vulnerable to complications over the first 72 hr post-operatively and careful monitoring should be performed during this period.

Monitoring the flap

Clinical
This remains the mainstay of flap observation. For the first 12 hr this should be done half-hourly then hourly. Possible parameters are colour, appearance, capillary refill, tissue turgor, dermal bleeding, and temperature difference. Observation is done through a window in the dressing, and this should be enlarged if there is any difficulty. Simple adhesive temperature probes are placed on the flap (skin flaps only) and the adjacent skin. Bleeding can be detected from a stab wound into the flap. Arterial problems are demonstrated by a pale flap with slow capillary return and an 'underfilled' appearance. A stab wound produces a slow ooze of dark red blood or nothing, and the flap will be cool with a temperature difference of $\geq 2°C$. Venous congestion is represented by an engorged bluish flap with brisk capillary refill and rapid bleeding of dark blood if pierced. Again, there will be a temperature difference and the tissue will be cool.

Doppler
Most commonly used is US Doppler, which uses the reflection of sound from pulsatile vessels to detect flow. This can be used for both artery and vein to detect pedicle and intra-flap flow. As well as the more common hand-held machines, implantable probes can be used. Laser Doppler measures the frequency shift of light, has limited depth penetration (1.5 mm^3), and is not widely used. Unfortunately, Doppler can give false-positive readings, probably because of reflected or transmitted pulse down an occluded vessel. Do not trust the Doppler if it disagrees with your clinical findings.

Other methods
- Vital dye measurements: usually a bolus injection of fluorescein and then visualization of the staining in the flap with a Woods UV lamp.
- Near-infrared spectroscopy: detects the changes in oxy, deoxy, and Hb concentrations in the flap.
- Photoplethysmography: detects fluid volume changes in a skin flap using variations in infrared absorption.
- The pulse oximeter has been used to effect, and there are many other methods which are mainly experimental at this stage.

Monitoring the patient
- Initial simple measures include ensuring there is no tourniquet effect from over-tight dressings or extraneous items, e.g. tracheostomy tapes in head and neck reconstruction. The patient should be suitably positioned in a warm quiet room and be pain free.

- Regular observation (half-hourly for the first 12 hr, then hourly) of temperature, pulse, blood pressure, urine output, and drainage. There are many parameters but a pulse <100 and systolic pressure >100 mmHg is desirable. Urine output should not fall below 30 mL/hr and ideally should average 50 mL/hour. Diuretics should NOT be used to maintain urine output. Rather, increase intravascular volume.
- A haemoglobin and haematocrit should be performed 4–5 hr post-operatively and daily for 3 days. The haematocrit should be ~30. If <25 give blood: if >35 give crystalloid. A Hb of 10 is optimum in terms of blood viscosity and oxygenation.

Anti-thrombotic therapy

Heparin, dextran, proteolytic enzymes (urokinase, streptokinase, tissue plasminogen activator), and prostacyclin have all been used. The routine use of these is not proven and may cause haematoma or allergic reaction. However, in situations where technical or patient factors dictate, or following re-exploration, their use may be prudent.

Heparin may be given as a one-off intra-operative bolus (3000–5000 units) or as formal anticoagulation with a loading dose of 5000 units and 2000 units/hr, adjusting with APTT to maintain at 1.5–2 greater than normal. Dextran 40 (10% solution) is occasionally given as a loading dose (50 ml) followed by IV infusion at 25–50 mL/hr using 500 mL/day. Proteolytics and prostacyclin have been used intra-operatively in flap salvage situations.

Leeches

These are useful for small flaps and areas of large flaps that exhibit venous congestion. They are not a substitute for a patent venous anastomosis.

Summary

Careful observation is essential. Early recognition of problems or any doubt prompt a return to theatre. Survival rates >50% can be expected in salvaged flaps, and are directly proportional to delay in detection of problems and return to theatre.

Advancement flaps

Definition
An advancement flap is a local flap which moves forward from donor to recipient site without rotation or lateral movement. The simplest form is an undermined wound for direct closure.

Principles
The flap is adjacent to the defect. It should be oriented to take advantage of the local vascular supply and skin elasticity. With the exception of the V–Y flap, these flaps can be based on a subdermal blood supply alone or on a subcutaneous pedicle.

Techniques
- **Single pedicle** Incise parallel lines from the defect, elevate the skin in a subcutaneous plane, and advance the rectangular flap into the defect. There is often excess skin at the base of these flaps which can be excised as two triangles (Burrow's) or incorporated with a Z-plasty as in a forehead rotation advancement flap.
- **Bi-pedicle** Incise on a line parallel to the defect, elevate the flap leaving it pedicled at either end, and advance it into the defect. This technique is used in cleft palate repair (Langenbeck) allowing the donor to heal by secondary intention. It is used infrequently on the skin because of the need to skin graft the donor site.
- **V–Y** This flap is based on a subcutaneous pedicle. The laxity in the subcutaneous tissues permits the flap advancement and the lateral elasticity in the skin permits closure of the tail (secondary defect). The V–Y principle is often used in design of other flaps to close the secondary defects.
  - **Deep pedicle** V–Y flaps can be based on tissues deep to the flap, relying on the depth and extensibility of the subcutaneous fat to allow forward movement. Following skin incision, deepen into the subcutaneous fat bevelling away from the flap to allow a broad base. Advance the flap. Extra advancement is achieved by 'swan-necking': undermine the leading edge of the flap and deep mine the base and trailing edge of the flap, allowing the pedicle to unfold. This is used mainly for cutaneous facial defects. Deep-based V–Y flaps can also be based on perforators and can include fascia or muscle (e.g. the biceps femoris to close pressure sores and fasciocutaneous V–Y on the lower limb).
  - **Lateral pedicle** Based on bilateral connecting subcutaneous tissue dividing the flap from its connection to the underlying facia. Gentle teasing with the scissors allows further advancement. Sometimes used as a unilateral pedicle as in a horn flap.
  - **V–Y variations** There are many variations of the V–Y flap. Occasionally the V–Y technique is used to close another flap defect, and combination flaps exist such as the Hatchet flap which has elements of advancement and rotation with V–Y closure of the secondary defect.

ADVANCEMENT FLAPS   751

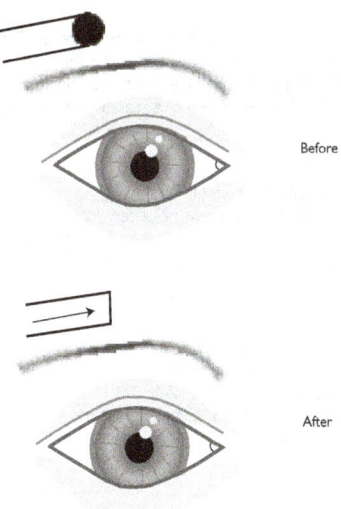

Fig. 22.4 Advancement flap: single pedicle.

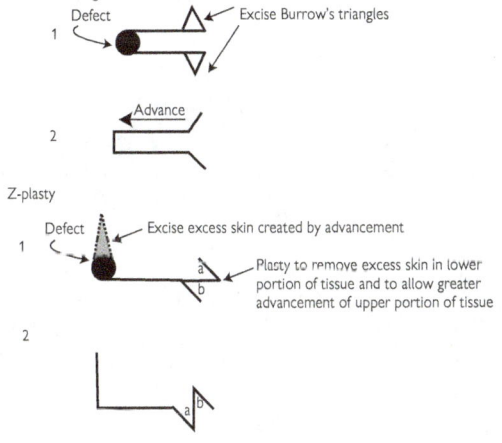

Fig. 22.5 Burrow's triangles and Z-plasties: methods of dealing with the excess skin at the base of advancement flaps.

Y–V

Often used to break up a scar in burns contracture or Dupuytren's closure. A line of adjacent Ys is drawn perpendicular to the scar axis. All are incised and the triangular flaps are advanced into the longitudinal limbs of the Y producing a zig-zag. This lengthens the scar by the additive width of all the triangular flaps.

Common errors
- Error 1: flap designed too small.
- Error 2: flap will not advance without tension. Usually due to error in design (too small) or insufficient dissection of the pedicle. Inset under tension will lead to flap tip necrosis or retraction.

How to excise a dog ear or Burrow's triangle
- Suture the dog ear into a corner.
- With a skin hook stretch the dog ear out flat.
- Cut along one border of the dog ear.
- Open out the dog ear.
- Trim the other side of the dog ear and suture. Can be excised in line or perpendicular to the original incision/excision.

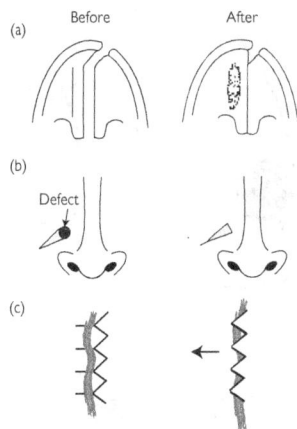

Fig. 22.6 Advancement flaps: (a) bipedicle (used here to close a cleft palate); (b) V–Y (used here to close a paranasal defect); (c) Y–V (used here to break up a scar).

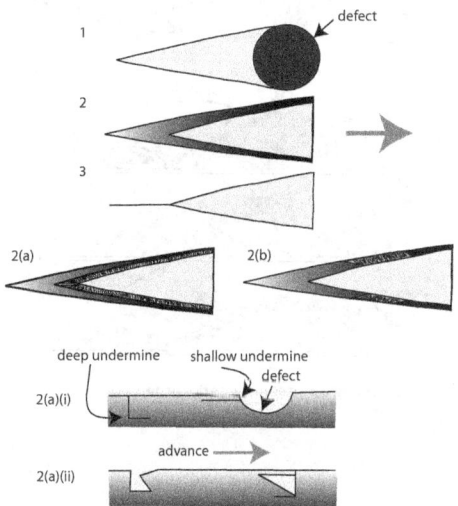

Fig. 22.7 V–Y flap: (1) design of V–Y flap; (2) advancement of the flap; (3) closure as a Y. Flap can be based on (2a) a deep pedicle or (2b) a lateral pedicle. 2(a)(i) A deep-pedicled V–Y flap can gain extra advancement by 'swan-necking' the flap. Undermine superficially at the leading edge and deeply at the trailing edge, allowing the flap to extend as in 2(a)(ii).

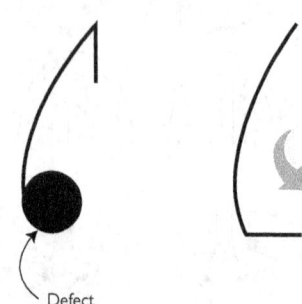

Fig. 22.8 Hatchet flap.

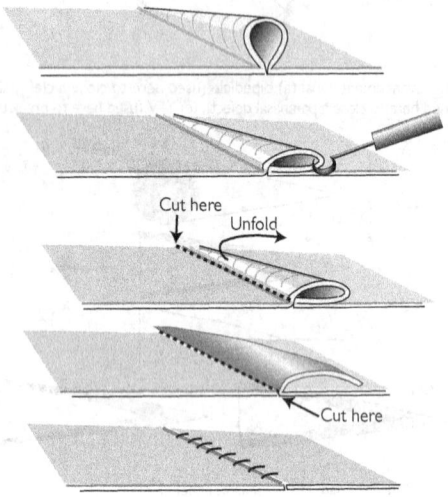

Fig. 22.9 Excision of dog ear or Burrow's triangle technique.

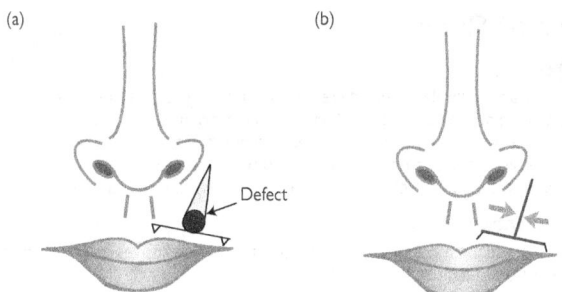

Fig. 22.10 AT flap: two advancement flaps with Burrow's triangles excised.

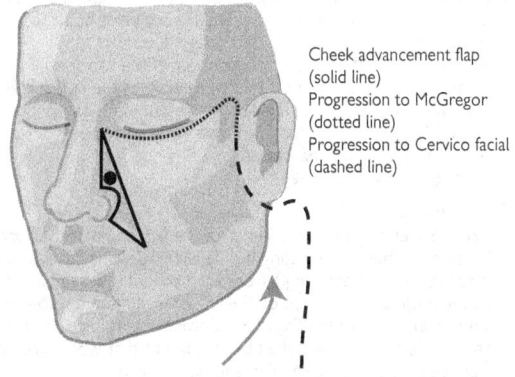

Cheek advancement flap (solid line)
Progression to McGregor (dotted line)
Progression to Cervico facial (dashed line)

Fig. 22.11 A cheek advancement flap demonstrating the range of advancement flaps. See section on cheek reconstruction.

Pivot flaps

Definition
These are local flaps that have an arc of movement about a fixed point (pivot point) to reach the defect. The pivot point is the point of origin of the line of maximum tension in the flap and the point on which it pivots. It is easy to mistakenly consider the apex of the defect as the pivot point. It is NOT. Incorrect choice of pivot point compromises flap design!

Transposition flap
This is usually a rectangular or square flap which moves laterally from a pivot point to close the defect.

Design
The defect is triangulated to excise excess skin at the base of the defect and flap. This excision can be performed after the flap is transposed in the manner one would use to excise a dog ear.
- **Rule 1** The length from the pivot point to the apex of the flap should be equal to or greater than the length from pivot point to the apex of the defect furthest from the flap.
- **Rule 2** The length of the leading border of the flap should be equal or greater than the length of the furthest edge of the defect.

The simplest way to design this flap is to use a piece of string and measure the flap dimensions needed from the proposed pivot point to fill the defect. The donor can be closed by using the V–Y principle, by utilizing another flap, or with an SSG.

Common errors
- **Error 1** Designing the distal ends of the flap and defect as parallel incisions. When triangulating the defect or designing the flap, the distal incisions should angle from each other by the same degree as the angle of movement or the line of maximum tension will move on transposition of the flap. The alternative is to increase the length of the flap relative to the defect by an amount that would create an angle between the apices of the flap and defect equal to the angle of movement of the line of maximum tension.
- **Error 2** Failure to follow the rules will result in a flap that is too short or will be inset under excess tension to fit.

Tips
- A back-cut can be employed to move the pivot point such as to reduce tension.
- Design the flap 20% larger than you think it should be.

Rotation flap

This is a semicircular flap that rotates about a pivot point to close the defect. It is an extension of the principles of the transposition flap and can be viewed as multiple contiguous transposition flaps each designed to close the secondary defect of the previous flap. Each flap gradually increases in size and the pivot point rotates and displaces further from the defect. The size of these contiguous flaps eventually increases sufficiently to be able to take advantage of skin elasticity to enable closure of the secondary defect.

Design
The defect should be converted to an isoceles triangle, with an angle of 30° at its apex. The diameter or base of the semicircle should be 3 times the length of side of the 30° triangle. The circumference of the flap should be 5–8 times greater than the width of the defect. Further rotation can be gained by a back-cut. Ideally, the donor should close primarily but a skin graft or second flap may be required.

Rules
- **Rule 1** The length from the pivot point to the apex of the flap should be equal to or greater than the length from pivot point to the apex of the defect furthest from the flap.
- **Rule 2** The length of the leading border of the flap should be equal or greater than the length of the furthest edge of the defect

Errors
Error 1 Failure to design a large enough flap.
Error 2 Failure to design a rotation with constant radius as this creates tension between pivot point and the points of closure along the circle.
Error 3 Failure to follow the rules.
Error 4 Failure to account for convexity of the body surface which gives some loss of rotation.

Tips
- A back-cut can be employed to move the pivot point so as to reduce tension. This will work for tension at the tip of the flap but not for tension along the line of closure, so ensure the flap is circular!
- Design the flap 20% larger than you think it should be.

Interpolation flap

This flap moves about a pivot point but the donor and recipient sites are not adjacent and hence the pedicle has to pass above or below the intervening skin to reach the defect. It is commonly considered a distant flap of the island type, rather than a local flap.

Design
The design is best done with a cloth template or string, ensuring that the length of pedicle and flap dimensions are sufficient to reach and close the defect without tension. Donor closure is directly, local flap, or graft. With an externalized pedicle, division and inset occurs ~2 weeks after the initial procedure.

Rotation flaps

Rotation flaps are useful when there are large surfaces of skin without significant anatomical landmarks to obstruct the rotation. The common teaching for rotation flaps is to design a flap 5–8 times the size of the defect. This can be proved geometrically, which can aid design, particularly as the most common error is to design the flap too small.

For a semicircular rotation flap, the radius of the semicircle needs to be twice or three times the arc of the circle subtended by the defect. This gives a segment of semicircle with an angle that roughly gives you five times the arc of the defect for the rotation flap.

Geometry

Arc length (s) is given by

$$s = r \times \theta$$

where r is the radius and θ is the central angle in radians.

We wish to choose an angle of 30° which would give us six segments in a semicircle (180°/6 =30°). A complete revolution is 2π radians (360°). Therefore half a revolution (a semicircle) is π radians (180°). Hence 30° = $\pi/6$ radians. Therefore the arc length for a central angle of 30° is

$$s = r \times \pi/6.$$

When a defect is excised, length of the arc (s) is generally equal to the width of the defect. We want to know the radius so that the rotation flap can be designed which, by rearranging the formula above, is given by

$$r = s/\theta$$

Thus for a six-segment semicircle

$$r = s \times 6/\pi$$

and since $\pi = 3.14$,

$$r \approx 2s.$$

If we want nine segments in a semicircle (perhaps because of inelastic skin or the need to rotate around a convexity as well), the angle is 180°/9 = 20° = $\pi/9$ radians. Therefore the radius required for a nine-segment semicircle is 3s.

For a quarter-circle rotation flap, we need to choose an angle which gives us six segments in as quarter-circle, i.e. 15° = $\pi/12$ radians. Therefore

$$s = r \times \pi/12$$

Since $\pi = 3.14$, the radius of a quarter-circle which will give six arcs is 4s, and the radius for a quarter circle which will give nine arcs is 6s. Thus the radius of the quarter-circle must be four to six times the defect width! This explains why a semicircular design is preferred!

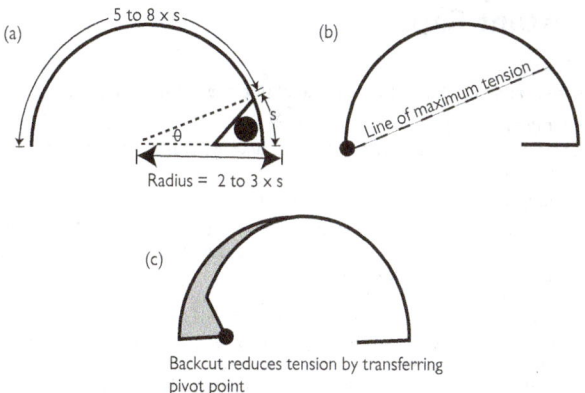

Fig. 22.12 Rotation flap geometry.

Practical considerations

In practice, the geometrical considerations mean that the defect, and the areas of skin laxity and availability around it, must be assessed. Measure the width of the defect which will form the segment of the circle requiring closure. Double or treble this measurement to calculate the radius of the rotation flap. Draw this radius along the long line of the defect to the centre of the flap. Draw a semicircle extending from the defect and pivoting around the centre point of the circle. The semi-circumference of this flap will be five to eight times the width of the defect. Note that the pivot point of this flap is not the centre point of the circle, but is the far point of the incision opposite the defect. Hence when the flap is raised and transposed the tension line extends from the pivot point to the furthest point on the semicircle. This tension line can be reduced by performing a back-cut. This brings the pivot point of the flap closer to the centre point of the circle; however, it also diminishes the blood supply entering the base of the flap.

If a back-cut is done, then it is cheated in to close the back-cut defect.

Distant flaps

Direct flaps
Donor and defect are at distant sites, but these can be approximated.

Examples
Groin to hand, cross-leg, cross-finger, and hypogastric or other truncal flaps to upper limb.

Technique
Usually random pattern flaps with length-to-breadth ratio of 1:1, although some are axial pattern (e.g. groin). The flap is raised, the flap and recipient sites are approximated, and the flap inset. Solid immobilization of the donor and defect areas without tension is the key to successful transfer. This may be by external fixation, POP, or sutures. The pedicle is divided 2–3 weeks following filling of the defect. The pedicle edge of the flap is usually then inset, but occasionally this has to occur as a third procedure if there is an excess of fibrous tissue at the defect.

Indications
Donor and defect can be approximated and immobilized for the required duration without ill effects

Advantages
Shorter surgical time; less functional loss at donor site; reliable, especially with limited resources; no microsurgery needed.

Disadvantages
Patient immobility often with the part dependent rather than elevated; joint stiffness; difficulty in wound care to the area; two or more procedures; less flexibility in flap inset; longer hospital stay.

Tubed pedicle flap
Strictly, a tubed pedicle flap is a direct distant flap whose bridging segment is made long in order to allow some movement between the donor and recipient sites. This bridge may be sufficiently long that it can be sutured into a tube. However, tubed pedicle flaps are more commonly understood to be the staged transfer of a distant flap using a carrier. This flap is mainly of historical interest.

Technique
Initially a bipedicled flap is raised and tubed. After 2–3 weeks one end of the tube is detached and inset on a created defect on the wrist. After a further 2–3 weeks the other end of the tube is detached and then attached to the recipient site. After another 2–3 weeks the wrist is released and the flap trimmed to size. An alternative to using the wrist/forearm as the carrier is to waltz the flap end over-end every 2–weeks until it reaches its recipient site.

Indications
Donor and defect cannot be approximated and a carrier is required. Other techniques or flaps are not available.

Advantages
No microsurgery required; no recipient vessels needed.

Disadvantages
Multiple stages; original wound/defect contracts or heals during this period; immobilization; lacks flexibility in design and inset; flap contracts in size before it reaches the defect.

Pedicled (island) flap

A distant flap that has its pedicle reduced in size, in some cases down to just the vessels. So called as this flap design resembles an island with a connecting bridge. This bridge can lie under the flap as in a perforator flap.

Technique
The design is usually based on axial vessels. The flap is designed and the skin incised (usually circumferentially), preserving the supplying vessels. The flap is elevated such that its sole connection to the body is the vessels and their surrounding connective tissue. The relative amount of preserved connective tissue inversely varies according to the calibre of the vessels. The flap pivots on the pedicle and is transposed into the defect, usually through a subcutaneous tunnel. Rarely, the pedicle is left externally, dressed, and excised after 2 weeks. The pedicle can be maintained with a strip of overlying skin to help cover it.

Indications:
Most common flap after local flaps; used when no local options or when local options are suboptimal, or their donor defects are difficult to close.

Advantages
No microsurgery required; no recipient vessels needed.

Disadvantages
Reach restrained by pedicle length; pedicle may become twisted or compressed; may involve sacrificing a main vessel to a limb (e.g. radial artery).

Fascio-cutaneous flaps

Definition
Fascio-cutaneous flaps are skin flaps which include the deep fascia to increase the reliability of skin circulation.

Anatomy
Predominantly the blood supply for fascio-cutaneous flaps is via the septo-cutaneous vessels which pass along the fascial septa between muscles to supply the pre- and sub-fascial plexi. The fascia itself is relatively avascular but its inclusion ensures the safety of the pre fascial plexus. The blood ascends from the fascial plexi to reach the skin. The orientation of vessels of the fascial plexus is usually longitudinal to the deep artery and flow may be multidirectional, hence allowing distally based flaps. Fascio-cutaneous flaps are more common on the extremities arising from the septa between the long muscles. The torso has broader muscles and more musculo-cutaneous perforators; however fascio-cutaneous flaps may be raised along a transverse or oblique axis. This contrasts with the longitudinal orientation of flaps raised on the limbs.

Classification (Cormack and Lamberty 1984) (see Fig. 22.2)
- Type A: multiple fascio-cutaneous perforators at the base of the flap and orientated along its long axis (e.g. Ponten super-flap in the lower leg).
- Type B: pedicled or free flap based on a single fascio-cutaneous perforator (e.g. medial arm flap and saphenous artery flap). A modification is to take the deep artery also, thus increasing pedicle length.
- Type C: pedicled or free flap reliant on multiple perforators which reach the fascia from the deep artery via the fascial septum between muscles. Hence it is necessary to include the deep artery in the flap (e.g. radial forearm flap).
- Type D: extension of the type C flap; the fascial septum is taken in continuity with adjacent muscle and bone which derive their blood supply from the same artery (e.g. radial forearm with FPL and bone from the radius).

Method of use
- Rotation: the point of rotation of a fascio-cutaneous flap is where the blood supply enters (e.g. scapular flap rotates on the circumflex vessel).
- Advancement: V–Y advancement or ordinary advancement flaps.
- Transposition: the flap is transposed to the defect.
- Turnover: usually fascia alone or adipofascial (e.g. de-epithelialized cross-finger flap.
- Reverse flow (retrograde): distally based flap requiring division of the main vessel like a reverse radial forearm flap Very expensive, and may compromise distal limb perfusion.
- Free: the pedicle is divided and re-attached to restore blood supply
- Neurotized: maintenance or reconnection of sensory supply can greatly improve outcome.

Advantages
- Reliable.
- Ease of elevation and transfer.
- Relatively thin.
- No functional deficit.
- Can be sensate.

Disadvantages
- SSG often required to close donor site.
- Less malleable and less volume for dead space filling.
- Size limitations.
- Donor site.

Surgical variations
- With the inclusion of the fascia (type A flaps) the length-to-width ratio of the flap can be increased from 1:1 in subcutaneous random flaps to 2–2.5:1.
- Fascial and adipofascial flaps can be designed to leave the skin component behind and hence reduce donor deformity.
- Fascio-cutaeous flaps can be raised without the fascia but with the preservation of the pre fascial plexus. The dissection is more difficult and the flap may be more unreliable.

Reference
Cormack GC, Lamberty BG (1984). *Br J Plast Surg* **37**, 80–87.

Muscle flaps

Flaps comprising muscle as their major component or utilizing muscle to carry the blood supply to skin require knowledge of the blood supply to each muscle and the intra-muscular network. The myocutaneous skin paddle is based on perforators ascending through the muscle to supply the skin. In general, the skin directly superficial to the muscle extending for 3–4 cm centrifugally can be reliably harvested with the muscle.

Classification

Mathes and Nahai (1981) classify muscle flaps according to their blood supply (see Fig. 22.1):
- Type 1: one vascular pedicle (tensor fascia lata, gastrocnemius, rectus femoris).
- Type 2: one dominant and minor pedicle(s) (gracilis, trapezius, soleus, biceps femoris, abductor digiti minimi).
- Type 3: two dominant pedicles from different sources, either of which can support the whole muscle (gluteus maximus, rectus abdominis, serratus anterior, temporalis).
- Type 4: segmental supply, each of which only supplies its and an immediately adjacent segment (sartorius, sternomastoid, tibialis anterior, flexor and extensor digitorum).
- Type 5: one dominant pedicle near the insertion which can supply the whole muscle and several minor pedicles near the origin which can also supply the muscle (latissumus dorsi).

A dominant pedicle can supply the muscle in the absence of any other vascular input. A minor pedicle can only maintain the viability of a portion of the muscle. Multiple blood supplies that only go to segments of muscle are termed segmental pedicles. Most muscles are type 2.

Method of use

- Rotation: the point of rotation of a muscle flap is where the blood supply enters (e.g. latissimus dorsi breast reconstruction). Type 5 muscles have two arcs of rotation one at the dominant pedicle, the other at the secondary pedicles.
- Advancement: V–Y advancement or ordinary advancement.

Musculo-cutaneous flaps can be used (e.g. biceps femoris to cover ischial sore).

- Turnover: usually segmentally supplied muscles such as sartorius to protect the femoral vessels after groin dissection, tibialis anterior to cover the tibia, or latissimus dorsi to cover the lumbo-sacral area.
- Reverse flow (retrograde): distally based muscle flap requiring division of the main vessel like a reverse radial forearm flap (e.g. reverse flow soleus for distal leg coverage with division of posterior tibial vessels). Very expensive, and may compromise distal limb perfusion. Not commonly used.
- Free: the pedicle is divided and re-attached to restore blood supply.
- Functional: the muscle remains innervated and can restore/preserve function (e.g. latissimus dorsi for biceps reconstruction).

Anatomy

The blood supply to muscles is shown in the classification. It should be remembered that there are other smaller sources of blood supply to a muscle, particularly at the origin and insertion. The venous drainage is via venae comitantes (VCs) that accompany the arteries. The motor nerve to a muscle generally accompanies the main pedicle. In a muscle supplied by more than one pedicle the territories are linked by 'choke' arteries that allow bidirectional flow.

Advantages

- Pliability and malleability, hence the ability to obliterate dead spaces of any shape or volume effectively.
- Greater vascularized surface area and higher flow rates allow effective delivery of leucocytes, oxygen, and antibiotics to a wound. More resistant to infection than fascio-cutaneous flaps.
- Dynamic functional transfers are possible.
- Inosculation of marginal tissue at the wound edge.
- More reliable vascular anatomy.
- Vessels often outside the zone of injury.
- A large flap can be taken, leaving little or no external contour deformity. Better donor site in muscle-only flaps.
- Can often be split longitudinally for different components.
- Can be contoured.

Disadvantages

- Functional deficit (potentially) at donor site.
- Donor site contour defect.
- Can be too bulky especially if musculo-cutaneous.
- Muscle can atrophy unless neurotized.

Reference

Mathes SJ, Nahai F (1981). *Plast Reconstruct Surg* **67**, 177–87.

Vascularized bone 'graft'

Vascularized bone 'graft' (VBG) is a misnomer. A graft has no intrinsic blood supply; it must gain a blood supply from its recipient bed. The words 'vascularized' and 'graft' are mutually exclusive, and the correct term is actually 'bone flap'. However, VBG is commonly used!

VBGs may be pedicled flaps or free flaps. The pedicles are often too short to permit transfer of the bone to the recipient site. Therefore the majority of procedures are done as free flaps.

VBG donor sites
- Calvarium on the superficial temporal vessels.
- Clavicle on the sternocleidomastoid muscle.
- Humerus on the posterior radial recurrent vessels.
- Radius on the radial artery or on the radial vessels of the volar carpal arch, or pronator quadratus of the dorsal carpal arch, or first or second supra-retinacular arteries.
- Metacarpal on the first or second dorsal metacarpal arteries.
- Scapula on the circumflex scapular vessels or with trapezius.
- Rib on the intercostal or thoracodorsal vessels, or with pectoralis major.
- Iliac crest on the deep circumflex iliac or superficial circumflex iliac vessels.
- Medial or femoral condyle on the descending genicular vessels.
- Fibula on the peroneal vessels.
- Second metatarsal on the dorsalis pedis vessels.
- Toes/joints on the first dorsal metatarsal artery.
- Chondro-epiphyses on the anterior tibial and peroneal vessels.

Blood supply of bone
- 16% of cardiac output goes to bone (same as kidneys).
- 5–20 ml/min/100 g of tissue.
- Wide regional differences between bones and between areas of individual bones.

The actual mechanics of bone blood flow is controversial, but the most widely accepted theory is that of Brookes (1971).

Arterial supply
- Nutrient artery (main supply).
- Periosteal (via overlying soft tissues).
- Metaphyseal (both via the circulosis articuli vasculosis).
- Epiphyseal (which is supplied by the articular vessels).

Microcirculation
There are two microcirculations which may or may not act as a portal circulation:
- Cortical: blood flows from capillaries towards the central canals of the Haversian system in a centrifugal manner and drains into the periosteal plexus of veins.

- Medullary: blood flows from capillaries toward the medullary sinusoids in a centripetal fashion and then on to veins, which finally drain into the central venous sinus.

Venous drainage
- Nutrient.
- Metaphyseal.
- Epiphyseal.
- Periosteal.

Effects of trauma and fixation on bone blood supply
- Fractures cause local damage to the blood supply of bone and this leads to ischaemia at the site of injury which is proportional to the velocity of the trauma.
- Plates and screws cause damage to the periosteal blood supply; especially the venous drainage.
- Intramedullary reaming damages the endosteal blood supply and may lead to some necrosis, but if the periosteal supply is intact this is not clinically significant (Trueta and Cadavias 1955; Smith et al. 1990).
- External fixation causes least amount of trauma and the least amount of compression of blood supply, and therefore the least amount of vascular impairment.

Types of bone graft
- Cancellous.
- Cortical.
- Cortico-cancellous.
- Vascularized.

Indications
- Enhancement of fracture healing.
- Reconstruction of bony defects.
- Enhancement of arthrodesis.
- Treatment of non-unions.
- AVN.
- Complex tissue loss vascularized.
- Physeal arrest.
- Congenital pseudarthrosis

Healing mechanisms
Differs for each type of graft:
- Cancellous: most cells die due to ischaemia but the large surface area and wide open pores of the trabecular bone allow rapid capillary ingrowth and osteoconduction. Osteo-induction follows due to the liberation of growth factors from dead osteoblasts in the graft. Healing is usually rapid. The graft is initially structurally very weak but gains strength with time. This technique is usually reserved for defects of 6 cm or less.

- Cortical: all the cells die and as the bone is hard lamellar bone revascularization is slow and incomplete. Up to 50% of the graft becomes necrotic and is never replaced by native bone. Initially the graft is structurally strong but this diminishes over time and the patients are at risk of stress fracture especially 6–12 months post-operatively. They need to protect the graft for up to 5 years. Therefore these grafts are reserved for defects greater than 6 cm (Enneking 1980).

Bone grafts in 7.5–12 cm defects, 68% union and 17% stress fracture; in 12–25 cm defects, 67% union and 58% stress fracture. This complication rate is the reason for using vascularized bone.

- Vascularized: the majority of cells survive and are capable of taking part in normal bone healing. Therefore the slow process of revascularization, osteoconduction, and osteo-induction is avoided. Structurally the bone is strong and gains strength with healing and hypertrophy. It is suitable for large defects where load bearing is important and can be combined with soft tissues to reconstruct complex defects. It can also be used where conventional bone grafting has failed or where the bed in unfavourable (e.g. post irradiation).

Disadvantages

Long operative times; potential donor site morbidity; partial or total vascular failure and the need for supplementary bone grafting in a number of cases. However, vascularized bone has been proved to be superior to non-vascularized bone in the experimental and clinical setting.

Further reading

De Boer HH, Wood MB (1989). *J Bone Joint Surg Br* **71**, 374–8.
Haw CS, O'Brien BM, Kurata T (1978). *J Bone Joint Surg Br* **60**, 266–9.
Shaffer JW, Field GA, Goldberg VM, Davy DT (1985). *Clin Orthop Relat Res* **197**, 32–43.
Zdeblick TA, Shaffer JW, Field GA (1988). *Clin Orthop Relat Res* **236**, 296–302.

References

Brookes M (1971). Growth cartilages. The blood supply of bone: an approach to bone biology. Butterworth, London.
Enneking WF, Eady JL, Burchardt H (1980). *J Bone Joint Surg Am* **62**, 1039–58.
Smith SR, Bronk JT, Kelly PJ (1990). *J Orthop Res* **8**, 471–8.
Trueta J, Cavadias AX (1955). *J Bone Joint Surg Br* **37**, 492–505.

Venous drainage in reverse flow flaps

The Chinese flap or radial forearm flap described in 1981 was instrumental in the design and expansion of distally based flaps. Previously the distally based flap was seemingly impossible because of the venous valves obstructing drainage. However, distally based flaps are successful and the venous drainage seems to occur despite the presence of valves.

Anatomy of venous system

Three planes of venous drainage: the superficial system such as the cephalic vein and the saphenous vein which clearly have valves, the deep system which generally are paired VCs running with each artery which have fewer valves, and the communicating venous system, which is also called perforating veins, running between the two.

There are several theories of the mechanism of venous drainage in reverse flow flaps:
- Ladder intervenous communications in the VCs, whereby multiple level venous anastomoses between parallel running VCs allow the blood to cross over and bypass the valves.
- Valve incompetence created by:
  - Increased blood pressure and flow.
  - Vein distension.
  - Sympathectomy and denervation of the vein and valves.
  - Antegrade flow caused by vein filling by arteriovenous channels, causing valves to open briefly and due to retrograde pressure the cumulative effect is retrograde flow.
- Drains via small veins with no valves, called avalvular oscillating veins.
- There are veins with valves directing flow peripherally first before connecting with veins that have proximal flow.

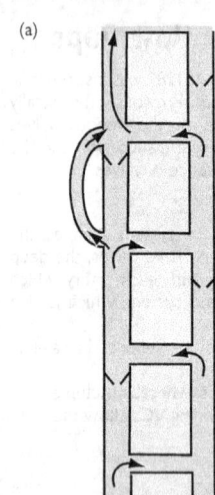
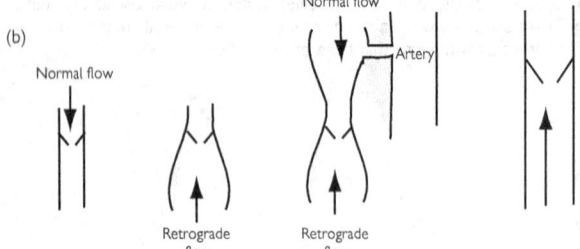

Fig. 22.13 (a) Retrograde venous flow by byassing valves using ladder communications; (b) retrograde venous flow by sympathectomy, denervation, and venous distention leading to valve incompetence.

Venous flaps

A relatively recent concept in flaps based on venous perfusion of skin. Pure venous flaps survive on deoxygenated blood passing through the flap within its venous system. How does this perfuse the skin? No one really knows. These flaps have a high failure rate.

Arterialized venous flaps, where an artery is anastomosed to the venous pedicle of an area of skin thus creating a arteriovenous fistula through the flap, seem to be more reliable. The mechanism of skin perfusion is unknown but proposed to be as follows:

- Retrograde flow from the arterialized vein back through the tiny arteriovenous communications into the artery and then forward flow through the capillary network, draining through the non-arterialized venous side (also called reverse shunting).
- High-pressure retrograde flow through the veins and retrograde through the capillary network. (also called reverse flow).
- Capillary bypass, in which the capillary network is completely bypassed and flap nutrition is supplied entirely by the blood in the larger vessels.

Classification (Thatte and Thatte 1993)

- Veno-venous:
  - Unipedicle.
  - Bipedicle.
- Arteriovenous types:
  - Arteriovenous shunt.
  - Arterialized venous flow-through flap (VFTF).

Advantages

- Many potential donor sites (forearm, dorsal foot, hand and digits, leg).
- No sacrifice of major artery.
- Simple elevation and dissection.
- Thin tissue.

Disadvantages

- Unreliable.
- Thin tissue.
- Skin only.
- Small size only.
- Microsurgery required.

Flap territory

Largest recorded veno-venous flap that survived was 10×8 cm. However, many smaller flaps (2×1) have necrosed. Arterialized venous flaps of size 3×3 cm can reliably survive.

Indications

- Small thin defect reconstruction on the digits and hand, preferably already requiring reconstruction of the artery and/or vein.

Method
- **Position** Patient supine, tourniquet.
- **Planning** Draw out the superficial veins of the palmar distal forearm. Choose the flap area where a vein passes through the flap and preferably has branches within the flap zone.
- **Incision** Incise around the flap.
- **Dissection** Leave the veins extending for 1 cm beyond the flap borders. Clip the branches and leave the chosen venous axis marked by two clips. Start distally and raise flap supra-fascially. Transfer flap and anastomose veins to artery and vein, or artery and artery.
- **Closure** Close donor site directly or by FTSG.

Complications and donor site morbidity
- Small flap size if wish to achieve primary closure; otherwise FTSG.
- Necrosis rate relatively high, especially in veno-venous flap.

Novelties and tips
Choose area with extensive network veins, close to dermis. Composite venous flaps have been reported (Inoue et al. 1990).

References
Inoue G, Maeda N, Suzuki K (1990). *Br J Plast Surg* **43**, 135–9.
Thatte MR, Thatte RL (1993). *Plast Reconstr Surg* **91**, 747–51.

Z-plasty

An extremely versatile technique to lengthen or break up a scar.

Principles
- Incise or excise scar or contracture.
- Design opposing triangular flaps sharing a common border along the scar.
- Transpose the two triangular flaps.

Indications
- Reorient linear scar to relaxed skin tension lines.
- Break up linear scar.
- Lengthen scar or contracted skin.
- Create or deepen web space, or obliterate depression.
- Swap tissues from one area to another.

Geometry
- The angle of the Z-plasty determines the potential gain in length.
- The geometric formula gives a 25% increase in length for every 15° increase in angle.
- The greater the angle the more lateral laxity is required to allow transposition of the flaps.

Table 22.1 Geometry of Z-plasty

Angle	Gain in length %
30°	25%
45°	50%
60°	75%
75°	100%
90°	Impossible to transpose

Method
- *Planning*
  - Draw along the scar or contracture to be corrected.
  - Mark the points where you would like the new scar to lie.
  - If possible, design it so that this will lie on the RSTLs.
  - Draw a line from the scar to the points, creating triangular flaps which share a common border along the scar line.
- *Incision* Incise the lines and elevate the flaps.
- *Closure* If well designed the flaps generally transpose themselves as the contracture relaxes; if not transpose the flaps and suture.

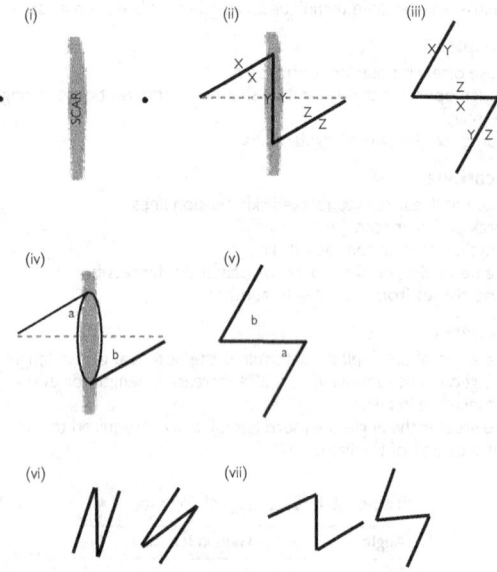

Fig. 22.14 Planning a Z-plasty. (i) Mark points where you would like the transverse limbs to be. (ii) Draw flaps; the lengths of x, y, and z should be the same. (iii) Complete the transposition. (iv) With scar excision, use the dotted line technique to mark the eventual position of the transverse limb. (v) Completed position. (vi) A narrow-angle Z-plasty does not give much gain in length. (vii) A wide-angle Z-plasty gives a marked gain in length.

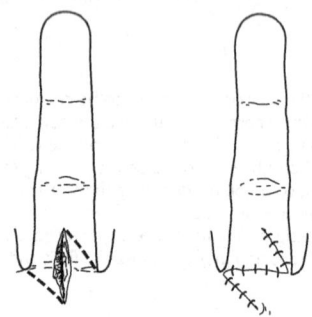

Fig. 22.15 Z-plasty closure of laceration crossing a flexor crease.

Complications
- Failing to transpose the flaps and re-suturing the Zs into their starting position.
- Tip necrosis (especially if sutured under tension; try to reduce tension by a tension-relieving suture halfway along the flap which runs obliquely towards the recipient apex).
- Inability to transpose flaps because of insufficient lateral laxity.

Novelties and tips
Use a pair of open forceps or calipers to determine the start points of your Z-plasty, as the position of the ends of these forceps will indicate the eventual lie of the transverse limb once the triangular flaps have transposed.

Variations
- Multiple, in series: good for long scars.
- Double opposing Z-plasties; good for web spaces.
- Skew Z-plasty (unequal flaps): good where anatomy dictates.
- Flying or jumping man flaps are a combination of Z-plasty with V–Y.

W-plasty

Described by Borges (1959), this technique of disguising a scar involves excising the scar with a zig-zag design of triangles on each side which interdigitate when closed.

Indications
- Reorient linear scar.
- Break up linear scar.
- Treat a trap-door scar.

Limitations
Can contract to present as a linear scar. Can end up as irregular surface scar requiring dermabrasion. Must have sufficient lateral laxity to allow excision and closure.

Method
- *Planning* Draw a continous line of triangles or zig-zags down one side of the scar with diminishing triangle size at the extremes of the scar. Repeat the exact size triangles on the opposite side but offset so that one triangle will sit inside its opposite member. The point of the triangle on one side corresponds to the midpoint of the base of the triangle on the opposite side. This increases lateral tension, therefore excess tissue is needed laterally. If possible, design it so that some of the limbs of the triangles lie on the RSTLs.
- *Incision* Incise around the design and excise the central skin and scar.
- *Closure* Close triangles.

Complications and donor site morbidity
- Scar contracts and becomes linear.
- Scar is ridged.

Novelties and tips
Can use a template to ensure matching triangles.

Reference
Borges AF (1959). *Br J Plast Surg* **12**, 29.

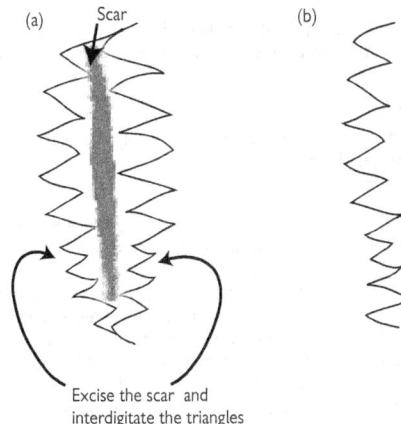

Fig. 22.16 W-plasty: (a) Draw matching triangles on either side of the scar. Excise the scar and interdigitate the triangles. (b) Final result.

Rhomboid flap
(Also known as Limberg flap)

Described by Limberg (1966) and therefore also known as a Limberg flap, this random pattern flap uses an easy geometric design to close defects with local tissue.

Indications
- Any defect where tissue laxity can be identified at least in one plane adjacent to the defect.

Method
- *Planning* Determine the RSTLs and the direction of maximal laxity. Design the flap by first drawing the V-shape (the two flap sides) that will allow easy closure and result in a donor scar in a RSTL. Move the V, maintaining its relationship to the RSTLs and the lax plane, until it centres on the defect. Draw a rhomboid around the defect so that one of its sides is parallel to one of the flap sides and the other flap side meets the junction of two sides of the rhomboid that have formed an angle of 120°. The rhomboid should have sides of equal length, two angles of 60°, and two angles of 120°, with the distance between the two 120° angles equal to the length of the sides. For any rhomboid, four potential rhomboid flaps can be planned by drawing lines parallel to the sides of the rhomboid and equal to their length. Choose one of the two rhomboid flaps that leaves the donor in RSTL.
- *Incision* Incise around the flap and around the rhomboid.
- *Dissection* Elevate the flap in the subcutaneous plane. Transpose into the defect.
- *Closure* Close the donor site directly. Inset flap.

Advantages
- Easy geometric design.

Complications
- Incorrect placement of flap to place donor site closure scar in RSTL.
- Flap designed too small.
- Most tension is in closure of the secondary defect and the furthest corner of the flap. This is reduced in the Dufourmental design.

Variation
Square peg into round hole. In this variation the defect is cut out as a circle and a rhomboid is raised from this and trimmed to size as necessary.

Reference
Limberg AA (1966). *Mod Trends Plast Surg* **2**, 38–61.

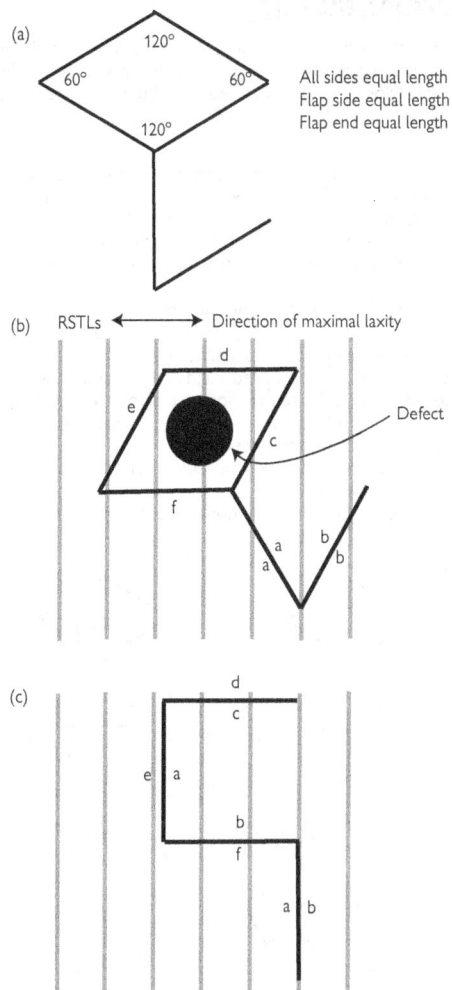

Fig. 22.17 Rhomboid flap: (a) general design; (b) design orientated against RSTLs so closure of secondary defects is in line of least tension; (c) flap transposition and closure.

Dufourmental flap

A variation of the rhomboid flap proposed by Dufourmental (1963), this flap reduces the tension required to close the rhomboid flap by angling the secondary closure away from the rhomboid. It is more difficult to design.

Method
- Before excision of the lesion draw a rhomboid around the defect. Unlike the rhomboid flap, this need not be a strict 120° and 60° rhomboid (some recommend angles of 30° and 150° angles). However, the rhomboid should have sides of equal length.
- Extend the side of the rhomboid in the chosen area of the flap with a line (dotted 1).
- Draw a dotted line connecting the angle of the rhomboid in the chosen area of the flap with the opposing angle of the rhomboid, and extend this line into the flap area for quite a distance (dotted 2).
- Bisect the angle formed by dotted 1 and dotted 2 and draw a line equal to the length of the sides of the rhomboid along this bisection (flap 1).
- Draw a line perpendicular to the dotted 2, joining the end of flap 1. Its length should be equal to the side of the rhomboid.
- Cut out the rhomboid and the flap, being careful that you do not cut on the planning lines
- Transpose the flap and close the donor site directly before insetting.

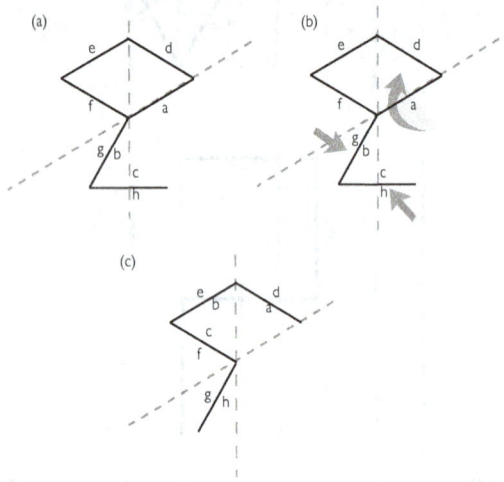

Fig. 22.18 Dufourmental flap: (a) design; (b) transposition; (c) end result.

Reference
Dufourmental C (1966).

Bi-lobed flap

A random pattern two-skin-flap design used to transfer the defect in two steps into an area with greater tissue laxity that allows direct closure. First described by Esser in 1918 and modified by Zitelli (1989).

Vascularity
Random.

Movement
Pivot flap by two transposition flaps.

Principles
This is a two-flap technique. The primary flap, which is adjacent to and slightly smaller than the defect, closes the defect. The secondary flap closes the first flap defect. It is designed to be half the size of the primary flap and should lie in an area of laxity which maybe adjacent to the first flap (transposition) or further away (interpolation).

Uses
Mainly facial defects, especially the nasal tip where there is an anatomical shortage of tissue directly around the defect but laxity close by, but can be used anywhere.

Planning
Assess defect size and the location of loose tissue. Mark the flap. In general, a laterally based design is used for the nasal tip and a medially based design for defects of the alar lobule. Try not to cross the nasal midline.

Geometry
- A vertical line is drawn through the centre of the defect. The location of the pivot point lies about one radius of the defect away from the defect. Avoid placing the pivot point close to the alar margin or medial canthus of the eye. The first flap is usually at an angle of 30°–45° to this line and adjacent to the defect. The width of the flap is slightly smaller than the defect.
- The second flap may be adjacent to the first, but more commonly there is a bridge of tissue between them.
- The angle of the second flap may be at 60°–180° from the line through the defect but is most commonly at 120°.
- The second flap is half the size of the first and pivots to the defect left by the first flap. The length of the flaps are designed to reach the end of the defect that they need to fill, but in practice they are designed to be longer. The pivot point for a bi-lobed flap is the centre of a circle at the convergence of the axis of the flaps.
- The flaps are incised and undermined. The first flap is placed into the defect. The second flap pivots into the donor left by the first flap and the donor for the second flap is closed directly.

Post-operative care
Nothing specific; ensure no haematoma.

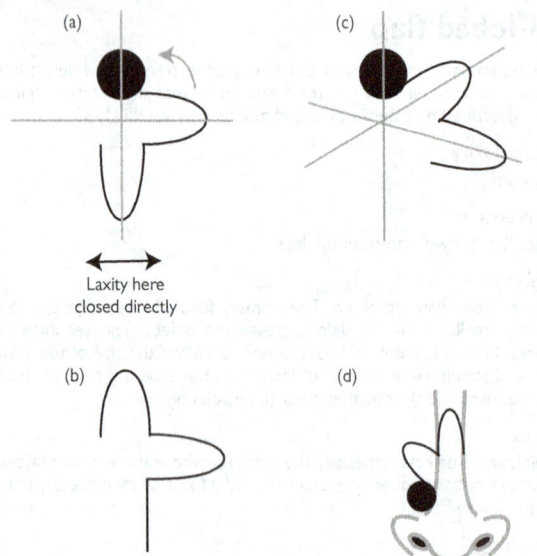

Fig. 22.19 Bi-lobed flap: (a) design; (b) closure; (c) alternative design; (d) example on the nose, note the tertiary defect closed directly along RSTL and in the area of loosest tissue.

Risks and complications
Can sometimes pin cushion especially on the nose. Poor design leads to poor results (small flaps, excess tension, damaged blood supply, inadequate haemostasis). Poor design can also lead to elevation or distortion of the alar margin.

Tips
Useful on the back based on paraspinal perforators. Also used to redistribute skin such as in correction of radial dysplasia (Evans) or deviated thumbs. Zitelli (1989).

Reference
Zitelli JA (1989). *Arch Dermatol* **125**, 157–9.

Horn flap

Another variation of the V–Y flap which advances and rotates. It relies on its blood supply coming through a unilateral subcutaneous pedicle.

Classification
Local island flap which is advanced in a V–Y fashion.

Composition
Cutaneous.

Dimensions
Horn-shaped flap corresponding to the arc of a circle, with a pedicle which is analogous to a radius of the same circle, allowing advancement of the flap around circumference. Pedicle enters flap on concave side, and dissection is more superficial on that side.

Uses
Face including side of nose and eyebrow, especially in medial canthal area. Also advocated in leg.

Anatomy
Radially (laterally) based subcutaneous pedicle. Random.

Method
- *Planning* Curvature/shape of flap is adjusted to accommodate exact position of defect, e.g. lesion excised near to medial canthus is reconstructed with a more curved flap than one excised from the side of nose, although both may originate in the glabellar area. A horn flap on the lower limb has a much larger radius and can be a larger flap.
- *Incision* Around flap down to subcutaneous fat only. Down to or through fascia on the convex side of the flap.
- *Procedure* The adjacent skin on the concave side of the flap is elevated subdermally to expose the pedicle. The leading edge of the flap and pedicle are incised. The flap is raised from convex side to concave in the subfascial plane. Raising is continued until the pivot point is reached under the fascia. The trailing edge of the pedicle is divided. The skin adjacent to the defect on the concave side of the flap is also undermined to allow rotational advancement of the flap pedicle. The flap and pedicle are advanced and the tip is trimmed to fit the defect.
- *Donor* Closed directly.
- *Post-operative* Routine.

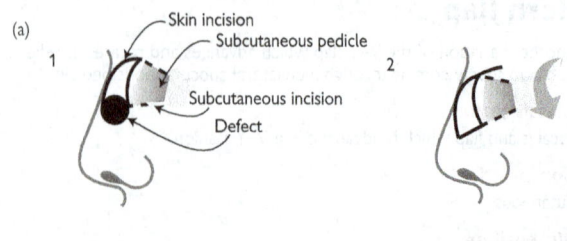

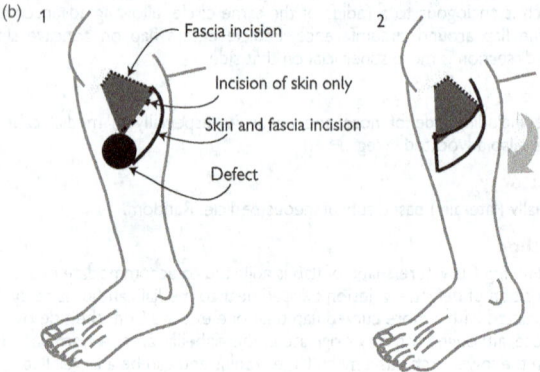

Fig. 22.20 (a) Nasal horn flap. (1) Defect and design of a unilateral pedicled V–Y flap. Dotted line indicates release of the subcutaneous tissue which is also released from the overlying skin and deep bone in the shaded area as well as deep to the flap. (2) Advanced and closed. (b) Leg horn flap. (1) Defect and design. The V flap is based on the fascia on one side of the flap. The bold dotted line should be through the skin and fat only leaving the fascia pedicle intact. The fine dotted line indicates the fascia release allowing flap to swing. (2) Advanced and closed.

Advantages
- Less 'trap-door' scarring (possibly due to curved shape of flap dispersing tendency to contracture along curve).
- Entry of pedicle on radial/concave side makes significant advancement possible.
- Easy to execute in the upper part of the nasal dorsum; also easy on the leg with a fascia-only pedicle (Pennington).

Disadvantages
- Quite extensive dissection relative to defect.
- More difficult to plan.

Banner flap

A random pattern local transposition flap consisting of a banner- or-bullet shaped skin flap, most commonly used around the nose and face for circular defects.

Composition
Cutaneous.

Dimensions
Limited by ability to close secondary defect without causing deformity, and by maximum length-to-breadth ratio of 2:1.

Uses
For small defects <1.5 cm diameter on nasal dorsum away from tip, or elsewhere on face especially forehead.

Anatomy
Random pattern blood supply.

Method
- *Planning* Long axis of the flap is significantly longer than the diameter of the defect to allow easy closure of secondary defect. The base of the flap is made narrower than the diameter of the defect. Plan in reverse from pivot point to ensure that flap length is adequate and will not cause deformity on closure of flap or donor site. Design donor site in zone of skin laxity along RSTLs.
- *Incision* Down to subcutaneous fat.
- *Procedure* Flap is transposed 90° and tip is trimmed to fit defect.
- *Donor* Closed directly.
- *Post-operative* Routine.

Advantages
Easy to execute in the upper part of the nasal dorsum.

Disadvantages
Unreliable in the lower third of the nose, often resulting in a prominent dog ear, which requires further operations to correct. Excision of dog ear during the first operation risks compromising flap blood supply. Asymmetrical elevation of the alar rim tends to occur when the flap is taken primarily from one side of the nose; this can be minimized by taking the flap from across the bridge of the nose, so that donor defect involves both sides of the nose. This may be more aesthetically obvious as the flap disturbs the dorsal nasal lines.

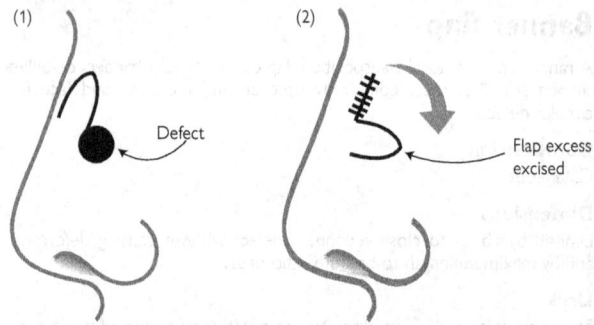

Fig. 22.21 Banner flap: (1) defect and design; (2) flap transposed and secondary defect closed directly in line of RSTL.

Dorsal nasal flap

A local flap consisting of the whole dorsal nasal skin raised as a flap based on the angular artery most commonly used for tip or alar defects on the nose. There are two possible designs ipsilateral or contralateral. The secondary defect is planned to sit in the glabella allowing closure as a V–Y. A very aesthetically pleasing flap.

Composition
Local, rotation advancement cutaneous.

Dimensions
Entire dorsum of nose.

Uses
For small defects <2 cm diameter on nasal tip and junctional defects between dorsum and alar.

Anatomy
Type A with a random pattern blood supply from tiny branches from the angular artery or with an axial blood supply from a branch of the angular artery that enters the skin of the nasal radix below the medial canthal ligament.

Types of dorsal nasal flap
- Contralateral (Marchac).
- Ipsilateral (Rieger).

Method
- *Planning* LA can be used. Decide on type of dorsal nasal flap according to defect site and shape. Draw flap design keeping incisions along aesthetic unit junctions, i.e. follows the junction of the nose and cheek, and then the alar groove, the tip and the other alar groove. In the ipsilateral there is a back cut along the nose–cheek junction.
- *Triangulate* the defect to fit the flap along aesthetic junctions. Try to extend flap along nasal tip borders rather than cut across the aesthetic unit; this may enlarge the defect but will be worth it. Do hydro-dissection with LA in the deep plane.
- *Incision* Excise the lesion and triangulate the defect. Incise around the flap down to the submuscular layer.
- *Procedure* Skin, subcutaneous tissue and muscle are elevated from the convex side towards the base of the flap, just above the periosteum and perichondrium of the nasal dorsum, in the deep subcutaneous plane just above the nasal bone and cartilage. This dissection is much easier after hydro-dissection with LA. Advance the flap secure with vicryl.
- *Donor* Closed directly, by V–Y closure at glabella.
- *Post-operative* Routine.

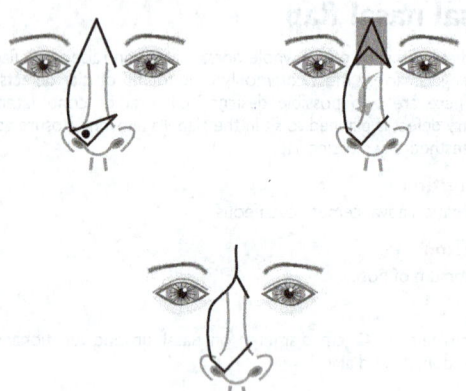

Fig. 22.22 Dorsal nasal flap: contralateral pedicle (Marchac).

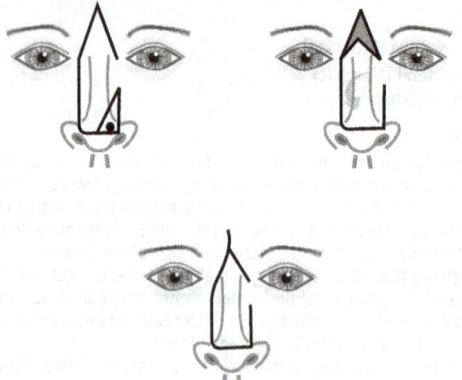

Fig. 22.23 Dorsal nasal flap: ipsilateral pedical (Reiger).

Advantages
Provides single unit of closely matching tissue with scars that coincide with aesthetic unit junctions, large flap so scars less easily seen and less trap-dooring of flap; donor closes directly, can be done under LA; same tissue so good colour and texture match.

Disadvantages
Can cause notching if used for infratip defects; seems like a big flap but it does look better than a small one, especially in the younger patient.

Nasalis flap

A local advancement myocutaneous flap consisting of a comet- or teardrop-shaped island of skin based on nasalis muscle perforators which is advanced as in a V–Y flap. Commonly used for reconstruction of alar defects on the nose.

Classification
Pedicled, island.

Composition
Myocutaneous.

Dimensions
Teardrop-shaped; lower incision right in the alar groove; upper incision is continued from the upper pole of the defect; longitudinal dimension variable.

Uses
For small defects (≤1.25 cm) of the lateral tip or nostril wing, paramedian lesions.

Anatomy
The nasalis muscle is a quadrilateral-shaped muscle with a thin origin along the piriform aperture, widening as it moves up the side of the nose and becoming aponeurotic as it continues medially and becomes associated with the dermis of the nasal tip and bridge. It is supplied by a branch of the superior labial artery at the muscle's base.

Method
- *Planning* The flap must extend all the way to the alar base, since the separation of skin from its muscle and blood supply occurs there. Plan in reverse from advancement point to ensure flap width is adequate and will not cause alar elevation or deformity on closure of flap or donor site.
- *Incision* Down to subcutaneous fat except at the alar base where only the skin is completely divided, creating an island. The flap base continues wider than the apex of the flap and is exposed by elevating the adjacent skin.
- *Procedure* Flap is elevated and its muscular attachments at the piriform base are detached, preserving the lateral subcutaneous attachments. Redundant corners of the flap are excised and flap is advanced.
- *Donor* Closed directly.
- *Post-operative* Routine.

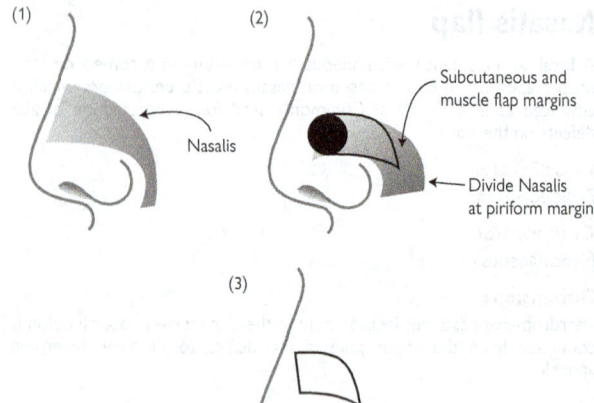

Fig. 22.24 Nasalis flap: (1) nasalis muscle outline; (2) defect and design of a deep-based V–Y flap advanced by advancing the majority of nasalis, preserving myocutaneous perforators; (3) advanced and closed.

Advantages
Distinct aesthetic advantage over rotation flap, i.e. scars at or parallel to natural lines of the lateral alar crus, no dog ears and oedema or trapdoor deformity. Bilateral flap can be used to resurface larger defects (2 cm). It has been used successfully for reconstruction of retracted nostrils following burns.

Disadvantages
Asymmetrical elevation of the alar rim can occur.

Nasolabial flap

A local flap consisting of the skin in the nasolabial fold, alar groove, and cheek–nose margin along the axis of the facial and the angular arteries. Most commonly used for tip or alar defects on the nose when proximally based and for lip reconstruction when inferiorly based. There are two possible designs, proximal or distally based. The secondary defect is planned to sit in the nasolabial fold or cheek nose junction. An aesthetically pleasing flap.

Composition
Local, transposition, cutaneous.

Dimensions
Can be 1–2 cm wide, especially if skin is taken from the nasolabial fold.

Uses
- Proximally based: for small defects (<2 cm diameter) on nasal tip; alar and junctional defects between dorsum and alar. Can reconstruct full-thickness defects by turning in the tip of the flap to form the alar rim and the mucosa.
- Distally based: alar and peri-alar reconstruction; lip and commissure reconstruction; intra-oral defects including tongue and floor of mouth.

Anatomy
Type B with axial pattern blood supply based on the angular artery and the termination of the facial artery, and which anastomoses with the ophthalmic artery at the medial orbital wall so can be proximally or distally based.

Method
- *Planning* LA can be used. Decide on type of nasolabial flap according to defect site and shape. Draw flap design, keeping incisions along or parallel to aesthetic unit junctions, i.e. follow the junction of the nose and cheek along the alar groove and the nasolabial fold. Triangulate the defect to fit flap along aesthetic junctions. Try to extend flap along cheek–nasal borders, making a very long nasolabial flap rather then a short flap that cuts across the aesthetic unit, especially the alar groove. Obliteration of this groove is very noticeable and is the most common error in performing this flap.
- *Incision* Excise the lesion and triangulate the defect. Incise around the flap down to the subcutaneous supramuscular layer (quite deep).
- *Procedure* Skin and subcutaneous tissue are elevated from superior towards the base of the flap. Transpose the flap.
- *Donor* Closed directly.
- *Post-operative* Routine.

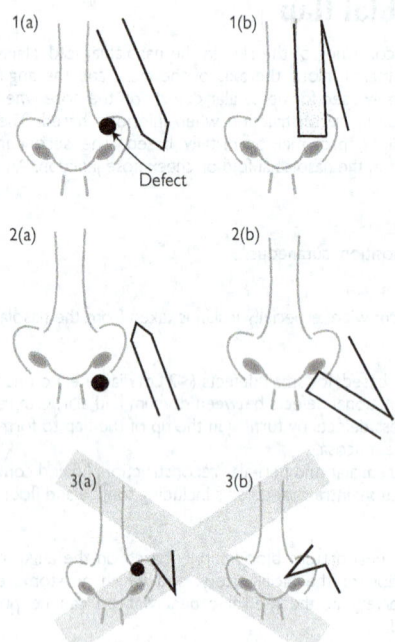

Fig. 22.25 Nasolabial flaps. 1(a) Raise the flap based high on the angular artery so that 1(b) when it is transferred it does not obliterate the alar groove. 2(a) An inferior based nasolabial fold applied to a nasal base defect; 2(b) closed: 3(a) Do *not* design the nasolabial flap like this as 3(b) it will obliterate the alar groove and be obvious.

Advantages
Provides single unit of closely matching tissue with scars that coincide with aesthetic unit junctions; donor closes directly; can be done under LA; same tissue so good colour and texture match.

Disadvantages
Can cause notching if too short. Can obliterate critical alar groove. Can be bulky if used for alar rim and mucosa.

Tips
Avoid obliterating alar groove by careful design and by taking the flap as high up the cheek–nose margin as the medial canthus. Alternative strategies are a two-stage exteriorized pedicle technique with division of pedicle after 2–3 weeks to ensure preservation of critical anatomical margins, or having a de-epithelialized pedicle that is buried.

Cervico-facial flap

A commonly used and versatile flap for cheek reconstruction. Raised in the deep subcutaneous plane just above platysma. It is a particularly useful flap as it can keep extending inferiorly until it provides sufficient tissue for tension-free closure.

Composition
Local rotation advancement flap.

Dimensions
Whole cheek.

Uses
Defects of any size on the cheek in any cheek zone.

Anatomy
The facial skin over the cheek is of fairly consistent thickness, greater than that of the eyelid and lips. The subcutaneous fat layer is also thicker and has more fascial connections. Deep to the subcutaneous fat lies the SMAS–platysma layer, which is indistinct in areas but is a continuous sheet of fascia. The plane is easiest found superficial to platysma and then followed superiorly. The facial nerve lies deep to the SMAS on the superficial aponeurosis of masseter. The skin is supplied by the facial artery medially and the external carotid terminal branches, the superficial temporal and maxillary, laterally.

Types
- Anteriorly and inferiorly based rotation advancement flap but extending much further down the neck (Juri and Juri 1979).
- Posteriorly (inferior lateral based).
- Cervico-pectoral flap: a variant of the above but extending onto the chest over pectoralis major in the delto-pectoral flap zone (Becker 1978).

Method
- *Planning* LA for small defects but GA is preferred for larger defects. Decide on type of cervicofacial flap according to defect site, size, and shape. Draw flap design, keeping incisions along aesthetic unit junctions, i.e. follow the junction of the nose and cheek, and then the eyelid cheek margin, pre-auricular margin, or nasolabial fold. Triangulate the defect to fit flap along aesthetic junctions.
- *Incision* Excise the lesion and triangulate the defect or leave this until after the flap has advanced. Incise around the flap down to subcutaneous fat or SMAS layer.

- **Procedure** Skin and subcutaneous tissue are elevated from the incision towards the base of the flap. Raise flap, and advance; if not sufficient extend the flap down into the neck, and if still insufficient extend onto chest. Advance the flap.
- **Donor** Closed directly.
- **Post-operative** Routine.

Advantages
Provides single unit of closely matching tissue with scars that coincide with aesthetic unit junctions; large flap so scars less easily seen and less trap-dooring of flap; donor closes directly; can be done under LA if small; same tissue so good colour and texture match.

Disadvantages
Seems like a big flap! However, it does look better than a small one, especially in the younger patient.

Complications
- Haematoma.
- Flap-edge necrosis.

References
Becker DW, Jr (1978). *Plast Reconstr Surg* **61**, 868–70.
Juri J, Juri C (1979). *Plast Reconstr Surg* **64**, 692–6.

Jejunal flap

Transplantation of the intestine was first described by Carrel in 1905. Gastric and colon have been used, but jejunum is the most popular because of its low complication rate.

Anatomy
Vascular anatomy: type 1 or 3 (if take two pedicles)
The jejunum comprises the proximal 40% of the small intestine. It commences at the duodenojejunal flexure and ends at the ileum. Jejunal arteries are branches of the superior mesenteric artery and travel within the mesentery towards the bowel. As they approach the jejunum, they form arcades which anastomose with each other. Branches from the arcades (vasa rectae) pass to the intestine wall. Veins correspond to the arteries.

Flap territory
Pedicle length up to 20 cm. The normal length of jejunum raised is 10–14 cm. Can take more using two vascular arcades.

Indications
- Pedicled proximally:
    - Lower oesophageal reconstruction; usually supercharged two-segment reconstruction of total oesophagus.
- Free:
    - Pharyngo-oesophagus replacement.
    - Oral cavity defects; it may be used as a tube or split along its anti mesenteric border and opened out.
    - Vaginal reconstruction.

Limitations
Intra-abdominal operation; lumen 3–5 cm; previous bowel surgery may complicate harvest.

Method
- **Position** patient supine.
- **Incision** midline laparotomy.
- **Dissection** mobilize the jejunum on its vessels. Identify the ligament of Treitz and take a segment of proximal jejunum ~50 cm distal to this. Ensure that the segment is longer than required and centred on a suitable artery and vein. Choose an arcade supplying sufficient length of bowel. Trace vessel to source vessel. Dissection commences from the root of the mesentery to the bowel, which is clamped and divided. Correctly mark proximal and distal ends of the bowel so that it can be placed in the correct direction of peristalsis in the neck. When in the neck do the proximal anastomosis, splitting along the antimesenteric border to spatulate the end in cases of size discrepancy.
Next do the microsurgery and finally the distal anastomosis, trimming the redundant jejunum to fit snugly. Remember that the neck is usually extended for the ablative surgery! Bleeding and peristalsis indicate that the flap is alive.

- *Closure* Anastomose bowel. Close donor site directly.
- *Donor* Monitor for bowel anastomotic problems.

Advantages
- Diameter of the jejunum similar to oesophagus.
- Replace mucosa with mucosa.
- Good pedicle length.

Disadvantages
- High fistula rate (up to 30%) especially if significant size discrepancy at the proximal end.
- Involvement of the abdominal cavity in an already sick patient.

Complications and donor site morbidity
- Hernia.
- Abdominal infection.
- Intra-abdominal complications.

Tips
- Get a general surgeon to help.
- Not for the casual case.
- In units where this is done routinely it is a good flap. In other places a tubed skin flap may be more appropriate.

Omental flap

Transfer of potentially large volumes of well vascularized fat with some unique macrophagic lymphocytic activity. Used as pedicle flap for mediastinal and head and neck reconstruction. First described as a free flap by MacLean and Buncke (1972).

Anatomy
The greater omentum is a double layer of peritoneum containing lymphatics and adipose tissue. It hangs down from the greater curvature of the stomach for ~25 cm and doubles back to attach to the transverse mesocolon.

Vascular anatomy: type 1 or 3 (if take two pedicles)
The gastro-epiploic vessels form a vascular arcade along the greater curvature of the stomach. The flap can be based on the right gastro-epiploic or the left gastro-epiploic The free flap is based on the right gastro-epiploic, a branch of the gastroduodenal. Pedicle length can be increased by dissecting it from the proximal flap tissue. The right gastro-epiploic vein accompanies the artery.

Flap territory
The entire omentum can be used (maximum size approx. 25 × 35 cm).

Suitability for free tissue transfer
Good pedicle length and vessel diameter. Can be used as a flow-through flap.

Indications
- Pedicled proximally (right gastro-epiploic):
  - Mediastinum.
- Pedicled distally (left gastro-epiploic):
  - Pelvic reconstruction.
  - Has been used for lymphoedema.
- Free:
  - Facial atrophy, Romberg's disease.
  - Scalp.
  - Cheek.
  - Back.
  - Radionecrosis.

Limitations
- Can change size with weight change.
- Flimsy tissue.
- Opens abdominal cavity with risk of infection when used for infective indication.

Method
- **Position** Patient supine.
- **Planning** Get a general surgeon to help.
- **Incision** Midline laparotomy.
- **Dissection** The omentum is found and lifted up under tension. The lesser sac is approached throught the underside of the omentum and separated from the transverse colon in this avascular plane. The vascular branches to the greater curvature of the stomach are divided, leaving the omentum on the right and left gastro-epiploic arteries. Divide the left artery and check perfusion.
- **Closure** Close donor site directly. Inset flap.

Complications and donor site morbidity
- Risks associated with any laparotomy.
- Gastric volvulus (minimized by suturing of greater curvature to transverse colon).
- Weight gain or loss is seen in the omentum.
- Does not incorporate into tissues; therefore must be secured in place or becomes gravitationally dependent.
- Donor site problems such as adhesions or volvulus.
- Minimal long-term morbidity.

Tips
- Can segmentalize the flap between arcades.
- Transillumination of the omentum allows identification of main segments.

Reference
McLean DH, Buncke HJ Jr (1972). *Plast Reconstr Surg* **49**, 268–74

Lateral arm flap

A fascio-cutaneous flap from the distal lateral arm based on the posterior radial collateral artery and its septocutaneous perforators (Song et al. 1982; Katsaros et al. 1984 (free lateral arm)).

Anatomy
Utilizes skin on the distal posterior lateral aspect of the lateral arm between the deltoid insertion and the lateral epicondyle of the humerus, centred over the axis of the lateral intermuscular septum.

Vascular anatomy: type C
The profunda brachii artery courses posterior to the humerus within the spiral groove and emerges at the deltoid insertion. Beyond the deltoid insertion the artery continues as the posterior radial collateral.

The flap receives its blood from numerous small perforators from the posterior radial collateral artery as it travels along the lateral intermuscular septum between triceps and brachialis. The perforators directly supply the skin coursing within the septum. There are perforators supplying the supracondylar ridge of the humerus. Distally the vessel splits into an anterior and posterior branch, allowing it to be distally based on either vessel. The anterior continues quite superficially as the radial recurrent artery (the first branch from the radial artery) between brachialis and brachioradialis (lateral to the radial nerve). The posterior has a distal anastomosis with the posterior recurrent interosseous artery (recurrent from the posterior interosseous artery) found between brachioradialis/lateral epicondyle and the olecranon.

Neural supply
The posterior radial collateral artery is accompanied in the septum by the posterior cutaneous nerves of the arm and forearm.

Flap territory
A skin ellipse 10 × 15 cm, with a central axis along the line deltoid insertion to lateral epicondyle. For direct closure keep width <5 cm.

Suitability for free tissue transfer
Yes. Avoids sacrifice of major vessel. The proximal posterior radial collateral vessels are ≥1 mm in diameter, with a pedicle length of 7–8 cm. This can be extended by harvesting profunda brachii. Usually thinner flap than groin, but can still have thick subcutaneous fat.

Indications
- Skin only.
- Neurotized skin.
- Osteofascio-cutaneous with supracondylar ridge humerus.
- Pedicled:
  - Distally used for elbow (olecranon or cubital fossa) soft tissue reconstruction.
  - Proximally can cover upper arm defects up to the acromion, coracoid, and axilla.

- Free can be used for any indication above and in addition:
  - Both lower and upper limb reconstruction.
  - Head and neck reconstruction.

Limitations
The pedicle is not as long as some other local flaps, such as the radial forearm flap. Some would not advocate this flap in women and children because of the cosmetic consequences. Donor cannot be closed if flap >6 cm wide. Bulky in some. Can be hairy.

Method
- *Position* Patient supine or lateral; tourniquet.
- *Incision* Skin: design ellipse longitudinally centred over line drawn over palpated intermuscular septum corresponding to line from deltoid insertion to lateral epicondyle. Apex of ellipse at deltoid insertion proximally and distally at lateral epicondyle. Design can alter along this line to fit according to the pivot point (proximally the deltoid insertion, distally approximately (depending on the vessel) the lateral epicondyle) and planning in reverse principles.
- *Dissection* Incise around the flap and longitudinally along the line towards the pivot point. Elevate the skin flap in the supra-fascial plane from anterior to posterior until the intermuscular septum is seen. Elevate the skin posterior to anterior until the intermuscular septum is seen. Retract brachialis anteriorly and triceps posteriorly to expose the septum. Visualize the perforators and the posterior radial collateral artery. Follow the vessel proximally or distally according to flap design plan. Keep the vessel and septum with the flap, leaving the radial nerve intact. Once the flap is bipedicled on the vessel, divide the unrequired end and pivot about the remaining vessel, or divide this also if using as a free flap.
- *Closure* Close donor site directly, if possible over drains. If tight it is preferable to SSG or FTSG the defect. Inset flap.

Complications and donor site morbidity
The radial nerve may be damaged in the spiral groove or by tight closure. Loss of sensation/hyperaesthesia in the lateral elbow/forearm. An aesthetically displeasing donor scar. However, when the donor can be closed primarily, it a favourable donor site compared with the radial forearm flap.

Novelties
Has been used as an extended flap by extending the ellipse of skin distally as far as the mid-forearm. Can be thinned quite radically, preserving the perforators.

References
Song R, Song Y, Yu Y, Song Y (1982). *Clin Plast Surg* **9**, 27–35.
Katsaros J, Schusterman M, Beppu M, Banis JC Jr, Acland RD (1984). *Ann Plast Surg* **12**, 489–500.

Medial arm flap

A fascio-cutaneous flap based on the medial upper arm skin which can be pedicled (Kaplan and Pearl 1980) or free (Newsom 1981) and can be sensate.

Anatomy
The medial arm skin in the distal half of the arm is supplied by an axial direct artery to the skin arising from a branch of the superior ulna collateral artery.

Vascular anatomy: type B
Based on the superior ulna collateral artery (SUCA) and the VCs. SUCA originates from the brachial artery about 6 cm from the pectoral insertion, which is roughly the mid-point of the arm, and sends a direct axial branch to skin. Distally the continuation of the superior ulna collateral artery pierces the intermuscular septum to join the ulnar nerve in the posterior compartment along the medial head of triceps. SUCA anastomoses with the inferior ulnar collateral artery (IUCA) proximal to the medial epicondyle and with the posterior ulnar collateral artery (PUCA), distally allowing the flap to be distally based but only if SUCA is taken with the flap more proximally than the cutaneous artery origin.

Neural supply
The medial arm skin is innervated by the medial cutaneous nerve of arm which can be harvested and the flap kept innervated (if proximally based) or re-innervated by neural anastomosis if distally based or free. The ulnar nerve travels with the artery and can be harvested with the flap to provide a vascularized ulnar nerve for brachial plexus reconstruction.

Flap territory
The medial arm skin of size 28 × 8 cm (pedicled) or 13 × 7 cm (free).

Suitability for free tissue transfer
Uncommonly used as it is difficult to raise, has variable anatomy, has only a moderate length pedicle (3–4 cm) and small vessels (<1–2 mm diameter). However, it does have thin pliable non-hairy pale skin and is in a very discreet area.

Indications
- Pedicled proximally:
    - Coverage of nose (Tagliocozzi)
    - Axilla (post burn contracture).
- Pedicled distally:
    - Antecubital fossa.
    - Elbow.
- Free:
    - Any small cutaneous defect requiring thin pliable skin, especially if the donor site needs to be well hidden.

Limitations
Minimal sensory supply; minimal volume of tissue; only moderate size if direct closure of donor site.

Method
- **Position** Patient supine; tourniquet; arm abducted on arm board.
- **Planning** Draw a line coracoid to medial epicondyle and posterior axilla to medial epicondyle. The flap will be designed within these two lines. Palpate the brachial artery in the mid-arm to locate the origin of the vessel. This is the proximal pivot point. The distal pivot point is 5 cm proximal to the medial epicondyle. Template the defect, and draw the outline of the flap, making it into an ellipse to aid direct closure.
- **Incision** Incise around the flap and longitudinally along the line towards the pivot point or point of origin of SUCA.
- **Dissection** Elevate the skin flap in the supra-fascial plane from lateral to medial until the intermuscular septum is seen; look for and preserve the cutaneous vessel(s). Beware the median nerve and the musculo-cutaneous nerve. Elevate the skin posterior to anterior until inter-muscular septum is seen. Retract triceps posteriorly to expose the SUCA and ulnar nerve. Follow the vessel proximally or distally according to flap design plan. Keep the vessel and septum with the flap, leaving the ulnar nerve behind. Other perforators to the skin may be seen from the SUCA and the IUCA lying anterior to brachialis. Once the flap is bipedicled on the vessel, divide the unrequired (usually distal end) and pivot about the remaining vessel, or divide this also if using as a free flap. For safety the entire dissection can be performed subfascially. However, the chance of injury to the nerves is then greater.
- **Closure** Close donor site directly, if possible over drains. If tight it is preferable to SSG or FTSG the defect. Inset flap.

Unusual complications
Sensory denervation of the medial arm and proximal ulnar forearm. Ulnar nerve symptoms usually due to tight closure and intra-operative manipulation.

Donor site morbidity
Ulnar nerve symptoms are usually temporary. Beware the musculo-cutaneous/lateral nerve of forearm and median nerve.

Novelties and tips
Could be raised as a vascularized ulnar nerve 'graft' including skin and soft tissue cover.

References
Kaplan EN, Pearl RM (1980). *Ann Plast Surg* **4**, 205–15.
Newsom HT (1981). *Plast Reconstr Surg* **67**, 63–6.

Radial forearm flap

Classic fascio-cutaneous flap sometimes called the Chinese flap (Yang et al. 1981). May be used pedicled proximally, distally, or as a free flap. Can include fascia, skin, nerve, muscle, tendon, and bone. Was immensely popular but use has decreased.

Anatomy
The skin of the entire forearm can be supplied by the radial artery (and has been used in this way in salvage procedures).

Vascular anatomy: type C
Based on the radial artery and either the VCs or a superficial vein (usually the cephalic vein). The radial artery travels under cover of the anterior margin of brachioradialis in the proximal forearm and distally under the deep fascia on the radial dorsal margin of FCR. On the deep surface the artery lies on FDS and distally FPL. Throughout its course the radial artery gives perforator branches to skin and fascia that pass along the septal plane. These perforators are more abundant in the distal third of the forearm. They supply the fascial plexus and perforate directly to skin and so the fascia need not be incorporated in the flap. There are similar branches that pass deep to supply the radius periosteum.

Neural supply
The radial forearm skin is innervated by the lateral cutaneous nerve of the forearm, which is a continuation of the musculo-cutaneous. This branch can be harvested and the flap kept innervated (if proximally based) or re-innervated by neural anastomosis if distally based or free. The superficial radial nerve travels with the artery and can be harvested with the flap to provide a vascularized nerve.

Flap territory
The entire forearm can survive on these perforators and the radial artery. However, the usual flap limitations are the ulna subcutaneous border and the dorsal border of brachioradialis. The smallest flap could be 1 cm^2 but at this size there are less wasteful alternatives. The entire length of the radial vessels, a 10 cm length of radius, and a similar length of FCR or PL tendon can be harvested with the flap.

Suitability for free tissue transfer
Easily and widely used as it has a long pedicle (up to 20 cm) with large vessels (3–5 mm diameter), is easy to raise, and is robust and reliable. Thin pliable skin or fascia, with unique versatility for reconstruction of multiple components.

Indications
- Pedicled proximally:
  - Elbow reconstruction (including tendon for triceps if needed).
- Pedicled distally:
  - Dorsum and palm of hand.
  - Coverage of proximal fingers/thumb.
  - Wrist.

- Free:
  - Any defect requiring thin pliable skin, especially if a long pedicle is also needed.

Limitations
Involves sacrifice of the radial artery; minimal sensory supply; minimal volume of tissue; may be hairy; donor site is ugly.

Method
- **Position** Patient supine; tourniquet; hand table or arm board.
- **Planning** Do Allen's test and outline superficial veins prior to surgery. Plan in reverse. The pivot point proximally is 3 cm below brachial artery at antecubital crease and distally is either the radial artery at radial styloid level or this can be extended to the radial artery at the snuff-box. Centre the flap over the radial artery.
- **Incision** Incise around the flap (preserving a superficial vein) and longitudinally along the line towards the pivot point.
- **Dissection** Elevate the skin flap in the sub-fascial plane from ulnar to radial until the FCR and the intermuscular septum is seen. Retract FCR ulnarwards to expose the septum, the radial artery and its VCs. Elevate the skin flap from radial dorsal to ulnar supra-fascially over brachioradialis until the septum. Visualize the perforators and the radial artery. Keep the vessel and septum with the flap, leaving the radial nerve behind. Once the flap is bipedicled on the vessel, divide the unrequired end and pivot about the remaining vessel, or divide this also if using as a free flap. Keep a superficial vein and follow in pivot point direction as a safety vein if possible. The entire dissection can safely be performed above the fascia, which reduces donor site morbidity.
- **Closure** Close donor site directly, if possible over drains. If tight it is preferable to SSG or FTSG the defect. Inset flap.

Unusual complications
- Rarely, because of compromise of blood supply to the hand, it is necessary to reconstruct the radial artery using a vein graft.
- Sensory denervation of the forearm and hypersensitivity in radial nerve distribution.

Donor site morbidity
Donor site is ugly as it almost always has to be skin grafted. Partial graft failure is high due to exposure of and movement of the tendons (FCR). Cold intolerance, reduced strength as a result of radial artery sacrifice.

Novelties and tips
Has been used as a flow-through flap, and also raised as a perforator flap, preserving the radial artery but basing it distally on one or more perforators. Can raise the flap, preserving a superficial vein as well as the VCs, by dissecting proximally into the antecubital fossa. The superficial vein will join the deep VC, allowing one vein anastomosis to drain both systems. If taking bone, take less than a third of the circumference, with bevelled

edges to avoid stress risers, and protect the ulna from fracture by casting/splinting for 6 weeks.

When raising as a free flap, design as an oblique ellipse across the radial artery (proximal end ulnar, distal end dorso-radial). This allows inclusion of cephalic vein and direct closure of the defect using a hatchet flap.

Reference

Yang GF, Gao YG, Chan BC, et al. (1981). *Natl Med J China* **61**, 139.

Ulnar forearm flap

A fascio-cutaneous flap based on the ulnar artery in the forearm (Lovie et al. 1984). May be used pedicled proximally, distally, or as a free flap. Can include fascia, skin, nerve, muscle, tendon, and bone.

Anatomy
The skin of the entire forearm can be supplied by the ulnar artery (and has been used in this way in salvage procedures).

Vascular anatomy: type C/D
Based on the ulnar artery and either the VCs or a superficial vein, usually the basilic vein. The ulnar artery originates from the brachial 1–2 cm distal to the cubital crease and travels under the median nerve, PT, FCR, PL, and FDS. It then proceeds distally, initially under the cover of FCU and later lying under the deep fascia between FCU and FDS. It is accompanied by the ulnar nerve on its lateral aspect. Throughout its course the ulnar artery gives off perforator branches to skin and fascia which pass along the septal plane between FCU and FDS. These perforators are more abundant in the proximal third of the forearm. They supply the fascial plexus and perforate directly to skin, and so the fascia need not be incorporated in the flap. There are similar branches that pass deep to supply the ulnar periosteum, enabling a bone flap to be taken.

Neural supply
The ulnar forearm skin is innervated by the medial cutaneous nerve of the forearm. These branches can be harvested and the flap kept innervated (if proximally based) or re-innervated by neural anastomosis if distally based or free. The ulnar nerve travels with the artery and could be harvested with the flap to provide a vascularized nerve.

Flap territory
The entire forearm can survive on these perforators and the ulnar artery. However, the usual flap limitations are the ulnar subcutaneous border and the ulnar border of brachioradialis. The entire length of ulnar nerve, a 10 cm length of ulna, and a similar length of FCU tendon can be harvested with the flap.

Suitability for free tissue transfer
Less commonly used than radial forearm, it has a long pedicle (up to 20 cm) with large vessels (3–5 mm diameter), is easy to raise, and is robust and reliable. Thin pliable skin (which may be less hairy than the radial skin) or fascia, with some versatility for reconstruction of multiple components.

Indications
- Pedicled proximally:
  - Elbow reconstruction (including tendon for triceps if needed).
- Pedicled distally:
  - Dorsum and palm of hand.
  - Coverage of proximal fingers/thumb.
  - Wrist.

- Free:
  - Any defect requiring thin pliable skin, especially if a long pedicle is also needed.

Limitations
Involves sacrifice of the ulnar artery; minimal sensory supply; may be hairy; donor site is a contact area when the forearm rests on objects.

Method
- *Position* Patient supine; tourniquet.
- *Planning* Do Allen's test and outline superficial veins prior to surgery. Plan in reverse. The pivot point proximally (and the maximum free flap pedicle) is 3 cm below brachial artery at antecubital crease and distally the pivot point is the ulnar artery at pisiform. Centre the flap over the ulnar artery.
- *Incision* Incise around the flap (preserving a superficial vein) and longitudinally along the line towards the pivot point.
- *Dissection* Elevate the skin flap in the supra-fascial plane from ulnar to radial over the FCU until the intermuscular septum is seen. Elevate the skin radial to ulnar until the FDS and the inter-muscular septum are seen. Retract the FCU ulnarwards to expose the septum and the ulnar artery and its VCs at distal margin. Visualize the perforators and the ulnar artery. Follow the vessel proximally according to flap design. Keep the vessel and septum with the flap, leaving the ulnar nerve behind. Once the flap is bipedicled on the vessel, divide the unrequired end, and pivot about the remaining vessel or divide this too if using as a free flap. Keep a superficial vein and follow in pivot point direction as a safety vein if possible. For safety the entire dissection can be performed sub-fascially.
- *Closure* Close donor site directly, if possible over drains. If tight it is preferable to SSG or FTSG the defect. Inset flap.

Complications
- Rarely, have to reconstruct the ulnar artery using a vein graft.
- Sensory denervation of the forearm and hypersensitivity in ulnar nerve distribution.

Donor site morbidity
Donor site is better than radial forearm flap as can close directly larger donor wounds, and graft failure is less common as the bed is muscle.

Novelties and tips
Has been used as a flow-through flap, and also raised as a perforator flap preserving the ulnar artery but basing it distally on one or more perforators. If taking bone, take less than a third circumference, with bevelled edges to avoid stress risers, and protect the ulna from fracture by casting/splinting for 6 weeks.

Reference
Lovie MJ, Duncan GM, Glasson DW (1984). *Br J Plast Surg* **37**, 486–492

Dorsal ulnar flap

A pedicled axial fascio-cutaneous flap, also known as the Becker flap (Becker and Gilbert 1988), utilizes the distal medial ulnar forearm skin based on a perforator vessel from the distal ulnar artery.

Anatomy
Vascular anatomy: type B
The medial ulnar forearm skin in the distal half of the forearm is supplied by an axial direct artery to the skin arising from a perpendicular perforating branch of the ulnar artery called the dorsal ulnar artery. This is a highly consistent artery which arises from the ulnar artery 2–5 cm proximal to the pisiform and is found with the dorsal branch of the ulnar nerve deep to the flexor carpi ulnaris. It arises at an angle of 90°–120° to the ulnar artery and runs obliquely to the deep surface of FCU. The dorsal ulnar artery divides into three branches, one going to the pisiform, one to the FCU, and one continuing as the cutaneous artery. The cutaneous branch reaches the level of the deep fascia and divides into distal and proximal branches. The distal branch passes onto the dorsal aspect of the hand, supplying the three ulnar metacarpals and the abductor digiti minimi. The proximal branch is often found close to the medial cutaneous nerve of the forearm, and runs towards the olecranon, giving branches to the skin overlying the ulnar border of the forearm from PL to EDC to ring finger. This artery supports a fascio-cutaneous flap 10–20 cm long and 5–9 cm wide on the ulnar side of the forearm.

Neural supply
The medial forearm skin is innervated by the medial cutaneous nerve of forearm which theoretically could be re-innervated by neural anastomosis.

Flap territory
The boundaries are the PL tendon anteriorly and the EDC tendons dorsally. Distally the pivot point is the medial ulnar neck, and proximally the flap can extend almost to the medial epicondyle.

Suitability for free tissue transfer
No, because the vessels are small and short.

Indications
Nice thin, usually hairless, skin: no large vessel sacrificied:
- Pedicled distally:
  - Wrist palmar and dorsal.
  - Ulnar side of palm and dorsum hand.
  - Fascia only for median and ulnar nerve re-vascularization.
  - Not recommended but can be osseocutaneous flap with a portion of ulnar cortex.

Limitations
Minimal sensory supply; minimal volume of tissue; only moderate size if direct closure of donor site.

Method
- *Position* Patient supine; tourniquet; arm abducted on arm board.
- *Planning* Palpate the distal fossa proximal to the pisiform at the medial ulna head between ECU and FCU (usually 2–3 cm proximal to the pisiform). This is the pivot point as the vessel emerges from the ulnar artery. Draw a line from this point to the medial side of the olecranon (along the groove between ulna and FCU). This line is the central axis of the flap. Plan in reverse, allowing a generous length for transposition. Draw the outline of the flap as a U-shape with the pivot point at the base of the U. A complete ellipse can be designed provided that the pivot point (and vessel) lie within the distal end of the ellipse.
- *Incision* Incise around the flap.
- *Dissection* Raise the flap from palmar to dorsum distally at the pivot point to confirm the location of the perforator. Elevate the skin flap in the supra- or subfascial plane from proximal elbow to distal wrist until the perforator is seen (retract FCU). This will involve division of the medial nerve of the forearm branches, especially if the flap extends proximally. Transpose the flap about the pivot point. It can be rotated through 180° especially if it is completely incised circumferentially and 'propellered' around. Inset flap.
- *Closure* Close donor site directly, if possible over drain. If tight it is preferable to SSG or FTSG the defect.

Complications and donor site morbidity
- Sensory denervation of the medial ulnar forearm.
- Temporary ulnar nerve symptoms usually due to tight closure.
- Beware the dorsal ulnar nerve branch.

Novelties and tips
- Could be raised as a fascia-only flap for re-vascularization of the median nerve in recalcitrant carpal tunnel syndrome.
- Could be raised as a skin island with a much larger fascial flap for reconstruction of gliding surface for extensor tendons.

Reference
Becker C, Gilbert A (1988). *Eur J. Plastic Surg* **11**, 79–82.

Posterior interosseous artery flap

A classic septocutaneous type fascio-cutaneous flap from the dorsal forearm which is usually pedicled proximally or distally (Penteado et al. 1981; Masquelet and Penteado 1987; Costa and Soutar 1988; Zancolli and Angrigiani 1988) and occasionally used as a free flap.

Anatomy

The dorsal distal two-thirds of forearm skin is supplied by numerous perforators to the skin arising from a branch of the posterior interosseous artery.

Vascular anatomy: type C

The posterior interosseous artery (PIA) flap is based on a descending branch of the PIA. The PIA arises from the common interosseous branch of the ulnar artery and enters the extensor compartment above the proximal end of the interosseous membrane between the heads of supinator and the abductor pollicis longus. Its surface marking on the pronated forearm is along the line between the lateral epicondyle of the humerus and the DRUJ. The artery enters the posterior compartment of the forearm at the junction of the upper and middle thirds of this line, between the supinator and the abductor pollicis longus and then courses between the deep and superficial layers of the extensor muscles. It lies on the dorsal surface of the APL and EPB accompanied by the posterior interosseous nerve in the valley between APL, EPB and EPL, EI on interosseous membrane leading to an anastomosis with the anterior interosseous artery (AIA) and then onto the floor of the fourth extensor compartment. This is not the artery on which the flap is based! There is another branch of the PIA that travels distally in the septum between the extensor carpi ulnaris and extensor digiti minimi muscles. As it does so, it branches to muscle and very small perforators to skin. The blood supply to the distally based flap relies on anastomoses between the AIA, the dorsal carpal arch, and the PIA. The PIA only enters the extensor compartment at the level of the junction of the proximal third and distal two-thirds of this axis. Hence, if designing a distally based flap, any of the flap extension that lies proximal to this point is randomly vascularized. The flap should be designed centred over this axial line along its middle third segment.

A proximally based segment has the entry point of the PIA as the pivot point and the flap can be designed from this point distally along the axis up to the DRUJ.

Neural supply

The dorsal ulnar skin of the forearm is supplied by medial cutaneous nerve of forearm and the posterior antebrachial nerve. Neither are large enough to neurotize the flap.

Flap territory

The dorsal forearm skin is of maximum size 20 × 10 cm. The longer the flap, the shorter the pedicle. Flap extension into the proximal third of the forearm (proximal to the point of perforation of the PIA through the interosseous membrane) is random.

Suitability for free tissue transfer
Uncommonly used, as it is difficult to raise because of the conglomeration of vessels and nerve branches at the emergence of the PIA into the dorsal compartment. The vessels are small (<1–2mm diameter) and the skin is hairy. However, it does have thin pliable skin and avoids sacrifice of a major vessel.

Indications

- Pedicled proximally:
  - Antecubital fossa.
  - Elbow—good for elbow coverage, especially olecranon. Donor is not so good as it is on dorsum of wrist and forearm and is very visible and cannot be closed directly, but can use a Becker flap!
- Pedicled distally:
  - Hand.
  - First web space.
  - Dorsum of digits to PIPJ.
- Free:
  - Any small cutaneous defect requiring thin pliable skin.

Limitations

Small size (4 cm wide) if direct closure of donor site. Often hairy. Small vessels. Large flaps often venously compromised.

Method

- *Position* Patient supine. Tourniquet. Do not over exsanguinate. Arm abducted on arm board.
- *Planning* Palpate the fossa just proximal to the DRUJ; this is the pivot point in a distally based flap. Draw a line lateral epicondyle to DRUJ with the elbow flexed. Confirm that this line corresponds to the palpable septum between EDM and ECU. If they do not correspond follow the latter. Split the line into thirds. The flap will be designed along this line. The proximal pivot point is at the junction of the proximal and middle thirds of this line. This is the point of the first most proximal perforator and the entrance of the PIA to the extensor compartment. Template the defect; plan in reverse, allowing adequate length of pedicle for the transposition. Draw the outline of the flap centred over the axis line and making it into an ellipse to aid direct closure.
- *Incision* Initially incise only longitudinally along the line from flap towards the pivot point.
- *Dissection* For a distally based flap, elevate the skin flaps in the suprafascial plane on either side of the distal longitudinal incision leading to nthe DRUJ. This exposes the deep fascia through which you can see the septum between the EDM and ECU. Incise through the fascia longitudinally 1 cm parallel to the septum on either side of the septum. Retract the EDM, looking towards the intermuscular septum. Look for the vessel running longitudinally in the septum at the junction of the septum and the deep afascia. The vessel is tiny. Once the vessel and axis of the flap is confirmed, incise around the flap, staying

supra-fascially. Elevate the flap skin supra-fascially from radial to ulnar until the septum is seen or you are over the EDM. Elevate the skin supra-fascially from ulnar to radial until the septum is seen or you are over the radial half of ECU. At this point incise through the fascia and connect this with the previous parallel lines. Look for the perforators and vessel in the septum and preserve. Follow the vessel from distal to proximal, dividing any muscular branches. Protect the neural branches to ECU and EDM. Ligate the PIA as it emerges through the interosseous membrane, and then transpose the flap distally usually through a subcutaneous tunnel.
- A proximally based is designed distally and is then elevated on either side until the septum is seen, and then the vessel is followed proximally.
- *Closure* Close donor site directly if possible over drains. If tight it is preferable to SSG or FTSG the defect. Inset flap.

Complications
Denervation of the EDM or ECU. Extensor lag In little finger.

Donor site morbidity
Scar visible on extensor aspect of forearm. Moderate to large flaps will need SSG or FTSG.

Novelties and tips
Could be inset with an exteriorized pedicle to gain extra reach. Preserve a subcutaneous superficial vein along the line of the pedicle if possible to improve venous drainage. Alternatively, keep a vein in the flap to supercharge it. Most common error is to have the flap axis too radial.

References
Costa H, Soutar DS (1988). *BR J Plast Surg* **41**, 221.
Masquelet AC, Penteado CV (1987). *Ann Chir Main* **6**, 131–9.
Penteado CV, Masquelet AC, Chevrel JP (1981). *Surg Rad Anat* **8**, 209–15
Zancolli EA, Angrigiani C (1988). *J Hand Surg (Br)* **13**, 130–5.

Fingertip flaps

Distal fingertip amputations, particularly palmar oblique amputations preserving nail, nailbed, and some distal phalanx, should be reconstructed rather then shortened. If sufficient pulp remains, healing by secondary intention or FTSG may be sufficient. If not, the two flaps described here or, for larger defects, the neurovascular island flap, the cross-finger flap, or the homodigital reverse island flap are options.

Anatomy
These are both neurovascular island flaps, albeit based on the fine terminal branches of the digital neurovascular bundles. The digital arteries divide at the level of the DIPJ into numerous branches that anastomose in various patterns (T, H, X, etc.) in the midline of the pulp. The V–Y palmar flap is based on these tiny branches which are unique to the distal phalanx and so the technique should not be used elsewhere. The lateral Kutler flaps are based on the digital vessels proper.

V–Y fingertip advancement flap
First described by Tranquilli-Leali in 1934. Modified by Atasoy *et al.* (1970).

Method
- *Planning* LA can be used. Debride the defect. With the cut distal end as the base draw an equilateral triangle with its apex at the DIPJ flexion crease. The distal width of the triangle should only be as wide as the nail matrix defect.
- *Incision* Incise the skin. Incise down to periosteum at the triangle base. Incise the apex down to the flexor sheath.
- *Procedure* Divide the fascial attachments from the distal phalanx to the pulp by sharp dissection in the palmar supraperiosteal plane under the flap, moving from distal to DIPJ. Blunt dissect the intervening third of the flap lateral borders, exposing the fine vessel and nerve branches. Anything that feels fibrous should be divided. A gap of at least 0.5–0.75 cm should open between the two sides. The flap should now be attached to the finger by only a very few neurovascular branches. Advance the flap and secure to the distal phalanx by inserting a K-wire or needle through the flap and into the distal end of the distal phalanx. This will reduce the tension on the distal end of the flap, allowing tension-free inset. The flap should be tension free, as tension will kill it. If it is not tension free, dissect some more of the fascial bands.
- *Donor* Closed directly in V–Y fashion.
- *Post-operative* Remove wire/needle at 2 weeks.

Advantages
This flap is better than the Kutler flap as there is no midline scar in the pulp. Can be done under LA. Like for like tissue, so good colour and texture match. Sensate.

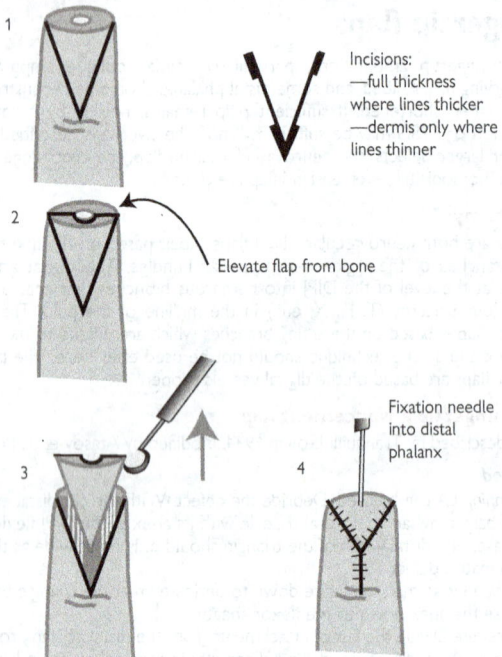

Fig. 22.26 Atasoy–Tranquill-Leali V–Y fingertip flap. (1) Full-thickness incision where the lines are thicker and superficial incision where lines are thinner. (2) Divide the periosteal attachments. (3) Traction with a skin hook and division of the fascial bands between the flap and finger. (4) Fixation of the flap to the distal phalanx with a needle or wire.

Disadvantages
Often done as a V–V flap, i.e. no advancement as insufficient dissection and release has been performed. This results in contracture and a beaked nail.

Kutler flap (Kutler 1947)
Two triangular lateral advancement flaps to provide sensibility and padding to the fingertip. Two triangles are fashioned such that their apices are on the DIPJ and their bases are on the border of the defect. Thus the V is converted into a Y on each side of the defect. The subcutaneous tissue upon which the flaps are based must be protected as it contains the feeding perforators.

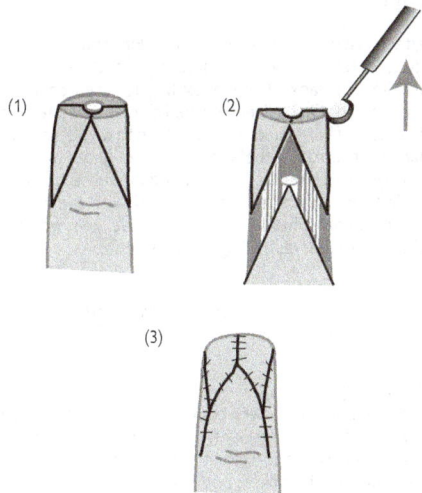

Fig. 22.27 Kutler flaps: (1) design; (2) flaps elevated and retracted distally; (3) inset.

Method
- *Planning* LA can be used. Debride the defect. With the cut distal end as the base draw two triangles with their apexes at the midlateral line at DIPJ flexion crease level. The triangles are not equilateral but have a short limb along the midlateral line and a longer limb from the midline of the defect to the apex. The apex can be extended to the mid-phalanx, becoming increasingly a neurovascular island flap proper.
- *Incision* Incise the skin. Incise down to periosteum in the midlateral line.
- *Procedure* Elevate the flap from lateral in the supra-periosteal flexor sheath plane. The neurovascular bundles should be seen on the deep surface of the flap. The midline border of the flap is then incised down to flexor sheath and periosteum. Repeat on the other side. Advance the flaps secure to the distal phalanx by inserting a K-wire or needle through the flap and into the distal end of the distal phalanx. This will reduce the tension on the distal end of the flap allowing tension free inset.
- *Donor* Closed directly in V–Y fashion.
- *Post-operative* Remove wire/needle at 2 weeks.

Advantages
Like for like tissue so good colour and texture match. Sensate.

References
Atasoy E, Ioakimidis E, Kasdan ML, Kutz JE, Kleinert HE (1970). *J Bone Joint Surg (Am)* **52**, 921–6.
Kutler W (1947). *JAMA* **133**, 29.

Kite flap

An axial pattern fascio-cutaneous flap using skin from the dorsum of the first web space extending over the dorsum of the metacarpophalangeal joint and proximal phalanx of the index finger, based on the first dorsal metacarpal artery. In 1952 Higenfield pedicled the whole first web and dorsum as a flap. Then Paneva Holevich narrowed the pedicle, and Foucher islanded it, creating the kite flap as we know it today (Foucher and Brown 1979). It is used as a pedicled flap with a pivot point at the base of the first web space, or distally based with a pivot point at the base of the proximal phalanx. It can include the dorsal superficial branches of the radial nerve, making it a sensate flap.

Anatomy

The skin over the thumb and index metacarpal and the intervening first web space are supplied by an axial vessel the first dorsal metacarpal artery.

Vascular anatomy: type B

The first dorsal metacarpal artery continues on from the radial artery in the snuff-box as the radial artery dives deep between the two heads of the first dorsal interosseous to enter the palm. The first dorsal metacarpal artery divides into two branches: one travels to supply the thumb metacarpal and splits to form the dorsal radial and ulnar thumb arteries (the ulnar of which is the basis of the Brunelli flap), and the other continues distally to supply the index metacarpal and the skin of the first web space. It continues over the index MCPJ and proximal phalanx up to the PIPJ. It travels radial parallel to the index metacarpal. The first dorsal metacarpal artery usually travels superficial to the fascia, but can sometimes be found deep to the aponeurosis/fascia. Sometimes there are two vessels, one deep and one superficial. The first dorsal metacarpal artery has an anastomosis with a palmar perforator from the palmar digital metacarpal or digital artery, at the level of the neck of the metacarpal.

The venous drainage is to VCs, fascial veins, and along superficial veins.

Neural supply

The skin is supplied by one or more dorsal superficial branches of the radial nerve which supply up to the neck of the proximal phalanx.

Flap territory

The primary flap territory lies over the first web space and the radial half of the MCPJ, but can be extended over the proximal phalanx to the level of the PIPJ, as a random extension.

Suitability for free tissue transfer

Rarely used; bad donor site.

Indications
Sensate, or not.
- Pedicled proximally:
  - Thumb reconstruction (especially sensate reconstruction of thumb pulp).
  - Cover of first web after release.
- Pedicled distally:
  - Cover of proximal and middle phalanges.
  - Cover of palmar aspect index MCPJ.

Limitations
Arc of rotation limits reach to IPJ of thumb, but this can be extended by taking extended flap and by flexing IPJ and adducting the thumb.

Method
Proximal flap
- *Position* Patient supine. Tourniquet.
- *Planning* Palpate the radial artery at base of first web space. This forms the pivot point. Draw a line from base of first web space along the side of index metacarpal to the level of the metacarpal neck. Plan in reverse to ensure adequate pedicle/flap length. Template the defect, and draw the outline of the defect on the distal end of the line. If the flap lies solely on the proximal phalanx, then some skin over the MCPJ should be included to ensure primary blood supply to the flap.
- *Incision* Incise around the flap and along the line of the pedicle.
- *Dissection* Elevate the dorsal first web skin over the pedicle. Incise around the flap to paratenon on the lateral and distal flap margins. Continue the lateral flap incisions proximally, creating the subcutaneous pedicle the same width as the flap. Start distally and raise flap subfascially, leaving paratenon behind. Continue raising in this plane, ligate or clip the palmar perforator at the MC neck, and continue proximally, until the base of the first web is reached. Transpose flap. Close pedicle incision.
- *Closure* Close donor site by FTSG, with the MCPJ flexed to 90°. Inset flap.

Distal flap
- *Planning* Palpate the radial artery at base of first web space. Draw a line from base of first web space along the side of index metacarpal to the level of the metacarpal neck. This is the flap axis, and the line of access to the pedicle in its distal half. The pivot point is the neck of the metacarpal or the MCPJ level. Plan in reverse to ensure adequate pedicle/flap length. Template the defect, and draw the outline of the defect on the proximal first web space at the proximal end of the line.
- *Incision* Incise around the flap and along the line of the pedicle.

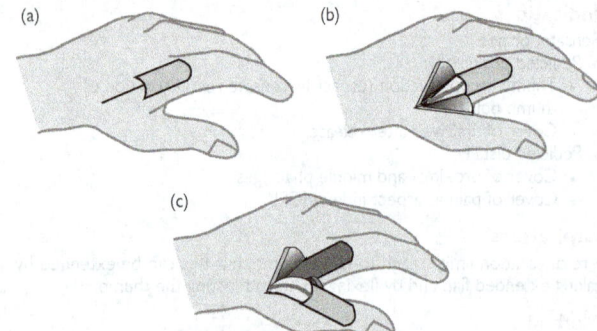

Fig. 22.28 Kite flap: (a) design; (b) elevate the dorsal first web skin superficially, exposing the deep soft tissues containing the vessel; (c) flap transposed. Note the wide pedicle.

- *Dissection* Elevate the dorsal first web skin on either side of the line. Incise around the flap to paratenon on the lateral and proximal flap margins. Find the first dorsal metacarpal artery originating from radial proximally and ligate. Start proximally and raise flap subfascially, leaving paratenon behind. Continue raising in this plane until the palmar perforator at the MC neck. If this gives adequate pedicle length stop here and transpose the flap. If not, ligate this perforator and continue distally until the base of the proximal phalanx is reached. The flap is now surviving on communication between the dorsal phalangeal branches and the dorsal metacarpal artery branches, which makes the flap less reliable. Transpose flap. Close pedicle incision.
- *Closure* Close donor site by FTSG, with the MCPJ flexed to 90°. Inset flap.

Advantages
- Reliable local flap

Complications and donor site morbidity
- Ugly donor site.
- Donor site is in a contact area for key grip.
- Donor site can be hypersensitive due to radial nerve neuromas.
- If used as a sensate flap, frequent failure to integrate and differentiate transferred index sensation at new position on thumb.

Tips
To reduce donor morbidity try to dorsalize the flap as much as possible, and avoid taking from key grip area. Can try to leave nerve behind. Can raise supra-fascially. Retain the pedicle in a good cuff of subcutaneous tissue.

Reference
Foucher G, Braun JB (1979). *Plast Reconstr Surg* **63**, 344.

Flag flap

An axial pattern fascio-cutaneous flap using skin from the dorsum of the proximal phalanx of the fingers, based on the dorsal metacarpal artery. Credited to Vilian and Iselin in 1973 (Iselin 1973; Vilain and Dupuis 1973), this flap was described as a random pattern flap from the dorsum of the middle phalanx with a narrowed pedicle on the basis that the subdermal vascular plexus was so rich as to be able to sustain a larger distal segment than the classic 1:1 random pattern ratio. This gave a design like a flag with a distal rectangle the full width of the digit and the pedicle one-third the width at one lateral edge. However, the design over the proximal phalanx is in fact an axial flap supplied by the continuation of the dorsal metacarpal artery after its anastomosis with the palmar supply at the level of the metacarpal neck. This continuation anastomoses with the dorsal digital artery branch from the true digital artery. It can be used as a pedicled flap with a pivot point at the base of the web space, or distally based with a pivot point at the neck of the proximal phalanx. Commonly, the more reliable axial proximally based proximal phalanx design is used and the pedicle is incorporated into the flap.

Anatomy

Vascular anatomy: type A/B
The skin over the metacarpals is supplied by axial vessels, the dorsal metacarpal arteries originating from the dorsal carpal arch. They travel parallel to the metacarpals in the interspace between them, deep to the deep fascia. At the level of the neck of the metacarpals the dorsal metacarpal arteries anastomose with a palmar perforator from the palmar digital metacarpal or digital artery. At this point they can be viewed as having three branches, one that dives deep to join the palmar supply, one that continues on to anastomose with the dorsal digital artery, and one that heads vertically superficially to the skin where it branches into an axial ascending branch (heading to the wrist) and descending branch (heading to the dorsum of the proximal phalanx). The venous drainage is to VCs, fascial veins, and along superficial veins.

Neural supply
The skin is supplied by dorsal superficial branches of the radial and ulnar nerves which supply up to the neck of the proximal phalanx.

Flap territory
The primary flap territory lies over the proximal phalanx to the level of the PIPJ, as a random extension the skin over the middle phalanx can be raised.

Indications

Homodigital or heterodigital.
- Pedicled proximally:
  - Cover of the dorsum of the MCPJ.
  - Cover of web.
  - Heterodigital cover of adjacent proximal phalanx.
- Pedicled distally:
  - Cover of proximal and middle phalanges.

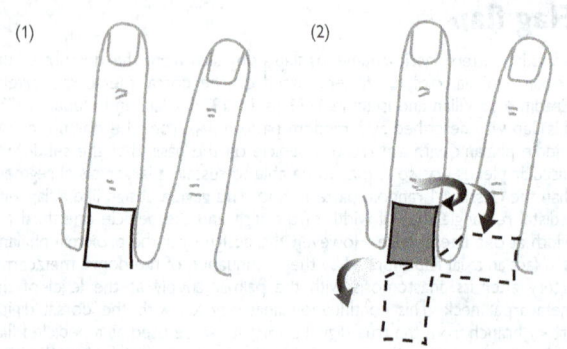

Fig. 22.29 Flag flap: (1) design; (2) arc of rotation.

Limitations
Arc of rotation limits reach. Vascularity can be compromised by the trauma necessitating the cover.

Method
- *Position* Patient supine. Tourniquet.
- *Planning* Draw a rectangular flap encompassing the whole dorsum of the proximal phalanx. Leave a one-third width pedicle at the web at which you plan to base the rotation. Plan in reverse to ensure adequate pedicle/flap length.
- *Incision* Incise around the flap.
- *Dissection* Elevate the flap skin from extensor paratenon starting distally and raise flap subfascially, leaving paratenon behind. Do not look for the padicle but leave it intact in the subcutaneous tissue. Transpose flap.
- *Closure* Close donor site by FTSG. Inset flap.

Complications and donor site morbidity
- Donor site needs FTSG.
- Donor site can be hypersensitive due to neuromas.

References
Iselin F (1973). *Plast Reconstr Surg* **52**, 374.
Vilain R, Dupuis JF (1973). *Plast Reconstr Surg* **51**, 397.

Brunelli dorsal ulnar thumb flap

A distally based axial pattern fascio-cutaneous flap using skin from the ulnar lateral dorsum of the thumb around the level of the metacarpophalangeal joint and base of proximal phalanx, based on the dorsal ulnar thumb artery. It is used as a distally pedicled flap with a pivot point at the IPJ or just beyond.

Anatomy

The skin over the thumb dorsum is supplied by two axial vessels: the radial and ulnar dorsal thumb arteries.

Vascular anatomy: type B

The first dorsal metacarpal artery continues on from the radial artery in the snuff-box as the radial artery dives deep between the two heads of the first dorsal interosseous to enter the palm. The first dorsal metacarpal artery divides into two branches: one travels to supply the thumb meatacarpal and splits to form the dorsal radial and ulnar thumb arteries (the ulnar of which is the basis of the Brunelli flap). This artery travels suprafascially to anastomose with the radial vessel through a distal arch at the level of the hyponychium. Along the way it also anastomoses with the palmar digital artery just before the IPJ and just after the IPJ. The venous drainage is to VCs and very fine fascial and subcutaneous veins. Rather than dissecting the artery, the pedicle consists of the subcutaneous tissue the width of the flap and containing the vessels, much like a de-epithelilized peninsula flap.

Neural supply

The skin is supplied by one or more dorsal superficial branches of the radial nerve nerves which supply up to the IPJ. However, as the flap is distally based it is insensate.

Flap territory

The primary flap territory lies over the first web space and the ulnar half of the MCPJ, but can be extended to over the proximal phalanx to the level of the PIPJ as a random extension.

Indications

- Pedicled distally:
    - Cover of palmar aspect IPJ and thumb pulp.
    - Cover of dorsal aspect IPJ and distal phalanx.

Method

- **Position** Patient supine. Tourniquet.
- **Planning** Pinch the dorsolateral skin at the level of the MCPJ and base of the proximal phalanx. This is the area of the flap. Draw a line from the corner of the nailbed to the point midway between the mid-lateral point and the dorsal ulnar condyle of the metacarpal head. This is the axis of the flap. Plan in reverse to ensure adequate pedicle/flap length. Template the defect, and draw the outline of the defect on the proximal end of the line, or as far proximal as the pedicle length requires.
- **Incision** Incise around the flap and along the line of the pedicle.

- ***Dissection*** Elevate the dorsal thumb skin in the subdermal plane on either side of the line to expose the subcutaneous tissue the width of the flap. Incise through the subcutaneous tissue down to extensor paratenon parallel to the axis to create tram tracks the width of the flap from the distal end of the flap to the IPJ. Incise around the flap to paratenon on the lateral and proximal flap margins. Raise the flap subfascially, leaving paratenon behind from proximal to distal until the IPJ is reached. The pedicle can be lengthened by basing the flap on the perforator distal to the IPJ or on the dorsal arch in the hyponychium. Transpose flap.
- ***Closure*** Close donor site and pedicle incision. At the pivot point the bulk of the pedicle may prevent closure of the skin, in which case leave it to heal by secondary intention. Inset flap.

Advantages
- Reliable local flap.
- Donor site closes directly.

Complications and donor site morbidity
- Scar can contract first web if flap is very proximal.
- Insensate flap.
- Pivot point can be bulky and need secondary revision.
- Can make the thumb look hour-glass shaped.

Neurovascular island flap

A reliable if somewhat intricate flap based on one of the neurovascular bundles of the digit.
- Composition: skin and subcutaneous tissue and the neurovascular bundle.
- Dimensions: triangular half of the middle and distal phalanx.
- Uses: neurovascular island flaps are used for larger defects of the fingertip.

Anatomy
The neurovascular bundle lies between Cleland's and Grayson's ligaments in the finger on the palmar aspect adjacent to the flexor sheath bilaterally. Release of the ligaments allows the vessels to centralize, which allows advancement of the distal flap. Further advancement comes from the straightening of the slightly tortuous path of the normal vessel. It supplies the skin and soft tissue by numerous branches which communicate freely with the opposite side of the digit allowing a retrograde flow flap to be used.

Types
- Neurovascular island flap (Venkataswami).
- Step advancement flap (Evans).
- Distally based island flap (not neurovascular just vascular!).

Method
- *Planning* GA or brachial block is preferred. Draw a midlateral line on the side chosen for the flap. If possible, use the non-contact side. Commencing at the PIPJ flexion crease draw an oblique line across to the opposite side of the defect, creating a triangular flap design as seen in Fig. 22.30.
- *Incision* Incise the midlateral line to the periosteum. Incise the oblique line but do not divide the neurovascular bundle! Elevate the proximal digital skin superficially from the midlateral line to the midline. From the contralateral corner of the flap elevate the flap from the flexor sheath and proceed proximally, the neurovascular bundle will remain in the elevated flap. The neurovascular bundle can then be lifted from the proximal finger to the level of the MCPJ. The flap is islanded.
- *Procedure* Advance the flap, secure with needle or K-wire through subterminal flap into distal phalanx open-end medullary canal, and suture inset flap.
- *Donor* Closed directly in a V–Y, this may give a slight hour-glass appearance to the middle phalanx. Replace the proximal skin.
- *Post-operative* Plaster digit to keep MCPJ at 90° and IPJs fully extended. Mobilize as soon as comfort allows, but splint PIPJ in extension for ≥2 months.

Advantages
Provides single unit of closely matching glaborous tissue with sensation; one stage.

Disadvantages
Difficult dissection unless experienced in digital anatomy.

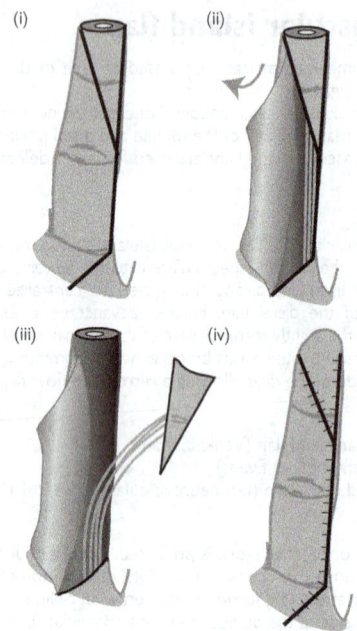

Fig. 22.30 Neurovascular island flap: (i) the design; (ii) elevate the proximal skin exposing the neurovascular bundle; (iii) elevate the flap from the flexor sheath and finger keeping the bundle in the flap; (iv) advance the flap, closing the donor site in a V–Y manner.

Complications
- Beware development of PIPJ flexion contracture.
- Tip of flap necrosis due to terminal tension.
- Scar contracture across DIPJ.

Evans stepped neurovascular island flap (Fig. 22.31)
In order to minimize the oblique scar contracture which sometimes occurs, this design converts the oblique line into a series of steps along which the flap climbs, leaving a broken scar which is less susceptible to contracture.

Distally based homodigital island flap (Fig. 22.32)
A similar flap can be based on the digital vessel retrograde flow. An area of skin from the lateral side of the proximal phalanx is raised with the digital artery and a good cuff of soft tissue to include the tiny venous drainage vessels. The proximal side of the vessel and soft tissue is divided and the vessel followed distally, maintaining its anastomosis with the contralateral vessel at the level of the DIPJ. This flap is not sensate.

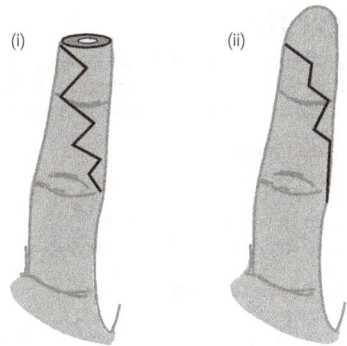

Fig. 22.31 Evans step advancement neurovascular island flap: (i) design using progressively larger steps to break up the oblique scar; (ii) advancement showing the steps taken distally by the flap.

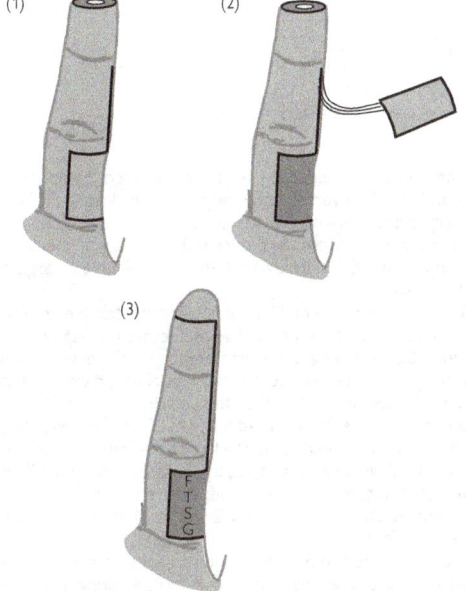

Fig. 22.32 Distally based neurovascular island flap: (1) design; (2) flap elevation maintaining the pedicle distally; (3) flap used to close the fingertip and the donor site closed with a FTSG.

Cross-finger flap

Proposed by Gurdin and Pangman (1950). A commonly used and versatile flap for digital reconstruction. Although supplanted in many circumstances by homodigital flaps, the cross-finger flap remains a very useful simple reliable procedure.
- Composition: distant cutaneous flap.
- Dimensions: whole dorsum of middle or proximal phalanx.
- Uses:
    - Defects of pulp, or palmar aspect of digit.
    - As reversed de-epithelialized flap useful for dorsal digital defects.
- Contraindications:
    - Older patients unable to tolerate the static fixed position of PIPJ flexion.
    - Other injury to the injured finger that may exacerbate stiffness.

Anatomy
The skin is supplied by dorsal branches from the digital arteries. At the proximal phalanx level there is an obliquely running vessel, whereas the middle phalanx has several smaller transverse vessels.

Types
- Standard lateral based.
- Standard proximal based.
- Standard neurotized.
- Reverse or de-epithelialized (Atasoy 1982).

Method
- *Planning* LA can be used, but GA/BPB is preferred. Template the defect and plan in reverse. Draw the flap design, keeping it between the interphalangeal joints. The distal edge of the flap should be along the opposing mid-lateral line. Ensure sufficient flap for the pedicle between the two digits. Its always better to make it too large rather then too small.
- *Incision* Incise along the mid-lateral line and the transverse edges of the flap, dividing the superficial veins. Elevate the flap in the supraparatenon plane, leaving the thin paratenon on the extensor tendon for grafting. Keep elevating to the mid-lateral line, dividing Cleland's ligaments if necessary to lengthen the pedicle.
- *Procedure* Once the flap is raised apply FTSG to the donor finger suturing it securely. Then apply the flap to the defect. A fixation suture between the fingers can ease the surgeon's concern of dehiscence or inadvertent flap tension in the uncooperative patient.
- *Post-operative* Dress and leave for 2 weeks. Mobilize all possible joints to reduce stiffness.
- *Stage 2* Divide the flap pedicle. Some surgeons do not inset the flap border for fear of creating tension and necrosis along this edge. However, tension can be avoided by excision of the fibrous tissue that accumulates and fills the elevated aspect of the flap pedicle prior to inset.

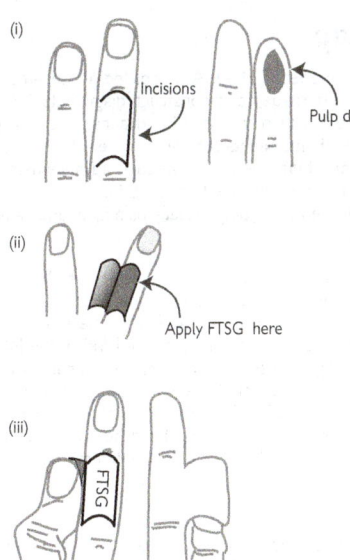

Fig. 22.33 Cross-finger flap: (i) dorsal and palmar view of index finger pulp defect and flap designed on middle finger; (ii) flap raised and FTSG to be applied to the donor site; (iii) dorsal and palmar view showing the flexion required in the index finger to inset the flap.

Advantages
Provides good tissue reliably, can be sensate and functional.

Disadvantages
Two-stage procedure with limited mobility of the digits in the intervening period. Not suitable for those liable to stiffness (old, injured). Not glaborous skin for pulp or palmar skin replacement.

Variation: de-epithelialized reverse cross-finger flap
In this variant the epithelium is removed from the donor site (in some cases keeping it pedicled on the far side of the digit), elevating the cross-finger flap as usual (although it comprises only subcutaneous tissue). As this flap does not have epithelium, either side of the flap can be applied to the defect. In the most common circumstance it is flipped over and the dermal surface is applied to a dorsal defect on the adjacent digit. The epidermis is replaced on the donor site, and FSTG covers the flap.

References
Gurdin M, Pangman WJ (1946). *Plast Reconstr Surg* **5**, 368–71.
Atasoy E (1982). *J Hand Surg (Am)* **7**, 481–3.

Moberg flap

First described by Moberg (1964). A bipedicled advancement flap of the palmar skin and soft tissue to reconstruct distal pulp loss. Particularly used in the thumb. Much of the gain in advancement is from flexion of the inter-phalangeal joint. Numerous variations exist.
- Composition: local bipedicled neurovascular advancement flap.
- Dimensions: whole palmar aspect thumb skin.
- Uses: defects of the thumb pulp, usually palmar oblique amputation.

Anatomy
The palmar skin is supplied by the digital vessels which are incorporated in the flap. This means that if the dorsal digital vessels are not preserved, dorsal digital necrosis can occur. In the fingers there is a separate dorsal vessel for the proximal phalanx arising at the level of the MCPJ but distal to this the dorsal digital vessels arise from the palmar digital vessels and hence the dorsum of the middle and distal phalanx is vulnerable to necrosis with this technique. The variation of incorporating only one palmar vessel in the flap and leaving the other to nourish the dorsum avoids this problem. The thumb has independent dorsal digital vessels that extend to the eponychium.

Method
- **Planning** LA can be used for small defects but GA/BPB is preferred for larger defects where the flap has to extend proximally. Draw flap design, keeping incisions along midlateral lines. The proximal flap has a number of variations in design.
- **Incision** Debride the wound. Incise the midlateral lines down to periosteum preserving the neurovascular bundles in the palmar flap.
- **Procedure** From the midlateral incision raise the flap in the plane superficial to the tendon sheath, and then progress from distal to proximal. Advance the flap and inset. Inset may be aided by using a K-wire or needle to penetrate through the flap and into the distal end of the distal phalanx, taking tension away from the leading edge of the flap.
- **O'Brien variation** To obtain further advancement incise the skin transversely at the level of the MCPJ and dissect the neurovascular bundles, without skeletonizing them. The secondary defect is full-thickness skin grafted.
- **Foucher variation** As for the O'Brien variation but the secondary defect is closed using a proximally based triangular transposition flap from the ulnar border of the thumb. (This lateral triangular transposition flap is also called a Gibraiel flap when used in other circumstances).
- **V–Y variation** The base of the flap is incised as for the O'Brien variation. However, the incision is not transverse but V-shaped allowing V–Y closure with advancement.
- **Post-operative** When healed therapy to regain IPJ extension.

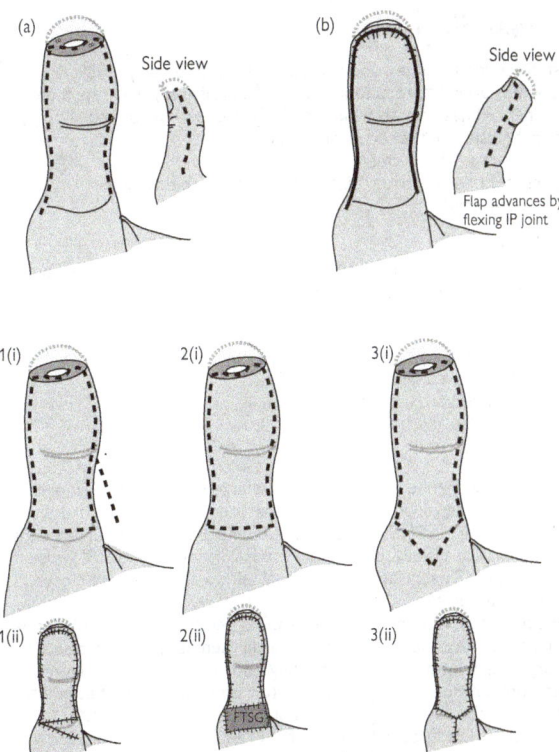

Fig. 22.34 Moberg advancement flap: (a) Midlateral incisions to MCPJ level, palmar and side view; (b) flap advanced mainly by flexion IPJ, palmar and side view. Other thumb advancement flaps (variations): 1(i) O'Brien with Foucher triangular transposition flap to close secondary defect; 1(ii) Foucher flap transposed and O'Brien flap inset; 2(i) O'Brien modification by transverse release at base of flap preserving neurovascular bundles; 2(ii) flap advanced and FTSG in secondary defect; 3(i) Moberg flap with V–Y base; 3(ii) Flap advanced and secondary defect closed as V–Y.

Advantages
Replaces like with like tissue. Replaces loss with immediately sensate glaborous skin.

Disadvantages
Causes IPJ flexion contracture.

Reference
Moberg E (1964). *J Bone Joint Surg (Am)* **46**, 817–25.

Thenar flap

First described by Gatewood (1926); modified by Beasley (1969).
- Composition: distant random pattern flap classically from the thenar eminence but currently from the MCPJ crease of the thumb allowing direct closure of the secondary defect.
- Dimensions: 1.5 × 1 cm.
- Uses: pulp defects of any size on the index or middle finger, especially children.

Anatomy
The skin over the thenar eminence is supplied by numerous perforators allowing a random pattern flap to be raised in any direction.

Types
- Ulnar-based U on thenar eminence (Gatewood).
- Proximally based distal inset (Beasley).
- Distally based proximal inset (Dellon).
- Thenar H-flap.

Method
- *Planning* LA can be used but GA is preferred for children. Template the defect after debridement. Draw flap design with mid-axis along the proximal MCPJ flexion crease of thumb. Base pedicle of flap either proximally or distally. Ensure that flap is 25% longer and 50% wider then defect. Triangulate the flap distal end to allow primary closure without a dog ear.
- *Procedure* Elevate the flap from distal to pedicle in the subcutaneous plane. (Beware the underlying nervacular bundles.) Close the secondary defect. Inset the flap on the fingertip. You may wish to insert another suture from finger to palm to restrain inadvertent attempts to avulse the flap by finger extension.
- *Post-operative* Dress with as much PIPJ extension as flap will allow.
- *Stage 2* About 10–14 days later divide the pedicle and either leave to heal or complete inset and tidy up donor site.

Advantages
Replaces glaborous skin.

Disadvantages
Not sensate; two-stage; bad scar if flap raised from thenar eminence. PIPJ contracture if done in adults, especially those with stiff hands.

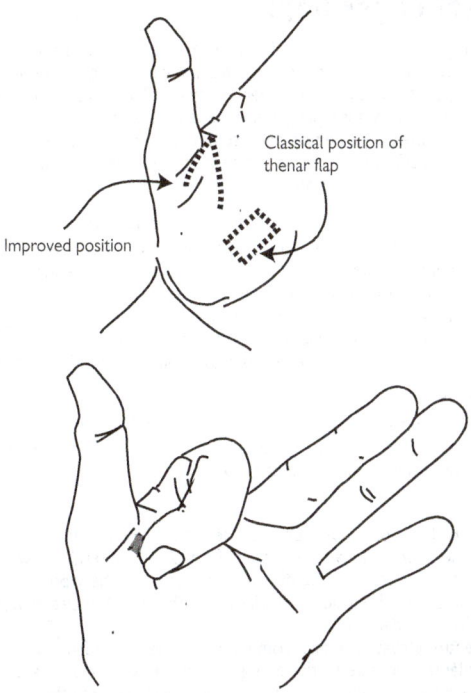

Fig. 22.35 Thenar flap showing the current recommended flap position rather than the classical area, and demonstrating the flexion of the finger required to inset the flap.

References

Beasley RW (1969). *Plast Reconstr Surg* **44**, 349–52.
Gatewood MD (1926). *JAMA* **87**, 1479.

Dorsal finger flaps

Dorsal digital defects can be difficult to manage. Because they are often due to abrading injuries, the zone of trauma can be large even if the area requiring full-thickness skin cover is small. The underlying extensor mechanism lies very superficial and is vulnerable to exposure and stiffness. Joint level injuries are common because of their protruberance. If paratenon is intact a FTSG can give a very nice aesthetic result. Exposed tendon, bone, or joint will need a flap.

Dorsal transposition flap (dorsal Hueston flap)

A transposition flap based along one lateral edge. It utilizes the lax skin over the joints to allow direct closure of the secondary defect.
- Composition: local rotation, advancement or transposition flap.
- Dimensions: whole dorsal skin over middle phalanx.
- Uses: DIP or PIP joint level injuries, if small. Distal phalangeal defects. Less useful for proximal defects unless small in longitudinal distance.

Anatomy

The dorsal skin is supplied by dorsal branches from the digital arteries which run transversely over the distal and proximal phalanx but are more longitudinal over the proximal phalanx.

Method

- *Planning* LA can be used for small defects. Draw a rectangular flap over the middle phalanx, extending from the midlateral line with transverse limbs along the dorsal IPJ creases, and the wound.
- *Incision* Excise the lesion and triangulate the defect. Incise around the flap down to paratenon.
- *Procedure* Elevate the flap from lateral border to midline in the paratenon plane. Continue to the opposite midline. Advance/transpose the flap. Inset the wound site first and then suture towards the base. Direct closure is usually possible with finger extension. If not, use FTSG.
- *Post-operative* Routine. Physiotherapy to mobilize IPJs.

Advantages

Provides single unit of closely matching tissue with scars that coincide with aesthetic unit junctions. Same tissue, so good colour and texture match.

Dorsal bipedicled flap

Bilateral transposition flap based proximally and distally and transposed along one lateral edge (wound edge), leaving the other lateral edge to heal by secondary intention or FTSG.
- Composition: local advancement flap.
- Dimensions: dorsal skin.
- Uses: longitudinal dorsal injuries.

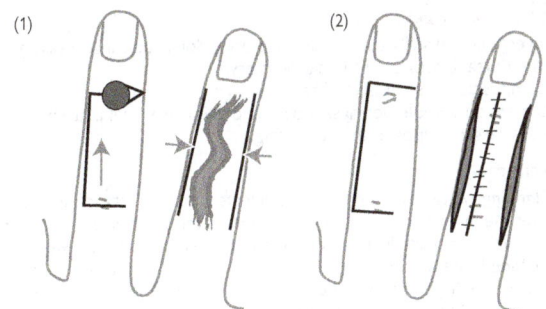

Fig. 22.36 Dorsal finger advancement flap and bipedicled flap: (1) middle finger with a DIPJ defect being closed with a dorsal transposition flap and the ring finger with a longitudinal midline injury being closed by bipedicled advancement flaps; (2) Following flap inset.

Method
- *Planning* LA can be used for small defects. Draw parallel bipedicled flaps on either side of the longitudinal wound.
- *Incision* Incise the lateral border of the flaps down to paratenon.
- *Procedure* Elevate the flap from lateral border to midline in the paratenon plane. Advance the flap. Inset flap.
- *Post-operative* Routine. Physiotherapy to mobilize IPJs.

Advantages
Simple and effective use of local tissue. Allows early mobilization despite lateral wounds.

Variations
It is possible to have these long flaps as unipedicled flaps allowing greater transposition at the distal tip if required.

Dorsal phalangeal flap

A reverse flow distally based island flap using dorsal phalangeal skin based on the dorsal branches of the digital artery.
- Composition: distant island flap.
- Dimensions: whole dorsal skin over middle or proximal phalanx.
- Uses: larger injuries of the dorsal finger.

Method
- *Planning* LA can be used for small defects. Draw a rectangular flap over the middle phalanx, extending from the midlateral line to midlateral line with transverse limbs along the dorsal IPJ creases, and the wound.
- *Incision* Incise around the four sides of the flap. The transverse and far side of the flap incisions should be down to paratenon. The pedicle side should be through skin only.
- *Procedure* Elevate the flap from the far lateral border to the pedicle midline in the paratenon plane, as you would raise a cross-finger flap. In the base of the flap view the digital artery passing longitudinally. Divide the artery at the proximal end. Dissect along the palmar aspect of the vessel leaving the artery supplying the flap dorsal and the nerve palmar. The flap will then be islanded on the artery alone at the distal lateral end. Preserve a cuff of soft tissue around the artery for venous drainage. For longer pedicle length dissect further distally along the vessel. Transpose the flap. Inset flap.
- *Closure* Close donor site with FTSG.
- *Post-operative* Routine. Physiotherapy to mobilize IPJs.

Advantages
Replaces like for like, no restriction on placement.

Disadvantages
Can become congested because of poor venous drainage. Can be bulky at the pedicle rotation point.

De-epithelialized reverse cross-finger flap
See cross-finger flap.

Free venous flap
See venous flap section.

Forehead flaps

Two main types of forehead flap exist based on different blood supplies. The first type is one of the original axial pattern cutaneous flaps using skin from the **lateral forehead**, possibly extending over the midline, and based on the superficial temporal artery. It was popular prior to free tissue transfer. It is generally used as a pedicled flap for forehead, lateral canthal, midface, and upper eyelid reconstruction.

The other is the **midline forehead** flap, utilizing the midline forehead skin based on the supratrochlear vessels or less commonly the supraorbital vessels. This pedicled flap is commonly used for nasal and medial canthal reconstruction.

Uncommon types of forehead flap are the **fronto-temporal flap**, a forehead flap based on the supratrochlear vessels but taking lateral supra-brow and temporal skin (needs delay), and the **fronto-parietal osseo-cutaneous flap**, a midline forehead flap which includes the outer table of the frontal bone, allowing bony reconstruction of the nose.

Anatomy

The five layers of tissue over the cranium are skin, subcutaneous tissue, (containing vessels and nerves), frontalis which becomes the galea over the scalp, sub-aponeurotic layer, and periosteum.

Vascular anatomy: type B

- Supraorbital artery is located by finding the supra-orbital foramen which lies above the midpoint of the pupil. This is a palpable bony landmark.
- Supratrochlear artery lies 0.5–1.5 cm medial to the supra-orbital.
- Anterior branch of the superficial temporal artery (lateral forehead flap) follows the course of the frontal branch of the facial nerve midway between the lateral eyebrow and the temporal hairline.

The venous drainage is to VCs. All the vessels anastomose together, allowing reliable raising of the forehead on any of these vessels.

Neural supply

The frontal facial muscles (frontalis, corrugator supercilli) are supplied by the temporal branch of the facial nerve, and skin sensation is supplied by the supratrochlear and supraorbital branches of the ophthalmic division of the trigeminal nerve. Hence the midline forehead flaps can remain sensate.

Flap territory

The whole forehead could be raised on the superficial temporal vessels and bilateral central forehead on the midline vessels. However, only 2–3 cm maximum width of forehead can be removed if direct closure is to succeed. However, most of the flap merely acts as a carrier for the distal portion that is required for defect reconstruction.

Suitability for free tissue transfer
Not really; bad donor site and central vessels are small. Superficial temporal vessels are used as basis of a free flap, but utilizing the temporalis fascia rather then the skin.

Indications
- Pedicled midline:
  - External nasal reconstruction.
  - Internal nasal reconstruction.
  - Medial canthus reconstruction.
  - Medial lower eyelid and midface reconstruction.
- Pedicled lateral:
  - Forehead reconstruction.
  - Cheek.
  - Lateral canthus, eyelid.
  - Cover of the skin on the neck and lower face.

Limitations
Arc of rotation limits reach. Forehead size limits flap size. The midline forehead flap can be extended by designing it as an up–down flap, obliquely across the forehead (gull wing design (Gillies)), dropping the pivot point by using the ophthalmic rather than the supratrochlear artery, with a back-cut into the medial canthus.

Pre-operative subgaleal tissue expansion can be used to augment the area and vascularity of the flap and facilitate primary closure of the donor site defect, although problems have been reported with secondary contraction of the transferred flap.

Method
Midline flap
- *Position* Patient supine.
- *Planning* Assess height of patient's forehead. Palpate the supratrochlear notch indicating site of vessel and mark. Draw a line vertically form this point; this is the axis of the flap. Plan in reverse to ensure adequate pedicle/flap length. Template the defect, and draw the outline of the defect on the distal end of the flap. If the flap extends into the hairline try to fit in obliquely or consider dropping the pivot point. Ensure an extra 15–20% in pedicle length for the pivot.
- *Incision* Incise around the flap.
- *Dissection* Start distally and raise flap under frontalis and aponeurosis. Be careful as you approach the base of the flap as the artery enters here and hence crosses the plane of dissection approximately 1 cm above the supra-orbital ridge. Easiest way to protect the vessel is to go sub-periosteal when you are about 1 cm superior to the supra-orbital rim, and continue the dissection in this plane. Rotate flap into defect and stitch in place. If tight or lifting the nose, then extend the pivot point or carefully debulk the pedicle to reduce the flap wastage as it pivots. The underside of the bridge can be grafted, tubed, or just dressed. The distal portion may be radically thinned to reduce bulk as the blood supply is in the subdermal plexus. (Be wary of doing this

if the patient is a smoker!) Inset flap. The deep surface can be left to re-mucosalize if the mucosal defect is small. Leave in place for 3–4 weeks. Divide pedicle, excise excess, or return to forehead and inset.
- *Closure* Close donor site directly (this can be facilitated by scoring the galea, undermining, and converting the lateral forehead into two lateral advancement (H flaps) or rotation flaps. Use SSG or leave to heal.

Lateral flap
- *Planning* Palpate the superficial temporal artery indicating site of vessel and mark. Plan in reverse to ensure adequate pedicle/flap length. Template the defect, and draw the outline of the defect on the distal end of the flap. Ensure an extra 15–20% in pedicle length for the pivot.
- *Incision* Incise around the flap.
- *Dissection* Start distally and raise flap under frontalis and aponeurosis. Be careful as you approach the base of the flap as the artery enters here and crosses the plane of dissection at the zygomatic arch. Rotate into defect and stitch in place. The underside of the bridge can be grafted, tubed, or dressed. The distal portion may be radically thinned to reduce bulk as the blood supply is in the subdermal plexus. Inset. Leave in place for 3–4 weeks. Divide pedicle and inset.
- *Closure* Close donor site by SSG. Inset flap.

Advantages
- Thin, large, and generally hairless flap.
- Good colour match for the head and neck, nose.

Complications and donor site morbidity
- Ugly donor site, especially if not closed directly.
- Two stage procedure; often lymphoedema after second stage. This is reduced if a longer period is allowed between stages.
- Insufficient length and contraction pulls up nose.
- Lateral forehead flap includes or divides the temporal branch of the facial nerve.
- Further adjustment of the pedicle base, columella, and alae may be required and delayed thinning of the flap may also be necessary.

Tips
Can be pre-expanded to allow greater flap size and length yet still allow direct closure. Pedicle can be de-epithelialized and inset to avoid second stage (but still bulky). Tip of flap can be turned up to provide lining but is bulky at alar rim. Can include outer table frontal bone. A midline forehead donor site scar is less visible than a para-median or oblique scar.

The gull-wing flap (Millard 1974) is a geometric modification of the midline forehead flap which incorporates raising of transverse 'wings' from the donor site which can usually be closed primarily and lie within the natural skin creases of the forehead. These lateral extensions are used to reconstruct the alae.

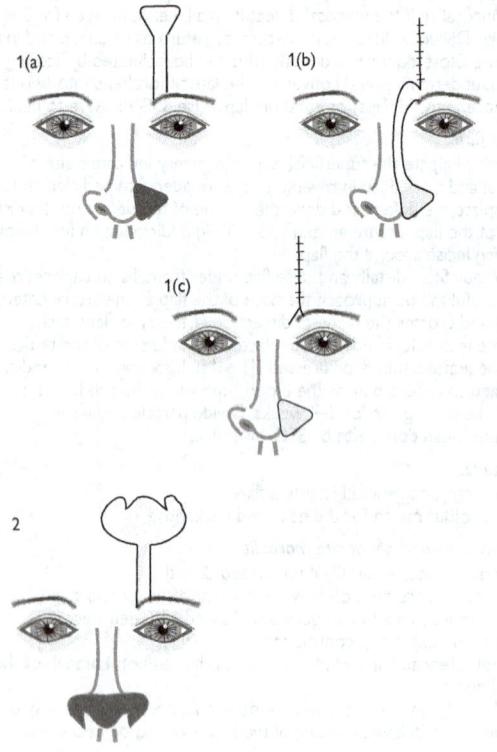

Fig. 22.37 Forehead flaps: 1(a) standard supratrochlear midline; 1(b) transposed; 1(c) pedicle divided and inset completed; 2 Millard gull-wing modification.

Reference

Millard DR, Jr (1974). *Plast Reconstr Surg* **53**, 133–9.

Temporalis flap

A muscular flap based on the superficial temporal artery. It is generally used as a pedicled flap for facial reanimation, or reconstruction of the face from orbit to mastoid.

Anatomy

The temporalis muscle, covered by the the deep temporal fascia, originates from the temporal fossa, the temporal fascia and the temporal line. It inserts onto the anterior coronoid and ramus of mandible. Two blood supplies enter the muscle. The main supply enters on its deep surface, at the level of the zygomatic arch, from the deep temporal artery (a terminal branch of the maxillary artery). A secondary supply to the posterior part of the muscle comes from the middle temporal artery (a terminal branch of the superficial temporal artery) which pierces the temporal fascia above the zygomatic arch to supply the muscle. Venous drainage is by corresponding veins of the same name.

Vascular anatomy: type B

The superficial temporal artery (a terminal branch of the external carotid) crosses the temporalis lying superficial to it and the temporo-parietal fascia. At the temporal line it comes to lie on the outer aspect of the galea (a continuation of the SMAS). At its origin it gives off a transverse facial branch travelling with the parotid duct; later it gives off the middle temporal artery. At the level of the lateral canthus the superficial temporal artery divides into two branches, an anterior frontal and posterior parietal. The anterior branch of the superficial temporal artery (lateral forehead flap) follows the course of the frontal branch of the facial nerve midway between the lateral eyebrow and the temporal hairline. The parietal branch courses almost vertically to the vertex lying superficial to the fascia. The venous drainage is to VCs.

Neural supply

Mandibular branch of the trigeminal nerve.

Flap territory

The temporalis can reach the orbit and cheek and by dividing the zygomatic arch can reach the mastoid or mandible.

Indications

- Pedicled:
  - Orbital or lateral canthal reconstruction.
  - Sinus obliteration.
  - Facial reanimation.

Method
- **Position** Patient supine.
- **Planning** Palpate or Doppler the superficial and parietal temporal arteries indicating site of vessels and mark. Palpate the temporalis.
- **Incision** Incise vertically as for one side of a bicoronal flap. This can be a zig-zag or T-shaped incision for better exposure.
- **Dissection** Start distally and raise the scalp flap in the supra-muscular plane. Detach the origin and elevate the muscle from the temporal fossa superior to inferior. If necessary the middle temporal artery can be divided to improve reach. The zygoma can also be divided, but cautious dissection is advised as the main pedicle enters the deep surface in this region and the zygomatic branch of the facial nerve crosses the zygoma. . A flap of the superficial layer of the deep temporal fascia can be taken to improve reach. Be careful not to be too subdermal or alopecia will result.
- **Closure** Close donor site directly. Inset flap.

Advantages
- Local flap of functioning muscle supplied by nerve other than facial nerve.
- No functional loss.

Complications and donor site morbidity
- Facial nerve palsy.
- Alopecia.
- Depression in temporal fossa.

Novelties and tips
Can include outer table parietal bone.

Temporo-parietal flap

Based on the superficial temporal artery. It was popular prior to free tissue transfer. It is generally used as a pedicled flap for frontal sinus or ear reconstruction or as a free flap to resurface the hand (Upton et al. 1986).

Anatomy
The temporo-parietal fascia overlies the temporalis muscle but is not the muscle fascia, which is called the deep temporal fascia. It can be seen as a continuation of the SMAS inferiorly, and the frontalis-occipitalis superiorly. The layers in this region are skin, connective tissue, temporo-parietal fascia, deep temporal fascia, and temporalis. It is supplied by the superficial temporal artery branches.

Vascular anatomy: type B
The superficial temporal artery (a terminal branch of the external carotid) crosses the temporalis lying superficial to it and the temporo-parietal fascia. At the temporal line it comes to lie on the outer aspect of the galea (a continuation of the SMAS). At its origin it gives off a transverse facial branch travelling with the parotid duct; later it gives off the middle temporal artery. At the level of the lateral canthus the superficial temporal artery divides into two branches, an anterior frontal and posterior parietal. The anterior branch of the superficial temporal artery (lateral forehead flap) follows the course of the frontal branch of the facial nerve midway between the lateral eyebrow and the temporal hairline. The parietal branch courses almost vertically to the vertex lying superficial to the fascia. The venous drainage is to VCs.

Neural supply
The auriculo temporal (sensory) nerve lies superficial to the fascia with the vessels, whereas the facial nerve branches lie deep to the fascia.

Flap territory
The temporo-parietal fascia has dimensions 12 × 10 cm.

Suitability for free tissue transfer
Hidden donor site, good vessels, but limited size and fascia only.

Indications
- Pedicled:
    - Ear reconstruction.
    - Sinus obliteration.
    - Bone reconstruction of zygoma, brow.
- Free:
    - Hand dorsum reconstruction.
    - Gliding tissue reconstruction.
    - Any defect or reconstruction requiring thin fascia.

Limitations
- Limited flap size.
- Fascia only so requires grafting.

Method
- **Position** Patient supine.
- **Planning** Palpate or Doppler the superficial and parietal temporal arteries indicating site of vessels and mark.
- **Incision** Incise vertically as for one side of a bicoronal flap. This can be a zig-zag or T-shaped incision for better exposure.
- **Dissection** Start distally and raise the scalp flap in the subfollicular plane. Be careful not to be too subdermal or alopecia will result. Do not be too deep as you may injure the superficial temporal vessels. Once the skin is elevated you can see the vessels and the fascia. Incise around the border of the fascia required and elevate off the temporalis fascia. Dissect the pedicle proximally (pre-auricular) if a longer pedicle is needed For a bone flap take overlying galea and periosteum in continuity with the outer table; then pedicle it with the superficial temporal protected by a cuff of fascia.
- **Closure** Close donor site directly. Inset flap.

Advantages
- Thin fascia-only flap.

Complications and donor site morbidity
- Facial nerve palsy.
- Alopecia.

Novelties and tips
Can include outer table parietal bone.

References
Upton J, Rogers C, Durham-Smith G, Swartz WM (1986). *J Hand Surg (Am)* **11**, 475–83.

Auriculo-temporal flap

A free flap of the anterior superior portion of the helix of the ear based on the superficial temporal artery used to resurface the alar nasae and nasal tip (Parkhouse and Evans 1985). Has been used as a pedicle flap.

Anatomy
The anterior part of the helix leading into the helix crus and the hairless skin lying immediately anterior to it in the pre-auricular temporal region can be used to reconstruct the nasal tip. The thin skin with cartilage support provides near-perfect like for like replacement of the nasal alar and rim. The pre-auricular/temporal skin and the post-auricular skin can cover the nasal dorsum and provide lining.

Vascular anatomy: type B
The superficial temporal artery as it passes anterior to the ear over the zygomatic arch gives off several branches that pass posteriorly to the helix. The venous drainage is to VCs.

Neural supply
The auriculo-temporal (sensory) nerve lies superficial to the fascia with the vessels and supplies the anterior ear.

Flap territory
The anterior superior ear and surrounding skin can be harvested on this vessel.

Suitability for free tissue transfer
This site has been used as a donor for composite graft but free vascularized transfer allows greater volume of tissue and better reliability. Superficial vessels are moderate in size; length is short.

Indications
- Pedicled:
  - Nose reconstruction.
- Free:
  - Nasal tip and alar reconstruction.

Limitations
Limited flap size; maximum defect would be hemi-nasal.

Method
- **Position** Patient supine.
- **Planning** Palpate the superficial temporal arteries in the pre-auricular region and mark. Template the nasal defect with foil and mark plan on helix and pre-auricular skin. The anterior extent of the flap should cover the palpable vessels.
- **Incision** Incise vertically along the pre-auricular skin following the ear contour and around the flap.

- ***Dissection*** Incise full thickness through the helical cartilage and distal margins of the flap. Elevate the anterior skin passing posterior to the superficial temporal vessels. Watch out for the facial nerve lying anteriorly. Divide the vessels superiorly. Follow the vessels inferiorly. Dissect the pedicle proximally (pre-auricular) if a longer pedicle is needed.
- ***Closure*** Close donor site directly by advancing pre-auricular skin and by closing the wedge excised from the helix. Inset flap and revascularize to facial vessels in the nasolabial fold.

Advantages
- Thin skin with cartilage support flap.
- Good colour match.

Complications and donor site morbidity
- Facial nerve palsy.
- Ear deformity.

Novelties and tips
Can be used for columella reconstruction.

Reference
Parkhouse N, Evans D (1985). *Br J Plast Surg* **38**, 306–13.

Delto-pectoral flap

Described by Bakamjian (1965), this flap dramatically altered concepts in flap surgery. It is an axial pattern cutaneous flap using skin from the anterior superior chest extending over the anterior deltoid, based on anterior thoracic perforators. It was popular prior to free tissue transfer. It is generally used as a pedicled flap after a delay procedure to increase length but can be taken as a free flap if the internal mammary artery is dissected out.

Anatomy

Vascular anatomy: type A

The superior border is the infra-clavicular line. The inferior border lies along the fourth rib to the apex of the axilla. It is possible to go as low as the fifth rib if that is required. The lateral margin is the delto-pectoral groove but a large random portion (10–15 cm) can be raised by extending over the deltoid region and raising beneath the deltoid fascia lateral to delto-pectoral groove if the flap is delayed. Medially dissection should be stopped 2 cm from the sternal edge. The blood supply is from the anterior perforating branches of the second and third (and sometimes fourth) intercostal spaces which arise from the internal mammary artery and penetrate the pectoralis fascia ~1 cm from the sternal edge. The venous drainage is to VCs.

Neural supply

The skin is supplied partly by intercostal nerves and can remain partially sensate. The superior portion is supplied by the supraclavicular nerves which have to be divided to mobilize the flap.

Flap territory

A flap of size 15–20 × 10–15 cm could be raised if delayed. However, most of the flap is not useful for closing the defect; it merely acts as a carrier for the distal portion that is required for defect reconstruction.

Suitability for free tissue transfer

Not really. Bad donor site and tedious vessel dissection to get adequate pedicle.

Indications

- Pedicled proximally:
  - Head and neck reconstruction.
  - Coverage of plexus in supraclavicular fossa as adipo-fascial flap.
  - Cover of the skin on the neck and lower face.

Limitations

Arc of rotation limits reach.

Method
- **Position** Patient supine.
- **Planning** Draw a line under the clavicle. Palpate the sternal edge and mark the intercostal spaces at the edge indicating site of perforators. The inferior border of the flap as it meets the sternal edge forms the pivot point. Plan in reverse to ensure adequate pedicle/flap length. Template the defect, and draw the outline of the defect on the distal end of the flap. If the flap extends onto the deltoid, consider delay.
- **Delay** Flap delay by incising around the skin of the flap and dividing the cutaneous branches of the thoraco-acromial trunk.
- **Incision** Incise around the flap.
- **Dissection** Start distally and raise flap subfascially. Avoid the cephalic vein in the delto-pectoral groove. Continue raising in this plane until 2 cm from the sternal edge to avoid injury to the perforators.
- **Closure** Close donor site by SSG. Inset flap.

Advantages
- Large thin hairless flap in women.
- Good colour match for the head and neck.
- Can be split and tailored.

Complications and donor site morbidity
- Ugly donor site, flap very visible and deforming over the clavicle.
- 10% tip necrosis especially if no delay.

Novelties and tips
Always delay the deltoid extension to ensure viability.

Reference
Bakamjian VY (1965). *Plast Reconstruct Surg* **36**, 173–84.

Pectoralis major flap

First described by Hueston and McConchie (1968) as a musculo-cutaneous flap and part of the delto-pectoral flap, this flap undergoes continual renaissance. Mainly used in head and neck reconstruction and in the closure of sternal wounds. Lesser uses in functional reconstruction of the upper arm (biceps). Can carry a rib segment for bone reconstruction.

Anatomy

A broad flat muscle with distinct segments:
- Origin: it arises by the aponeurosis of the external oblique, anterior sternum, second to sixth costal cartilages, and the medial half of the clavicle.
- Insertion is the lateral lip of the bicipital groove by a flat trilaminar tendon.
- Action adducts, flexes, and internally rotates the arm; external respiratory muscle.

Vascular anatomy: type 5

The dominant blood supply is the thoraco-acromial trunk (from the second part of the axillary artery) which divides into a deltoid branch to the clavicular head and pectoral branch to the sternocostal head. The pectoralis major is also supplied segmentally by segmental perforators from the internal mammary artery and lateral thoracic artery. The skin overlying the muscle is supplied by numerous perforators, sufficiently dispersed to allow almost an infinite variety of skin flap designs. The main reliable perforators from the pectoral branch are concentrated at the site of penetration of the muscle by the pedicle and along the sternal border of the muscle.

Neural supply

Pectoralis major is innervated by the medial and lateral pectoral nerves, branches of the medial and lateral cords, respectively. The skin is supplied segmentally by intercostals.

Flap territory

The muscle roughly forms a triangle from the axilla, along the clavicle down the sternum edge, and then along the fifth rib interspace. The skin over this area and extending 10 cm inferiorly over the rectus can be utilized.

Suitability for free tissue transfer

Possible, but in practice rarely used.

Indications

- Muscle only.
- Neurotized muscle (functioning muscle transfer).
- Myocutaneous.
- Osteomyocutaneous.
- Pedicled proximally (thoraco-acromial):
  - Used for head and neck reconstruction (to zygomatic arch).
  - Mandibular reconstruction.

- Sternal and mediastinal defects.
- Can functionally reconstruct elbow flexion/extension, winging scapula.
- Can cover axillary, chest wall and breast defects.
- Pedicled distally (sternal internal mammary perforators):
  - Sternal and mediastinal defects.
- Free can be used for any indication above and in addition:
  - Both lower and upper limb reconstruction.
  - Head and neck reconstruction.
  - Chest and trunk reconstruction.

Limitations
Arc of rotation; turnover flap cannot be used if IMAs used; skin donor cannot easily be closed directly unless narrow flap.

Sternocostal pedicled myocutaneous flap for head and neck
- **Position** Patient supine. Arm on table/support and prepared.
- **Planning** Surface markings of artery are a line from acromion to xiphi sternum and a vertical line from the midpoint of the clavicle to this The pivot point is the infra-clavicular midpoint. Plan in reverse. The pedicle will increase in length when dissected free of the muscle, so the usual 20% need not be added. The skin paddle is ideally based over the muscle on the distal portion of this line. It can be 50% greater than muscle to be harvested. Design as a vertical, oblique, or transverse ellipse to aid direct closure.
- **Incision** Incise around the flap until muscle, and incise along the third rib to the anterior axillary line in a defensive line which gives a rotation flap to aid closure.
- **Dissection** Raise the adjacent skin flaps to expose and find the lateral and inferior edge of the pectoralis major. Raise the skin paddle incontinuity with the underlying pectoralis major in a submuscular plane from inferior to superior until the pedicle is seen. Dissect the pedicle from the clavicular head of the muscle. Once the pedicle is dissected cut through the muscle around the flap, leaving the pedicle intact. The flap is then completely islanded on the pedicle, giving extra length and preserving the clavicular head; alternatively a cuff of muscle can be preserved around the pedicle, or the whole pectoralis major muscle raised. If islanding try and leave the acromial branch to the clavicular head. Separate clavicular head from the clavicle near the pivot point; pass the flap through this aperture. Usually pedicle goes over the clavicle; in rare cases when extra length is required the clavicle can be split.
- **Closure** Close donor site directly over drains if possible; if not graft. inset flap.

Pedicled muscle-only flap for sternal
- **Position** Patient supine.
- **Planning** If IMAs used for CABG must use thoraco-acromial axis. If not can potentially use as turnover flap based on sternal perforators.
- **Incision** Incise around the sternal edge (usually open wound!) until pectoralis major seen.

- *Dissection* Raise the skin supra-muscularly to expose the lateral and inferior edge of the pectoralis major. Release the inferior and superior edge of pectoralis major. Dissect pectoralis major in submuscular plane from lateral to medial. The pedicle need not be seen. Advance the muscle into the sternal defect. If more muscle is required divide the insertion of the muscle to the humerus. Attach the muscle to both sides of the sternum to give chest wall and respiratory support. Both pecs can be used to increase the support, one (completely detached) in the defect and the other (still attached to humerus and functional) to double breast over the top to the contralateral sternum
- *Closure* Close donor site directly over drains.

Complications and donor site morbidity

Clinically there is no functional defect. Scar can be obvious. Pedicle can be bulky and obvious. Nipple or breast distortion.

Novelties

Can raise with rib where the muscle originates to reconstruct mandible, clavicle.

Pectoralis minor

A free muscle flap used for facial reanimation. Nice small flat muscle which can be split longitudinally for different insets. Short small pedicle but suitable for facial reanimation.

- *Anatomy* A small muscle arising from the third, fourth, and fifth ribs and inserting on the coracoid along with short head of biceps and coraco-brachialis. The superior border is skirted by the thoraco-acromial trunk and the inferior border by the lateral thoracic artery that supplies branches to it.
- *Action* Assists serratus anterior in protraction of the scapula and adduction of the abducted arm; external respiratory muscle.
- *Vascular anatomy: type 1*
- *Neural supply* Pectoralis minor is innervated by the medial pectoral nerve (a branch of the medial cord) as it passes to pectoralis major. The skin is supplied segmentally by intercostals.
- *Indications* Used as a free flap.
- *Neurotized muscle* Free functioning muscle transfer.
- *Method*
  - *Position* Patient supine. Arm on table/support.
  - *Incision* Incise along delto-pectoral groove/anterior axillary border.
  - *Dissection* Expose pectoralis minor; free up the lateral and superior borders, preserving the pedicle and the medial pectoral nerve. Detach from the ribs then the coracoid.
  - *Closure* Close donor site directly over drains. Inset flap.
- *Complications and donor site morbidity* Clinically there is no functional defect.

Reference

Hueston JT, McConchie IH (1968). *Aust NZ J Surg* **38**, 61–3.

Scapular flap

First described by Fonseca (1978). Large pliable axial pattern fasciocutaneous flap with good pedicle length. May be combined with a parascapular flap and/or a latissimus dorsi, on subscapular vessels. It is generally used as a pedicled flap but can be taken as a free flap (Hamilton and Morrison (1982). Usually skin only but can include bone at border of scapular).

Anatomy

Vascular anatomy: type B

The scapular flap consists of skin lying transversely over the scapula below the spine of the scapula. The skin is supplied axially by a cutaneous vessel (transverse scapular cutaneous artery) originating from the circumflex scapular branch of the subscapular which passes through the triangular space and divides into two terminal branches, the transverse scapular cutaneous artery and the vertical parascapular artery. The transverse scapular artery courses in a plane above the muscular aponeurosis parallel to the spine of the scapular terminating 2 cm from the midline of the back. Venous drainage is by the accompanying VCs. The vertical parascapular artery supplies the parascapular skin and has osseous branches supplying the lateral border of the scapula It forms the vascular axis for the parascapular and the scapular bone flap. The scapular flap can be designed such that the entry point of the vessel corresponding to the triangular space (palpable as the depression below the glenoid, lateral to the scapula between teres minor/subscapularis superiorly and teres major inferiorly and the long head of triceps laterally) is under one end of an ellipse which extends as far medially as the spine. The superior border is the top of the scapula. The inferior border can be as far as the tip of the scapula. However, to achieve direct closure maximal flap width is likely to be 10 cm. The triangular space or omotricipital space can also be found using the formula $D = (L - 2)/2$, where L (cm) is scapula spine to inferior angle and D (cm) is scapula spine to pedicle (Dos Santos 1984). This approximates the pedicle 68% of the time.

Neural supply

The skin is supplied by intercostal nerves and cannot be innervated.

Flap territory

Skin up to 10 cm wide for direct closure by 24 cm length (to or across midline). Pedicle 5–14 cm, including the subscapular artery which involves tedious dissection through the triangular space or separately through the axilla. There are many small branches to divide here and it is easy to confuse a branch with the main vessel, so double check before cutting any branches! Large vessel diameter.

Indications
- Pedicled:
    - Axillary coverage.
    - Coverage of dorsum shoulder.
- Free:
    - Hand reconstruction.
    - Foot cover.
    - Facial or other contour correction (de-epithelialized).

Limitations
Arc of rotation limits reach. Limited size.

Method
- *Position* Patient prone or midlateral. Re-check markings once positioned as scapula is very mobile.
- *Planning* Palpate the triangular space and check with the formula to determine site of emergence of pedicle. This is the pivot point for a pedicled flap. Draw a line from this point 1 cm parallel to and beneath the spine of the scapula, extending to the vertebral column. This is the central axis of the flap. The flap ellipse should overlie the pivot point. Plan in reverse to ensure adequate pedicle/flap length. Template the defect, and draw the outline of the defect on the flap. A pedicled flap will 'propeller' around the pivot point. A free flap will have a short pedicle enabling the anastomosis to be beyond the limits of the cutaneous flap.
- *Incision* Incise around the flap.
- *Dissection* Start medially and raise flap supra-fascially. Continue raising in this plane until the perforator is seen. Chase the pedicle as it decends deep into the triangular space. Will need to divide the muscular branches and the vertical parascapular branch to achieve 6 cm pedicle length. For bone (2–3 × 11 cm) need to retain muscle periosteum branches from vertical para scapular artery.
- *Closure* Close donor site directly by undermining skin edges. Inset flap.

Advantages
- Hairless flap in women, with moderate thickness, thick dermis.
- Large vessels but fairly short pedicle.
- Hidden scar.
- No sacrifice of major vessel unless pedicle is chased proximal to thoracodorsal.

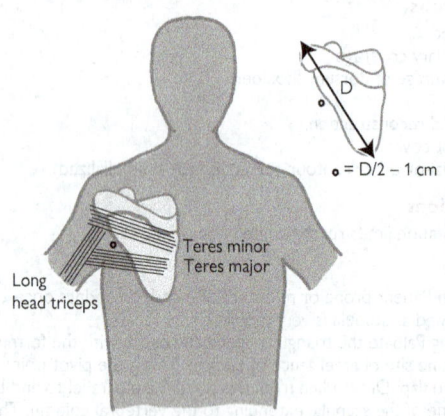

Fig. 22.38 Surface marking for the scapular and the parascapular flaps. Note that the position of the pedicle is half the length of the scapula minus 1 cm.

Complications
- Limited size if plan to close directly.
- To obtain longer pedicle requires tedious dissection through the space and/or into axilla.

Tips
- Raise supra-fascially to avoid getting lost in all the different fascial intersections and layers around the shoulder.
- Can raise scapular and parascapular combined if large defects.

References
Dos Santos (1984). *Plast Recon Surg* **73**: 599–604.
Hamilton SG, Morrison WA (1982). *Br J Plast Surg* **35**, 2–7.

Parascapular flap

Fascio-cutaneous flap from the back suitable for transfer pedicled or free (Nassif et al. 1982). Can include lateral border of the scapula.

Anatomy
The skin of the back is very thick and durable. Hence it provides robust cover. Generally the adipose layer is less thick than the abdomen. The flap uses skin overlying the lateral border of the scapula extending from the axilla to 10–15 cm beyond the tip of the scapula.

Vascular anatomy: type B
The parascapular flap pedicle is the parascapular branch of the circumflex scapular artery. The vascular bundle emerges from the omotricipital space with the transverse scapular artery the majority of the time; rarely it emerges separately below teres major. The triangular or omotricipital space is found using the formula $D = (L - 2)/2$, where L (cm) is scapula spine to inferior angle and D (cm) is scapula spine to pedicle (Dos Santos 1980). This approximates the pedicle 68% of the time. The venous drainage is to VCs.

Neural supply
The skin is supplied by intercostal nerves and cannot be innervated.

Flap territory
A flap of size 30 × 15 cm could be raised. A bone segment of up to 8 cm long and 1 cm wide but only a few millimetres thick can be raised.

Suitability for free tissue transfer
Adequate pedicle length of 7–10 cm with large diameter (2.5–3.5 mm). The pedicle length can be extended to 15 cm with thoracodorsal sacrifice.

Indications
- Pedicled:
  - Axillary coverage.
  - Coverage of dorsum shoulder.
- Free:
  - Hand reconstruction.
  - Foot cover.

Limitations
Arc of rotation limits reach.

Method
- ***Position*** Patient prone or midlateral. Re-check markings once positioned as scapula is very mobile.
- ***Planning*** Palpate the triangular space and check with the formula to determine site of emergence of pedicle. This is the pivot point for a pedicled flap. Draw a line from this point 1 cm parallel to the lateral border of the scapula. This is the central axis of the flap. The flap ellipse should overlie the pivot point. Plan in reverse to ensure adequate pedicle/flap length. Template the defect, and draw the

outline of the defect on the flap. A pedicled flap will most likely 'propeller' around the pivot point. A free flap will have a short pedicle, enabling the anastomosis to be beyond the limits of the cutaneous flap.
- *Incision* Incise around the flap.
- *Dissection* Start distally and raise flap supra-fascially. Continue raising in this plane until the perforator is seen. Chase the pedicle as it decends deep into the triangular space. There are many small branches to divide here and it is easy to confuse a branch with the main vessel, so double check before cutting any branches!
- *Closure* Close donor site directly by undermining skin edges. Inset flap.

Advantages
- Hairless flap in women, with moderate thickness, thick dermis.
- Large vessels but farly short pedicle.
- Hidden scar.

Complications
- Limited size if plan to close directly.
- To obtain longer pedicle requires tedious dissection through the space and/or into axilla.

Tips
Raise supra-fascially to avoid getting lost in all the different fascial intersections and layers around the shoulder.

References
Dos Santos (1984). *Plast Recon Surg* **73**: 599–604.
Nassif TM, Vidal L, Bovet JL, Baudet J (1982). *Plast Reconstr Surg* **69**, 591–600.

Trapezius flap

This used to be a very popular flap, but is used infrequently now. It is based on the trapezius, a large flat triangular superficial muscle of the upper back (28 × 34 cm in the adult male). A skin paddle can be taken with the muscle, the dimensions of which are governed by the ability to achieve primary closure or accepting a skin grafted donor. The skin paddle is generally oriented either vertically over the inferior muscle fibres or laterally which will incorporate the superior fibres and can be extended to include cervico-humoral flap. Flap can be muscle, musculo-cutaneous, osseomuscular, osseomusculo-cutaneous, or a neurotized functional muscle transfer. Wider arc of rotation and more hidden donor site (cf. pectoralis major).

Anatomy
Muscle originates from the external occipital protuberance, nuchal line, ligamentum nuchae, and spinous processes of seventh cervical and all thoracic vertebrae. Insertion is of superior fibres to the lateral third of clavicle posterior surface, middle fibres to the acromion and scapular spine, and inferior fibres to the medial base of scapular spine. Action of the muscle is in stabilizing the scapula with rotation such that the glenoid points superiorly. Denervation or loss of whole muscle unit leads to shoulder droop deformity, winging of the scapula, and malrotation of the scapula. Therefore it is important to maintain innervation to some portion of residual muscle via the accessory nerve.

Vascular anatomy: type 2
The blood supply is from a dominant pedicle, the transverse cervical artery, itself a branch of the thyrocervical trunk (80%), or direct from subclavian (20%). The transverse cervical artery courses between the sternocleidomastoid and scalenius muscles, crosses the brachial plexus and then the anterior margin of trapezius to enter its deep surface at the base of the neck before it divides into ascending and descending branches giving rise to flap orientation over either. Pedicle length 4 cm, diameter 1.8 mm. Minor pedicles comprise posterior intercostal perforators adjacent to cervical and thoracic vertebral bodies, and the largest minor pedicle is the occipital artery which is 3 cm long and has a diameter of 1 millimetre. The venous drainage is to VCs.

Neural supply
Innervation by the spinal accessory as primary motor nerve, which enters the deep surface of the muscle 5 cm above the clavicle. Cervical nerves 3 and 4 provide proprioception. Cutaneous sensation is via cervical nerves anteriorly and posterior intercostals posteriorly; therefore the flap not sensate unless neurorraphy at recipient site

Flap territory
A skin flap of size 30–40 cm long × 10–15 cm wide could be raised if designed vertically with the inferior extent of the skin paddle able to extend 5–10 cm below the distal edge of the muscle at T12. Vertical skin paddle is based over the middle or inferior fibres, with the superior preserved. Therefore there is no shoulder droop. The lateral skin paddle,

based over the superior fibres, with dimensions 6–10 cm wide × 8–30 cm long is centred over the acromion. Bone transferred can be lateral clavicle or spine of scapula.

Suitability for free tissue transfer
Not really; tedious vessel dissection to obtain adequate pedicle. Much better options exist.

Indications
Muscle, musculo-cutaneous, osseomuscular, or osseomusculo-cutaneous.
- Pedicled proximally:
  - Head and neck reconstruction, including occiput and temporal regions.
  - Mandibular reconstruction.
  - Coverage of plexus in supraclavicular fossa.
  - Back reconstruction.
  - Chest reconstruction.
  - Facial reconstruction, especially orbits, ear, and parotid.
  - For OBPP shoulder functional transfer.
- Pedicled distally:
  - Back reconstruction.

Method
- **Position** Patient prone.
- **Planning** The skin paddle is marked with the patient sitting or standing with arms neutral as when lateral the scapula will rotate according to arm position. For a vertical skin paddle or muscle-only transfer, draw a line from the midpoint of the clavicle vertically backwards to run parallel between the scapula and spine. This is the axis of the descending vessel. Draw a vertical paddle skin island or superiorly based pedicle such that it runs between scapula and spine centrally over the axis. The posterior supraclavicular fossa forms the pivot point. Plan in reverse to ensure adequate pedicle/flap length. Template the defect, and draw the outline of the defect on the distal end of the flap. For a transverse skin paddle palpate the anterior border of the trapezius to the acromion and mark; this forms the axis of the flap. The skin paddle can then be drawn centred over this axis and can extend onto the lateral arm.
- **Incision** Incise around the flap down to muscle or if muscle only down drawn axis.
- **Dissection** Start distally. Raise skin paddle from latissimus dorsi if extends beyond trapezius. Then raise surrounding skin until trapezius can be identified. Delineate the edge of trapezius and elevate. Separate from spine. Elevate myocutaneous unit in submuscular plane from distal to proximal. Take care at level of scapular not to raise rhomboid muscles. Continue raising in this plane until pedicle is seen on underside of muscle. Then can follow and protect pedicle. The muscle is divided laterally at the level of the skin paddle, taking care to preserve superior fibres and hence avoid shoulder droop.
- **Closure** Close donor site directly if on back; if transverse style, will probably need grafting. Inset flap.

Advantages
- Good local coverage for occipital or cervical spine defects.
- Can be a functional transfer.

Complications
- Ugly donor site if transverse flap.
- Pedicle can be bulky.
- Morbidity greater than for latissimus dorsi, and leads to severe shoulder dysfunction.
- Muscle is quite thin for dead-space defect filling.

Further reading
Demergasso F, Piazza MV (1979). *Am J Surg* **138**, 533–6.
Jaques DA, Hovey LM, Chambers RG (1971) *Am J Surg* **122**, 744–7.

Gluteus maximus flap

An important muscle in ambulation and hence used mainly in paraplegics. Mainly a musculo-cutaneous rotation flap or V–Y advancement flap for treatment of ischial or sacral pressure sores. Gluteus can be used partially preserving some function. Occasionally used as a free flap for breast reconstruction (Fujino et al. 1976). Forms the basis of the superior gluteal artery perforator (SGAP) flap.

Anatomy

Thick broad rectangular muscle superficial to gluteus medius and minimus. Originates from the gluteal line of ilium, iliac crest, and sacrum. Runs obliquely at 45° inferiorly laterally. Inserts a quarter on the gluteal line inferior to the greater tuberosity of femur and three-quarters on the iliotibial tract. Its action is to extend and laterally rotate the hip and extend the knee.

Vascular anatomy: type 3

The two dominant blood supplies are the superior and inferior gluteal arteries, supplying the superior and inferior portion of muscle, respectively. They are branches of the internal iliac artery. They enter the deep surface of the muscle, the superior above the piriformis and the inferior below via the sciatic foramen. Corresponding veins of the same name drain into the external iliac vein. The skin overlying the gluteus maximus on the buttock is supplied by musculo-cutaneous perforators from the same vessels. Because of good subdermal vascular plexi large areas of the buttock skin can survive on one perforator.

Neural supply

Inferior gluteal nerve (L5, S1–2) a branch of the sacral plexus that runs in close proximity to the inferior gluteal artery. The skin in the natal cleft is supplied by the posterior primary rami of all five sacral segments. The upper three lumbar segments supply the upper buttock skin and the lateral buttock is supplied by the subcostal, ilio-hypogastric and lateral femoral cutaneous nerve of thigh. The inferior buttock is supplied by the posterior cutaneous nerve of thigh which penetrates the muscle.

Flap territory

The muscle forms a quadrilateral shape from sacrum to greater tuberosity and proximal femur. The skin over this area can be utilized. The gluteal crease does not represent the lower border of the muscle but is caused by hip joint flexion and extension. However, it is a useful crease for designing rotation flaps. For breast reconstruction use the superior gluteal skin and fat as a free flap. The quantity available depends on the patient's habitus.

Suitability for free tissue transfer

Yes, but uncommonly used. Main use is as an SGAP flap. The pedicle is short (2–3 cm) but the vessels are of large diameter. A free perforator flap 10–15 cm wide × 25–30cm long can be harvested with direct closure.

Indications
- Muscle only.
- Myocutaneous (pedicled or free).
- Skin only as an SGAP flap.
- Pedicled:
  - Used for sacral and ischial pressure sore reconstruction.
- Free:
  - Breast reconstruction.

Limitations
Long scar on the buttock; may need to reposition patient intra-operatively.

Method
- *Position* Patient prone.
- *Planning* Myocutaneous rotation flap: as large a rotation flap as possible should be designed as this allows re-elevation and re-use in the future. The rotation can be inferiorly or superiorly based. Superior avoids injury to posterior thigh vessels and nerve.
- *Incision* Along the rotation design.
- *Dissection* Deepen incision to the muscle locating the superior and inferior borders. Divide the insertion and elevate the muscle from the gluteus medius via the trochanteric bursa with blunt dissection. Arteries come into view ~5 cm from sacral edge on the deep surface of the muscle. The origin may also need to be divided to cover sacral pressure sores effectively. The leading edge of the rotation can be separated into cutaneous and muscular elements to fill the dead space better and to provide skin cover whilst avoiding scars in pressure-bearing areas.
- *Closure* Close donor site directly over drains. Inset flap.
- *Free flap* Plan ellipse transverse over the superior gluteal vessels with the vessels entering the medial quarter to apex of the flap, elevate skin and fat, and include a segment of the underlying gluteus including the superior gluteal vessel. In SGAP dissect pedicle through the muscle.

Complications
Injury to superior gluteal nerve in the ambulant. Injury to the posterior nerve and vessels of thigh resulting in inability to use posterior thigh flap for reconstruction in future.

Donor site morbidity
Excellent in the paraplegic patient. In the ambulant, loss of abduction and extension of the thigh. Possible nerve damage unless careful dissection; short vascular pedicle. As a perforator flap, the dissection is difficult with a significant failure rate

Tips
In an ambulant patient this flap can still be used with partial division of the origin to give more movement. The large buttock rotation flap can also be designed to cover pressure sores on the trochanter, sacrum, and ischium simultaneously.

Reference
Fujino T, Harashina T, Enomoto K (1976). *Plast Reconstr Surg* **58**, 371–4.

Rectus abdominis flap

This is a muscle only or myocutaneous flap based on the rectus abdominis muscle and its blood supply, perforators from which (found centred around the umbilicus) supply the abdominal skin. The skin paddle, if required, can be designed longitudinally as in a vertical rectus abdominis myocutaneous (VRAM) flap or transverse as in a transverse rectus abdominis myocutaneous (TRAM). This section deals with the muscle-only flap.

Anatomy

Rectus abdominis is a paired long flat muscle which is traversed by three tendinous intersections. It is ensheathed by the anterior and posterior rectus sheaths and extends the whole length of the anterior abdominal wall. The muscle has two heads of origin: the lateral head from the pubic crest, and the medial head from the front of the symphysis pubis. The muscle is broad at its insertion. It is inserted by three slips (which lie deep to the pectoralis major) into the costal cartilage of the fifth, sixth, and seventh ribs.

Vascular anatomy: type 3

The rectus abdominis has two major pedicles, superior and inferior. The superior pedicle is a continuation of the internal mammary artery after it has divided into the superior epigastric and the musculophrenic branches at the level of the sixth intercostal space. The superior epigastric lies between the muscle and the posterior rectus sheath for a variable distance before coursing deep in the muscle. The inferior pedicle is a branch of the external iliac artery. The deep inferior epigastric artery commences just proximal to the inguinal ligament, runs up along the medial wall of the internal inguinal ring, and pierces the posterior rectus sheath to reach the rectus abdominis. Each pedicle supplies more than its own half of the muscle, and there are numerous anastomotic branches between the terminal branches of the two pedicles. There are also minor vascular contribution from terminal branches of the segmental intercostals.

Neural supply

Rectus abdominis is innervated segmentally by intercostal nerves from T6 to T12.

Flap territory

The whole muscle can be raised on either its superior or inferior pedicle. In cases of sternal dehiscence with loss of the internal mammary vessels the flap can still survive when raised superiorly on retrograde flow from the musculophrenic division.

Suitability for free tissue transfer

Ideal, since it leaves an acceptable donor site with no loss of function, a good scar (a simultaneous abdominoplasty can be performed with a Pfannanstiel incision), there are large-calibre vessels for anastomosis, it can be harvested with the patient supine, and in many cases allows a two team approach.

Indications
- Pedicled:
  - Superior: sternal/mediastinal, breast, lower chest, upper abdomen.
  - Inferior: groin, perineum, superior hip and thigh.
- Free: coverage anywhere.

Limitations
Cannot maintain neurotization. If pedicled, limited by arc of rotation.

Method
- **Position** Patient supine.
- **Incision** Longitudinal para-median incision or Pfannanstiel incision
- **Dissection** Elevate the abdominal skin, dividing perforators as seen. Incise the anterior rectus sheath longitudinally and elevate from the muscle (this may be tricky at the intersections). Easily lift the muscle from the deep rectus sheath. See the inferior and superior pedicle on the deep surface of the muscle and follow the appropriate one, dividing the other. Divide the muscle at the opposite side to the pedicle. You may leave the muscle pedicled proximally and transpose the distal end of muscle medially around to cover the defect, or divide the pedicle end of the muscle as well to aid transposition by reducing bulk at the point of rotation.
- **Closure** Close the rectus sheath in layers with a strong loop nylon. Close the skin directly over drain. Inset flap; cover with SSG.

Complications
- Abdominal bulges or hernias (~5%).
- Decreased abdominal strength.
- Necrosis of abdominoplasty flap if this approach used.
- Umbilical necrosis.

Free tissue transfer
- Large muscle flap available for transfer.
- Robust large arteries.
- Reliable anatomy.
- Quick to raise.
- Good subdermal fat perfusion.

Donor site morbidity
The rectus abdominis is a relatively expendable muscle, and hence donor site morbidity is minimal. Abdominal scar can be hidden if a Pfannanstiel incision and an abdominoplasty flap approach are used. Hernia can be avoided by careful closure of the fascia, and in cases where fascia is taken with the flap (i.e. VRAM or TRAM) use mesh for support.

Novelties and tips
- Has been used as a flow-through flap to reconstruct vascular supply to a limb as well as simultaneous muscle cover.
- Ideally, two teams of appropriately trained staff required to reduce the operative time. In perineal reconstruction can pass flap and pedicle intra-pelvic to increase the range of reach.

VRAM (vertical rectus abdominis myocutaneous) flap

This is a myocutaneous flap based on the rectus abdominis muscle and its blood supply, perforators from which (found centred around the umbilicus) supply the abdominal skin. The skin paddle can be designed longitudinally as in a VRAM flap or transverse as in a TRAM flap.

Anatomy
See rectus abdominis flap.

Vascular anatomy
See rectus abdominis flap.

Vascular anatomy of the VRAM skin
Perforating vessels from the epigastric arteries as they course through the rectus muscle. They are predominantly found in the peri-umbilical region along the line of the epigastric vessels. There are also some perforators from the segmental intercostals which tend to be found along the lateral rectus edge. These can be sacrificed. The flap can be raised on a single epigastric artery and vein.

Neural supply
Rectus abdominis and the abdominal skin are innervated segmentally by intercostal nerves from T6 to T12.

Flap territory
In a VRAM the skin directly over the rectus is harvested in a longitudinal design. This is usually a long ellipse to aid direct closure. The perforators supplying this flap have a far greater territory, as detailed in the section on the TRAM flap.

Suitability for free tissue transfer
Yes, since it leaves an acceptable donor site which can be directly closed, a large volume of tissue can be taken on a single pedicle, and there are large-calibre vessels for anastomosis.

Indications
- Pedicled:
  - Superior: sternal, breast, lower chest, upper abdomen.
  - Inferior: abdomen, groin, perineum, superior hip and thigh.
- Free: coverage anywhere.

Limitations
Too bulky a flap to be used on the limbs. If pedicled, limited by arc of rotation. Cannot be neurotized.

Method
- **Position** Patient supine.
- **Incision** An incision outlining the skin flap design which should include the peri-umbilical perforators. The skin flap can be central, superior, or inferior. The skin flap can extend over the midline but becomes less reliable as it extends beyond the lateral border of the contralateral rectus.

On the ipsilateral side the flap can extend to the mid-lateral line. Most VRAMs are simple ellipses the width of the rectus, allowing direct closure. If more tissue is required, a TRAM is preferred to allow direct closure.
- *Dissection* Partial elevation of the skin from the superior and inferior aspects of the anterior rectus sheath can be performed as well. The central perforators must be preserved. The largest are those found peri-umbilical and arise directly from the epigastric arteries as they course through the rectus. To preserve these perforators safely a quadrant of rectus sheath and the width of underlying rectus muscle is harvested as well as the skin and subcutaneous tissue. If muscle volume is needed, the entire rectus is harvested. If not, just a segment of rectus bearing the perforators is taken and islanded on the chosen epigastric vessels. Incise the anterior rectus sheath transversely above and below the perforators and longitudinally from this level towards the origin of the chosen epigastric artery. Elevate the sheath from the muscle (this may be tricky at the intersections) and lift the muscle from the deep rectus sheath. See the inferior and superior pedicle on the deep surface of the muscle and follow the appropriate one. The rectus muscle and the epigastric vessel within it can be divided at the opposite end to the pedicle at the level of the preserved quadrant of sheath. You can leave the muscle pedicled proximally and transpose the distal end of muscle (and the skin/fat it is supplying) around to cover the defect or divide the pedicle end of the muscle at the level of the proximal end of the quadrant, being careful to preserve the epigastric vessels which are then dissected free of the remaining proximal muscle to island the flap completely on its vascular pedicle. This can also be divided if free transfer is planned.
- *Closure* Close the rectus sheath in layers with strong loop nylon. If the rectus defect cannot be closed use mesh. Close the skin directly over drains; undermining the skin at the supra-fascial plane may aid closure. Inset flap.

Complications
- Abdominal bulges or hernias (~5%).
- Decreased abdominal strength.
- Necrosis of skin flaps.
- Umbilical necrosis.

Free tissue transfer
- Large surface area and volume available for transfer.
- Robust reliable large arteries.
- Good subdermal fat perfusion.

Donor site morbidity
See rectus abdominis flap.

Novelties
Rectus-preserving techniques can be used to reduce the donor morbidity by leaving some lateral and medial strips of rectus, or by dissecting the perforator and epigastric vessel from the rectus muscle (DIEP flap).

TRAM (transverse rectus abdominis myocutaneous) flap

This is a myocutaneous flap based on the rectus abdominis muscle and its blood supply, perforators from which (found centred around the umbilicus) supply the abdominal skin. The skin paddle can be designed longitudinally as in a VRAM flap or transverse as in a TRAM flap.

Anatomy
📖 See rectus abdominis flap.

Vascular anatomy
📖 See rectus abdominis flap.

Vascular anatomy of the TRAM skin
The TRAM skin is supplied by perforators from the epigastric arteries as they course through the rectus. These perforators are found along the line of the vessels and especially around the umbilicus. The perforators penetrate the skin and supply the subcutaneous and sub-dermal plexus. The vascular territories are named zone 1–4 according to reducing quality of perfusion and increasing distance from principle blood supply. Zone 1 directly overlies the rectus and epigastric supply, zone 2 is the adjacent territory over external oblique, zone 3 is the contralateral territory over rectus, and zone 4 is the contralateral territory over external oblique.

Neural supply
Rectus abdominis and the abdominal skin are innervated segmentally by intercostal nerves from T6 to T12.

Suitability for free tissue transfer
Yes, since it leaves an acceptable donor site, a large volume of tissue can be taken on a single long pedicle, a simultaneous abdominoplasty can be performed to enable direct closure, and there are large-calibre vessels for anastomosis.

Indications
- Pedicled:
  - Superior: sternal, breast, lower chest, upper abdomen.
  - Inferior: abdomen, groin, perineum, superior hip and thigh.
- Free: coverage anywhere.

Limitations
Too bulky a flap to be used on the limbs. If pedicled, limited by arc of rotation. Cannot be neurotized.

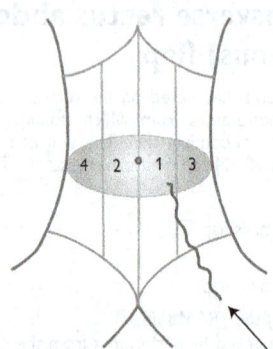

Fig. 22.39 The vascular perfusion zones of a TRAM flap.

Method
- **Position** Patient supine.
- **Incision** An incision outlining the elliptical flap design which should include the peri-umbilical perforators. The flap can be central, superior, or inferior. The flap can extend over the midline but becomes less reliable as it extends beyond the lateral border of the contralateral rectus. On the ipsilateral side the flap can extend to the scapula tip.
- **Dissection** Elevate the abdominal skin on the contralateral side to the proposed pedicle in the supra-fascial plane to the midline. Elevate the ipsilateral flap skin from lateral to medial where it overlies the external oblique, dividing peforators as seen. Partial elevation of the skin from the superior and inferior aspects of the anterior rectus sheath can also be performed. The central perforators must be preserved. The largest are those found peri-umbilical and arise directly from the epigastric arteries as they course through the rectus. To preserve these perforators safely a quadrant of rectus sheath the width of underlying rectus muscle is harvested as well as the skin and subcutaneous tissue. Incise the anterior rectus sheath transversly above and below the perforators and longitudinally from this level towards the origin of the chosen epigastric artery. Elevate the sheath from the muscle (this may be tricky at the intersections) and lift the muscle from the deep rectus sheath. See the inferior and superior pedicle on the deep surface of the muscle and follow the appropriate one. The rectus muscle and the epigastric vessel within it can be divided at the opposite end to the pedicle at the level of the preserved quadrant of sheath. You can leave the muscle pedicled proximally and transpose the distal end of muscle and the skin and fat it is supplying around to cover the defect or divide the pedicle end of the muscle at the level of the proximal end of the quadrant, being careful to preserve the epigastric vessels which are then dissected free of the remaining proximal muscle to island the flap completely on its vascular pedicle. This can also be divided if free transfer is planned.

- *Closure* Close the rectus sheath in layers with strong loop nylon. If the rectus defect cannot be closed use mesh. Close the skin directly over drains. Undermining the skin at the supra-fascial plane may aid closure. Inset flap.

Complications and donor morbidity
- Abdominal bulges or hernias (~5%).
- Decreased abdominal strength.
- Necrosis of skin flaps.
- Umbilical necrosis.

Variations
Has been used as a bi-pedicled flap on both SEAs to increase the size and volume of transferred tissue. Has also been used as a supercharged flap whereby it has been pedicled superiorly for breast reconstruction, and to augment the blood supply and drainage the deep inferior epigastric vessels are anastomosed in the axilla.

Rectus-sparing techniques to reduce the donor site mobidity include leaving lateral and medial muscle strips, or dissecting out the perforators and the epigastric vessels leaving the entire muscle behind (DIEP flap).

DIEP (deep inferior epigastric perforator) flap

Anatomy
📖 See rectus abdominis flap.

A variation of the TRAM flap which preserves rectus muscle by dissecting the cutaneous perforators retrogradely through the muscle to the inferior epigastric artery. The vascular basis of the flap is the same as the TRAM except the volume of flap is reduced by virtue of carrying it on a reduced number of perforators or even on a single perforator.

Vascular anatomy
📖 See TRAM flap.

Indications
Free: mainly used for breast reconstruction.

Advantages
Rectus sparing leading to less hernia and abdominal wall bulging, retention of abdominal strength, and symmetry.

Limitations
Reduced volume of tissue of primary vascularity, and greater areas of marginal vascularity.

Method
- **Position** Patient supine.
- **Planning** Preoperative Doppler, either hand-held or duplex, can aid perforator location and guide flap planning. A standard TRAM flap is marked.
- **Incision** An incision outlining the elliptical flap design, which should include the peri-umbilical perforators. The flap can extend over the midline but becomes less reliable as it extends beyond the lateral border of the contralateral rectus. On the ipsilateral side the flap can extend to the mid-lateral line.
- **Dissection** Incise down to the rectus fascia around the flap, taking care to preserve the superficial inferior epigastric veins. Elevate the contralateral skin and fat in the supra-fascial plane until the midline. If a significant perforator is encountered on the contralateral side, it may be prudent to adjust the plan intra-operatively and base the flap on this, as the length of pedicle with a DIEP permits this. If not continue dissection until the medial row of perforators are seen. Elevate the ipsilateral skin and fat from lateral to medial until the lateral row of perforators is encountered. Decide on whether to use the lateral or medial row of perforators. If there is one dominant perforator than the flap can be based on this or with one or two others in the same row for security. Divide the remaining perforators. The chosen perforators are followed retrogradely through the rectus by incising the anterior rectus sheath and then longitudinally splitting the muscle in the line of its fibres. The side branches are divided with

bipolar or ligaclips and the perforator is followed back to its origin from the lateral or medial branch of the deep inferior epigastric vessels. The branch is double clipped superior to the perforator. The inferior epigastric artery is found deep to the rectus below the arcuate line, and followed antegradely to join the superficial trans-muscular dissection. Branches of the intercostal nerves that run anterior to the vessels are kept intact to avoid denervation. The inferior epigastric artery and vein are divided at their origin and delivered through the muscle from deep along the perforator pathway.
- *Closure* Close the rectus sheath in layers with strong loop nylon. Standard abdominoplasty closure. Inset flap.

Specific complications
- Abdominal bulges or hernias (~1%).
- Necrosis of skin flaps.
- Umbilical necrosis.
- Partial necrosis of flap.
- Fat necrosis.

Donor site morbidity
Less morbidity reported.

Further reading
Allen RJ, Treece P (1994). *Ann Plast Surg* **32**, 32–8.
Koshima I, Soeda S (1989). *Br J Plast Surg* **42**, 645–8.

Latissimus dorsi flap (and TAP flap)

First performed by Tansini in 1892, but rediscovered and popularized by Olivari (1976). A muscle only or myocutaneous flap, which can be muscle sparing by taking only a segment of muscle or more recently by dissecting the skin perforators through the muscle creating a thoracodorsal artery perforator (TAP) flap. It can also be used as a functioning muscle transfer.

Anatomy

A broad flat muscle connecting the humerus to the ilium and back. It arises by tendinous fibres from the spinous process of the six lower thoracic vertebrae, from the posterior layer of the thoraco-lumbar fascia, from the outer lip of the ilium, and by fleshy interdigitations with the lower three or four ribs where it interdigitates with serratus posterior inferior. There is frequently a slip arising from the scapula tip.

It winds around the teres major to insert as a quadrilateral bilaminar tendon into the crest of the bicipital groove medially. At its insertion the tendon is crossed anteriorly by the axillary vessels and the cords/branches of the brachial plexus. Its superficial dorsal surface is subcutaneous; however, it is covered by trapezius in its posterior superior medial corner. Deep to the muscle is serratus posterior inferior and the rhomboids (superiorly).

Vascular anatomy: type 2

The dominant blood supply is the thoracodorsal artery, a continuation of the subscapular artery arising from the third part of the axillary artery. At about 3 cm from its origin the subscapular artery divides into the circumflex scapular artery (which escapes the axilla through the triangular space) and the thoracodorsal artery. The latissimus dorsi is also supplied segmentally by intercostal and lumbar perforators. The skin overlying the muscle is supplied by numerous perforators sufficiently dispersed to allow an almost infinite variety of skin flap designs. The main reliable perforators from the thoracodorsal artery are concentrated at the site of penetration of the muscle by the pedicle and along the anterior border of the muscle. The perforators penetrating the muscle to supply the skin just as the thoracodorsal artery enters the muscle, or soon after that, form the basis for the TAP flap. If the the thoracodorsal artery has been divided, the flap may survive on retrograde flow from the serratus anterior branch.

Neural supply

Latissimus dorsi is innervated by the thoracodorsal nerve, a branch of the posterior cord. The skin is supplied segmentally by intercostals.

Flap territory

The muscle forms a triangle from axilla to T7, T7 to ileum, and ileum to axilla. The skin over this area and extending 10 cm anteriorly can be utilized. The distal end of the muscle may be poorly vascularized by the thoracodorsal artery.

Suitability for free tissue transfer

The workhorse for reconstruction in plastic surgery. A very reliable free flap. The pedicle is long and the vessels are of large diameter.

Indications
- Muscle only.
- Neurotized muscle (functioning muscle transfer).
- Myocutaneous.
- Skin only as a TAP flap.
- Pedicled:
  - Used for axillary or shoulder soft tissue reconstruction.
  - It can cover upper limb defects up to and including the elbow.
  - It can functionally reconstruct elbow flexion/extension, shoulder external rotation.
  - It can cover chest wall, spinal, and breast defects.
  - It can be used in head and neck reconstruction.
- Free can be used for any indication above, and in addition:
  - Both lower and upper limb reconstruction.
  - Head and neck reconstruction.
  - Chest and trunk reconstruction.

Limitations
- Long scar on the back.
- May have to reposition patient intra-operatively.
- Distal end of muscle unreliable as is a secondary territory primarily supplied by the lumbar perforators.

Method
- *Position* Patient on side or prone. Can be supine if experienced.
- *Incision* Muscle only: oblique longitudinal incision 5 cm posterior parallel to the palpable anterior muscle edge from posterior border axilla to ileum. Skin: design ellipse either transverse or oblique (following anterior border) with apex of ellipse at posterior border axilla.
- *Dissection* Elevate the skin in the supra-muscular plane anteriorly until the anterior edge is seen. Elevate the skin posteriorly to the spine. Incise along the anterior edge. Find the plane between latissimus dorsi and ribs and divide the perforators passing through this plane. Distally this plane blends with serratus posterior inferior. Divide the aponeurotic origin from the spine and pelvis, and the muscular slips from the ribs. Incise along the superior edge which may have attachment to scapula and trapezius. Follow the insertion superficially proximally to the humerus. On the deep surface view the pedicle and dissect from distal to proximal. Divide the branches to serratus anterior. Pedicle or divide for free flap. Divide insertion as required for extra mobility if pedicled.
- *Closure* Close donor site directly over drains. Inset flap.

Complications
Seroma common; can be minimized by quilting the skin flaps to the back on closing.

Donor site morbidity
Clinically there is no functional defect (due to pectoralis major and teres major). Scar can be obvious.

Novelties
- Has been used as a distally based flap on the distal perforators to cover lumbar and sacral wounds.
- Used as a perforator flap (free or pedicled).

Reference
Olivari N (1976). *Br J Plast Surg* **29**, 126–8.

Serratus anterior flap

A muscle-only flap, which can be muscle sparing by taking only a segment of muscle. It can also be used as a functioning muscle transfer.

Anatomy

A broad flat multipennate muscle connecting ribs 1–8 to the scapula. The first two digitations originate from the outer aspects of the first and second ribs. They form the floor off the posterior triangle of the neck. The third and fourth digitations originate from the third and fourth ribs. The final four digitations originate by fleshy interdigitations from the anterior angles of the fifth, sixth, seventh, and eighth ribs. Serratus inter-digitates with the external oblique.

The first two digitations insert on the upper angle of the scapula. The third and fourth digitations insert on the vertebral border of the scapula on its costal surface. The final four digitations insert on the inferior angle of the scapula.

The muscle protracts the scapula and keeps it opposed against the chest wall. The lower four digitations help the trapezius to rotate the scapula so that the glenoid points upwards and laterally. Denervation results in winging and malrotation.

Vascular anatomy: type 3

There are two dominant blood supplies. The first is the serratus branch of the thoracodorsal artery, itself a continuation of the subscapular artery arising from the third part of the axillary artery. At about 3 cm from its origin the subscapular artery divides into the circumflex scapular artery (which escapes the axilla through the triangular space) and the thoracodorsal artery. The thoracodorsal artery splits into the thoracodorsal and serratus branch approximately 5–8 cm from its origin. The serratus branch heads posteriorly, lying just superficial to the fascia of serratus before entering the muscle, usually after splitting into several branches. It mainly supplies the lower four slips. The serratus is also supplied by the lateral thoracic artery. This vessel is a branch from the second part of the axillary artery. It follows the lateral border of the pectoralis minor and mainly supplies the upper four slips. If the thoracodorsal artery has been divided proximal to the serratus branch, the flap may survive on retrograde flow along the thoracodorsal branch from the latissimus dorsi.

Neural supply

The first two digitations are by C5, the third and fourth digitations are by C6, and the final four digitations are by C7. All nerve supplies reach the muscle along the long thoracic nerve. The C5 and C6 contributions join together within the scalenius medius and the C7 branch joins at the inferior posterior border of the scalenius medius over the first digitations of the serratus anterior. The nerve then continues on the superficial surface of the muscle deep to its fascia. It lies posterior to the mid-axillary line and is vulnerable in axillary dissections, transthoracic sympathectomies, and posterior triangle of neck procedures.

Flap territory
The muscle forms a roughly rectangular shape from the axilla (10 × 15 cm).

Suitability for free tissue transfer
A very reliable free flap. The pedicle is long and the vessels of large diameter. Donor site morbidity can be minimized by only harvesting three or four slips and preserving the nerve supply to the remaining muscle.

Indications
- Muscle only.
- Neurotized muscle (functioning muscle transfer).
- Pedicled:
  - Used for axillary or shoulder soft tissue reconstruction.
  - it can cover small local chest wall defects.
- Free can be used for any indication above and in addition:
  - Both lower and upper limb reconstruction.
  - Head and neck reconstruction.

Limitations
- Fear of causing scapula and upper limb morbidity.
- Small thin muscle.

Method
- **Position** Patient on side or supine if experienced.
- **Planning** Examine and record shoulder function and scapula posture. The scapula is tested by asking the patient to flex the shoulder and push against the wall, and to abduct the shoulder to 90°. Observe for winging or malrotation.
- **Incision** An axillary midline longitudinal incision.
- **Dissection** Incise the skin and find the anterior edge of the latissimus dorsi. Retract the latissimus dorsi anteriorly. Locate the thoracodorsal vessel and its serratus branch on the medial wall of the axilla and the thoracodorsal and long thoracic nerves. Divide the lower three or four muscular slips from the ribs, working from inferior to superior. There is a nice plane deep to the serratus; it can be helpful if you find this plane first and then place a finger in it to help delineate the attachment of the ribs. Elevate the serratus vessels off the upper four slips, dividing any small branches. Divide the serratus between the fifth and sixth or the fourth and fifth slips. Leave the nerve attached to the remaining slips unless planning a neurotized flap, in which case do an intra-neural dissection taking only those fascicles supplying the segments of muscle being harvested. Follow the muscle posteriorly to its insertion and divide from scapula. Divide the branches to latissimus dorsi if a longer pedicle is needed. Try to avoid this so that the latissimus can be used later if the serratus fails! Pedicle or divide for free flap.
- **Closure** Close donor site directly over drains. Inset flap.

Complications
Seroma is common.

Donor site morbidity
Functional defect can be marked if you take the whole serratus anterior or clumsily denervate the remaining muscle.

Novelties
Has been used as a serratus fascial flap for gliding tissue reconstruction or when a super-thin flap is required.

Gracilis

Anatomy
Gracilis is a strap muscle lying superficially on the inner aspect of the thigh. It originates by a thin flat aponeurosis from the lower half of the margin of the symphysis and the anterior half of the pubic arch. It inserts into the medial tibia (pes anserinus) and some fibres go to the patella on the medial side.

Vascular anatomy: type 2
The medial circumflex femoral artery (a branch of the profunda femoris) passes superficial to adductor brevis and deep to adductor longus to enter gracilis about 8–10 cm below the pubic tubercle, on the muscle's deep antero-lateral aspect. There are two distal pedicles which are branches from the superficial femoral artery. All branches enter on the deep surface.

Neural supply
Gracilis is innervated by a branch of the obturator nerve.

Flap territory
The entire muscle can be raised on the main pedicle. The cutaneous territory is not reliable, but some skin can be based on the cutaneous perforator which is found at the penetration site of the pedicle.

Suitability for free tissue transfer
Personal favourite free muscle transfer. Pedicle length 10 cm. Easy harvest. Moderate-sized vessels.

Indications
- Pedicled muscle or myocutaneous:
  - Reconstruction of genitalia.
  - Reconstruction of groin.
  - Coverage of perineum, pubis, groin, abdominal wall, ischium.
- Free flap:
  - Muscle flap for any suitable defect.
  - Functional unit for biceps, finger flexors, facial reconstruction.

Limitations
The cutaneous territory is not as reliable as other flaps. Maximum size is 8–10 cm wide × 20–30 long × 1 cm deep.

Method
- **Position** Patient supine, hip abducted and externally rotated.
- **Incision** Incise down to muscle from pubic ramus to mid-thigh longitudinally, 3 cm behind a line drawn from adductor longus tendon insertion on pubic ramus and medial femoral condyle. Most common error is incising too anterior and elevating adductor longus!

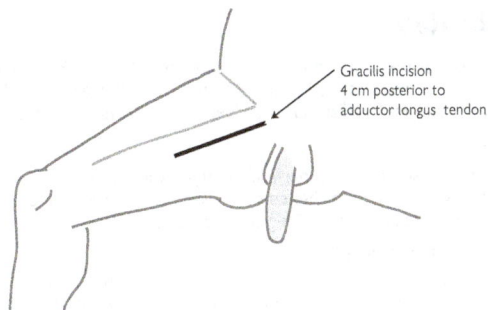

Fig. 22.40 Gracilis incision 4 cm posterior and longitudinal to the adductor longus tendon.

- *Dissection* Incise through the fascia longitudinally. Elevate the fascia anteriorly and posteriorly. Incise along the posterior muscle edge and elevate the deep plane by retracting the muscle, folding it anteriorly. See the pedicle entering the deep anterior aspect. Divide the other perforators passing into the muscle distally. Incise along the anterior muscle edge avoiding the anterior passage of the pedicle. Distal to the pedicle incise the fascia between adductor longus and brevis (magnus distally); insert a self-retainer in this groove and expand it to retract these muscles. The pedicle travels in this plane and can now be dissected. Divide the vessel branches to the adductors, liberating the pedicle. The nerve enters separately at an oblique angle proximal to the vessels. The muscle should now be free, apart from the origin, insertion, and pedicle. Divide the insertion by retracting on the muscle and dividing the tendinous junction. For a pedicled flap divide origin completely but leave pedicled on the vessels and transpose the distal end of muscle. For a free flap divide the posterior three-quarters of the origin from the inferior pubis ramus (there is small vascular pedicle to be diathermied here) to protect the pedicle while you divide them. Then complete the proximal muscle origin release.
- *Closure* Close donor site directly over drain. Inset flap and cover flap with SSG as required.

Complications

The pedicle enters the muscle at an angle and care must be taken on planning and inset to avoid undue kinking.

Donor site morbidity

Donor site heals with a well hidden scar when closed primarily. No functional loss.

Variations

Functional reconstruction of anal sphincters. Has been split longitudinally to provide two separate limbs of muscle, especially for facial reanimation.

Groin flap

The first axial pattern pedicled flap, performed by Wood in 1862! However, it was not properly described until 1972 (McGregor and Jackson 1972) and the basis of the first free flap was described in 1973 (O'Brien et al. 1973).

Anatomy

Utilizes skin based on the superficial circumflex iliac artery (SCIA), longitudinally aligned, lateral to the femoral vessels, along the groin crease in a line inferior and parallel to the inguinal ligament.

Vascular anatomy: Type B

The SCIA arises from the common femoral artery in the femoral triangle, 2–3 cm below the inguinal ligament, close to the origin of the superficial epigastric, circumflex femoral, and profunda femoris arteries. Considerable variations in the exact pattern of origin of these vessels are found. The SCIA runs deep to the deep fascia laterally inferior and parallel to the inguinal ligament until the medial border of sartorius. Here the vessel divides into the deep and superficial branches. The superficial branch continues more superficially just supra-fascial, supplying the skin beyond the ASIS and heading obliquely cranially towards the midline. The SCIV drains into the femoral vein 1–2 cm medial to the artery and can be proximal or distal to the arterial origin.

Neural supply

The skin is supplied by the lateral intercostal branch from T12, which crosses the iliac crest 5 cm posterior to the ASIS. The lateral femoral cutaneous nerve as it emerges medial to the ASIS passes just deep to the flap. Care must be taken to preserve it.

Flap territory

The flap extends from just medial to the femoral vein almost as far superio-laterally as the spine (35–40 cm). It may extend up to 10–12 cm in width; it is usually elliptical with the long axis parallel to the inguinal ligament, centred on a line 2–3 cm below the inguinal ligament which continues superiorly as it follows the skin creases around the trunk.

Suitability for free tissue transfer

Excellent. Short pedicle. The artery is rather small, usually 1–2 mm in diameter. No donor functional defect. Well-hidden scar. Large flap. Can include other territories (superficial epigastric, DCIA).

Indications

- Skin only.
- Osteofascio-cutaneous with iliac crest.
- Pedicled:
  - To cover hand, forearm, and elbow defects.
  - To cover lower abdomen, perineum.
- Free can be used for any indication above and in addition:
  - Any reconstruction requiring good-quality skin and subcutaneous tissue with or without volume.

Limitations
Can be bulky when used as a free flap because of preservation of the subcutaneous fat at the pedicle. Can be thinned radically once lateral to sartorius. The pedicle is short and the diameter and anatomy of the SCIA tend to vary. The pedicle dissection can be difficult. Can be hairy. As a pedicled distant flap for the hand, makes hand elevation and therapy difficult.

Method
- *Position* Patient supine.
- *Planning* Skin: design ellipse longitudinally centred over line drawn 2–3 cm below the inguinal ligament from the femoral vessels to the ASIS and continue the line as required around the trunk maintaining the direction. The medial apex of the ellipse is medial to the femoral vessels such that the width of the flap is reached as the femoral vessels are palpable. Use planning in reverse patterns to design the flap.
- *Incision* Incise around the flap from the femoral vessels laterally superiorly and inferiorly to the lateral apex. Superiorly you will divide the superficial epigastric vessels.
- *Dissection* Elevate the flap from lateral to medial. Stay in the supra-fascial plane until sartorius is reached. Slow down and proceed over sartorius supra-fascially until the medial border is reached. The vessel should be visible through the fascia, and at the medial border the deep branch passing into sartorius or medial to sartorius can be seen. Dissect around this vessel to ensure that you can visualize the medial continuation of the SCIA, and then divide the deep branch. Follow the SCIA on the deep surface of the flap until the origin of the artery is seen. This distance is much shorter than you would imagine. Dissect around the arterial origin and follow the vein medially and isolate. Continue the skin incision on the medial aspect of the flap and divide the vessels if it is to be free; leave medial skin and vessels intact if pedicled.
- *Closure* Close donor site directly if possible over drains. If tight, flex the hip. Inset flap.

Complications and donor site morbidity
Seroma in donor site. Hyperpigmentation has been noted as a complication. Venous drainage is more likely to be a problem in free transfer than arterial supply, so keep a safety vein laterally in the flap to supercharge the drainage if required. Can be hard to monitor as the skin is very pale. Excellent inconspicuous scar in the line of the groin crease.

Novelties
Flap can be split longitudinally laterally to cover two adjacent defects (fingers). Can take a cuff of the femoral artery with the origin of the SCIA if the arterial lumen is too narrow.

References
McGregor IA, Jackson IT (1972). *Br J Plast Surg* **25**, 3–16.
O'Brien BM, MacLeod AM, Hayhurst JW, Morrison WA (1973). *Plast Reconstr Surg* **52**, 271–8.

DCIA (deep circumflex iliac artery) flap

The DCIA is an axial pattern osseous flap named after its vessel of supply; it is aso called 'vascularized iliac bone graft' or 'iliac crest bone flap' after the segment of bone used. Almost always used as a free tissue transfer. Described by Taylor and Watson (1978). Was most popular for mandibular reconstruction because of the similar shape of the iliac bone.

Anatomy

The deep circumflex iliac artery flap is used as a vascularized bone 'graft'. The internal oblique muscle may be included. An osteocutaneous DCIA flap can be used in appropriate reconstructions, but the blood supply to the skin is considered less reliable than that to the bone.

Vascular anatomy

The DCIA originates from the external iliac artery just superior to the inguinal ligament. It then runs parallel to the ligament deep to the inguinal canal running in the junction of transversalis and the iliac fascia, towards the ASIS; 1 cm medial to the ASIS it gives off a large ascending branch and it also anastomoses with an ascending branch from the lateral circumflex femoral artery. The DCIA then pierces the transversalis fascia to run 2 cm below the iliac crest in the groove between the iliacus and transversalis fascia. The artery ends at the midpoint of the crest ~8 cm beyond the ASIS where it anastomoses with the superior gluteal and iliolumbar arteries within the transversus abdominis. Throughout its course musculo-cutaneous perforators arise from the DCIA. The bone vessels come through iliacus, so it is necessary to include a cuff of iliacus in the flap. The anatomy of the DCIA is consistent. The pedicle of the flap is around 6 cm long and 3 mm in diameter. Venae commitantes run with the artery and drain into the external iliac vein.

Flap territory

The iliac crest from ASIS and extending posteriorly for up to 18 cm.

Suitability for free tissue transfer

Good contour; good bone for osteo-integrated implants for mandible reconstruction.

Indications

- Pedicled:
  - For acetabular reconstruction.
- Free:
  - Reconstruction of the mandible.
  - Any bony defect requiring good-quality thick bone.

Limitations

Difficult to harvest; too curved for long-bone reconstruction; skin paddle unreliable unless SCIA taken as well (but this leaves a bad donor site).

Method

- **Position** Patient supine.
- **Planning** Draw a line starting medial to the mid-point of the inguinal ligament which then runs along the upper edge of the ligament and the iliac crest. Its posterior extent depends on the requirements of the reconstruction.
- **Incision** Incise along the line. The incision can be extended medially or along the course of the femoral vessels. Expose the inguinal ligament and the ASIS.
- **Dissection** The inguinal ligament and the external oblique, internal oblique and transversalis are released from the ASIS, avoiding injury to the lateral femoral cutaneous nerve and the ascending branch of the DCIA which is found 1 cm above and lateral to the ASIS. The origin of the DCIA is identified by exploring the external iliac vessels at the level of the origin of the large inferior epigastric artery (IEA). The ascending branch is ligated unless it is planned to include a portion of the internal oblique muscle. The ascending branch of the circumflex femoral is also ligated. The muscles of the abdominal wall and the inguinal ligament are retracted, exposing the DCIA on the iliacus muscle. The DCIA is traced laterally around the inner aspect of the iliac crest. Note that the lateral cutaneous nerve runs between the pedicle and iliacus. A cuff of iliacus muscle a minimum of 1 cm below the vessels is kept with the iliac crest. An oscillating saw is then used to divide the iliac bone as required for the reconstruction. In some cases only the inner cortex is required, which allows a cosmetically more satisfactory donor site. Where both cortices are required the tensor fascia lata and the gluteus maximus are detached from the outer aspect of the iliac crest. The ASIS is preserved for better cosmesis and functional stability. A large skin paddle centred on the iliac crest nourished by perforators can be included in the flap, but the presence of the perforators may be unreliable.
- **Closure** Close donor in layers in order to lessen the risk of post-operative herniation. Inset flap.

Complications

Hernia, femoral nerve palsy, lateral cutaneous nerve of thigh palsy.

Donor site morbidity

Lateral iliac pain and bulging common; loss of hip contour if take ASIS; nerve palsies as above; hernia.

Novelties and tips

- Could be raised including skin and soft tissue cover, or with whole iliacus muscle and periosteum which can be entubulated. The outer table can be osteotomized to contour the bone whilst maintaining bone perfusion.
- One-stage repair of compound leg defects with free revascularized flaps of groin skin and iliac bone.

Reference

Taylor GI, Watson N (1978). *Plast Reconstr Surg* **61**, 494–506.

TFL (tensor fascia lata) flap

Anatomy
This muscle with its long fascial extension arises from the anterior part of the outer lip of the iliac crest and from the outer aspect of the anterior superior iliac spine. It lies between gluteus medius and sartorius. The muscle is inserted between the two layers of the fascia lata about a quarter of the way down the thigh, forming the ilio-tibial tract which continues to the outer tuberosity of the tibia.

Vascular anatomy: type 1
Pedicle: transverse branches of the lateral femoral circumflex artery, a branch of the profunda femoris about 10 cm below the anterior superior iliac spine. Musculo-cutaneous perforators are given off proximally and supply the skin over the ilio tibial tract as far distally as the knee. However, note that the distal skin is really an adjacent territory as it is primarily supplied distally by perforators direct from the profunda femoris artery.

Neural supply
Vascular and neural supply are from different origins. The motor nerve supply is from the sciatic nerve via the superior gluteal nerve. The skin overlying the TFL and ilio-tibial tract is supplied segmentally by the continuation of T12 intercostal and the lateral femoral cutaneous nerve.

Suitability for free tissue transfer
Yes, as a muscular, myocutaneous, fascial or composite osteomyocutaneous flap (using anterior 5–8 cm of iliac crest).

Indications
- Anterior abdominal wall.
- Suprapubic defects.
- Groin and perineal defects.
- Trochanteric defects.
- Acetabular defects.
- When strong vascularized fascia is required such as abdominal wall defects and chest wall defects.

Limitations
The working portion is primarily fascio-cutaneous and hence is not ideal for the volume filling of major defects. Short pedicle for free flap transfer. Donor site problems. Limitations of arc of rotation as pedicled transfer.

Method
- *Position* Patient on side or supine.
- *Incision* If muscle and fascia only, a longitudinal incision along the mid-lateral line which curves anteriorly proximally. If musculo-fascio-cutaneous, draw a line from ASIS to lateral femoral condyle. The muscle and flap lie posterior to this line. Design the skin paddle over the TFL or the junction of TFL and ilio-tibial tract. This can be designed as an elliptical island of skin or as a U-shape, leaving it pedicled proximally as a transposition flap. In this case the apex

of the U can approximate the knee, though this distal segment is random. Incise around the skin flap.
- *Dissection* Find the plane between sartorius and TFL and follow distally, this will lead you to the plane under the ilio-tibial tract. Follow and divide as distally as required. Divide the perforators from the profunda femoris passing through this plane. Dissect the posterior border between TFL and gluteus. Divide the origin of TFL from the iliac crest. As the muscle falls from the crest, retract away from sartorius and find the pedicle and preserve. Leave pedicled proximally and transpose the distal end of the flap around to cover defect.
- *Closure* Close donor site directly over drain, unless a large skin paddle is taken, in which case a graft will be needed. Inset flap.

Complications
- The distal third may not be reliable without a delay procedure. Bulky at rotation point.
- There may be lateral knee instability in athletic patients.

Donor site morbidity
- When cutaneous can be difficult to primarily close donor.
- Can be functionally disturbing, so mainly reserved for pressure sore management in paraplegics, hole filling in complicated hip replacement, and when large vascularized fascia required.

Anterolateral thigh flap

A fascio-cutaneous flap of anterior lateral thigh skin based on perforators from the descending branch of the lateral circumflex artery. This flap is gaining in popularity because of its good donor site and variation of uses. Usually used as a free flap.

Anatomy

Vascular anatomy: type B/C

It is classified as a type B if one perforator is included and as type C if multiple perforators are included.

The lateral circumflex artery comes off the profunda femoris and passes under the rectus femoris muscle. It branches into an ascending, transverse (to TFL) and descending branch. The descending branch is the main artery for this flap. At the midpoint of a line joining the ASIS to the lateral side of the patella, the artery splits into a medial and a lateral branch. The medial returns under the rectus femoris and the lateral supplies the perforators for this flap. The venous drainage is by paired VCs which empty into either the femoral or profunda femoris veins.

Neural supply

Lateral femoral cutaneous nerve which can be used to neurotize the flap.

Flap territory

Up to 15 cm wide × 38 cm long. Pedicle length is ≥10 cm. Vessel diameter is 1–3 mm.

Suitability for free tissue transfer

Thin pliable hairy skin, with a long pedicle of moderate size.

Indications

- Pedicled proximally:
  - Thigh and hip defects.
  - Lower abdominal wall.
- Pedicled distally:
  - Knee defects.
- Free:
  - Any cutaneous defect requiring thin pliable skin.
  - Head and neck, intra oral and skull base reconstruction.

Limitations

Minimal sensory supply. Only moderate size if direct closure of donor site. Donor site can be impossible to close in youthful or obese Caucasians. Tedious dissection. Hair-bearing area.

Advantages
Large amount of tissue. Accessible and expendable donor. No functional loss. Neurosensory. Can give more bulk or be thinned where necessary.

Method
- *Position* Patient supine. Sandbag under the ipsilateral hip.
- *Planning* Draw from ASIS to the lateral border of the patella. Draw a circle of radius 3 cm at the midpoint of this line. Doppler out the perforators in the infero-lateral quadrant. Occasionally the more dominant perforators are medial to the rectus femoris from the medial branch. In this case an anteromedial thigh flap should be considered. Template the defect, and draw the outline of the flap with its long axis centred over the line on the thigh and with the chosen perforator under the junction of proximal and middle third. Make it into an ellipse to aid direct closure, if possible.
- *Incision* Incise around the medial side of the flap and incise longitudinally along the line towards the ASIS.
- *Dissection* Deepen the incision on the medial side through the deep fascia. Raise in a subfascial plane until the perforator(s) are seen. If you are lucky, they will be septal coming between the vastus lateralis and the rectus femoris (20%). However, they are usually found coming through the vastus lateralis muscle (80%). Having defined the perforator, retract the rectus femoris and the descending branch (pedicle) should be visible in the intermuscular space. Check for any other perforators, and then design the final flap. Incise the other three margins of the flap and raise in a subfascial plane. The perforators should be dissected out of the vastus lateralis or a thin cuff of muscle can be taken. Generally only one perforator is needed, but a large flap is better with two. The vascular pedicle should be carefully separated from the nerve to the vastus lateralis (motor) which lies lateral to the artery. To make the flap sensory, the lateral femoral cutaneous nerve can be identified superficial to the deep fascia at the superior incision. Follow the descending branch of the lateral circumflex femoral artery proximally until sufficient pedicle length is obtained.
- *Closure* Close donor site directly if possible over drains. If tight it is preferable to SSG the defect. Inset flap.

Complications and donor site morbidity
Inability to close donor site necessitiating graft. Reportedly defects up to 15 cm wide have been closed primarily with no functional deficit. However, this is mainly possible in older patients or those with weight loss such as head and neck patients.

Novelties and tips
This flap can be thinned to make it a cutaneous flap and can be raised in the supra-fascial plane. Thinning is best done whilst still attached on the leg as there may be some edge necrosis. Check for the perforator position before too much flap incision as the Doppler is often wrong!

Biceps femoris flap

A muscular or musculo-cutaneous flap of posterior thigh skin based on perforators from the profunda femoris artery. This flap is a pedicle flap used for ischial pressure sores as either an advancement musculo-cutaneous flap (usually V–Y) or a muscle rotation flap (Tobin et al. 1981).

Anatomy

Biceps femoris originates from two heads, the long head from the ischial tuberosity and the short head from the linea aspera of the femur. It inserts on the head of the fibula.

Vascular anatomy: type 2 muscle

The posterior thigh skin is supplied by multiple perforators arising from the profunda femoris artery, which pass through the biceps femoris to the skin. The proximal are the most important and are within 5–8 cm of the origin. Venous drainage is via VCs. The biceps femoris is supplied by two main branches from the profunda femoris and can survive on the proximal branch alone.

Neural supply

Biceps femoris is supplied direct from the sciatic nerve into the deep surface or the proximal half of the muscle. The proximal posterior thigh skin is supplied by the posterior femoral cutaneous nerve.

Flap territory

Up to 12 cm wide × 30–40 cm long.

Indications

- Pedicled proximally:
  - Ischial pressure sores especially if failed posterior (gluteal) thigh flap.
  - Buttock, trochanter, and perianal reconstruction.

Limitations

Transects the inferior gluteal artery and its branches that supply the posterior (gluteal) thigh flap rendering it inutile in the future. Sensory supply. Donor site.

Advantages

Large amount of tissue. Muscle can be inset separate from skin to some degree. Accessible and expendable donor. No functional loss in paraplegics, and acceptable in others. Sensate if sensation present. Can be re-used by re-advancement.

Method: V–Y advancement flap

- **Position** Patient prone.
- **Planning** Draw a line from ischium to fibula head giving axis of muscle. Mark skin pedicle over the proximal half of the muscle, usually immediately adjacent to the defect. A strict V is not necessary Because the laxity of the surrounding skin will permit direct closure.
- **Incision** Around skin paddle and extend distally down the line towards knee.

- **Dissection** Deepen incision to muscle. Spare the posterior cutaneous nerve of thigh. Dissect muscle from vastus lateralis laterally and semitendinosus medially until pedicled deep on its vessels. Divide the tendinous insertion, watching out for the common peroneal nerve that is medial over the head of the fibula. Elevate distal to proximal, dividing the short head from the femur. The sciatic nerve lies just deep to the muscle at this point. Stop dissection 10 cm from the origin to ensure that the proximal perforators remain undamaged. If any of the origin remains intact, divide it and advance flap into the defect using the proximal muscle to fill the dead space. Some undermining of the leading edge of the flap can be done to help muscle and skin inset.
- **Closure** Close donor site directly over drains.

Method: muscle turnover

- **Position** Patient prone.
- **Planning** Draw a line from ischium to fibula head giving axis of muscle.
- **Incision** Incise down the line towards knee.
- **Dissection** Deepen incision to muscle. Spare the posterior cutaneous nerve of thigh. Dissect muscle from vastus lateralis laterally and semi-tendinosus medially until pedicled deep on its vessels. Divide the tendinous insertion, watching out for the common peroneal nerve that is medial over the head of the fibula. Elevate distal to proximal, dividing the short head from the femur. The sciatic nerve lies just deep to the muscle at this point. Divide the distal perforators. Stop dissection 10 cm from the origin when the proximal perforators are seen. If any of the origin remains intact, divide it and rotate the flap into the defect like turning the pages of a book.
- **Closure** Close donor site directly over drains.

Complications and donor site morbidity

Some loss of knee flexion in the non-paraplegic.

Novelties and tips

Design the V flap sufficiently large to avoid pressure on any junction.

Reference

Tobin GR, Sanders BP, Man D, Weiner LJ (1981). *Ann Plast Surg* **6**, 396–401.

Soleus

Anatomy
Originates at the posterior aspect of the upper third of the fibula, popliteal line, and posterior aspect of tibia in the middle third. Flexor hallucis longus lies deep together with flexor digitorum longus. The posterior tibial vessels and nerve are separated by deep fascia from the muscle. It is safer to lift the flap from the distal portion first. Not all of the muscle need be used. Muscle inserts into the middle third of the posterior aspect of the calcaneus.

Vascular anatomy: type 2
Fibular origin: dominant proximal pedicle based on the peroneal artery
Tibial origin: dominant proximal pedicle and three or more distal pedicles which are branches from the posterior tibial artery and travel in the inter-muscular septum. The branches enter on the deep surface.
Either of these pedicles will support the whole muscle.

Neural supply
Soleus is innervated proximally by a branch of the sciatic nerve-posterior tibial division.

Flap territory
Large broad flat muscle which lies deep to the gastrocnemius muscle. Not usually used as a myocutaneous flap.

Suitability for free tissue transfer
Not commonly used for free tissue transfer.

Indications
Transposed as a local flap medially or laterally to cover the middle third of the leg in compound tibial fracture or osteomyelitis. Beware in either scenario of flap damage at the time of the original injury.

Limitations
Robust flap with limitations from pre-existing injury from original trauma, arc of rotation, unsightly bulky flap, and lack of skin. Cannot cover the distal third of the tibia and around the ankle joint if proximally based. Needs SSG to cover the muscle flap.

Method
- **Position** Patient on side or prone. Tourniquet.
- **Incision** A longitudinal incision halfway between medial mid-lateral and posterior midline, or a direct posterior midline. A pre-exisitng anterior defect can be extended obliquely posteriorly.

- *Dissection* Find the plane between gastrocnemius and soleus and divide the perforators passing through this plane. Divide the origin of soleus from the medial tibia. As the muscle falls from the tibia, find the pedicle and preserve. If hemi-soleus split the muscle longitudinally. If whole soleus continue dissection, releasing fibula origin. Divide the distal peforators from posterior tibial artery. Distally release muscle attachment to triceps surae/Achilles tendon preserving the tendon and gastrocnemius. Leave pedicled proximally and transpose the distal end of muscle medially around leg to cover defect in subcutaneous tunnel.
- *Closure* Close donor site directly over drain. Inset flap. Cover with SSG.

Complications

With the robust proximal vascular basis this flap has few complications. Slightly bulky initially, but this usually settles with time. Bloody dissection in hemi-soleus flaps.

Donor site morbidity

Obvious decreased power of plantar flexion, but the donor site heals well when closed primarily.

Novelties

Has been used as a distally based flap on the distal perforators of the posterior tibial artery, to cover distal third and ankle defects.

Medial and lateral gastrocnemius flaps

Anatomy
The two heads of the gastrocnemius insert on the inner aspects of the medial and lateral femoral condyles, respectively, by thick tendons. The medial head is larger and extends to a greater distance inferiorly. The heads fuse in the midline with the sural nerve running between and together with the soleus muscle form the triceps surae or Achilles tendon which inserts on the posterior calcaneum. The popliteal vessels lie deep superiorly as they travel between the two heads before heading deep to the soleus. A bursa on the inner aspect of the medial head of gastrocnemius communicates with the knee joint. Located on the medial aspect of the medial head are the tendons of semi-membranosus and semi-tendinosus, and the biceps femoris curls around the lateral aspect of the lateral head along with the common peroneal nerve. Dissection should be from distal to proximal.

Vascular anatomy: type 1
The medial and lateral sural arteries, which are branches of the popliteal artery, enter proximally close to the insertion to the femoral condyles at the level of the knee joint. The vessels arborize within the muscle and travel along its fibres longitudinally. Each head has an independent vascular network. A small number of musculo-cutaneous perforators supply the overlying skin.

Neural supply
Each muscle is innervated by a branch of the posterior tibial division of the sciatic nerve.

Suitability for free tissue transfer
Not commonly used for free tissue transfer, but can be utilized.

Indications
The medial head is the first choice flap because of its greater bulk and length, and hence greater covering capacity. Muscular or myocutaneous cover for knee and upper third of the leg. Also useful in covering proximal third compound fractures of the tibia and osteomyelitis.

Limitations
A pair of robust flaps with limitations with respect to arc of rotation and width of coverage. The lateral head cannot cover the middle third of the tibia, especially anteriorly, and the medial head cannot cover the distal third of the tibia and the anterior aspect of the middle third.

Method
- **Position** Patient on side or prone. Tourniquet.
- **Incision** A longitudinal incision halfway between mid-lateral and posterior midline, or a direct posterior midline. A pre-exisitng anterior defect can be extended obliquely posteriorly.

- *Dissection* Find the plane between gastrocnemius and soleus. Find the plane between gastrocnemius and deep fascia and divide the perforators passing through this plane. Find the plane between the two heads of gastrocnemius. This is easiest from the superficial proximal aspect and is marked by the sural nerve. The plane lies oblique in the saggital plane, and becomes less distinct distally. The deep plane is a continuous sheet of aponeurosis. Split the two heads apart. Distally release the muscle attachment to triceps surae/Achilles tendon preserving the tendon, other gastrocnemius, and soleus. Proximally follow the muscle superficially until it becomes tendinous. Encircle the tendon as it inserts into the femur and divide here. The pedicle lies distal to this point and deep and so remains protected. The muscle is now attached solely by its neurovascular pedicle. Leave pedicled proximally and transpose the distal end of muscle medially around leg to cover defect, through a subcutaneous tunnel.
- *Closure* Close donor site directly over drain, inset flap, cover with SSG. If a myo-cutaneous flap is raised, the perforators from gastrocnemius to skin are preserved. It is difficult to design the skin paddle on the muscle so that it transposes to the required position. The skin is frequently thicker then the anterior knee skin. The donor site usually needs skin grafting.

Complications

As long as the proximal blood supply is maintained, few complications will be encountered. Venous engorgement is the most likely complication and is caused by compression of the flap as it passes under the skin and fascia to reach the anterior aspect of the leg. Avoid this by ensuring a capacious tunnel, dividing the deep fascia, and avoiding tight compressive bandages and POP. Monitor the flap and release as necessary. Lateral gastrocnemius transfer can cause peroneal nerve compression.

Donor site morbidity

Slightly decreased plantar flexion with little donor site morbidity if closed primarily. There may be a bulky contour and some ache/stiffness in the calf.

Tips

Has been used as a neurotized free flap for functional muscle transfer.

Medial plantar flap

A fascio-cutaneous flap based on the medial plantar skin supplied by perforators from the medial plantar vessels from which it can be pedicled or transferred free. It can be sensate and include muscle. It is specialized glaborous skin and therefore is perfect for reconstruction of the palm and sole.

Anatomy

The medial plantar skin on the instep of the foot is non-weight-bearing.

Vascular anatomy: type C

The medial plantar flap can be raised on the medial plantar artery, the lateral plantar artery, or both arteries. The medial and lateral plantar arteries are the terminal branches of the posterior tibial artery which bifurcates deep to the abductor hallucis (AH) muscle. The medial plantar artery is the smaller branch. It runs between the AH and the flexor digitorum brevis (FDB) before anastomosing with the first plantar metatarsal artery. The larger terminal branch of the posterior tibial artery (the lateral plantar artery) travels beneath the proximal part of the FDB and then runs between it and the abductor digiti minimi to join the dorsalis pedis artery and so form the plantar arch. It is based on perforators that branch along the length of the medial plantar artery and the VCs. The perforators and the neural branches to skin from the medial plantar nerve travel between the AH and the FDB.

Neural supply

The medial and lateral plantar nerves, which are the terminal branches of the tibial nerve, accompany the corresponding arteries and supply the skin of the sole. The larger medial plantar nerve supplies the medial two-thirds of the sole and toes, and the lateral plantar nerve supplies the lateral third. The medial plantar flap skin can be innervated by raising it along with fascicles and branches from the medial plantar nerve.

Flap territory

The medial plantar flap can encompass the entire non-weight-bearing area of the sole of the foot.

Suitability for free tissue transfer

Rarely used as it is uncommon to need glaborous skin. Also difficult to raise and has variable anatomy, with only a moderate length pedicle (3–4 cm) and small vessels (<1–2 mm in diameter), unless it is harvested with posterior tibial vessels in which case pedicle length and diameter are much larger. However, it does have thin pliable non-hairy glaborous sensate skin.

Indications

- Pedicled proximally:
  - Coverage of heel, weight-bearing sole defects.
  - Cover of Achilles, lateral ankle.
- Pedicled distally:
  - Coverage of toes, metacarpal heads.

- Free:
  - Any small cutaneous defect requiring thin pliable glaborous skin, especially palm, contralateral foot.

Limitations

Limited supply of tissue. Minimal volume of tissue. Donor site cannot be directly closed, but needs closure by rotation flap (vascularized by plantar subdermal plexus) or FTSG.

Method

- **Position** Patient supine, lateral, or prone depending on recipient site. Tourniquet.
- **Planning** Draw the axis line of the flap which is a line from medial calcaneum to great toe metatarsal head. Confirm this axis by palpating the posterior tibial artery in the medial ankle to locate the origin of the vessel, and trace towards the AH. This is the proximal pivot point. Palpate the junction beween AH and FDB. The distal pivot point is the metatarsal head of the great toe. Template the defect, and draw the outline of the flap, ensuring that it lies over the axis of the vessel and remains in the non-weight-bearing region.
- **Incision** Incise around the flap and incise longitudinally along the line towards the pivot point or point of origin of the medial plantar artery or posterior tibial artery. This could be zig-zag to improve the scar,
- **Dissection** Elevate the skin flap in the supra-fascial plane from lateral to medial until the intermuscular septum with its perforators is seen. Preserve the plantar fascia. Elevate the skin over AH from medial to lateral until the same intermuscular septum is seen. Retract AH medially to expose the medial plantar artery and nerve. Alternatively find the vessel at the distal limit of the flap first. Divide the distal end of the vessels. Follow the vessel proximally or distally according to flap design plan. Divide the muscular branches and the anastomoses with the dorsal supply. Keep the vessel and septum with the flap, leaving the medial plantar nerve behind. If a neurotized flap is required, preserve a superficial nerve branch and follow proximally. This may require intra-neural fasicular dissection. Pivot about the vessel or divide this also if using as a free flap, once required length is dissected. For safety the entire dissection can be performed sub-fascially. However, this is more difficult as there are many septa and planes in which to lose one's way.
- **Closure** Close donor site by rotation flap, if possible over drains. If not, it is preferable to FTSG the defect. Inset flap.

Complications

Sensory denervation of the medial toes. Flap can become venously congested on VCs alone so keep superficial vein as a safety vein to supercharge if necessary.

Donor site morbidity

Failure to heal primarily, especially if grafted. Not too bad if FTSG, but can be problematic if SSG due to hypertrophy, cracking, and instability. Try to preserve medial plantar nerve to prevent forefoot and toe numbness.

Toe transfer

Versatile technique, based on the dorsalis pedis vessels allowing creation of composite flaps (of either the great or second toe or both second and third toes), cutaneous flaps of first web space, metatarsal bone flaps, and vascularized joint transfers.

Anatomy

Vascular anatomy

The toe can be harvested on either the plantar or dorsal systems but the dorsal is more easily used. Based on the dorsalis pedis artery and the VCs. The dorsalis pedis is the continuation of the anterior tibial artery. It continues deep to the extensor retinaculum midway between the malleoli with EHL medially and the EDL and deep peroneal nerve laterally. Before dorsalis pedis passes under EHB it branches as the medial and lateral tarsal artery. Under EHB it branches to form the dorsal arch. At the proximal limit of the first intermetatarsal space it dives deep as the deep plantar artery (plantar interosseous (metatarsal) artery) to join the plantar arch in the sole. The dorsalis pedis or the deep plantar artery gives origin to the first dorsal (interosseous) metatarsal artery. The first dorsal metatarsal artery (FDMA) runs distally between the first and second metatarsals in the variations listed below; 80% are type 1 or 2, and hence dissectable from dorsum.

- Type 1A: single vessel FDMA superficial dorsal to muscle.
- Type 1B: single vessel FDMA intramuscular.
- Type 2A: duplicated vessel FDMA one superficial and the other deep.
- Type 2B: single vessel FDMA deep.
- Type 3: FDMA absent, use the plantar interosseous artery.

At the web the FDMA anastomoses with the plantar supply and splits to supply the adjacent toes lying next to the digital nerves. The venous drainage is through the superficial dorsal venous system which communicate with the long saphenous system.

Neural supply

The dorsal foot skin is innervated by the superficial peroneal nerve, the first web by the deep peroneal, and the toes by the medial and lateral plantar terminal branches. The toes are innervated by anastomosis with the digital nerves.

Flap territory

Dorsalis pedis vessels can supply great and/or second toe, partial toe, first web space, and MCP or IP joints for vascularized transfer.

Indications

- Free:
  - Reconstruction of thumb.
  - Reconstruction of finger.
  - Pulp reconstruction.
  - Joint replacement.

Limitations
Dissection can be difficult because of anatomical variations and vascular branching. Limited skin can be taken, necessitating another flap or SSG for skin cover in some cases.

Method
- *Position* Patient supine. Tourniquet.
- *Planning* Palpate the dorsalis pedis artery in the mid-ankle and lateral to the navicular and mark. Mark the superficial veins, to be preserved with some length as the vein for transfers. Draw a V-shaped incision on the dorsum of the foot around the toe and another on the plantar surface, creating an ellipsoidal racquet incision around the base of the toe. The apex of the V should lie over the dorsalis pedis at the proximal metatarsal level.
- *Incision* Incise around the flap and incise longitudinally along the line of the artery towards the ankle. Alternatively the vessel access incision can be a zig-zag with elevation of the flaps.
- *Dissection* Elevate the skin from the access incision. Split the extensor retinaculum to expose the tibialis anterior or dorsalis pedis lying lateral to the EHL. Beware the superficial peroneal nerve, and deep peroneal nerve. Incise around the toe; dissect along the superficial veins proximally until they become the long saphenous. Dissect from dorsum to plantar between the second and third toes (if taking the second), so as to separate them, and to preview the level of the connecting vessels. Divide the intermetatarsal ligament. Dissect the lateral digital nerve. Approach the FDMA from the dorsum of the first web space, viewing initially the inter-toe connecting vessel. Follow the FDMA proximally, dividing the muscular and plantar interosseous artery branches, until it becomes the dorsalis pedis. This requires division of the EDB contribution to the great toe extensor mechanism, and the extensor retinaculum. Divide the extensor to the chosen toe at the needed length. Dissect the interosseii from the metatarsal and divide the intermetatarsal ligament, finding the digital nerve deep to it. Divide the metatarsal at its base. Elevate the metatarsal and then the flexor tendon at the required length. The toe will then be pedicled solely on the artery and vein. Release tourniquet and check reperfusion.
- *Closure* Close donor site directly, after approximating first and third metatarsals, reconstructing inter-metatarsal ligament by circumferential suture around both metatarsal necks, and suturing ligament remnants. Inset flap.

Complications and donor site morbidity
Sensory denervation of the dorsum of foot and first web space. Donor site of second toe is excellent.

Novelties and tips
Sometimes dissection described as proximal to distal , but is easier distal to proximal. Vessels are very susceptible to spasm, so avoid tension and vessel contact, and ensure that branches are clipped or carefully diathermied.

Great toe wrap around flap

A variation of the toe transfer used for thumb reconstruction that minimizes the donor defect by using only part of the great toe. Described using the lateral soft tissues, nail with perionychium, and the distal half of the distal phalanx (Morrison and MacLeod 1980), its use has been extended by either using the whole phalanx for bony support or limiting the flap to toe pulp alone.

Anatomy
Vascular anatomy
📖 See toe transfer.

Neural supply
The toe is innervated by the medial plantar terminal branches, and the dorsum proximally by the deep peroneal nerve. The toe is innervated by anastomosis with the digital nerve.

Indications
- Free:
  - Reconstruction of thumb where skeleton is intact, or the level of amputation is distal to MCPJ.

Limitations
Dissection can be difficult because of anatomical variations and vascular branching. Limited skin and bone can be taken, if more is needed do a whole toe transfer. If partial distal phalanx taken, the epiphysis is left behind and so it may not grow in children.

Method
- **Position** Patient supine. Tourniquet. No Esmarch.
- **Planning** Palpate the dorsalis pedis artery in the mid-ankle and lateral to the navicular and mark. Mark the superficial veins from the base of the toe. Plan in reverse the flap required. Measure the circumference of the normal thumb at the base of the proximal phalanx and at the midpoint of the distal phalanx. Plan those measurements on the great toe, allowing an extra 5 mm for secondary contraction. Mark the outlines of the flap on the lateral side of the great toe, leaving the surplus as a skin bridge on the medial aspect of the toe. Try to remove as little skin from the foot as possible. Consider alternative means of supplying skin if more is required on the hand or thumb. Draw an extension from this flap (can be a zig-zag) to access the vessels.
- **Incision** Incise around the flap and incise longitudinally along the line of the artery towards the ankle.
- **Dissection** Elevate the skin from the access incision. Split the extensor retinaculum to expose the dorsalis pedis artery lying lateral to the EHL. Beware the superficial peroneal nerve, and deep peroneal nerve. Incise around the toe flap. Identify the dorsal venous network, which lies just subcutaneously, and trace it to the long saphenous vein. Approach the FDMA from the dorsum of the first web space, viewing initially the inter-toe connecting vessel. Follow the FDMA retrograde

dividing the muscular and plantar interosseous artery branches until it becomes the dorsalis pedis. Incise round flap and elevate from medial to lateral off the paratenon of the extensor tendon. Distal to the extensor tendon insertion raise subperiosteally to the proximal edge of the eponychial fold. Plantarly raise off the flexor sheath. Divide the medial cutaneous nerve well proximally (unless not in flap and can be preserved with remaining toe); continue to the lateral bundle and divide the lateral nerve. Osteotomy is performed at the level of the proximal eponychial fold. If taking the whole distal phalanx, divide the extensor and flexor tendons and disarticulate the IPJ. The toe will then be pedicled solely on the artery and vein. Release tourniquet and check reperfusion. Narrowing of the nail can be achieved by excision of the germinal matrix at the lateral aspects of the nail fold. Narrow the distal phalanx as needed. If required, bone graft is harvested from the iliac crest and fixed with cross K-wires via the distal phalanx in the flap and into the residual thumb bone. Wrap the skin flaps around the bone, and anastomose the vessels and nerve(s).

- *Closure* Nibble the toe stump to create a rounded surface and decorticate any exposed bone for FTSG application. Close donor site by FTSG or by cross toe flap from second toe to cover plantar defect and FTSG to cover dorsal defect both toes.

Complications and donor site morbidity

Sensory denervation of the dorsum of foot and first web space. Donor site of great and second toe is reasonable but rather scarred and deformed. Healing can be delayed. Toe can be stiff. Iliac crest bone graft resorption.

Novelties and tips

Vessels are very susceptible to spasm, so avoid tension, vessel contact and ensure branches are clipped or carefully diathermied. Harvest the artery with a cuff of connective tissue.

Reference

Morrison WA, MacLeod AM (1980). *J Hand Surg (Am)* **5**, 575–83.

Fibula flap

This is the most versatile flap for bone reconstruction. Osseous or osseocutaneous or osteomusculocutaneous with the hemi-soleus.

Anatomy
The fibula bears 10–15% of the load through the lower leg and can be removed without functional impairment provided that sufficient fibula is left distally to preserve the syndesmosis in adults or to do a fibula–tibia osteosynthesis in children to maintain ankle stability.

Vascular anatomy
The fibula is nourished by the peroneal artery via a nutrient artery and by periosteal branches. The peroneal artery arises from the posterior tibial and heads laterally to join and then follow the medial side of the fibula between the tibialis posterior and the flexor hallucis longus. In the same plane lying medially is the posterior tibial neurovascular bundle. The nutrient branch enters the fibula between the junction of proximal third and middle third and the centre of the bone. The periosteal blood supply is sufficient to vascularize the bone. The distance and septum beween the peroneal and the fibula allow multiple level osteotomies to be performed yet maintain blood supply. This gives great versatility to the flap to be contoured or double-barrelled. The fibula head and neck are supplied by a circumferential branch from the anterior tibial artery. The skin paddle is based on the septocutaneous perforators via the lateral intermuscular septum or musculo-cutaneous perforators via the peroneal or soleus muscles. An 8 × 18 cm paddle can be marked out centred on the middle-distal third junction of the leg or over Dopplered perforators. The venous drainage is to VCs.

Flap territory
Up to 26 cm of bone. Skin 8 × 18 cm.

Suitability for free tissue transfer
Pedicle 2–4 cm (up to 10 cm if distal bone taken, therefore elongating pedicle). Large vessels. Many branches proximally.

Indications
- Pedicled proximally:
  - Ipsilateral tibial defect.
- Pedicled distally:
  - Ipsilateral tibial defect.
- Free:
  - Bony reconstruction.
  - Whole mandibular reconstruction is possible with suitable osteotomies to permit shaping of the bone.
  - Tibial defects.
  - Long bone replacement in any limb.
  - Avascular necrosis of the femoral head.
  - Osteomyelitis.

Limitations
Arc of rotation limits reach. If fibula head and physis required, needs separate vascular anastomosis for the anterior tibial circumflex branch.

Method
- *Position* Patient supine. Sandbag under the buttock. Flex knee and brace with foot support. Tourniquet.
- *Planning* Consider pre-operative angiogram or duplex Doppler. This is essential if circulation is compromised in the limb. Doppler is used for the perforators. Draw a line from the fibula head to the lateral malleolus. Mark the nutrient vessel at the midpoint of the line. Palpate the peroneal intermuscular septum indicating site of perforators. For an osseo-cutaneous flap, base the centre axis of the flap over the peroneal inter-muscular septum and try to plan the flap as distal as possible, maintaining the perforator in the proximal third of the flap.
- *Incision* Incise around the anterior flap, or if bone only along lateral inter-muscular septum.
- *Dissection* If skin being taken, elevate the skin flap anterior to posterior, looking for the perforators in the septum. Once found, incise posterior flap edge and elevate to find the same perforators. Follow perforators between the posterior and lateral compartments down to the lateral aspect of the fibula where they will pass around it, then deep. If no skin is to be taken, access the fibula via the lateral intermuscular septum between the peroneal and soleus muscles. Watch out for the superficial peroneal nerve. Dissection from this point is similar. Clear the peroneal and soleus muscles off the fibula. Continue anteriorly around the fibula and detach the anterior intermuscular septum and extensor muscles off the fibula. Leave a 1–2 mm cuff of muscle on the bone anteriorly and laterally. The osteotomy sites should be chosen leaving 6 cm of fibula proximally (watch for common peroneal nerve) and distally (preferably 10 cm to preserve the ankle syndesmosis). Place a malleable retractor adjacent to the fibula to protect the peroneal vessels and divide the bone. Retract the bone and find and divide peroneal vessels distally. Dissect the vessels proximally retaining a minimal cuff (1–2 mm) of muscle (tibialis posterior and flexor hallucis longus) to ensure that nutrient vessel and segmental periosteal vessels remain intact. Trace the peroneal vessels to their origin from the posterior tibial artery.
- *Closure* Do not close the deep fascia. Close donor site directly unless skin paddle large, too much tension or risk of compartment syndrome; then use SSG. POP to support foot and ankle in dorsiflexed position until patient mobile. Inset flap.

Advantages
- Long straight cortical bone.
- Can be contoured, doubled up.
- Little donor morbidity.

Complications and donor site morbidity
- Superficial peroneal nerve palsy.
- Compartment syndrome.
- Denervation of flexor hallucis longus.
- Contracture of flexor hallucis longus.
- Lateral deviation of ankle, especially in children.
- Skin paddle can be unreliable.

Tips
Take slightly more bone than you need and strip off the periosteum at each end then trim to fit. The periosteum can then be used to cover the osteosynthesis site to improve healing.

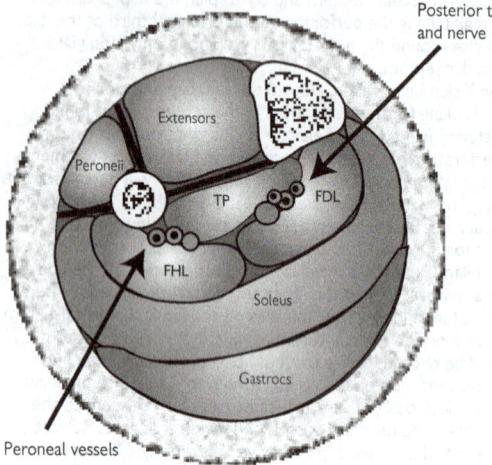

Fig. 20.41 Cross section through middle leg to show relationships.

Further reading
Taylor GI, Miller GD, Ham FJ (1975). *Plast Reconstr Surg* **55**, 533–44.

Sural flap

An axial pattern neurocutaneous flap using skin from the posterior calf, distally based on the sural artery. It is generally used as a distally based pedicled flap for coverage of the posterior aspect of the heel and the lateral malleolus, but can be proximally based.

Anatomy

The flap is based on the course of the sural nerve in the posterior calf. The nerve commences its descent deep to fascia between the heads of gastrocnemius, and at the level of the midcalf it pierces the deep fascia to lie superficial to it. At this point it receives contributions from the common peroneal nerve.

Vascular anatomy: type B

The sural nerve is accompanied by a small artery (the sural artery or short saphenous artery) which arises from the medial sural artery and has distal anastomoses with the peroneal artery. The most distal anastomosis is three finger-breadths proximal to the lateral malleolus and represents the pivot point of this flap. The venous drainage is retrograde along the short saphenous vein which accompanies the nerve as well as via VCs.

Neural supply

The skin is supplied by the sural nerve but is not sensate as it is distally based.

Flap territory

A flap of size 15–20 × 10 cm could be raised, from the superior calf. However, this cannot be closed directly. Most sural flaps are much smaller (usually 6 × 5 cm), allowing direct closure.

Indications

- Pedicled distally:
  - Heel and lateral malleolus cover.
- Pedicled proximally (rare):
  - Tibial tuberosity or anterior knee coverage.

Limitations

Arc of rotation limits reach. Size limited if direct closure required. Insensate if distally based.

Method

- **Position** Patient prone or on side.
- **Planning** Find the midpoint between the lateral malleolus and the posterior aspect of the Achilles tendon. Draw a line from this point, along the sural nerve heading obliquely up the calf to join the midline about halfway up the calf. Then ascend in the midline in the palpable groove between the two heads of gastrocnemius (this is occasionally visible as the short saphenous vein). This line forms the axis of the flap. It forms the pivot point three finger-breadths from the bottom of the line. Plan in reverse to ensure adequate pedicle/flap length. Template the defect, and draw the outline of the defect on the line over the gastrocnemius.

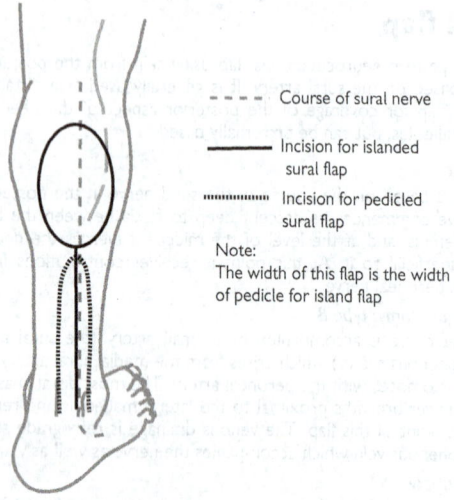

Fig. 22.42 Sural artery flap designs.

- *Incision* Incise around the flap and down the line of the pedicle.
- *Dissection* Elevate the skin subdermally on either side of the pedicle line to expose 4–5 cm wide strip of subcutaneous tissue containing the sural nerve, artery, and short saphenous vein. Incise through the subcutaneous tissue and deep fascia on either side of the pedicle and around the flap. Start proximally and raise the flap subfascially. Divide the little perforators from the peroneal artery as they enter the flap and pedicle. Continue raising in this plane until the pivot point to avoid injury to the anastomosis.
- *Closure* Close donor site by direct closure, FTSG or SSG. Inset flap.

Advantages
- Thin local flap.

Complications
- Ugly donor site if not directly closed.
- The pedicle can be very bulky and may require secondary revision.
- Insensate flap if distally based.

Leg fascio-cutaneous flaps

These encompass numerous flaps not based on any named axial vessel but on vascular perforators from the main vessels. These feed fascial vascular plexi, enabling the raising and transfer of pedicled flaps for closure of skin defects. As these perforators are concentrated around the joints, these flaps tend to be proximally based for cover of proximal defects and distally based for coverage of distal defects. They are relatively unreliable and suffer partial necrosis (of the most critical portion!). The initial flaps had multiple basal perforators (Pontén 1981). Distally based septocutaneous type C flaps similar in principle to the distally based radial forearm flap were designed on the peroneal (Dousky), anterior tibial (Wee), and posterior tibial (Hong) arteries, as were less destructive type B flaps using direct perforators and axial vessels (Amarante et al. 1986).

Anatomy

Musculo-cutaneous and septo-cutaneous perforators from named vessels pass towards the skin and subcutaneous tissues via the fascial septa between muscle groups or via the muscle. At the level of the deep fascia the perforators divide into multiple small vessels which pass centrifugally to supply the superficial tissues. They connect with each other over the convex surfaces of the muscles. They follow a more axial course in relation to the nerves (sural and saphenous). Most of these flaps are based solely on the perforators and do not involve the sacrifice of the main vessel, i.e. they are type A or B rather then type C so as to minimize disturbance of lower limb vascularity.

Vascular anatomy: type A(most)/B(lateral malleolar flap, sural, saphenous)

Perforators from the anterior tibial artery pass in the septum dividing the peroneal muscles and those of the anterior compartment. Peroneal artery perforators are found in the septum dividing the peroneal muscles from the posterior compartment. Perforators from the posterior tibial artery reach the deep fascia via the medial septum separating the superficial and deep posterior compartment muscles. Most flaps are based on the posterior tibial perforators. These are found behind the tibia and connect with the saphenous branch of the descending genicular artery travelling with the saphenous nerve and vein. They are found along the line of the posterior tibial artery and are more numerous closer to the ankle. Venous drainage is along the superficial and fascial veins and VCs.

Neural supply

The skin is supplied by the sural, saphenous, and superficial peroneal nerves. Some proximally based flaps can be sensate but distally based flaps cannot.

Flap territory

Flap size depends on the number of perforators retained. A cross-leg flap designed to use the entire hemi-circumference of the leg requires maintenance of all the posterior tibia perforators as they come around the tibia. However, to be able to transpose or rotate, most flaps require a narrowed pedicle and a reduced number of perforators or even a single perforator. These flaps are necessarily smaller (up to 20 × 6–8 cm). They comprise skin, subcutaneous tissue and fascia only.

Indications

- Pedicled distally:
  - Heel and lateral malleolus cover.
  - Distal third tibia and ankle cover.
- Pedicled proximally (rare):
  - Tibial tuberosity or anterior knee coverage.
  - Popliteal cover.

Limitations

Arc of rotation limits reach. Size limited. No bulk for dead-space filling. Insensate if distally based. Ugly—so avoid in young women. Bulky pedicle, especially at pivot point. Need to graft donor. Unreliable tip of flap. Not suitable for complex defects. Not suitable in degloving injuries or large zones of trauma.

Method

- **Position** Patient supine, prone, or on side. Doppler perforators.
- **Planning** Find the midpoint between the medial malleolus and the posterior aspect of the Achilles tendon. Draw a line from this point parallel to the posterior border of the tibia along the intermuscular septum. Follow the saphenous vein if visible. This line forms the axis of the flap. It forms the pivot point three finger-breadths from the bottom of the line. Plan in reverse to ensure adequate pedicle/flap length; add 20% for rotation/transposition. Template the defect, and draw its outline on the line proximally; continue the width of the flap distally to the pivot point.
- **Incision** Incise around the posterior edge of the flap.
- **Dissection** Elevate the skin flap posterior to anterior subfascially until the perforator pivot point is seen. Check the length of the pedicle now that the pivot point is confirmed. Raise the flap from distal to proximal including the saphenous nerve, artery, and long saphenous vein.
- **Closure** Close donor site by FTSG or SSG. Inset flap.

Advantages

- Thin local flap.
- Quicker than free flaps.
- No microsurgical skills needed.

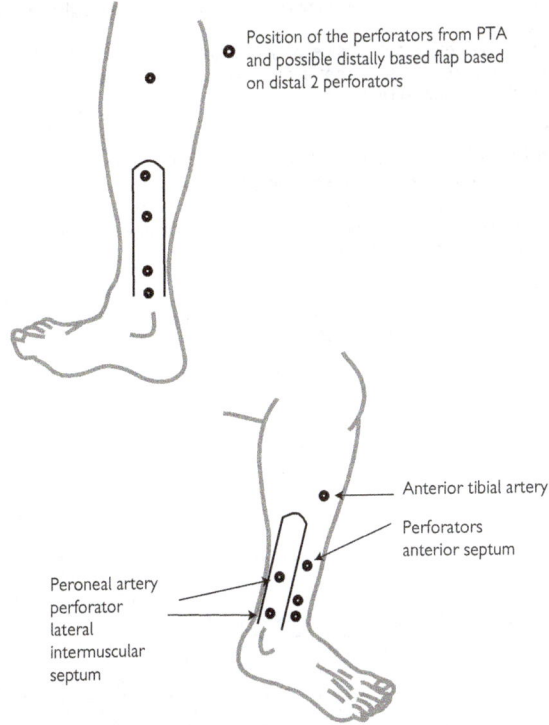

Fig. 22.43 Leg perforators are sited along the course of the major vessels and their overlying septum. They are more numerous closer to the joints. On this basis flaps should be raised with their base towards the closet joint.

Complications and donor site morbidity

- Ugly donor site if not directly closed.
- The pedicle can be very bulky and may require secondary revision.
- Insensate flap if distally based.
- Harder to design properly.
- High incidence of necrosis: major necrosis 7.5% and minor necrosis 30% (Quaba); 15% major complications and 37.5% minor complications (Hallock).
- Greater infection rate when used for open fractures.
- Re-operation often required.

- Delay in healing caused by complications delays time to weight-bearing and union.
- Necrosis often partial, thus delaying or allowing avoidance of decision to redo flap. By contrast free flap failure is complete and the decision to redo is easy.

Tips
- Make the flap much larger and longer (at least 25%) than you think; the usual error is making it too small and then closing under tension.
- Include the saphenous nerve, vein, and artery to make these safer.
- If flap fails to achieve operative aim of primary closure of defect with good well-vascularized cover, do another flap.

Reference
Amarante J, Costa H, Reis J, Soares R (1986). *Br J Plast Surg* **39**, 338–40.
Pontén B (1981). *Br J Plast Surg* **34**, 215–20.

Chapter 23

Appendices

Classifications *908*
Staging and survival of common cancers *914*
Eponymous syndromes *915*
Eponymous procedures *923*
Flap bibliography *924*
Bibliography *925*
Major plastic set *927*

Classifications

Fitzgerald skin types
- Type 1 Sensitive   Burns easily without tanning, freckly, dry thin skin.
- Type 2 Sensitive   Burns easily, tans a little, freckly skin.
- Type 3 Normal   Slowly tanning skin.
- Type 4 Normal   Tans easily, non-freckly, thick greasy skin.
- Type 5 Insensitive Dark skin.
- Type 6 Insensitive Black or dark brown skin.

(The lower the skin type the greater likelihood of skin cancer).

Flaps
- Component: e.g. fasciocutaneous.
- Circulation: e.g. random, axial.
- Contiguity: e.g. local, free.
- Contouring: flaps that move along an axis or pivot around a point.
- Conditioning: e.g. delayed flaps.

Musculocutaneous flaps (Mathes and Nahai)
- Type I: single vascular pedicle, e.g. gastrocnemius, tensor fascia lata.
- Type II: dominant and minor vascular pedicles. Survives on dominant only, e.g. gracilis, soleus, rectus femoris.
- Type III: dominant pedicles (usually two), e.g. rectus abdominis, gluteus maximus.
- Type IV: segmental vascular pedicles, e.g. sternocleidomastoid, extensor and flexor hallucis longus.
- Type V: dominant vascular pedicle and secondary segmental vascular pedicles, survives on either, e.g. pectoralis major, latissimus dorsi.

Boutonnière deformity
- Type I: passively correctable PIPJ and DIPJ not involved.
- Type II: passively not correctable PIPJ and DIPJ has intrinsic-intrinsic plus.
- Type III: passively not correctable PIPJ and DIPJ full passive range flexion.
- Type IV: fixed flexion PIPJ and fixed extension DIPJ.
- Type V: secondary joint changes.

Swan-neck deformity
- Type I: PIP joint flexion present in all positions of the hand.
- Type II: PIP joint flexion limited in some positions MCPJ.
- Type III: PIP joint flexion limited in all positions MCPJ.
- Type IV: Stiff PIP joint with radiological changes of damage.

Rheumatoid arthritis (Larsen)
0 Normal.
1 Osteoporosis, soft tissue swelling, minimal joint narrowing.
2 Bony erosions; normal architecture maintained.
3 Bony erosions; signs of deranged bony architecture.
4 Severe joint destruction; joint line visible.
5 Arthritis mutilans; joint line not visible.

Z deformity of the thumb (Nalebuff)
- Type I: Boutonnière deformity starting at MCPJ.
- Type II: Boutonnière deformity (starting with subluxation of CMCJ, and Type I metacarpal adduction).
- Type III: swan-neck deformity starting at CMCJ.
- Type IV: gamekeeper's thumb.
- Type V: swan-neck deformity with CMCJ normal.
- Type VI: arthritis mutilans.

Radiological changes in osteoarthritis
- Narrowing of joint space (loss of articular cartilage).
- Sclerosis of the bones (when bones become denuded of cartilage along with an increase in density).
- Cystic erosions in bone ends.
- Building up of bone spurs, osteophytes, or exostoses.

Mallet deformity
- Type I: closed injury ± associated chip fracture of the distal phalanx.
- Type II: open injury with a laceration only.
- Type III: open injury with skin and tendon loss.
- Type IV: intra-articular injury.
  - IVA: in children.
  - IVB: adults 20–50% articular area.
  - IVC: adults >50% articular area.

Trigger finger
- Type I: pain and nodularity.
- Type II: triggering present but self-correctable.
- Type III: triggering correctable only manually.
- Type IV: locked trigger digit.

Ring avulsion injury (Urbaniak)
- Type I: circulation adequate.
- Type II: circulation inadequate.
  - IIA: arterial repair required.
  - IIB: arteries and bone, tendon, and/or joint injuries require attention.
  - IIC: venous involvement only.
- Type III: complete degloving of skin or complete digital amputation.

Flexor digitorum profundus avulsion (Leddy and Packer)
- Type 1: tendon avulsion which retracts all the way into the palm no blood supply.
- Type 2: tendon avulsion with or without small bone fragment caught at PIPJ; hence maintains PIPJ vinculum and blood supply.
- Type 3: bone fragment caught at A4 pulley; maintains all blood supply and no tendon retraction.

Classification of neuroma (Herndon)
1. Neuroma in continuity.
2. End neuroma.
3. Neuroma associated with amputation stump.

Congenital hand (IFSSH–Swanson)
- Failure of formation:
  - Transverse (upper third of arm, metacarpal, phalangeal, carpal, etc.).
  - Longitudinal (radial and ulnar club hands).
  - Intercalated (phocomelia).
- Failure of differentiation:
  - Syndactyly, clinodactyly, camptodactyly, etc.
- Duplication:
  - Polydactyly, ulnar and thumb duplication.
- Overgrowth:
  - Macrodactyly (NTOM).
- Undergrowth:
  - Thumb hypoplasia.
- Constriction ring syndrome.
- Generalized skeletal abnormalities.

Radial dysplasia (Bayne and Klug 1987)
- Type I: short distal radius.
- Type II: hypoplastic radius.
- Type III: partial absence.
- Type IV: complete absence.

Syndactyly
- Simple, incomplete.
- Simple, complete (no bony fusion).
- Complex (bony fusions).
- Complicated (disarray of bony elements of rays, missing bony elements etc.).

Thumb duplication (Wassel)
- Type I: bifid distal phalanx.
- Type II: duplicated distal phalanx.
- Type III: bifid proximal phalanx.
- Type IV: duplicated proximal phalanx.
- Type V: bifid metacarpal.
- Type VI: duplicated metacarpal.
- Type VII: triphalangia.

Ulnar duplication—polydactyly (Stelling)
Type I: duplication ending in soft tissue only (no bony articulation).
Type II: digit articulates with normal or bifid metacarpal or phalanx.
Type III: duplicated digit with a separate metacarpal.

Polydactyly (Temtamy)
- Preaxial:
  - Type I: bony duplication (Wassel I–VI).
  - Type II: triphalangia (Wassel VII).
  - Type III: duplication? polydactyly of index finger.
  - Type IV: synpolydactyly (defined as syndactyly of third/fourth fingers and toes ± polydactyly of the same fingers and toes.
- Postaxial:
  - Type I: fully developed extra ray.
  - Type II: rudimentary extra ray.

Thumb hypoplasia (Blauth)
- Type I: minor hypoplasia (thumb smaller but essentially normal).
- Type II: adduction contracture of the thumb, thenar hypoplasia but normal skeleton.
- Type III: significant hypoplasia; skeletal hypoplasia especially at the CMC joint, intrinsic muscle hypoplasia, rudimentary extrinsic tendons.
  - IIIa: CMCJ OK.
  - IIIb: CMCJ absent.
- Type IV: floating thumb (pouce flottant).
- Type V: total absence of thumb.

Clasp thumb (Weckesser)
- Type I: deficient thumb extension.
- Type II: deficient extension of the thumb (flexion contracture).
- Type III: thumb hypoplasia.
- Type IV: pre-axial polydactyly with deficient extension.

Macrodactyly
- Type I: digital macrodactyly with lipofibromatous hamartoma.
- Type II: NTOM (neurofibroma type).
- Type III: hyperostotic macrodactyly (skeletal hypertrophy).

Constriction ring syndrome (Patterson)
- Type I: constriction band with no distal deficit.
- Type II: constriction band with distal lymphoedema.
- Type III: constriction band with distal acrosyndactyly.
- Type IV: distal auto-amputation.

Camptodactyly (modified Adams)
- Type 1: flexion contracture PIPJ.
- Type 2: partially fixed.
- Type 3: arthrographically fixed:
  - 3a: with no X-ray changes.
  - 3b: with X-ray changes.
- Type 4: more than one digit involved.

Vascular cutaneous catastrophe of the newborn (Carter)
- Type 1: skin only — dressings.
- Type 2: skin and superficial muscles — dressings/SSG.
- Type 3: skin and one compartment — emergency fasciotomy.
- Type 4: both compartments — as above or amputation.

Volkmann's contracture (Lipscomb)
- Mild: no nerve, minimal muscle deficit, treat by flexor slide.
- Moderate: no nerve, some dysfunction muscle treat by flexor slide.
- Severe: nerve deficit and little residual muscle function, treat by resection, neurolysis, transfers.
- Very severe: complete nerve deficit with no residual muscle function, treat by free functioning muscle transfer.

Lower limb trauma (tibial fractures)
Open tibial fractures (Gustilo and Anderson 1976)
- Type I: wound <1 cm.
- Type II: wound >1 cm without extensive soft tissue damage, flaps and avulsions.
- Type III: open segmental fracture or with extensive soft tissue damage or traumatic amputation:
  - IIIA: adequate soft tissue cover.
  - IIIB: soft tissue injury with periosteal stripping and bony exposure.
  - IIIC: associated arterial injury.

Open tibial fractures (Byrd et al. 1985)
- Type I: low energy–spiral/oblique fracture with a clean <2 cm wound.
- Type II: moderate energy—comminuted or displaced fracture with >2 cm skin laceration, with moderate muscle contusion but no non-viable muscle.
- Type III: high energy—severely displaced and comminuted fracture/segmental fracture or bony defect with extensive skin loss and devitalized muscle.
- Type IV: extreme energy—type III with degloving, crush injuries, or vascular damage.

Sternal dehiscence
- Type I: 2–3 days post-operative:
  - Serosanguinous discharge.
  - Usually no cellulitis, osteomyelitis, or costochondritis.
  - Negative wound cultures.
- Rx: Re-exploration:
  - Minimal debridement.
  - Rewiring of sternum with discharge.
- Type II: 2–3 weeks post-operative:
  - Purulent discharge.
  - Cellulitis with positive wound cultures.
  - Underlying costochondritis/osteomyelitis.
- Rx: Thorough debridement:
  - ?Open dressings.
  - Vascularized tissue cover.

- Type III: 2–3 years post-operative:
    - Chronic discharging sinus.
    - Positive wound culture.
    - Chondritis/osteomyelitis.
- Rx: As for Type II.

Waterlow pressure sore prevention/treatment policy

This scoring system considers the following categories appointing scores from zero upwards in each category.

- Body build:
    - Average/above-average/obese/below average.
- Skin type:
    - Healthy/tissue paper/dry/oedematous/clammy/discoloured/broken.
- Sex and age:
    - Male/female.
    - 14 to 49/50 to 64/65 to 74/75 to 80/over 81.
- Continence:
    - Complete/occasionally incontinent of urine or faeces/doubly incontinent.
- Mobility:
    - Fully mobile/restless/apathetic/restricted/inert/chair bound.
- Appetite:
    - Average/poor/nasogastric tube/nil by mouth or anorexic.
- Special risks:
    - Tissue malnutrition (smoking/anaemia/PVD/cardiac failure/cachexia).
    - Neurological deficit (diabetes/MS/CVA/paraplegia).
    - Major surgery/trauma (orthopaedic/on table > 2 hr).
    - Medication (cytotoxics/steroids/antiinflammatories).

Score >10 indicates that the patient is at risk of developing pressure sores. Use of barrier creams should be considered. Patient should have frequent changes of position. Consider special mattresses. An increasing score indicates that an increasing amount of pressure sore prevention should be instituted.

Staging and survival of common cancers

AJCC staging of common plastic surgery malignancies

Stage	Breast	Melanoma	Head & neck	Parotid
1	T1 <2 cm	1a) <0.75 mm 1b) 0.75 mm–1.5 cm	T1 <2 cm	T1 <2 cm T2 2–4 cm
2	T2 2–5 cm N1	2a) 1.5–4 cm 2b) >4 cm	T2 2–4 cm	T3 4–6 cm
3	T3 >5 cm T4 fixed N2 (fixed or supra-clavicular)	N1 <5 in transit metastases	T3 >4 cm	T4 > 6 cm, N0 or T1, T2, N1
4	Metastases	Metastases or >5 in transit	T4 (invasion) N1 or > M1	T3, N1, N2 M1

Five-year survival (%)

Stage	Breast	Melanoma	Head and neck	Parotid
1	80	94–98	70	59
2	65	78–42	50	
3	40	<50	30	
4	10	12	20	9

Eponymous syndromes

Ainhum
A fissure develops at an interphalangeal joint (usually the fifth toe). This heals as a fibrous band causing distal gangrene. It can be treated by division and Z-plasty of the hand but may need amputation. Occurs in people of African origin.

Albright syndrome
Pseudo-hyperparathyroidism. Polyostotic fibrous dysplasia. Short stature, round face, short metacarpals and metatarsals, ectopic ossification subcutaneous, parathyroid normal. Skin pigmentation.

Angel's kisses
Flat pale pink lesions on the nape of the neck which fade slowly. Also known as macular stains, salmon patches and stork marks.

Apert's syndrome
Bicoronal synostosis, midface hypoplasia, small beaked nose, class 3 occlusion, cleft palate (20% of cases) and complex syndactyly.

Baker's cyst
Herniation of the knee joint capsule posteriorly. Can be aspirated but will commonly recur.

Barton's fracture
A displaced articular fracture-subluxation of the distal radius. The carpus is displaced with the articular fracture fragment. The fracture may be dorsal or volar.

Baze–Dupre–Christol syndrome
X-linked follicular atrophoderma, BCCs, hypotrichosis, hypohidrosis.

Bazin's disease
Tuberculosis of the skin. Localized areas with fat necrosis and ulceration and an indurated rash (called erythema induratum). Especially common in adolescent girl's legs.

Bean syndrome
Also known as 'blue rubber bleb syndrome'. There are multiple venous malformations of the skin (especially hands and feet) and gastrointestinal tract.

Beau's lines
Transverse depressions in the nails seen after systemic or local disease due to temporary arrest in nail growth.

Becker naevus syndrome
An epidermal naevus developing on the shoulder or upper trunk in children or adolescents, especially males.

Hypertrichosis
Hyperpigmentation. Hamartomous augmentation of smooth muscle fibres, and other developmental defects such as ipsilateral hypoplasia of the breast. Skeletal abnormalities.

Beckwith–Wiedemann syndrome
Overgrowth disorder. May have exophthalmos, macroglossia, and gigantism. Abdominal wall defects.

Behçet's disease
Autoimmune progressive disease with painful ulcers of the mouth, scrotum, and labia. Ulcers heal by scaring. Also affects the joints and eyes.

Bell's palsy
Paralysis of facial nerve. Occurs equally on both sides. First noted in monkey.

Bennett's fracture
Fracture of the palmar articular surface of the base of the first metacarpal.

Binder's syndrome
Failure of nasal development.

Blaschko's lines
Lines of embryonic epidermal cell migration. They are linear on the limbs; S-shaped on the abdomen, and V-shaped on the chest and back.

Blepharochalasis
Recurrent bouts of eyelid oedema leading to excess eyelid skin and laxity of the canthi and lids.

Bouchard's nodes
Bony swellings or a hyaluronate-filled cyst at the proximal interphalangeal joint in osteoarthritis.

Boutonnière deformity
Disruption of the central slip of the extensor tendon at the level of the proximal interphalangeal joint along with volar movement of the lateral bands. Results in loss of extension at the proximal interphalangeal joint and hyperextension at the distal interphalangeal joint.

Bowen's disease
Intra-epidermal carcinoma *in situ*. Initially slow-growing red scaly plaque. Later it may change into a squamous cell epithelioma.

Caput ulnae syndrome
Wrist deformity in rheumatoid arthritis. Volar subluxation of the carpus from the ulna. Volar subluxation of the extensor carpi ulnaris and supination of the carpus.

Carpenter syndrome
Cranial synostosis with partial syndactyly of the fingers and preaxial polydactyly.

Charcot disease
Neuropathic arthritis. Rapid progressive destruction of a joint that lacks proprioception and sensation.

Charcot–Marie–Tooth disease
Perineal muscle atrophy at puberty or early adulthood. Spreads to hands and the arms. Sensation and reflexes usually diminished.

Colles' fracture
Fractured distal radius with dorsal comminution, dorsal angulation, dorsal displacement and radial shortening.

Cowden's syndrome
Multiple facial tricholemmomas. Keratoses of the palms and soles. Oral polyps and 50% develop breast cancer.

Crouzon syndrome
Bicoronal synostosis, midfacial hypoplasia with exorbitism and normal hands.

Dupuytren's contracture
Progressive fibroproliferative disorder of palmar fascia producing fascial fibrosis and contracture.

Eagle–Barret syndrome
Also known as prune belly syndrome. Absent or hypoplastic abdominal wall muscles, bilateral cryptorchism, urinary tract dilatation.

EEC syndrome
Ectrodactyly, ectodermal dysplasia, and cleft lip and palate.

Ehlers–Danlos syndrome
Connective tissue disorders resulting from defective collagen. Hypermobile fingers, hyper-extensible skin, fragile connective tissues, and poor wound healing.

Fanconi's anaemia
Radial club hand and aplastic anaemia.

Frey's syndrome
After surgery or injury around the parotid gland, salivation is accompanied by flushing and sweating of the skin.

Gardner's syndrome
Multiple premalignant colonic polyps, benign exostoses of bone, dermoid tumours, epidermal cysts, fibromas, and neurofibromas. Fundoscopy reveals black spots and can detect carriers of the gene before symptoms develop.

Goldenhar's syndrome
Hemifacial microsomia, epibulbar dermoids, and sometimes an abnormal facial nerve.

Gorlin's syndrome
Multiple BCCs, palmar pits, mandible cysts (odontogenic keratocysts), bifid or fused ribs, calcification of falx cerebri, cataracts, frontal bossing, pseudo-hypertelorism, syndactyly, spina bifida.

Heberden's nodes
Bony swellings or a hyaluronate-filled cyst at the distal interphalangeal joint in osteoarthritis.

Holt–Oram syndrome
Radial club hand and cardiac abnormalities.

Horner's syndrome
Disruption of the sympathetic supply to the eye. Ptosis, miosis, dilation lag. May also be impaired flushing and sweating ipsilaterally, and anhydrosis.

Hurler syndrome
Deficiency of α-L-iduronidase blocking degradation of dermatan sulphate and heparin sulphate causing excretion of mucopolysaccharides in the urine, cartilage, periosteum, tendons, heart valves, meninges, and cornea. Have thickened skin, coax valga, nodules over scapula, and mental deterioration.

Jadassohn naevus
Linear sebaceous naevus. Occurs mainly on the face.

Kaposi's sarcoma
Purple plaques or papules on the skin and mucosa caused by human γ-herpes virus. Metastasizes to lymph nodes. Common in central Africa, HIV-positive patients, and may occur in some ethnic groups and transplant patients.

Kasabach–Merritt phenomenon
Thrombocytopenia due to platelet consumption within a massive congenital haemangioma, or vascular malformation, usually in rare aggressive forms such as haemangio-endothelioma, pericytoma, and tufted angioma.

Kienbock's syndrome
Idiopathic avascular necrosis of the lunate.

Kleeblattschädel
Cloverleaf skull deformity. Trilobular cranial vault deformity due to stenosed sutures. Often accompanied by severe intracranial hypertension.

Klinefelter's syndrome
Gynaecomastia, psychopathy, decreased libido, sparse facial hair, small firm testes. Arm span greater than height. Genetic defect XXY or XXYY.

Klippel-Trenaunay syndrome
Port wine stain of an extremity. Beneath this is a slow flow venous or lymphatic malformation.

Lederhosen disease
Plantar fibromatosis.

Le Fort I fracture
The tooth-bearing portion of the maxilla is severed from the upper maxilla.

Le Fort II fracture
The middle third of the facial skeleton is driven back and downwards.

Le Fort III fracture
The fracture extends into the anterior fossa via the superior orbital margins.

Maffucci syndrome
Venous vascular malformations in conjunction with multiple enchondromas, typically in the limbs. Develop malignancies and painful spindle cell haemangio-endotheliomas.

Marcus Gunn syndrome
At rest eyelid in ptosis. On opening jaw ptosis converted to lid retraction. This is due to aberrant congenital nerve cross-over between the trigeminal and oculomotor cranial nerves.

Marjolin ulcer
Malignant transformation in a chronic wound, e.g. ulcer or osteomyelitic sinus.

Mayer–Rokitansky–Küster–Hauser syndrome
Vaginal agenesis.

Melkersson–Rosenthal syndrome
Recurrent alternating facial nerve palsy, furrowed tongue (lingua plicata) and faciolabial oedema.

Möbius syndrome
Congenital paralysis of cranial nerves VI and VII with bilateral facial paralysis. Cranial nerves III, V, IX, and XII may also be involved. Occasionally have limb and trunk abnormalities.

Morel–Lavallée syndrome
Closed internal degloving injury associated with pelvic fractures. Creates a cavity filled with bloody serous fluid.

Morton's neuroma
Neuroma of plantar interdigital nerve caused by chronic compression.

Muir–Torre syndrome
Multiple internal malignancies, sebaceous lesions, kerato-acanthomas, SCCs and BCCs.

Nagar syndrome
Looks like Treacher Collins syndrome but with upper limb anomalies (syndactyly, absent digits, and radius).

Notta's node
Nodular thickening of the flexor tendon in trigger thumb.

Ollier's disease
Multiple enchondromas; 25% malignant transformation risk.

Osler–Weber–Rendu syndrome
Also known as 'hereditary haemorrhagic telangiectasia'. Bright red arteriovenous malformations in the skin, mucous membranes, lungs, and abdominal viscera.

Paget's disease of the nipple
A red scaly lesion around the nipple. It is an intradermal intraductal carcinoma.

Parkes–Weber syndrome
As Klippel–Trenaunay syndrome but affected patients also have an arteriovenous fistula. Usually in limbs.

Parsonage–Turner syndrome
Brachial plexitis in which symptoms usually resolve spontaneously.

Peyronie's disease
Local fibrosis of the shaft of the penis causing angulation. May make coitus difficult. Associated with Dupuytren's contracture and premature atherosclerosis.

Pfeiffer syndrome
Similar facies to Apert's syndrome with broad toes and thumbs.

Pierre Robin sequence
Micrognathia, glossoptosis, cleft palate, and respiratory obstruction.

Poland's syndrome
Unilateral chest wall and upper limb abnormalities. The deformity can range from very mild to severe.

Preiser's syndrome
Idiopathic avascular necrosis of the scaphoid.

Proteus syndrome
Symmetrical overgrowth of bone and soft tissue, and development of vascular malformations.

Queyrat's erythroplasia
Penile Bowen's disease.

Ramsay-Hunt syndrome
Facial palsy, vestibulocochlear dysfunction, herpes vesicles in the skin of the ear canal and/or auricle.

Rolando fracture
Comminuted intraarticular fracture of the base of the thumb metacarpal.

Romberg's disease
Spontaneous hemifacial atrophy of unknown aetiology.

Saethre–Chotzen syndrome
Bicornal synostosis, low-set hairline, ptosis, small posteriorly displaced ears. Simple syndactyly of the hands and feet.

Secretan's syndrome
Self-inflicted dorsal oedema and fibrosis of the dorsum of the hand or foot.

Seymour fracture
Type 1 physeal distal phalanx fracture with dislocation of the proximal nail plate over the nailfold.

Sjögren's syndrome
Triad of dry eyes (keratoconjunctivitis sicca), dry mouth (xerostomia) and rheumatoid arthritis.

Smith's fracture
Reverse Colles' fracture.

Stahl's ear
Abnormal third crus which radially transverses the superior third of the ear.

Stener lesion
Complete rupture of the ulnar collateral ligament of the thumb with interposition of the adductor aponeurosis between the end of the avulsed ligament and its insertion into the base of the proximal phalanx.

Stewart–Treves syndrome
Malignancy within a lymphoedematous area of arm following mastectomy for breast cancer.

Stickler syndrome
Cleft palate with eye abnormalities (retinal detachment, cataracts, severe myopia), flat midface; hearing loss, and mild spondylo-epiphyseal dysplasia.

Sturge–Weber syndrome
Facial haemangioma and contralateral focal fits. The fits are caused by a capillary haemangioma in the brain. Also have low IQ and eye abnormalities.

TAR syndrome
Thrombocytopenia and absent radius.

Treacher Collins syndrome
Hypoplastic condition affecting the lateral part of the face due to abnormal development of the first and second brachial arches.

Turner's syndrome
Short stature, wide carrying angle, wide-spaced nipples, webbed neck, coarctation of the aorta, and lymphoedema of the legs.

van der Woude syndrome
Cleft lip or palate and/or distinctive pits of the lower lips. May also have hypodentia (absent teeth).

VATER syndrome
Vertebral anomalies, anal atresia, tracheo-oesophageal fistula, renal and radial abnormalities.

Vaughan–Jackson syndrome
Disruption of the digital extensor tendons in rheumatoid arthritis which may lead to their rupture.

Velocardiofacial syndrome
Also known as DiGeorge syndrome and CATCH 22 syndrome. Have cardiac anomalies, abnormal (long) face, thymic aplasia, cleft palate, hypocalcaemia, and chromosome 22 abnormality.

Volkmann's contracture
Muscle contracture and paralysis following trauma of the upper limb.

Wartenburg's syndrome
Compression of the superficial radial nerve at the wrist.

Watson syndrome
Crush injury to palm leading to adhesions and contracture of the intrinsics, causing pain on tight gripping.

Weber–Christian disease
Fever and panniculitis. Development of crops of painful subcutaneous fatty nodules resulting in atrophy of the subcutaneous fatty layer of the skin.

Werner syndrome
Autosomal recessive condition with similar skin changes to scleroderma. Age prematurely and have poor wound healing, diabetes, and cataracts.

Eponymous procedures

Carlioz procedure
Treatment of internal rotation contracture of the shoulder from OBPP by release of origin of subscapularis.

Gaenslan osteotomy
Technique of longitudinal split of calcaneal soft tissues and calcaneus excision allowing direct closure of posterior heel defects.

Gibson procedure
Technique of scoring one surface of cartilage releasing the surface stresses and causing the cartilage to warp or bend away.

Hoffer procedure
Treatment of inadequate recovery of external rotation and abduction in OBPP by transfer of latissimus dorsi (± teres major) insertion to external rotators and greater tuberosity of humerus.

Nirschl procedure
Treatment of tennis elbow by release of ECRB origin from lateral epicondyle.

Oberlin transfer
Method of re-innervating the biceps muscle in brachial plexus palsy by nerve transfer from intact ulnar to biceps in upper arm. Use fascicles going to FCU. Do not use if C7 injured.

Pontén flap
Fasciocutaneous flaps proximally based around the knee for lower limb cover.

Routledge procedure
Lip adhesion in Pierre Robin sequence. The tongue is sutured forward to the lower lip and alveolus to prevent it falling back and obstructing the airway.

Skoog procedure
Undermining adjacent tissue in subdermal plane to denervate sweat glands through cruciate or two parallel (modified) incisions.

Snow–Littler procedure
Method of reconstruction of first web space in cleft hand by transposing the cleft web skin palmarly based to the first web while simultaneously closing the cleft by index transposition ulnarly.

Weber–Fergusson incision
Subciliary paranasal upper lip incision for maxillary access.

Flap bibliography

Books

Aston SJ, Beasley RW, Thorne CHM (eds) (1997). *Grabb and Smith's Plastic Surgery* 5th edn. Lippincott–Raven, Philadelphia, PA.

Cormack GC, Lamberty BGH (1994). *The Arterial Anatomy of Skin Flaps*. 2nd edn. Churchill Livingston, London.

Masquelet AC, Gilbert A (2003). *An Atlas of Flaps of the Musculoskeletal System*. Martin Dunitz, Paris.

Strauch B, Yu HL (1993). *Atlas of Microvascular Surgery: Anatomy and Operative Approaches*. Thieme, Stuttgart.

Strauch B, Vasconez LO, Hall-Findlay E (1990). *Grabb's Encyclopedia of Flaps*. Little, Brown, Boston, MA.

Articles

Atasoy E, Ioakimidis E, Kasdan ML, Kutz JE, Kleinert HE. (1970). Reconstruction of the amputated finger tip with a triangular volar flap. *J Bone Joint Surg (Am)* **52**, 921.

Bakamjian VY (1965). A two stage method for pharyngoesophageal reconstruction with a primary pectoral skin flap. *Plast Reconstr Surg* **36**, 173.

Baker GL, Newton ED, Franklin JD (1990). Fasciocutaneous island flap based on the medial plantar artery: clinical applications for the leg ankle and forefoot. *Plast Reconstr Surg* **85**, 47.

Becker C, Gilbert A (1998). Le lambeau cubital. Ann Chirurg Main **7**, 136–42.

Costa H, Soutar DS (1988). The distally based island posterior interosseous flap. *Br J Plast Surg* **41**, 221.

Demergasso F, Piazza MV (1979). Trapezius myocutaneous flap in reconstructive surgery for head and neck cancer: an original technique. *Am J Surg* **138**, 533–6.

Foucher G, Braun JB (1979). A new island flap transfer from the dorsum of the index to the thumb. *Plast Reconstr Surg* **63**, 344.

Iselin F (1973). The flag flap. *Plast Reconstr Surg* **52**, 374.

Kaplan EN, Pearl RM (1980). An arterial medial arm flap-vascular anatomy and clinical applications. *Ann Plast Surg* **4**, 205–15.

Katsaros J, Schusterman M, Beppu M, Banis JC, Jr, Acland RD (1984). The lateral arm flap: anatomy and clinical applications. *Ann Plast Surg* **12**, 489.

Kutler W (1947). A new method for fingertip reconstruction. *JAMA* **133**, 29.

Lovie MJ, Duncan GM (1984). The ulnar artery forearm flap. *Br J Plast Surg* **37**, 486–92.

McCraw JB, Furlow LT (1975). The dorsalis pedis arterialized flap: a clinical study. *Plast Reconstr Surg* **55**, 177–85.

McGregor IA, Jackson IT (1972). The groin flap. *Br J Plast Surg* **25**, 3–16.

Morrison WA, MacLeod AM (1980). Thumb reconstruction with a free neurovascular wrap-around flap from the big toe. *J Hand Surg* **5**, 575.

Nassif TM, Vidal L, Bovet JL, Baudet J (1982). The parascapular flap: a new cutaneous microsurgical free flap. *Plast Reconstr Surg* **69**, 591–600.

Olivari N (1976). The latissimus dorsi flap. *Br J Plast Surg* **29**, 126.

Pontén B (1981). The fasciocutaneous flap: Its use in soft tissue defects of the lower le.g. *Br J Plast Surg* **34**, 215–20.

Song R, Gao Y, Song Y, Yu Y, Song Y (1982). The forearm flap. *Clin Plast Surg* **9**, 21.

Taylor GI, Watson N (1978). One-stage repair of compound leg defects with free, revascularized flaps of groin skin and iliac bone. *Plast Reconstr Surg* **61**, 494–506.

Taylor GI, Miller GD, Ham FJ (1975). The free vascularised bone graft: clinical extension of microvascular techniques. *Plast Reconstr Surg* **55**, 533.

Taylor GI, Townsend P, Corlett R (1979). Superiority of the deep circumflex iliac vessels as supply for free groin flaps. *Plast Reconstr Surg* **64**, 745.

Upton J, Rogers C, Durham-Smith G, Swartz WM (1986). Clinical applications of temperoparietal flaps in hand reconstruction. *J Hand Surg (Am)* **11**, 475.

Vilain R, Dupuis JF (1973). Use of the flag flap for coverage of a small area on a finger or the palm. *Plast Reconstr Surg* **51**, 397.

Zancolli EA, Angrigiani C (1988). Posterior interosseous island forearm flap. *J Hand Surg (Br)* **13**, 130.

Bibliography

Achauer BM, Eriksson E, Guyuron B, Coleman JJ, 3rd, Russell RC, Vander Kolk CA (2000). *Plastic Surgery Indications, Operations, and Outcomes*. Mosby, St Louis, MO.
Aston SJ, Beasley RW, Thorne CHM (eds) (1997). *Grabb & Smith's Plastic Surgery*, 5th edn. Lippincott–Raven, Philadelphia, PA.
Bailey H, Love RJM, Williams NS, Bulstrode CJK (2000). *Bailey & Love's Short Practice of Surgery*, 23rd edn. Arnold, London.
Baron S (ed.) (1996). *Medical Microbiology*, 4th edn. University of Texas Medical Branch, Galveston, TX.
Beard JD, Gaines PA (eds) (2001). *A Companion to Specialist Surgical Practice: Vascular and Endovascular Surgery*, 2nd edn. W.B. Saunders, Philadelphia, PA.
Block JA, Sequeira W (2001). Raynaud's phenomenon. *Lancet* 357, 2042–8.
Bowen TE, Bellamy R (1988). *Emergency War Surgery, Second United States Revision of the Emergency War Surgery NATO Handbook*. US Government Printing Office, Washington, DC.
Bradley L (2001). Pretibial lacerations in older patients: the treatment options. *J Wound Care* 10, 521–3.
Bremnes RM, Kvamme JM, Stalsberg H, Jacobsen EA (1999). Pilomatrix carcinoma with multiple metastases: report of a case and review of the literature. *Eur J Cancer* 35, 433–7.
Burget GC, Menick FJ (1994). *Aesthetic Reconstruction of the Nose*. Mosby, St Louis, MO.
Burnand K, Young AE (1998). *The New Aird's Companion in Surgical Studies* 2nd edn, Churchill Livingstone, London.
DeFranzo AJ, Marks MW, Argenta LC, Genecov DG (1990). Vacuum-assisted closure for the treatment of degloving injuries. *Plast Reconstr Surg* 104, 2145–8.
Dibbell DG, Jr, Mixter, RC, Dibbell, DG, Sr. (1991). Abdominal wall reconstruction (the 'mutton chop' flap). *Plast Reconstr Surg* 87, 60–5.
Doolabh N, Horswell S, Williams M, *et al.* (2004). Thoracic sympathectomy for hyperhidrosis: indications and results. *Ann Thorac Surg* 77, 410–14.
Du Vivier A (2002). *Atlas of Clinical Dermatology*, 3rd edn. Churchill Livingstone, London.
Dunkin C, Elfleet D, Ling C-A, Brown TLH (2003). A step-by-step guide to classifying and managing pretibial injuries. *J Wound Care* 99, 58–61.
Elliott DC, Kufera JA, Myers RAM. (1996). Necrotising soft tissue infections: risk factors for mortality and strategies for management *Ann Surg* 224, 672–83.
emedicine (www.emedicine.com).
Gorbatch SL (1993). Clostridia. In *Mechanisms of Microbial Disease*, 2nd edn. (eds M Schaechter, G Medoff, BI Eisenstein). Williams & Wilkins, Baltimore, MD.
Haiart DC, Paul AB, Chalmers R, Griffiths JMT (1990). Pretibial lacerations: a comparison of primary excision and grafting with 'defatting' the flap. *Br J Plast Surg* 43, 312–14.
Hak DJ, Olson SA, Matta JM (1997). Diagnosis and management of closed internal degloving injuries associated with pelvic and acetabular fractures: the Morel-Lavallée lesion. *J Trauma* 42, 1046–51.
Holzheimer RG, Mannick JA (2001). *Surgical Treatment: Evidence-Based and Problem-Oriented*. Zuckschwerdt, Munich.
Josty IC, Ramaswamy R, Laing JHE (2001). Vacuum-assisted closure: an alternative strategy in the management of degloving injuries of the foot. *Br J Plast Surg* 54, 363–5.
Julian CG, Bowers PW (1998). A clinical review of 209 pilomatricomas. *J Am Acad Dermatol* 39, 191–5.
King RA, Hearing VJ, Creel DJ, Oetting WS (2001). Albinism. In *The Metabolic and Molecular Basis of Inherited Disease*, 8th edn (eds CR Scriver, AL Beaudet, WS Sly, D Valle), pp. 5587–627. McGraw-Hill, New York.
Kokoska ER, Kokoska MS, Collins BT, Mackay B (1997). Early aggressive treatment for Merkel cell carcinoma improves outcome. *Am J Surg* 174, 688–93.
Kudsk KA, Sheldon GF, Walton RL (1981). Degloving injuries of the extremities and torso. *J Trauma* 21, 835–9.
Lau YS, Yeung JMC, Lingam MK. (2003). Vascular disease of the upper limb. *Mod Hypertens Manage* 5, 9–12.
Meleney FL (1924). Hemolytic streptococcus gangrene. *Arch Surg* 9, 317–31.
Moore K (1992). *Clinically Orientated Anatomy*, 3rd edn. Williams & Wilkins, Baltimore, MD.
Moore K, Agur A (eds) (1995). *Essential Clinical Anatomy*. Williams & Wilkins, Baltimore, MD.
Nahai F, Rand RP, Hester TR, *et al.* (1989). Primary treatment of the infected sternotomy wound with muscle flaps: a review of 211 consecutive cases. *Plast Reconstr Surg* 84, 439.

Nyamekye IK (2004). Current therapeutic options for treating primary hyperhidrosis. *Eur J Vasc Endovasc Surg* **27**, 571–6.

O'Donnell M, Briggs PC, Condon KC (1992). The horn flap: a curved advancement flap with lateral pedicle. *Br J Plast Surg* **45**, 42–3.

Ojimba TA, Cameron AEP (2004). Drawbacks of endoscopic thoracic sympathectomy. *Br J Surg* **91**, 264–9.

Ramirez OM, Ruas E, Dellon AL (1990). 'Components separation' method for closure of abdominal wall defects: an anatomic and clinical study. *Plast Reconstr Surg* **86**, 519–26.

Rang HP, Dale MM, Ritter JM (1995). *Pharmacology*, 3rd edn. Churchill Livingstone, London.

Ravitch MM (1977). *Congenital Deformities of the Chest Wall and Their Operative Correction*. W.B. Saunders, Philadelphia, PA.

Rybka FJ (1982). Reconstruction of the nasal tip using the nasalis myocutaneous sliding flaps. *Plast Reconstr Surg* **71**, 40–4.

Scottish Intercollegiate Guidelines Network (SIGN) (1998). *Drug Therapy for Peripheral Vascular Disease. SIGN Publication No. 27.* SIGN, Edinburgh.

Silk J (2001). A new approach to the management of pretibial lacerations. *Injury* **32**, 373–6.

Simon DA, Dix FP, McCollum CN (2004). Management of venous leg ulcers. *BMJ* **328**,1358–62.

Sinnatamby CS (ed.) *Last's Anatomy: Regional and Applied* 10th edn. Churchill Livingstone, London.

Slade DE, Powell BW, Mortimer PS (2003). Hidradenitis suppurativa: pathogenesis and management. *Br J Plast Surg* **56**, 451–61.

Smith AL (1993). Central nervous system. In *Mechanisms of Microbial Disease*, 2nd edn. (eds M Schaechter, G Medoff, BI Eisenstein). Williams & Wilkins, Baltimore, MD.

Smith J, Greaves I (2003). Crush injury and crush syndrome: a review. *J Trauma* **54**(Suppl), S226–30.

Stark RB (ed.) (1987). *Plastic Surgery of the Head and Neck*, Vols 1 and 2. Churchill Livingstone, London.

Stewart C (2004). Crush injuries. In *The Emergency Medicine Reports Textbook of Adult and Pediatric Emergency Medicine* (ed. G. Bosker). Thomson American Health Consultants.

Strauch B, Vasconez LO, Hall-Findlay EJ (1990). *Grabb's Encyclopedia of Flaps*, Vol. 1. Little, Brown, Boston, MA.

Suit HD, Mankin HJ, Wood WC, *et al*. (1988). Treatment of the patient with stage M0 soft tissue sarcoma, *J Clin Oncol* **6**, 854.

Thompson IM (1934). The diagnostic application of our knowledge of the normal variability of cutaneous nerve areas, exemplified by the median and ulnar nerves. *J Anat* **69**, 159–64.

Trott A (ed.) (1997). *Wounds and Lacerations: Emergency Care and Closure*, 2nd edn. Mosby, St Louis, MO.

Veves A, Giurini JM, LoGerfo FW (eds) (2002). *The Diabetic Foot: Medical and Surgical Management*. Humana Press, totowa, NJ.

Weinzweig J (ed.) (1999). *Plastic Surgery Secrets*. Hanley & Belfus, Philadelphia, PA.

Weinzweig N, Yetman R (1995). Transposition of the greater omentum for recalcitrant sternotomy wound infections. *Ann Plast Surg* **34**, 471.

Weiss SW, Goldblum JR (2001). *Enzinger and Weiss's Soft Tissue Tumors* 4th edn. Mosby, St Louis, MO.

Major plastic set

Artery forceps

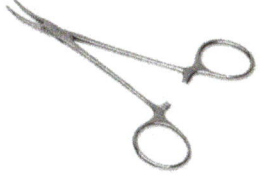

Fig. 23.1 Halsted.

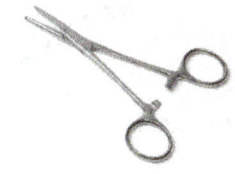

Fig. 23.2 Spencer–Wells.

Elevators

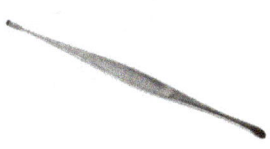

Fig. 23.3 Howarth.

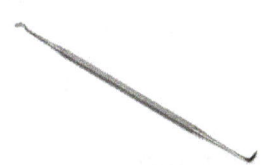

Fig. 23.4 Mitchell's trimmer.

Dissecting forceps

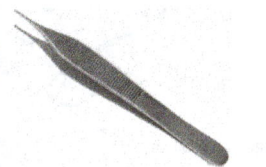

Fig. 23.5 Adson.

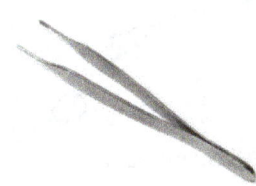

Fig. 23.6 Adson–Browne.

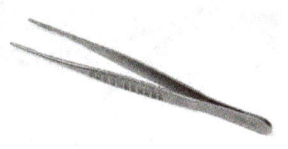

Fig. 23.7 DeBakey.

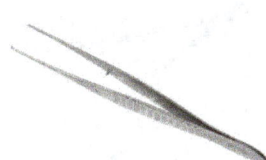

Fig. 23.8 Gillies.

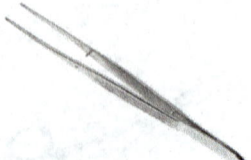

Fig. 23.9 McIndoe.

Tissue forceps

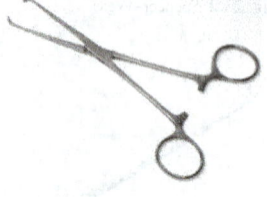

Fig. 23.10 Allis.

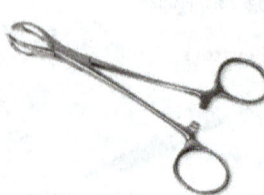

Fig. 23.11 Lanes.

Sponge holding/dressing forceps

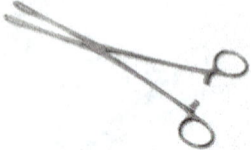

Fig. 23.12 Rampley.

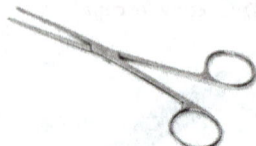

Fig. 23.13 Sinus.

Needle holders

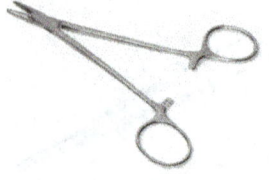

Fig. 23.14 Crile Wood.

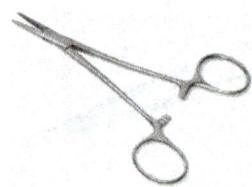

Fig. 23.15 Halsey.

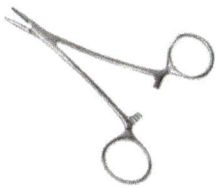

Fig. 23.16 Neivert.

Pens

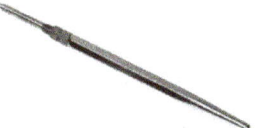

Fig. 23.17 Eckhoff.

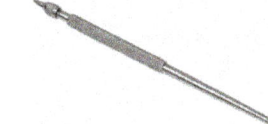

Fig. 23.18 Sommerlad.

Retractors

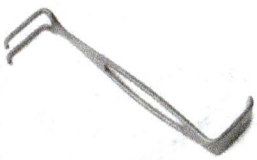

Fig. 23.19 Czerny.

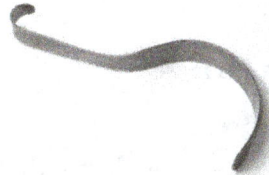

Fig. 23.20 Deaver.

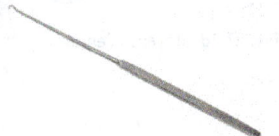

Fig. 23.21 Gillies.

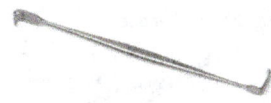

Fig. 23.22 Kilner (Senn).

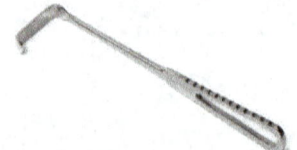

Fig. 23.23 Langenbeck.

Scalpel handle

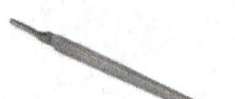

Fig. 23.24 Barron.

Scissors

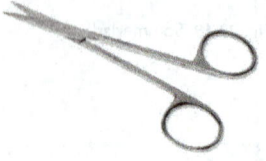

Fig. 23.25 Iris.

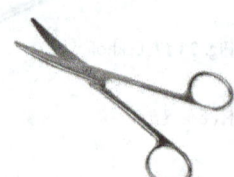

Fig. 23.26 Mayo.

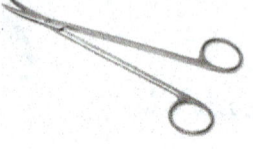

Fig. 23.27 McIndoe.

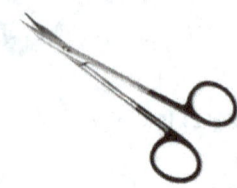

Fig. 23.28 Stevens (Tenotomy).

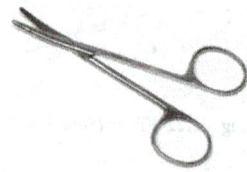

Fig. 23.29 Strabismus.

Index

A

abdominal wall reconstruction 384–6
abdominoplasty 713–6
acid burns 626
acrochordon 273
advancement flaps 751, 753, 754, 755, 795–6, 818
aesthetic surgery 655–726
  autologous fillers 683
  body contouring 709–10
    abdominoplasty 713–6, 716
    arm reduction 711–2
    calf augmentation 720–1
    liposuction 722–5
    medial thigh lift 719
    thigh and buttock contouring 717–8
  botulinum toxin 684
  breast
    assessment 662
    augmentation 670–3
    bra and breast sizing 661
    gynaecomastia 681, 679–81
    inverted nipples 677
    ptosis 674–6, 675, 676
    reduction 664–6, 667, 669
    tuberous breast 678
  carbon dioxide laser 682
  chemical peels 682
  definition 656
  dermabrasion 682
  facial
    augmentation of facial skeleton 704–5
    blepharoplasty 686–90, 691
    brow lift 692–3
    facelift 700–3, 702
    genioplasty 706–8
    rhinoplasty 694–7
    submucous resection 698–9
  facial ageing 660
  hydroquinones 683
  non-autologous fillers 683
  patient assessment 657–9
  procedures 656
  retin A 682
  skin lightening 685
  see also individual procedures
aggressive fibromatosis 480
ainhum 916
albinism 237, 236–7
Albright syndrome 916
alkali burns 627
alloplastic materials 120
alveolar bone grafting 187–8
amniotic band syndrome 223
amputations
  above-knee 448
  below-knee 445–7, 446
  external ear 316
  ray 420
  upper limb 418–9
    proximal 421
    ray 420
anaplasia 48
anatomy 71–104
  external ear 84–6
  eyelids 82–3
  facial nerve 87–9
  hand 90–6
  head and neck 74–7
  nose 78–81
  parasympathetic nervous system 103–4
  penis 101–2
  skin vascular 72–3
  wrist 99–100
aneurysmal bone cyst 415
angel's kisses 916
angiosomes 72–3
anophthalmos 291–2
anterolateral thigh flaps 884–5
antibiotic prophylaxis 114–5, 115
  leech therapy 126
  prevention of endocarditis 114
  surgical site infection 114
Apert's syndrome 144, 916
aphorisms 4–5
apocrine hidrocystoma 275
areolar complex reconstruction 373
arm see upper limb
arterial ulcers 433, 434
arteries
  radial 92
  ulnar 92
artery forceps 928
arthrogryposis 224–5
auriculo-temporal flaps 843–4
autogenous tissue implants 120
autologous fillers 683
avulsion
  external ear 316
  flexor digitorum profundus 909
  flexor tendon 544–5, 545
  ring avulsion injury 548, 909
axillary dissection 497–9
azathioprine (Imuran) 110

B

Baker's cyst 916
balloon naevus 243
banner flaps 786, 785–6
Barton's fracture 916
basal cell carcinoma 258–9
Baze-Dupre-Christol syndrome 916
Bazin's disease 916
Bean syndrome 916
Beau's lines 539, 916
Becker naevus syndrome 916
Becker's disease 240
Beckwith-Wiedemann syndrome 917
Behçet's disease 917
Bell's palsy 917
Bennett's fracture 566–7, 577, 917
bi-lobed flaps 781–2, 782
biceps femoris flaps 886–7
Binder's syndrome 917
bitumen burns 627
bladder exstrophy 139
Blaschko's lines 917
blast injuries 523
blepharochalasis 917
blepharophimosis 290
blepharoplasty 686–90, 691
blood transfusion 108–9
  administration 108
  blood products 109
  consent 108
  indications 108

side effects 108, 109
blue naevus 241
blue rubber bleb syndrome 916
body contouring 709–10
  abdominoplasty 713–6, 716
  arm reduction 711–2
  calf augmentation 720–1
  liposuction 722–5
  medial thigh lift 719
  thigh and buttock contouring 717–8
bone 24–5
  blood supply 24
  composition 24
  healing 24–5
  physiology 24
  types of 24
  zones 24
bone grafts 26–7
  alveolar 187–8
  cancellous 26
  classification 26
  cortical 26
  cortico-cancellous 26
  membranous 26
  survival of 27
  vascularized flaps 26
bone substitutes 27
bone tumours of hand 412–6
botulinum toxin 112–3, 684
Bouchard's nodes 917
boutonnière deformity 549–50, 550, 908, 917
Bowen's disease 250–1, 917
bra and breast sizing 661
brachial plexus injuries 589–92
  aetiology 589
  anatomy 589
  classification 589
  clinical presentation 589
  controversies 592
  definition 589
  diagnosis 590
  examination 590
  incidence 589
  management 591
  natural history 591
brachial plexus palsy, obstetric 593–4
  sequelae 595
brachydactyly 216–7
branchial clefts 155
breast
  aesthetic surgery assessment 662
  augmentation 670–3
  bra and breast sizing 661
  gynaecomastia 681, 679–81

  inverted nipples 677
  ptosis 674–6, 675, 676
  reduction 664–6, 667, 669
  tuberous breast 678
  burns 621
  see also nipple
breast cancer 364–6
  classification 364
  clinical features 364
  diagnosis 364
  epidemiology 364
  management 365
  pathophysiology 364
  risk factors 364
  staging and survival 366
  TNM classification 366
breast reconstruction 367–72
  aims 367
  choice of method 370, 371, 372
  examination 367–8
  history 367
  options for 368–9, 369
  secondary surgery 371
  timing of 368
brow lift 692–3
Brunelli dorsal ulnar thumb flap 821
burns
  assessment 606, 606–9
  breast 621
  chemical 626–7
  ear 622
  electrical 628
  emergency care 602–3
  escharotomy 610–1, 612
  external ear 315–7
  eyelids 621, 622
  fluid resuscitation 604–5
  foot 625
  hand 623–4
  head and neck 621
  hypermetabolic response 614–5
  immune effects 614
  infection 616–7
  Lund-Browder charts 608–9
  mouth and lips 622
  non-accidental injury 630
  nose 622
  oedema 614
  perineum 621
  reconstruction 620
  scalp alopecia 622
  shock 614
  treatment 615, 618–9
  Wallace rule of nines 607
  wound pathophysiology 613–5

C

calcifying epithelioma of Malherbe 276
calf augmentation 720–1
Campbell de Morgan spot 277
camptodactyly 200–1, 911
cancellous bone grafts 26
cancer
  basal cell carcinoma 258–9
  breast 364–6
  melanoma see melanoma
  squamous cell carcinoma 260–1
    staging 262, 262–3, 915
  staging 914
  survival 914
  see also tumours
caput ulnae syndrome 917
carbon dioxide laser 682
Carlioz procedure 924
carpal instability 576–8, 577, 578
Carpenter syndrome 918
cartilage 32–3
  composition 32
  growth 32
  healing 32
  nutrition 32
  types 32
cartilage grafts 32, 33
causalgia 647–8
cellulitis of hand 395
cement burns 627
ceramic implants 121
cervical plexus 77
cervico-facial flaps 793–4
Charcot disease 918
Charcot foot 439–40
Charcot-Marie-Tooth disease 918
cheek reconstruction 323–6
  aesthetic subunits 324
  aetiology 324
  aims and principles 324
  anatomy 323
  classification 323
  controversies 326
  options 325, 326
  selection 326
cheek repair 526
chemical burns 626–7
chemical peels 682
chest 363–82
  breast cancer 364–6
  breast reconstruction 367–72
  nipple-areolar complex reconstruction 373–4
chest wall deformity 232

chest wall reconstruction 375–7
chondrocytes 32
chondrodermatitis nodularis helicis 252
chondroitin sulphate 8
chromic acid burns 626
clasp thumb 204, 911
cleft hand 197–9
  aetiology 197
  associations 197
  classification 197–8, 198
  clinical presentation 198
  definition 197
  incidence 197
  indications for surgery 199
  management and prognosis 198, 199
  operative options 199
  synonyms 197
cleft lip/palate 152–3, 156
  aetiology 158
  antenatal care 159
  cleft lip repair
    bilateral 166–7, 167
    unilateral 162–5, 164, 165
  cleft palate repair 168–74
    anatomy 168, 169
    double opposing Z-plasty 170–1, 173
    midfacial growth 169
    post-operative complications 174
    post-operative recovery 174
    submucous 174
    surgical techniques 169–70, 300
    timing of repair 168
  embryology 158–9, 159
  familial association 159
  hearing 160–1
  multidisciplinary team 159
  neonatal care 159–60
  prenatal diagnosis 159
  striped Y classification 157
  submucous 156
  surgical management 160
  Veau's classification 157, 156–8
cleft rhinoplasty 175–7
  aims of 175
  anatomy 175, 176
  bilateral 177
  secondary 177
  timing of surgery 175
  unilateral 176
clinodactyly 202–3
cloacal exstrophy 139

Clostridium spp. 59, 468–70
Clostridium botulinum 58, 469
Clostridium difficile 59, 470
Clostridium tetani 57–8, 468–9
Clostridium welchii 57, 468
coagulation 7, 6–7
colchicine 7–8
collagen 7–8
  injectable 112
Colles' fracture 918
compartment syndrome 514, 515–7
complex regional pain syndrome 647–8
composite grafts 38
  classification 38
  definition 38
  graft take 38
  indications 38
  technical factors 38
congenital naevus 244
constriction ring syndrome 911
cortical bone grafts 26
cortico-cancellous bone grafts 26
cosmetic surgery see aesthetic surgery
Cowden's syndrome 918
cranial fronto-nasal dysplasia 145
craniofacial surgery 31
craniosynostosis 141
  aetiology 141
  classification 141
  definition 141
  incidence 141
  non-syndromic 142–3
    bicoronal synostosis 143
    metopic synostosis 142
    sagittal synostosis 142
    unicoronal synostosis 142–3
    unilambdoid synostosis 143
  pathogenesis 141
  surgery 147
  syndromic 144–5
    Apert's syndrome 144
    cranial fronto-nasal dysplasia 145
    Crouzon's syndrome 144
    Muenke's syndrome 145
    Pfeiffer's syndrome 144–5
    Saethre–Chotzen syndrome 145
creeping substitution 26–7

CREST syndrome 636
cross-finger flaps 827, 826–7
Crouzon syndrome 144, 918
crush injuries 513–4
cutaneous horn 252–3
cyclophosphamide (Cytoxan) 110
cylindroma 274
cystadenoma 275
cysts
  aneurysmal bone 415
  Baker's 916
  dermoid 269
  epidermoid 268
  tricholemmal (pilar) 268
  unicameral bone 415

D

deep circumflex iliac artery flaps 880–1
deep inferior epigastric perforator flaps 868–9
degloving injuries 511–2
  closed internal (Morel–Lavallée syndrome) 512
delay phenomenon 46
  mechanism of delay 46
delto-pectoral flaps 845–6
dermabrasion 682
dermal lesions 241
dermatin sulphate 8
dermatofibroma 270
dermatofibrosarcoma protruberans 267
dermis 13
dermoid cysts 269
desmoid tumours 480
diabetic foot 437–41
  reconstruction 440–1
DiGeorge syndrome 923
digital arthrodesis 424, 423–4
digital extensor mechanism 390–1, 391
  defects and assessment 390–1, 392–3
dissecting forceps 928, 929
distal radio-ulnar joint
  disorders 582
  instability 583
  instability test 426
distal radius fractures 579–81
distant flaps 760–1
distraction osteogenesis 28–31
  advantages 30
  bone generation 28
  complications 30–1

contraindications 30
craniofacial surgery 31
disadvantages 30
factors affecting new bone formation 29–30
hand 31
indications 30
steps in 28–9
techniques 28
dorsal finger flaps 832, 833
dorsal nasal flaps 788, 787–8
dorsal ulnar flaps 808–9
dressings 118, 118–9
indications for 119
drooling 327–8
aetiology 327
classification 327
clinical features 327
complications 328
definition 327
incidence 327
investigations 328
management 328
pathogenesis 327
post-operative care 328
Dufourmental flaps 780
Dupuytren's contracture 918
dysplasia 48
dysplastic naevus 245
dystonia 400

E

Eagle-Barret syndrome 918
ear
burns 622
embryology 67
external
anatomy 84–6, 85, 86
arterial supply 85
functions of 315
lymphatics 85
muscles and ligaments 84
sensory nerve supply 86, 86
venous supply 85
repair 526
Stahl's 922
ear reconstruction 315–7
aetiology of defects 315
treatment 315–7
eccondroma 413
ectropion 284–7, 287
EEC syndrome 918
Ehlers-Danlos syndrome 7–8, 918
electrical burns 628
elevators 928
embryology 61–70
ear 67

external genitalia 62
face 63–4, 64
hand 68–9
lip and palate 66
nose 65
enchondroma 412–3
entropion 288–9, 289
ephelides 240
epicanthus 293, 294
epicanthus inversus syndrome 290
epidermal growth factor 7
epidermal lesions 240
epidermal tumours 272–3
epidermis 12
epidermoid cysts 268
epidermolysis bullosa 234–5
epispadias-exstrophy complex 138–40
aetiology 138
classification 138
clinical features 138–9
complications 140
contentious issues 140
definition 138
incidence 138
pathogenesis 138
presentation 139
surgical management 139
Erb's palsy 589–92
erythema 52–3
escharotomy 610–1, 612
exostosis 414
external genitalia, embryology 62
extravasation 506–7
eyebrow repair 525–6
eyelids 283–304
anatomy 82–3, 83
anophthalmos 291–2
blepharophimosis 290
burns 621, 622
ectropion 284–7, 287
entropion 288–9, 289
epicanthus 293–4
epicanthus inversus syndrome 290
hypertelorism 293–4
hypotelorism 293–4
lacrimal pump mechanism 82
levator palpebrae superioris and Muller's muscle 83
lower lid 83
microphthalmia 291–2
orbicularis oculi 82
orbital septum 82–3
ptosis 290, 295–6, 296
reconstruction 297–301, 298, 299, 300, 301

in facial nerve palsy 302
repair 525–6
telecanthus 293–4

F

face
aesthetic surgery
augmentation of facial skeleton 704–5
blepharoplasty 686–90, 691
brow lift 692–3
facelift 700–3, 702
genioplasty 706–8
rhinoplasty 694–7
submucous resection 698–9
embryology 63–4, 64
facelift 700–3, 702
facial ageing 660
facial injuries, middle-third 527–32
facial lacerations 524–6
'windshield' injury 525
facial nerve palsy 318–22
acute facial nerve injury 320
aetiology of paralysis 318
chronic facial nerve injury 320
cross-facial nerve graft 321
to functional free muscle transfer 322
diagnosis and examination 319
direct nerve repair 321
dynamic muscle transposition 322
eyelid reconstruction 302
goals of reconstruction 319–20
interposition nerve graft 321
investigations 319
management 320
myoneurotization 321
nerve transfer 321–2
problems of 318–9
static procedures 320–1
static support procedures 322
Fanconi's anaemia 918
fascio-cutaneous flaps 762–3
lower limb 903–6, 905
fasciotomy 518–21, 519, 521
fat grafts 39–41
autogenous 39
complications 41
flaps 40–1

free dermal 40
healing 39
injection 41
felon 395–6, 396
fetal wound healing 42
extrinsic factors 42
intrinsic factors 42
fibroblast growth factors 7
fibrohistiocytic tumours 270–1
fibromatoses 480
definition 480
desmoid tumours 480
nodular pseudosarcomatous fasciitis 480
fibronectin 6–7
fibroplasia 6
fibula flaps 898–900
Fiche-Canniéu variant 98
fillers
autologous 683
non-autologous 683
fingertip flaps 813–5, 814, 815
Fitzgerald skin types 908
flag flaps 819–20, 820
flaps 735–906
advancement 751, 753, 754, 755, 795–6, 818
anterolateral thigh 884–5
auriculo-temporal 843–4
banner 785–6, 786
bi-lobed 781–2, 782
biceps femoris 886–7
Brunelli dorsal ulnar thumb flap 821
cervico-facial 793–4
chimeric 739
choice of 738
classification 736, 741–2, 742, 908
'crane' principle 739
cross-finger 826–7, 827
deep circumflex iliac artery 880–1
deep inferior epigastric perforator 868–9
definition 736
delto-pectoral 845–6
design and incisions 737
distant 760–1
dorsal finger 832, 833
dorsal nasal 787–8, 788
dorsal ulnar 808–9
Dufourmental 780
fascio-cutaneous 762–3
fibula 898–900
fingertip 813–5, 814, 815
flag 819–20, 852
flow-through 739
forehead 835–8, 838
free style 739
free tissue transfer 743–5

lessons in 746–7
gluteus maximus 858–60
gracilis 877, 876–3
great toe wrap around 896–7
groin 878–9
horn 783–4, 784
jejunal 795–6
kite 816–8
lateral arm 799–800
latissimus dorsi 870–2
leg fascio-cutaneous 903–6, 905
medial arm 801–2
medial and lateral gastrocnemius 890–1
medial plantar 892–3
Moberg 764–5
monitoring 748–9
muscle 764–5
musculocutaneous 908
nasalis 789–90, 790
nasolabial 791–2, 792
neurocutaneous 740
neurovascular island 823–9, 824, 825,
omental 797–8
parascapular 853–4
pectoralis major 847–9
pedicle 740
pin cushioning 739
pivot 756–7
posterior interosseous artery 810–2
prefabrication 739
prelamination 739
radial forearm 803–5
rectus abdominis 861–2
reverse flow, venous drainage 769–70, 770–2
rhomboid 778–9, 779
rotation 758–9, 759
scapular 850–2, 852
serratus anterior 873–5
soleus 888–9
sub-fascial 740
super-charged 740
super-drained 740
supra-fascial 740
sural 791–2, 902
temporalis 839–40
temporo-parietal 841–2
tensor fascia lata 882–3
thenar 830–1, 831
toe transfer 894–5
transverse rectus abdominis myocutaneous 865–7, 866
trapezius 855–7
ulnar forearm 806–7
vascularized bone 'graft' 766–8

venous 771
vertical rectus abdominis myocutaneous 863–4
W-plasty 776–7, 777
Z-plasty 773, 773–5, 774
flexor digitorum profundus avulsion 909
flexor sheath infection 397
flexor tendon
avulsion 544–5, 545
injuries 540–1
repair 542–3, 543
rehabilitation 546–7
delayed mobilization 546
early active mobilization 547
Kleinart 546–7
passive mobilization 547
fluid resuscitation, burns 604–5
5-fluorouracil 111
foot
burns 625
Charcot 439–40
diabetic 437–41, 440–1
fasciotomy 520
reconstruction 444
ulceration 438–9
forehead
flaps 835–8, 838
repair 525–6
fractures
distal radial 579–81
facial 527–32
hand 555–69
complications 570–2, 571
maxillary 531, 529
naso-orbital ethmoid 528–9, 530–2
orbital floor 528–9, 531
scaphoid 573–5
tibial 430
zygomatic 528–9, 531
free tissue transfer 743–5
lessons in 746–7
Frey's syndrome 918
Froment-Rober variant 98
frostbite 508–9
external ear 315–7
full thickness skin grafts 18–9

G

Gaenslan osteotomy 924
ganglia 405–6
Gardner's syndrome 918
gender reassignment 653–4
genioplasty 706–8
giant cell tumour of bone 416

INDEX

Gibson procedure 924
Gillies' principles 3
gingivoperiosteoplasty 187
glomus tumours 410
glossoptosis 152–3
gluteus maximus flaps 858–60
glycosaminoglycans 8
Goldenhar's syndrome 919
Gorlin's syndrome 255–7, 919
gout 640–1
gracilis flaps 876–7, 877
granuloma 411
granuloma telangiectatum 277
great toe wrap around flaps 896–7
Grenz layer 13
groin dissection 500–2
groin flaps 878–9
growth factors in wound healing 7, 9–10, 10–1
gunshot injuries 522
Guyon's canal 91–2
gynaecomastia 679–81, 681

H

haemangioma 249, 457, 459–60
haematoma of external ear 315–7
hair follicles 13
  tumours of 276
halo naevus 243
hamartoma 48
hand
  anatomical snuffbox 92
  anatomy 90–6
  arteries 92
  burns 623–4
  congenital deformities 910
  distraction osteogenesis 31
  embryology 68–9
  extrinsic muscles 93–6, 95
  fasciae 90–1
  fasciotomy 519
  fractures 555–69
    Bennett's 566–7, 577
    classification 555, 556
    complications 570–2, 571
    conservative management 557–8
    dynamic compression 561–3, 562
    external fixation 563–4
    incidence 555

internal fixation 559–60, 560
intra-articular phalangeal 564–5
metacarpal 566–7, 568, 569
outcome 565–6
pathomechanics 555
Rolando 567
surgical management 558–9
infections of 394–9
intrinsic muscles 96
nerve supply 91–2, 93, 97, 97–8, 98
  anatomical variants 98
ray amputations 420
skeleton 91, 90
trauma 534, 533–6
tumours of 248, 403, 401–4, 404
  bone 412–6
  metastatic 417
Hartmann's solution 604
head and neck 339–62
  anatomy 74–7
  burns 621
  cancer reconstruction 351–3
  neck 75
    dissection 359–62
    fascial planes 75
    lymphatic drainage 77
    nerves 77
    superficial muscles 75
    triangles of 75, 76
  parasympathetic nervous system 103
  superficial parotidectomy 357–8
  tumours
    maxillary carcinoma 341–2
    nasal cavity 340–1, 342
    nasopharyngeal carcinoma 342–3
    oral cavity, oropharynx and hypopharynx 344–50
    paranasal sinuses 340–1
    salivary gland 354–6
Heberden's nodes 919
hemifacial microsomia 148–9
  aetiopathogenesis 148
  genetics 148
  incidence 148
  pathology 148–9
herpetic whitlow 396
hidradenitis 649–50
high-flow arteriovenous malformations 463–4
Hoffer procedure 924

Holt-Oram syndrome 919
hormone replacement therapy, and deep vein thrombosis 117
horn flaps 783–4, 784
Horner's syndrome 919
Hurler syndrome 919
hyaluronic acid 8
hydrochloric acid burns 626
hydrofluoric acid burns 626
hydroquinone 683
  skin lightening 685
hyperhidrosis 651–2
hyperplasia 48
hypertelorism 293
hypertrichosis 917
hypertrophic scars 21
hypopharyngeal tumours 350
hypospadias 134–7
  aetiology 134
  classification 134
  clinical features 134–5
  complications 136
  contentious issues 137
  definition 134
  incidence 134
  medical management 135
  pathogenesis 134
  surgical management 135
hypotelorism 293

I

imiquimod 111
immunoglobulins, intravenous 110
implantation dermoid 407
implants 120–2
  alloplastic material 120
  autogenous tissue 120
  ceramics 121
  complications 122
  materials 120
  metals 121
  monomers 121
  polymers 121
infection 465–78
  burns 616–7
  Clostridia spp. 468–70
  flexor sheath 397
  hand 394–9
  microbiology 466–7
  necrotizing soft tissue 476–7
  osteomyelitis 471–4
  palmar space 398–9
  prosthesis-related 475
  surgical site 114
  web space 398
  see also individual infections

inflammation 6–7
infliximab (Remicade) 110
injectables 112–3
interferon 111
interleukins 7

J

Jadassohn naevus 919
jejunal flaps 795–6
joint infections, hand 398
juvenile digital fibromatosis 480
juvenile xanthogranuloma 270–1

K

Kaposi sarcoma 265–6, 919
Kasabach-Merritt phenomenon 919
keloid scars 21–2
keratin 12
keratoacanthoma 251
Kienbock's syndrome 919
kite flaps 816–8, 818
kleeblattschädel 919
Klinefelter's syndrome 919
Klippel-Trenaunay syndrome 920, 463
knee reconstruction 444

L

lacerations of external ear 316
lagophthalmos 286
lasers 130–1
 effects 131
 energy concepts 130
 laser machine 130
 mechanism of action 131
 properties 130
lateral arm flaps 799–800
lathyrogens 7–8
latissimus dorsi flaps 870–2
Le Fort fracture patterns 3, 530, 920,
Lederhosen disease 920
leech therapy 125–6
 contraindications 125
 definition 125
 history 125
 indications 125
 leech care 125
 method of use 125–6
 physiology 125
 prophylactic antibiotics 126
leg see lower limb

leiomyosarcoma 267
lentigo maligna 245
lentigo senilis 240
lentigo simplex 240
leprosy 55
 microbiology 466
leukoplakia 344
linear epidermal (sebaceous) naevus 254–5
lip
 burns 622
 embryology 66
 repair 526
lip reconstruction 329–35
 aetiology of lip defects 329
 aims 329
 anatomy 329, 330
 flap techniques 332, 334, 335
  Abbé flap 331–3
  Abbé-Estlander flap 331–3
  Gillies fan flap 331–3
  Karapandzic technique 333
  McGregor-Nakajima flap 333
  Webster-Bernard technique 333
 free flaps 333
 function of lips 329
 lower lip 330
 primary closure 331–3, 332
 upper lip 330
 vermilion 330
lipoma 408, 495–6
liposuction 722–5
local anaesthesia 106–7
 definition 106
 dosage 106–7
 pharmacology 106
 toxic effects 107
lower limb 429–48
 above-knee amputation 448
 below-knee amputation 445–7, 446
 diabetic feet 437–41
 fascio-cutaneous flaps 903–6, 905
 fasciotomy 520, 521
 pretibial laceration 435–6, 436
 reconstruction 442–4
 trauma 912, 430–2
 ulceration 433–4
Lund-Browder charts 608–9
lunotriquetral ballotement 426

lymphatic vascular malformation 463
lymphoedema 453–6

M

macrodactyly 220–2, 911
 aetiology 220
 classification 220
 clinical presentation 221
 definition 220
 incidence 220
 indications for surgery 222
 management 221
 operative options 222
 outcome 222
 pathology 221
 surgical principles 222
Madelung's deformity 226–7
Maffucci syndrome 409, 464, 920
mallet deformity 909
Marcus Gunn syndrome 920
Marjolin ulcer 920
Martin–Gruber variant 98
mast cell tumours 278
mastocytoma 278
maxillary carcinoma 341–2
maxillary fractures 529, 531
Mayer-Rokitansky-Küster-Hauser syndrome 920
medial arm flaps 801–2
medial and lateral gastrocnemius flaps 890–1
medial plantar flaps 892–3
medial thigh lift 719
Meige's disease 454
melanocytes 238, 240
melanoma 246–9
 adjuvant therapy 249
 classification 247
 clinical features 247
 definition 246
 follow-up 249
 incidence 246
 investigation 247
 local recurrence 249
 metastatic disease 249
 pathology 246–7
 prognosis 249
 regional lymph nodes 249
 risk factors 246
 staging 248
 treatment 247
melanoma in situ 245
Melkersson–Rosenthal syndrome 920

membranous bone grafts 26
Merkel cell carcinoma 263–5, 914
  staging 264
mesh grafts 17
metal implants 121
methotrexate 110
methylmethacrylate 121
microbiology 55–6, 466–7
microcystic adnexal carcinoma 266
micrognathia 152–3
microphthalmia 291–2
microsurgery 127–9
  definition 127
  instruments 128
  microvascular anatomy 127
  microvascular physiology 127
  technique 128–9
  uses 127
  vessel wall healing 127
microtia 154–5
midcarpal clunk 426
midcarpal shift test 426
Milroy's disease 453–4
Moberg flaps 828–9, 829
Möbius syndrome 920
molluscum sebaceum 251
Mongolian blue spot 241
monomer implants 121
Morel-Lavallée syndrome 512, 920
Morton's neuroma 920
mouth see oral cavity
Muehrcke's lines 539
Muenke's syndrome 145
Muir-Torre syndrome 921
muscle flaps 764–5
muscles
  levator palpebrae superioris 83
  Muller's muscle 83
  orbicularis oculi 82
  platysma 75
  sternocleidomastoid 75
  trapezius 75

N

naevus
  balloon 243
  blue 241
  congenital 244
  dysplastic 245
  flammeus 463
  halo 243
  of Ito 241
  Jadassohn 919
  linear epidermal (sebaceous) 254–5

organoid 254–5
of Ota 241
spindle 243
Spitz 243
naevus cells 238
  lesions of 242
Nagar syndrome 921
nail deformity 539
nailbed injuries 537–9, 538
nasal cavity tumours 340–1, 342
nasal dermoid 155
nasal reconstruction 306–13
  aesthetic subunits 307
  aetiology 306
  aims of 306
  anatomy 306
  choice of 310
  columella 312
  hemi-nasal 312
  history 306
  nasal alar 311, 312
  nasal dorsum 310
  nasal lining 308
  nasal sides 310
  nasal tip 311
  prosthetic 312
  skeletal support 309–10
  techniques 307–8
  tips 312–3
  total 312
nasal valves 80
nasalis flaps 789–90, 790
naso-orbital ethmoid fractures 528–9, 530–2
nasolabial flaps 791–2, 792
nasopharyngeal carcinoma 342–3
neck see head and neck
necrotizing soft tissue infection 476–7
needle holders 929, 930
nerves
  accessory (XI) 77
  facial 87–9
    danger zones 88, 89
    how to find 88
    see also facial nerve palsy
  infra-orbital 323
  median 91–2
  phrenic 77
  radial 92
  trigeminal 323
  ulnar 91–2
  zygomatico-facial 323
  zygomatico-temporal 323
neurilemmoma 407–8, 488–9
neurofibroma 490–1
neurofibromatosis 492–4
  type 1 492–4

type 2 494
neuroma 910
neuropathic ulcers 433
neurovascular island flaps 823–5, 824, 825
nipple
  inverted 677
  Paget's disease 921
  reconstruction 373, 374
Nirschl procedure 924
nitric acid burns 626
nodular pseudosarcomatous fasciitis 480
non-accidental injury 630
non-autologous fillers 683
nose
  anatomy 78–81, 79, 80
  burns 622
  embryology 65
  innervation 79
  internal nasal valve 80
  musculature 78
  primary components 78
  repair 526
  subunits/aesthetic units 80, 81
  vasculature 78
  see also nasal
Notta's node 921

O

Oberlin transfer 924
Ollier's disease 921
omental flaps 797–8
oncological drugs 111
operations, classification of 115
oral cavity, burns 622
oral cavity tumours 344–50
  anatomy 344
  classification 344
  clinical features 344
  diagnosis 345
  epidemiology 344
  investigations 345
  management 346
    chemotherapy 348
    excision margins 346
    neck nodes 347
    primary tumours 346
    radiotherapy 346–7
    surgical approach 346
  pathology 344
  premalignant lesions 344
  prognostic factors 347
  recurrence 347, 348
  risk factors 344
  staging 346
  survival 347
  TNM definitions 345

oral contraceptives, and deep vein thrombosis 117
orbital floor fractures 528–9, 531
organoid naevus 254–5
oropharyngeal tumours 350
orthodontics 184–6
 anatomy 184
 Angle's classification of occlusion 185–6, 186
 definitions 184
 infancy 184
 multidisciplinary team 184
 permanent dentition 185
 primary dentition 184
 transitional dentition 185
orthognathics 184
Osler-Weber-Rendu syndrome 464, 921
osteoarthritis 638–9
 radiological changes 909
osteochondroma 413
osteoconductive materials 27
osteoid osteoma 414–5
osteoinductive materials 27
osteomyelitis 471–4
 aetiology 471
 bacteriology 472
 classification 471–2, 472
 clinical features 473
 complications 474
 definition 471
 investigations 473
 management 473–4
 prevalence 471
 surgical treatment 474

P

Paget's disease
 of nipple 921
 of skin 253–4
palatal embryology 66
palatal fistula 182–3
palmar space infections 398–9
papillary eccrine adenoma 274
paranasal sinus tumours 340–1
parascapular flaps 853–4
parasympathetic nervous system 103–4
 anatomy 103
 clinical relevance 104
 head and neck 103
 neurotransmitters 104
 pelvic 104
 physiology 104

vagus 103–5
Parkes-Weber syndrome 464, 921
paronychia 396
parotidectomy, superficial 357–8
Parsonage-Turner syndrome 921
Pasteurella multocida 55, 466
pathology 48
pectoralis major flaps 847–9
penis
 anatomy 101–2
 arterial supply 101
 lymphatics 102
 nerve supply 102
 skin and fascial layers 101
 venous drainage 101
pens 930
perineal burns 621
perionychial injuries 537–9, 538
peripheral nerve 36–7
 anatomy 36
 healing 37
  factors affecting 37
  management 37
  postoperative care 37
  speed of 37
peripheral nerve injury 598–9
 classification 598
 consequences 598
 diagnosis 598
 nerve healing 598
peripheral neuropathy 437–8
Peyronie's disease 921
Pfeiffer syndrome 144–5, 921
phenol burns 626
photo-ageing 53
photo-sensitivity 52–3
photocarcinogenesis 53
Pierre Robin sequence 152–3, 921
pigmented melanocytic lesions 238
 benign 238
 malignant 238
pigmented villonodular synovitis/synovioma 406–7
pilomatrixoma 276
Pinkus tumour 253
pivot flaps 756–7
plagiocephaly without synostosis 146
 natural history 146
plantar fibromatosis 480

Poland syndrome 228–9, 921
pollicization 231–2
polydactyly 209, 910, 911
polymer implants 121
polymorphonuclear leucocytes 6–7
Pontén flap 924
porokeratosis 252
port wine stain 279–80
posterior interosseous artery flaps 810–2
potassium hydroxide burns 627
prednisone 110
Preiser's syndrome 921
pressure sores 644–6
 Waterlow prevention/treatment policy 913
pretibial laceration 435–6, 436
prostheses
 infection related to 475
 upper limb 422
Proteus syndrome 921
Pseudomonas aeruginosa 55–6, 466–7
ptosis 290, 295–6, 296
pyoderma gangrenosum 281–2
pyogenic granuloma 277

Q

Queyrat's erythroplasia 922

R

radial dysplasia 191–4, 910
 aetiology 191
 aims of correction 192
 associated disorders 191
 classification 191
 clinical presentation 192
 complications 194
 definition 191
 incidence 191
 management 192
 surgical options 193–4
 timing of surgery 193
radial forearm flaps 803–5
radial head, congenital dislocation 211
radio-ulnar synostosis 212–3
radiotherapy 49–51
 accelerated 51
 basis of 49
 CHART 51
 complications 50
 definition 49

hyperfractionation 51
physics 49
planning 50
radiation effects 51
role of 50
Ramsay-Hunt syndrome 922
ray amputations of hand 420
Raynaud's phenomenon 450–2
conditions associated with 451
screening tests 452
reconstruction 727–34
direct closure (primary intention) 729–33, 730, 732
reconstructive ladder 728
secondary intention 734
rectus abdominis flaps 861–2
vertical myocutaneous 863–4
transverse myocutaneous 865–7, 866
reflex sympathetic dystrophy 647–8
remodelling 6
retin A 682
retractors 930, 931
reverse flow flaps, venous drainage 769–70, 770–2
rheumatoid arthritis 632–5
aetiology 632
classification 632, 908
clinical features 633
diagnosis 633
incidence 632
investigations 634
management 634
pathogenesis 633
thumb deformity 632
rhinophyma 314
rhinoplasty 694–7
rhomboid flaps 778–9, 779
ring avulsion injury 548, 909
Rolando fracture 567, 922
Romberg's disease 149, 922
rotation flaps 758–9, 759
Routledge procedure 924

S

Saethre-Chotzen syndrome 145, 922
salivary gland tumours 354–6
adenoid cystic carcinoma 355
clinical features 355
incidence 354
investigations 355
muco-epidermoid carcinoma 355
pleomorphic adenoma 354
prognosis 356
staging 355
TNM classification 355
treatment 356
Warthin's tumour 354
WHO classification 354
scalp 74
arterial supply 74
clinical relevance 74
lymph drainage 74
nerve supply 74
venous drainage 74
scalpel handle 931
scaphoid fracture 573–5
scapholunate dissociation 576
scapular flaps 850–2, 852
scars 20–3
definition 20
hypertrophic 21
keloid 21–2
management 22–3
minimization 11, 15
pathophysiology 20
symptomatic 20–1
schwannoma, benign 407–8, 488–9
scissors 931
scleroderma 636
sebaceous carcinoma 266
seborrhoeic keratosis 272
Secretan's syndrome 922
senile haemangioma 277
sentinel lymph node biopsy 503–4
septal deviation 698
serratus anterior flaps 873–5
Seymour fracture 922
shock 614
Sjögren's syndrome 922
skin 12–3
conditions of 233–82
malignant 258–67
premalignant 245
see also individual conditions
dermis 13
epidermis 12
glands 13
hair follicles 13
layers of 12
solar damage 13
vascular anatomy 72–3
skin grafts 16–9
anaesthetist 16
classification 16
definition 16
donor site 16
full thickness 18–9
indications 16
superficial 16–8
uses 16
skin healing see wound healing
skin lightening 685
skin tumours 239
melanocytic 239
non-melanocytic 239
Skoog procedure 924
Smith's fracture 922
smoking 123–4
pathophysiology 124
quitting 123
relevance to plastic surgery 123–4
Snow-Littler procedure 924
sodium hydroxide burns 627
soft tissue sarcoma 481–7
aetiology 481
classification 481–2, 482
clinical features 481
definition 481
incidence 481
investigations 483–5
prognosis 486, 487
staging 482, 484
treatment 485–6
soft tissue tumours 405–8
solar damage 13, 52–4
photo-ageing 53
photocarcinogenesis 53
radiation 52, 52–3
severity of 53–4
sun protection factor 54
sunscreens 54
solar keratosis 250
soleus flaps 888–9
spinal closure 387–8
spindle naevus 243
Spitz naevus 243
sponge holding/dressing forceps 929
squamous cell carcinoma 260–1
staging 262, 262–3, 915
Stahl's ear 922
Staphylococcus spp. 56, 467
Stener lesion 922
sternal dehiscence 912–3
sternum reconstruction 378–81
Stewart-Treves syndrome 922

Stickler syndrome 922
Streptococcus spp. 56, 467
Sturge-Weber syndrome 464, 922
submucous resection 698–9
Sudek's atrophy 647–8
sulphuric acid burns 626
sun protection factor 54
sunscreens 54
superficial skin grafts 16–8
sural flaps 901–2, 902
sural nerve harvest 599
swallowing 336–7
swan-neck deformity 551–2, 908
sweat glands 13
 tumours of 274–5
symbrachydactyly 218–9
syndactyly 206–8, 910
 aetiology 206
 associated disorders 206
 classification 206–7
 clinical presentation 207
 complications 208
 definition 206
 incidence 206
 operative options 208
 surgical principles 207
 timing of surgery 207
syringoma 274
systemic sclerosis 636

T

TAR syndrome 923
tarsorrhaphy 302, 303
telecanthus 293, 294
temporalis flaps 839–40
temporo-parietal flaps 841–2
tendon healing 34–5
 blood supply 34
 healing 34
 nutrition 34
tendon transfers 600–1
tensor fascia lata flaps 882–3
thenar flaps 830–1, 831
thigh and buttock contouring 717–8
thigh reconstruction 443–4
thoracic outlet 599
thromboprophylaxis 116–7
 methods 116
 oral contraceptives and HRT 117
 risk factors 116
 spinal/epidural block 116–7

thumb
 clasp 911
 duplication 210, 910
 hypoplasia 214–5, 911
 in rheumatoid arthritis 632
 ulnar collateral ligament injury 553–4, 554
 Z deformity 909
 see also digital
tibial fractures 430
tibial reconstruction 444
tissue expansion 43–5
 definition 43
 indications 43
 physiology 43
 technique 43–5
 tissues used 43
 uses 43
tissue forceps 929
toe phalanx non-vascularized transfer 230
toe transfer 894–5
topical negative pressure 47–8
transformiong growth factor beta 7
transverse rectus abdominis myocutaneous flaps 865–7, 866
trapezius flaps 855–7
trauma 505–630
 boutonnière deformity 549–50, 550, 908, 917
 brachial plexus injuries 589–92
 burns
  assessment 606, 606–9
  breast 621
  chemical 626–7
  ear 622
  electrical 628
  emergency care 602–3
  escharotomy 610–1, 612
  eyelids 621, 622
  fluid resuscitation 604–5
  foot 625
  hand 623–4
  head and neck 621
  hypermetabolic response 614–5
  immune effects 614
  infection 616–7
  Lund-Browder charts 608–9
  mouth and lips 622
  non-accidental injury 630
  nose 622
  oedema 614

  perineum 621
  reconstruction 620
  scalp alopecia 622
  shock 614
  treatment 615, 618–9
  Wallace rule of nines 607
  wound pathophysiology 613–5
 carpal instability 576–8, 577, 578
 compartment syndrome 514, 515–7
 crush injuries 513–14
 degloving injuries 511–12
 distal radio-ulnar joint
  disorders 582
  instability 583
 distal radius fractures 579–81
 extravasation 506–7
 eyelids, burns 621, 622
 facial lacerations 524–6
 fasciotomy 518–21, 519, 521
 flexor digitorum profundus avulsion 909
 flexor tendon avulsion 544–5, 545
 flexor tendon injuries 540–1
  repair 542–3, 543
 frostbite 508–9
 gunshot and blast injuries 522–3
 hand assessment 534, 533–6
 hand fractures 555–69
  complications 570–2, 571
 lower limb 430–2, 912
 middle-third facial injuries 527–32
 nailbed and perionychial injuries 537–9
 obstetrical brachial plexus palsy 593–4
  sequelae 595
 peripheral nerve injury 598–9
 ring avulsion injury 548, 909
 scaphoid fracture 573–5
 swan-neck deformity 551–2
 tendon transfers 600–1
 triangular fibrocartilaginous complex disorders 585–6
 ulnar collateral ligament injury of thumb 553–4, 554

INDEX

ulnar head procedures 584
ulnocarpal abutment syndrome 587–8
Volkmann's ischaemic contracture 596–7, 912, 923
traumatic tattooing 510
Treacher Collins syndrome 150–1, 923
  aetiology and embryology 150
  classification 150
  clinical presentation 150
  genetics 150
  incidence 150
  investigation 151
  treatment 151
triangular fibro-cartilaginous complex disorders 585–6
tricholemmal (pilar) cysts 268
trigger finger 205, 909
tropocollagen 7–8
tumours 479–504
  bone 412–6
  epidermal 272–3
  fibrohistiocytic 270–1
  fibromatoses 480
  glomus 410
  hair follicles 276
  hand 401–4, 403, 404
  hypopharyngeal 350
  lipoma 408, 495–6
  mast cell 278
  nasal cavity 340–1, 342
  neurilemmoma 407–8, 488–9
  neurofibroma 490–1
  neurofibromatosis 492–4
  oral cavity 344–50
  oropharyngeal 350
  paranasal sinus 340–1
  salivary gland 354–6
  skin 239
  soft tissue sarcoma 481–7
  sweat glands 274–5
  vascular 277, 409–11
tumour necrosis factors 7
turban tumour 274
Turner's syndrome 923

U

ulcers
  arterial 433, 434
  leg 433–4
  Marjolin 920
  neuropathic 433

ulna carpal stress test 426
ulnar collateral ligament injury of thumb 527–32, 553–4
ulnar duplication 910
ulnar dysplasia 195–6
ulnar forearm flaps 806–7
ulnar head procedures 584
ulnocarpal abutment syndrome 587–8
unicameral bone cyst 415
upper limb 389–428
  amputations 418–9
    proximal 421
    ray 420
  congenital anomalies 189–90
  prostheses 422
  reduction 711–2
  see also various parts

V

van der Woude syndrome 923
vascular anomalies 457–8
vascular cutaneous catastrophe of newborn 912
vascular endothelial growth factor 7
vascular malformations 409, 442–4, 457, 458
vascular tumours 277, 409–11
vascularized bone 'graft' 766–8
VATERR syndrome 923
Vaughan-Jackson syndrome 923
velocardiofacial syndrome 923
velopharyngeal incompetence 178–81
  aetiology 178
  assessment 178
  closure pattern 179, 181
  complications 180
  definition 178
  management 179
  outcome 180
  posterior pharyngeal flap 180
  sphincter pharyngoplasty 179–80, 181
venous flaps 771
venous ulcers 433, 434
vertical rectus abdominis myocutaneous flaps 863–4

Volkmann's ischaemic contracture 596–7, 912, 923

W

W-plasty 776–7, 777
Wallace rule of nines 607
Wartenburg's syndrome 923
Watson scaphoid shift test 426
Watson syndrome 923
web space infections 398
Weber-Christian disease 923
Weber-Fergusson incision 924
Werner syndrome 923
wound healing 6–8, 14
  collagen synthesis, deposition, cross-linking and remodelling 7–8
  contraction 14
  definition 6, 14
  dermal repair 14
  epithelialization 14
  factors affecting 9–11
    general factors 9
    growth factors 9–10, 10–11
    local factors 9
    rate of wound healing 11
  growth factors 7
  mechanisms of 6–7
  phases of 6, 14
  scar minimization 11, 15
  systems involved 6
  types of 6, 14
  wound strength 14
wrist
  anatomy 99–100
  biomechanics 100
  differential diagnosis 427
  examination 425–7
  ligaments 99
  skeleton 99
  surface anatomy 100

X

xeroderma pigmentosum 253

Z

Z-plasty 773, 773–5, 774
zygomatic fractures 528–9, 531

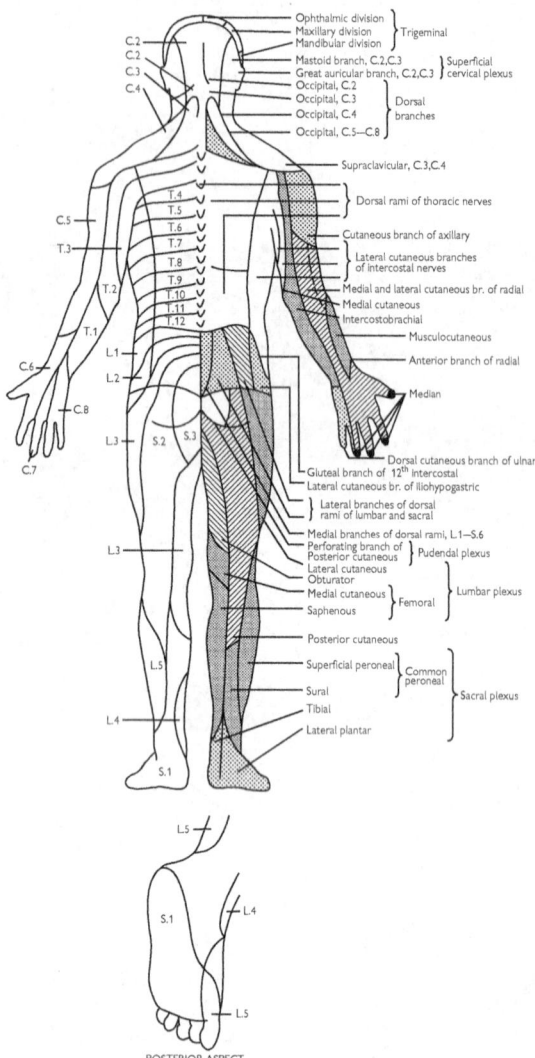

Dermatomes and peripheral nerve distribution. Reproduced with permission from Longmore, Wilkinson, and Rajagopalan (2004). *Oxford Handbook of Clinical Medicine 6e*, Oxford University Press.

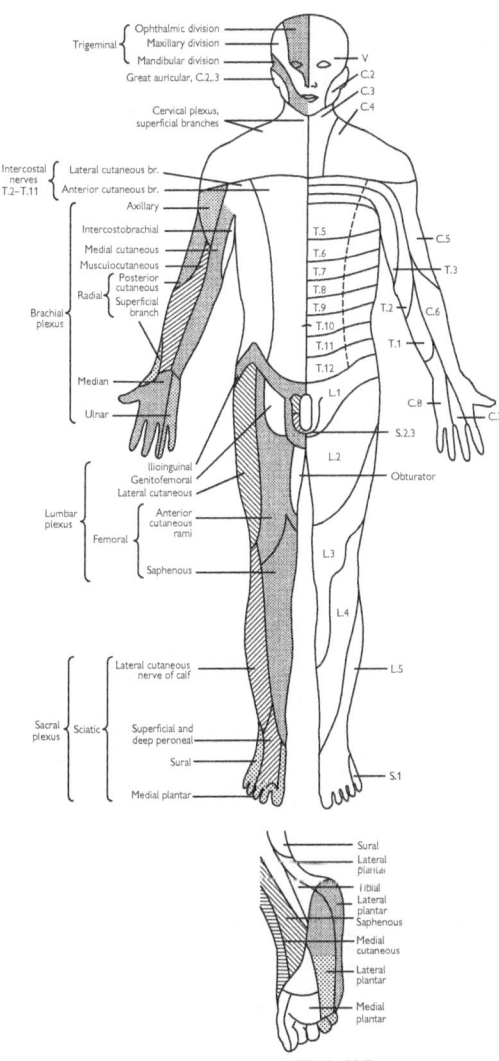

ANTERIOR ASPECT